# Medical Oncology

# Medical Oncology

Editor: Georgia Cassidy

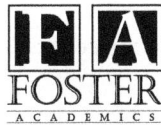

**FA**
**FOSTER**
A C A D E M I C S

www.fosteracademics.com

www.fosteracademics.com

FA FOSTER
ACADEMICS

Cataloging-in-Publication Data

Medical oncology / edited by Georgia Cassidy.
    p. cm.
Includes bibliographical references and index.
ISBN 978-1-63242-938-4
1. Cancer. 2. Oncology. 3. Cancer--Treatment. I. Cassidy, Georgia.
RC2684 .M43 2020
616.994--dc23

Foster Academics,
118-35 Queens Blvd., Suite 400,
Forest Hills, NY 11375, USA

ISBN 978-1-63242-938-4 (Hardback)

# Contents

# Preface

This book was inspired by the evolution of our times; to answer the curiosity of inquisitive minds. Many developments have occurred across the globe in the recent past which has transformed the progress in the field.

The branch of medicine that involves the prevention, diagnosis and treatment of cancer is known as oncology. Medical oncology, surgical oncology and radiation oncology are the three main divisions of oncology. Medical oncology is a mode of treatment of cancer through hormonal therapy, targeted therapy, chemotherapy and immunotherapy. It is mostly used in conjunction with radiation oncology and surgical oncology. Hormonal therapy is a cancer treatment that reduces or blocks the amount of hormones in the body to slow or stop the growth of cancer that uses hormones to grow. In chemotherapy treatment, drugs are used to destroy the cancer cells. Targeted therapy treatment also involves the use of drugs. It focuses on restricting the spread of cancer to other organs. Immunotherapy treatment activates the immune cells to fight against the cancer cells. The aim of this book is to present researches that have transformed this discipline and aided its advancement. It presents the complex subject of medical oncology in the most comprehensible and easy to understand language. It is an essential guide for both academicians and those who wish to pursue this discipline further.

This book was developed from a mere concept to drafts to chapters and finally compiled together as a complete text to benefit the readers across all nations. To ensure the quality of the content we instilled two significant steps in our procedure. The first was to appoint an editorial team that would verify the data and statistics provided in the book and also select the most appropriate and valuable contributions from the plentiful contributions we received from authors worldwide. The next step was to appoint an expert of the topic as the Editor-in-Chief, who would head the project and finally make the necessary amendments and modifications to make the text reader-friendly. I was then commissioned to examine all the material to present the topics in the most comprehensible and productive format.

I would like to take this opportunity to thank all the contributing authors who were supportive enough to contribute their time and knowledge to this project. I also wish to convey my regards to my family who have been extremely supportive during the entire project.

**Editor**

# Characterisation of microbial communities within aggressive prostate cancer tissues

Melissa A. Yow[1], Sepehr N. Tabrizi[2,3,4], Gianluca Severi[9], Damien M. Bolton[7], John Pedersen[8], Australian Prostate Cancer BioResource[10], Graham G. Giles[5,6] and Melissa C. Southey[1*]

## Abstract

**Background:** An infectious aetiology for prostate cancer has been conjectured for decades but the evidence gained from questionnaire-based and sero-epidemiological studies is weak and inconsistent, and a causal association with any infectious agent is not established. We describe and evaluate the application of new technology to detect bacterial and viral agents in high-grade prostate cancer tissues. The potential of targeted 16S rRNA gene sequencing and total RNA sequencing was evaluated in terms of its utility to characterise microbial communities within high-grade prostate tumours.

**Methods:** Two different Massively Parallel Sequencing (MPS) approaches were applied. First, to capture and enrich for possible bacterial species, targeted-MPS of the V2-V3 hypervariable regions of the 16S rRNA gene was performed on DNA extracted from 20 snap-frozen prostate tissue cores from ten "aggressive" prostate cancer cases. Second, total RNA extracted from the same prostate tissue samples was also sequenced to capture the sequence profile of both bacterial and viral transcripts present.

**Results:** Overall, 16S rRNA sequencing identified *Enterobacteriaceae* species common to all samples and *P. acnes* in 95% of analyzed samples. Total RNA sequencing detected endogenous retroviruses providing proof of concept but there was no evidence of bacterial or viral transcripts suggesting active infection, although it does not rule out a previous 'hit and run' scenario.

**Conclusions:** As these new investigative methods and protocols become more refined, MPS approaches may be found to have significant utility in identifying potential pathogens involved in disease aetiology. Further studies, specifically designed to detect associations between the disease phenotype and aetiological agents, are required.

**Keywords:** Prostate cancer, Sexually transmitted infection, Infection, 16S rRNA, RNA, cDNA, *Propionibacterium acnes*

## Background

First proposed in the early 1950s, an infectious aetiology for prostate cancer has since been widely investigated using conventional and serology-based case–control designs and some cohort studies but the evidence from these has been generally weak and inconsistent. A causal association is yet to be established.

Recent support for a role of infection in prostate cancer risk came from the detection of a novel candidate, *Propionibacterium acnes*, within prostate cancer tissues [1, 2]. There is also evidence of association between prostate cancer risk and gene variants of COX-2 [3], RNASEL [4] and TLR4 [5], identified in cases of hereditary

prostate cancer, indicating that infection and the host response to infection may be involved in the development of prostate cancer.

Studies that have investigated the role of infectious agents in the aetiology of prostate cancer have adopted single organism targeted approaches or have identified microbial constituents based on amplification of various hypervariable regions of the 16S rRNA gene in concert with traditional cloning and sequencing methods [6–9]. Single organism targeted approaches are limited by their specificity while traditional broad-range 16S rRNA gene amplification, cloning and Sanger sequencing can be laborious and costly, depending on the scale of the study, number and complexity of samples. When compared with conventional sequencing methods, cyclic array-based massively parallel sequencing (MPS) methods, albeit with shorter read length capability and less

* Correspondence: msouthey@unimelb.edu.au
[1]Genetic Epidemiology Laboratory, Department of Pathology, Faculty of Medicine, Dentistry and Health Sciences, University of Melbourne, VIC, Australia 3010
Full list of author information is available at the end of the article

accuracy in base calling, offer efficiencies in terms of cost, time and scalability.

The principal hypothesis that guided the direction of the work presented in this study was that persistent, rather than transient, infection of the prostate gland by a sexually transmitted or other infectious agent would be associated with risk. Thus, evidence of infection at the tissue level was sought by utilising two different molecular approaches, targeted partial 16S rRNA gene sequencing and total RNA sequencing using MPS. The overall objective of this study was to investigate the presence of infectious agent(s) in histopathologically determined aggressive prostate cancer cases (Gleason score ≥ 8).

## Methods
### Samples
Fresh-frozen scalpel-excised prostate tissue from males that had undergone radical prostatectomy with a Gleason score of ≥ 8 and tumour stage ranging from pT2c to pT3b (inclusive) were obtained from the Australian Prostate Cancer Bioresource [10] ($n = 10$). Tumour and benign tissues were provided for each case and the presence/absence of malignant tissue was confirmed by histopathology by a single pathologist (JP).

### Nucleic acid extraction
Frozen tissue was disrupted by freeze fracture, Buffer RLT Plus (Qiagen, Hilden, Germany) containing β-mercaptoethanol was added. The lysate was further homogenised using a QIAshredder® (Qiagen, Hilden, Germany) column and then underwent enzymatic digestion and nucleic acid extraction with the AllPrep DNA/RNA Mini Kit (Qiagen, Hilden, Germany) according to the manufacturer's instructions. Both DNA and RNA isolates were stored at −80 °C (Additional file 1).

### Quantitative and qualitative assessment of extracted DNA and RNA
The concentration and integrity of sample RNA was assessed with the Bioanalyzer 2100 instrument (Agilent Technologies) using RNA 6000 Nano Kit (Agilent Technologies). The concentration of sample DNA was assessed by Qubit® 1.0 Fluorometer (Life Technologies, Carlsbad, California, USA) and the Qubit® dsDNA BR Assay Kit (Life Technologies, Carlsbad, California, USA).

### Quantification, normalisation and pooling of libraries
Each RNA sample was normalised to 100 µg/µL in UltraPure™ DNAse/RNAse-Free Distilled Water (Invitrogen™, Burlington, USA). Normalised RNA samples were pooled in equimolar amounts according to tissue type i.e. "malignant" or "benign".

## 16S rRNA amplicon sequencing
### 16S rRNA polymerase chain reaction
Each PCR reaction contained 1X GeneAmp® PCR Buffer II (Roche Molecular Systems, Inc. Branchburg Township, USA), 10 µM (each) forward and reverse primer, 0.1 U AmpliTaq Gold® DNA polymerase (ThermoFisher Scientific, Waltham, Massachusetts, USA), 2.5 µM MgCl$_2$, 400 µM dNTPs, 2 µL of template DNA in a final volume of 20 µL with UltraPure™ DNAse/RNAse-Free Distilled Water (Invitrogen™, Burlington, USA). Amplification of each sample was performed in triplicate using a Veriti® 96-well Thermal Cycler (Applied Biosystems, Forster City, CA, USA). Negative amplification controls included dH$_2$O and TE buffer and the positive amplification control was *Salmonella typhimurium* (0.5 ng/µL). Cycling conditions were as follows: 95 °C for 5 min, 35 cycles at 95 °C for 45 s, 56 °C for 60 s and 72 °C for 90 s, with a final extension at 72 °C for five minutes.

### Primers
Universal primers 101F/534R and 515F/806R were used to amplify the V2-V3 and V4 hypervariable region of the 16S rRNA gene, respectively. The V4 region primer constructs were taken from Caporaso et al. (2011) [11] (supplementary methods). The V2-V3 region primer constructs were modified from [11] using V2-V3 region specific primers [12] to target the 16S rRNA V2-V3 hypervariable region (Additional file 1). Reverse primers were barcoded to enable multiplexing of samples.

### Purification of PCR products
Replicate wells were combined for each sample and excess primers, primer dimers and extraneous products were removed using a double-sided size selection/cleanup with Agencourt® AMPure® XP beads (Beckman Coulter, Inc., Massachusetts, U.S.A). Purified product was eluted in 30 µL dH$_2$O.

### Quantification and normalization of library pools
Library size and quantity were assessed using the Bioanalyzer 2100 using the High Sensitivity DNA kit (Agilent Technologies Inc., Waldbronn, Germany). Individual samples were combined in equimolar quantities for sequencing.

### Sequencing
Three custom primers were used for sequencing of the 16S rRNA V4 region amplicons as described in [11] and the 16S rRNA V2-V3 region amplicons as adapted from Caporaso et al. (2011) [11]. The libraries were sequenced by using the MiSeq® 500 cycle Reagent Kit v2 (Illumina, Inc., San Diego, CA, USA).

### Data analysis

The quality of raw reads was assessed using FastQC v0.10.1 [13]. Paired-end reads were then stitched using FLASh (Fast Length Adjustment of Short reads) v1.2.6 [14] to generate full length reads of the of the sequenced amplicons. The quality of the FLASh-stitched reads were again assessed using FastQC v0.10.1 [13].

The QIIME (Quantitative Insights Into Microbial Ecology) pipeline and software package (version 1.7.0) [15] were used for data analyses using Closed-reference Operational Taxonomic Unit (OTU) picking. The sequences were clustered against a reference sequence collection [16] (Greengenes 12_10 reference collection) and any reads that did not hit a sequence at 97% sequence similarity to the reference sequence collection were excluded from downstream analysis.

### Total RNA/cDNA sequencing
#### Library preparation and sequencing

Library preparation was performed using the Illumina® TruSeq® Stranded Total RNA Sample Preparation Kit in accordance with the manufacturer's instructions, however, did not include the initial poly(A) purification step (supplementary methods). The libraries were assessed with the Bioanalyser 2100 using the Bioanalyser DNA 1000 kit (Agilent). Individual libraries (tumour and cancer-unaffected prostate pools) were normalised to 2 nM. Sequencing was performed on the HiSeq™ 2000.

### Data analysis

Raw data underwent quality control and sequencing adapters were removed using Nesoni [17]. The full data set was queried for specific viral genomes (including human papillomaviruses 16 and 18, Herpes simplex virus 2 and Polyomaviruses) using human endogenous retroviruses (HERVs) as internal control as HERVs are remnant ancient retroviral sequences integrated into human germline DNA, some of which are actively transcribed. Reads were mapped to human rRNA (and other non-coding RNA) and to human mRNA using the SHort Read Mapping Package (SHRiMP) [18] and Burrows-Wheeler Aligner (BWA) [19], respectively. Aligned reads were removed from the dataset. Unmapped reads were assembled into contiguous sequences using the *de novo* assembler Velvet [20], under kmer values of 55, 65, 75 and 85. The assemblies were queried with Easy-Web-BLAST+ [21] for 16S rRNA sequences and the presence of viral proteins (specifically all viral polymerases within the NCBI's RefSeq viral protein reference database [22]).

## Results
### Characteristics of the case series

The mean age at radical prostatectomy of patients was 64.5 years. Three cases underwent radical laparoscopic robotic prostatectomy while the remaining seven cases had open radical retropubic prostatectomy. All cases were considered to be of an aggressive nature and were selected on the basis of a Gleason score of ≥ 8 and a TNM stage of at least PT2c (Table 1).

### 16S rRNA V4 hypervariable region

One thousand three hundred and twenty four unique OTUs were identified in all 20 prostate tissue samples combined. Per sample, the mean number of OTUs present was 231.55 (SD 48.45) and ranged from 151 to 314. Community composition was reasonably complex.

Overall, the most abundant taxa identified were assigned to the family *Enterobacteriaceae* (70.1%) and the genus *Escherichia* (6.9%). There were five other unique OTUs that represented ≥ 1% of the microbial community observed across all samples. These taxa included *Pseudomonadaceae* (1.2%), *Comamonadaceae* (1.2%), *Ralstonia* (1.7%), *Pseudomonas* (1.3%) and *Acinetobacter* (1.1%). There were five OTUs that represented $0.5 < 1\%$ of the microbial community observed and these included *Corynebacterium* (0.8%), *Caulobacteriaceae* (0.7%), *Curvibacter* (0.7%) *Aerococcus* (0.6%) and *Bradyrhizobium* (0.6%) The remaining 13.7% of sequences were assigned to 308 other unique OTUs (Additional file 2).

The greatest proportion of sequences, ranging from 37.2 to 81.2%, for each individual sample was represented by the family *Enterobacteriaceae.*. The prevalence of *Escherichia* ranged from 3.1 to 10.3% in the samples. Both taxa were represented in every sample. While there was up to a two-fold difference in the number of observed OTUs (151 to 314) among samples, the community composition of the most abundant samples (abundance > 0.5%) was reasonably consistent across individual samples, however, some taxa including *Pseudomonadaceae, Aerococcus, Corynebacterium* and *Actinobacter lwoffii* were overrepresented in a number of samples when compared to their contribution to overall abundance (Additional file 2).

A group of 18 OTUs was found to be present in 95% of samples (Table 2). While these 18 OTUs only represented a small proportion (on average 7.8%) of the overall membership of prostatic microbial community, they contributed to a large proportion (84.6%) of the relative abundance of the total communities of the 20 samples sequenced. The relative contribution of each 'core' OTU was reasonably consistent across samples (Fig. 1) with *Enterobacteriacae* (84.4%) and *Escherichia* (8.3%) the most abundant taxa contributing the 'core' community.

### 16S rRNA V2-V3 hypervariable region

Six hundred and thirty four unique OTUs were present in all 20 prostate tissue samples combined. On a per

**Table 1** Histopathological features (Gleason score and TNM stage), age at radical prostatectomy and pre-operative PSA (ng/μL) for ten prostate cancer cases obtained from the Australian Prostate Cancer BioResource

| Patient ID | Gleason Score | TNM Stage | Age (years) at resection | Surgical type | Pre-operative PSA (ng/μL) |
|---|---|---|---|---|---|
| PI | 8 | PT3AN0 | 67.6 | Open | 26.7 |
| P2 | 9 | PT3B | 68.9 | Open | 6.2 |
| P3 | 9 | PT3AN1MX | 73.3 | Open | 1.9 |
| P4 | 9 | PT2CN0 | 61.5 | Open | 3.1 |
| P5 | 9 | PT2C | 59.2 | Robot | 5.7 |
| P6 | 9 | PT3BN0 | 64.4 | Robot | n/a |
| P7 | 8 | PT3AN0 | 68.1 | Open | 13.9 |
| P8 | 9 | PT3A | 61.1 | Open | 9.2 |
| P9 | 9 | PT3AN0 | 53.4 | Open | n/a |
| P10 | 8 | PT3AN0 | 67.8 | Robot | 8.8 |

sample basis, the mean number of OTUs present was 117.95 (SD 23.95) and ranged from 71 to 160.

All samples combined, *Enterobacteriaceae* was dominant taxon (55.4%), followed by *Escherichia* (20.9%). There were seven additional OTUs with an abundance ≥ 1% including *Comamonadaceae* (1.8%), *Hyphomonadaceae* (1.5%), *Pseudomonas* (3.4%), *Corynebacterium* (1.3%), *Tepidimonas* (1.2%), *P. acnes* (1.1%) and *Acinetobacter*

(1.0%). *Ralstonia* and *Lutemonas* represented 0.8 and 0.6% of the total microbial community, respectively. The remaining 11% of sequences comprised of the 194 other OTUs (Additional file 3).

The highest proportion of sequences for each individual sample was assigned to *Enterobacteriaceae* with an abundance ranging from 21.9 to 69.4% followed by *Escherichia* with an abundance ranging from 6.5 to

**Table 2** Taxonomic assignments of the 18 OTUs present in 95% of samples (*n* = 20) that underwent sequencing of the V4 hypervariable region of the 16S rRNA gene and their relative abundance

| Core OTUs shared by 95% of samples | Relative abundance of OTU within the total community |
|---|---|
| | % |
| k_Bacteria; p_Proteobacteria; c_Gammaproteobacteria; o_Enterobacteriales; f_Enterobacteriaceae; g_; s_ | 70.1% |
| k_Bacteria; p_Proteobacteria; c_Gammaproteobacteria; o_Enterobacteriales; f_Enterobacteriaceae; g_Escherichia; s_ | 6.9% |
| k_Bacteria; p_Proteobacteria; c_Betaproteobacteria; o_Burkholderiales; f_Oxalobacteraceae; g_Ralstonia; s_ | 1.7% |
| k_Bacteria; p_Proteobacteria; c_Gammaproteobacteria; o_Pseudomonadales; f_Pseudomonadaceae; g_Pseudomonas; s_ | 1.3% |
| k_Bacteria; p_Actinobacteria; c_Actinobacteria; o_Actinomycetales; f_Corynebacteriaceae; g_Corynebacterium; s_ | 0.8% |
| k_Bacteria; p_Proteobacteria; c_Betaproteobacteria; o_Burkholderiales; f_Comamonadaceae; g_Curvibacter; s_ | 0.7% |
| k_Bacteria; p_Proteobacteria; c_Alphaproteobacteria; o_Caulobacterales; f_Caulobacteraceae; g_; s_ | 0.7% |
| k_Bacteria; p_Firmicutes; c_Bacilli; o_Lactobacillales; f_Aerococcaceae; g_Aerococcus; s_ | 0.6% |
| k_Bacteria; p_Firmicutes; c_Bacilli; o_Bacillales; f_Staphylococcaceae; g_Staphylococcus; s_ | 0.4% |
| k_Bacteria; p_Actinobacteria; c_Actinobacteria; o_Actinomycetales; f_Microbacteriaceae; g_; s_ | 0.4% |
| k_Bacteria; p_Firmicutes; c_Bacilli; o_Bacillales; f_Staphylococcaceae; g_; s_ | 0.3% |
| k_Bacteria; p_Proteobacteria; c_Gammaproteobacteria; o_Enterobacteriales; f_Enterobacteriaceae; g_Enterobacter; s_hormaechei | 0.3% |
| k_Bacteria; p_Proteobacteria; c_Gammaproteobacteria; o_Pseudomonadales; f_Moraxellaceae; g_; s_ | 0.2% |
| k_Bacteria; p_Proteobacteria; c_Gammaproteobacteria; o_Enterobacteriales; f_Enterobacteriaceae; g_Plesiomonas; s_ | 0.1% |
| k_Bacteria; p_Firmicutes; c_Bacilli; o_Lactobacillales; f_Streptococcaceae; g_Streptococcus; s_ | 0.1% |
| k_Bacteria; p_Proteobacteria; c_Gammaproteobacteria; o_Enterobacteriales; f_Enterobacteriaceae; g_Erwinia; s_ | <0.1% |
| k_Bacteria; p_Proteobacteria; c_Gammaproteobacteria; o_Enterobacteriales; f_Enterobacteriaceae; g_Serratia; s_marcescens | <0.1% |
| k_Bacteria; p_Proteobacteria; c_Gammaproteobacteria; o_Pseudomonadales; f_Moraxellaceae; g_Moraxella; s_ | <0.1% |
| Sum of "core" OTUs (across 95% of samples) | 84.6% |

The letters in the taxonomy column refer to k – kingdom, p – phylum, c –class, o –order, f – family, g – genus, s – species

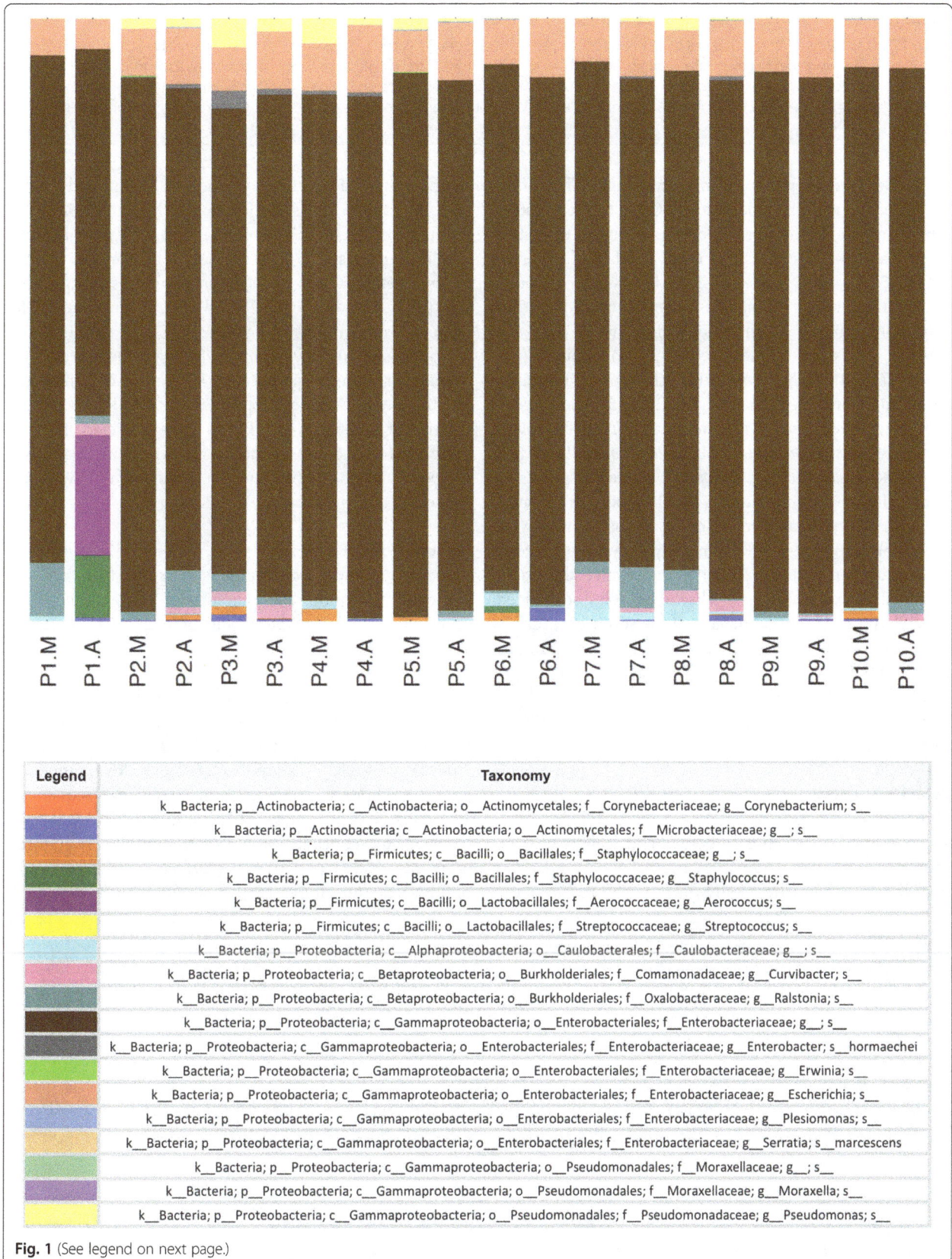

| Legend | Taxonomy |
|---|---|
| | k__Bacteria; p__Actinobacteria; c__Actinobacteria; o__Actinomycetales; f__Corynebacteriaceae; g__Corynebacterium; s__ |
| | k__Bacteria; p__Actinobacteria; c__Actinobacteria; o__Actinomycetales; f__Microbacteriaceae; g__; s__ |
| | k__Bacteria; p__Firmicutes; c__Bacilli; o__Bacillales; f__Staphylococcaceae; g__; s__ |
| | k__Bacteria; p__Firmicutes; c__Bacilli; o__Bacillales; f__Staphylococcaceae; g__Staphylococcus; s__ |
| | k__Bacteria; p__Firmicutes; c__Bacilli; o__Lactobacillales; f__Aerococcaceae; g__Aerococcus; s__ |
| | k__Bacteria; p__Firmicutes; c__Bacilli; o__Lactobacillales; f__Streptococcaceae; g__Streptococcus; s__ |
| | k__Bacteria; p__Proteobacteria; c__Alphaproteobacteria; o__Caulobacterales; f__Caulobacteraceae; g__; s__ |
| | k__Bacteria; p__Proteobacteria; c__Betaproteobacteria; o__Burkholderiales; f__Comamonadaceae; g__Curvibacter; s__ |
| | k__Bacteria; p__Proteobacteria; c__Betaproteobacteria; o__Burkholderiales; f__Oxalobacteraceae; g__Ralstonia; s__ |
| | k__Bacteria; p__Proteobacteria; c__Gammaproteobacteria; o__Enterobacteriales; f__Enterobacteriaceae; g__; s__ |
| | k__Bacteria; p__Proteobacteria; c__Gammaproteobacteria; o__Enterobacteriales; f__Enterobacteriaceae; g__Enterobacter; s__hormaechei |
| | k__Bacteria; p__Proteobacteria; c__Gammaproteobacteria; o__Enterobacteriales; f__Enterobacteriaceae; g__Erwinia; s__ |
| | k__Bacteria; p__Proteobacteria; c__Gammaproteobacteria; o__Enterobacteriales; f__Enterobacteriaceae; g__Escherichia; s__ |
| | k__Bacteria; p__Proteobacteria; c__Gammaproteobacteria; o__Enterobacteriales; f__Enterobacteriaceae; g__Plesiomonas; s__ |
| | k__Bacteria; p__Proteobacteria; c__Gammaproteobacteria; o__Enterobacteriales; f__Enterobacteriaceae; g__Serratia; s__marcescens |
| | k__Bacteria; p__Proteobacteria; c__Gammaproteobacteria; o__Pseudomonadales; f__Moraxellaceae; g__; s__ |
| | k__Bacteria; p__Proteobacteria; c__Gammaproteobacteria; o__Pseudomonadales; f__Moraxellaceae; g__Moraxella; s__ |
| | k__Bacteria; p__Proteobacteria; c__Gammaproteobacteria; o__Pseudomonadales; f__Pseudomonadaceae; g__Pseudomonas; s__ |

**Fig. 1** (See legend on next page.)

29.9%. Both were represented in every sample. The contribution of the most abundant taxa (>0.5%) to the community composition of each sample was reasonably consistent despite a two-fold difference in the number of observed OTUs (71 to 160). However, some taxa were overrepresented in a number of samples when compared to their contribution to overall abundance (Additional file 3).

Seven OTUs were represented in 95% of samples (*n* = 20) and together they constituted the 'core' community within these prostate tissue samples (Table 3). These OTUs were assigned to *Enterobacteriaceae* and *Streptococcaceae*, *Staphylococcus*, *Escherichia*, *Moraxella*, *Propionibacterium acnes* and *Streptococcus pseudopneumoniae*. Despite these 'core' OTUs representing only a small proportion (on average 5.9%) of the mean number of OTUs that comprise the overall prostatic microbial community, they contributed to a very large proportion (77.9%) of the relative abundance of the total communities of the 20 samples sequenced. The relative contribution of each of the seven 'core' OTUs was reasonably consistent across individual samples (Fig. 2). *Enterobacteriaceae* and *Escherichia* were observed to be the most abundant taxa contributing to the 'core' community with a relative abundance of 72.2 and 26.6% respectively.

### Total RNA sequencing
Human endogenous retroviral sequences (HERVs) were successfully detected in both benign and malignant datasets. After removing human ribosomal RNA and other non-coding read pairs, approximately 20 million read

pairs remained for each of the malignant and benign prostate tissue datasets. Removing human mRNA left approximately 2.8 million unmapped read pairs for both the malignant and benign datasets. The unmapped reads were assembled into contiguous sequences using Velvet at kmer values of 55, 65, 75 and 85 and were queried for sequences of interest using BLAST. Sequences identified as belonging to *Pseudomonas* spp. were detected in the benign prostate tissue dataset. No sequences analogous to the NCBI RefSeq [22] library of viral polymerases (with the exception of HERVs) were detected. No specific viral sequences including human papillomaviruses, polyomaviruses, herpes simplex virus 1 and 2, were detected in either dataset.

### Discussion
We used broad-range methods (one targeted and one agnostic) to explore and characterise microbial constituents within the prostate tissue of men with aggressive prostate cancer.

Previous studies have investigated the presence of bacterial, viral and prokaryotic organisms and their association with prostate cancer [9, 23, 24] using other methodologies including traditional bacterial culture, specific, targeted PCR and bacterial 16S rRNA amplification, traditional cloning and capillary sequencing methods. The advantage of MPS, in this context, is the capacity to sequence the entire genomic/transcriptomic content of samples without *a priori* knowledge of specific genes and targets [25], in addition to its sensitivity

**Table 3** Taxonomic assignments of the 7 OTUs present in 95% of samples (*n* = 20) that underwent sequencing of the V2-V3 region of the 16S rRNA gene and their relative abundance

| Core OTUs shared by 95% of samples | Relative abundance of OTU within the total community % |
|---|---|
| k_Bacteria; p_Proteobacteria; c_Gammaproteobacteria; o_Enterobacteriales; f_Enterobacteriaceae; g_; s_ | 55.4% |
| k_Bacteria; p_Proteobacteria; c_Gammaproteobacteria; o_Enterobacteriales; f_Enterobacteriaceae; g_Escherichia; s_ | 20.9% |
| k_Bacteria; p_Actinobacteria; c_Actinobacteria; o_Actinomycetales; f_Propionibacteriaceae; g_Propionibacterium; s_acnes | 1.1% |
| k_Bacteria; p_Firmicutes; c_Bacilli; o_Bacillales; f_Staphylococcaceae; g_Staphylococcus; s_ | 0.4% |
| k_Bacteria; p_Firmicutes; c_Bacilli; o_Lactobacillales; f_Streptococcaceae; g_; s_ | 0.1% |
| k_Bacteria; p_Firmicutes; c_Bacilli; o_Lactobacillales; f_Streptococcaceae; g_Streptococcus; s_pseudopneumoniae | <0.1% |
| k_Bacteria; p_Proteobacteria; c_Gammaproteobacteria; o_Pseudomonadales; f_Moraxellaceae; g_Moraxella; s_ | <0.1% |
| Sum of "core" OTUs (across 95% of samples) | 77.90% |

The letters in the taxonomy column refer to k – kingdom, p – phylum, c –class, o –order, f – family, g – genus, s – species

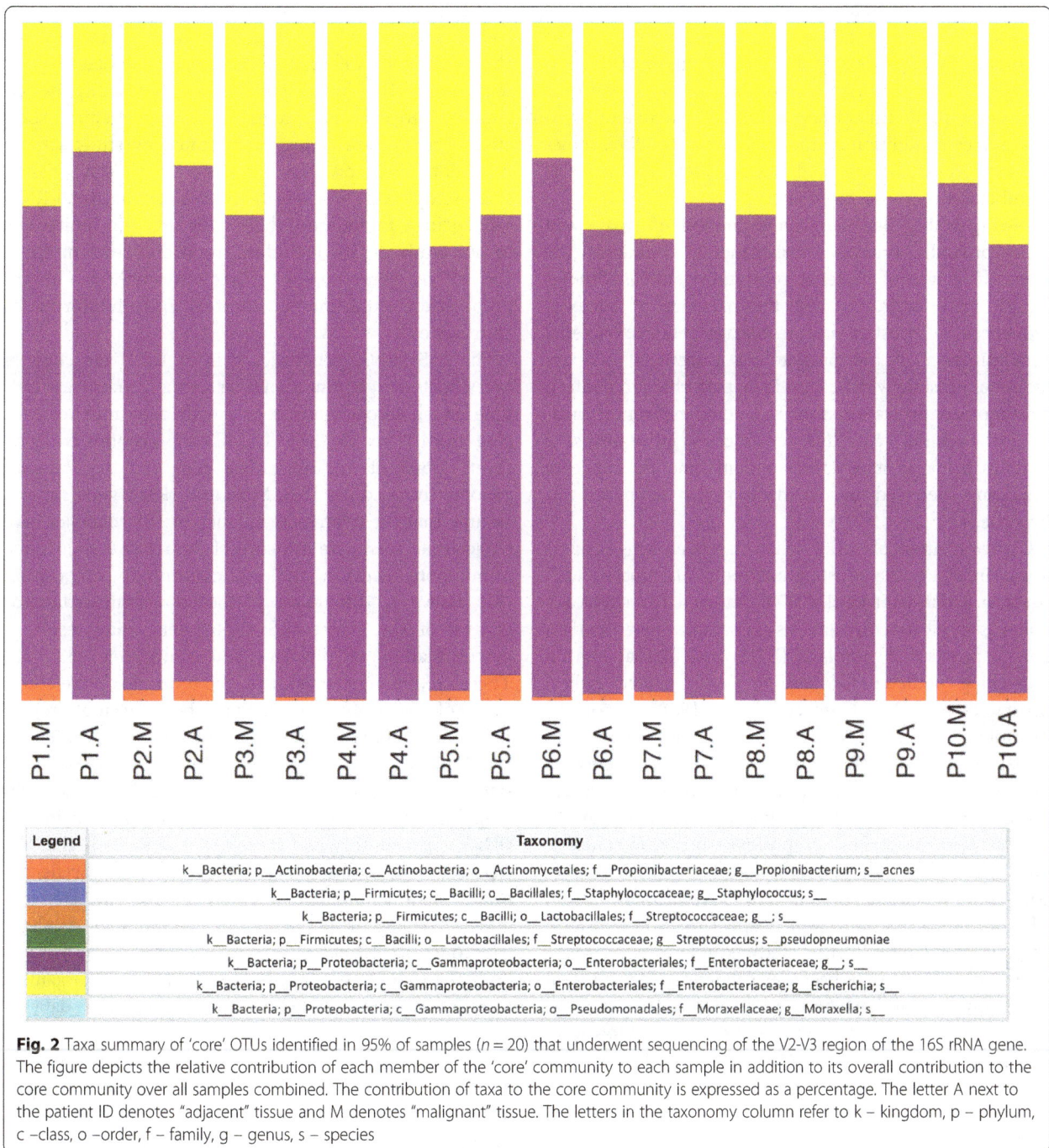

**Fig. 2** Taxa summary of 'core' OTUs identified in 95% of samples ($n = 20$) that underwent sequencing of the V2-V3 region of the 16S rRNA gene. The figure depicts the relative contribution of each member of the 'core' community to each sample in addition to its overall contribution to the core community over all samples combined. The contribution of taxa to the core community is expressed as a percentage. The letter A next to the patient ID denotes "adjacent" tissue and M denotes "malignant" tissue. The letters in the taxonomy column refer to k – kingdom, p – phylum, c –class, o –order, f – family, g – genus, s – species

and high-throughput capability. However, despite the advantages of applying new technology to a decades-old question, the data generated and the methods used for data analysis were still in early development. As this field evolves, the methods, data, analytical tools and strategies will become more refined and enable further elucidation of these study questions.

To date, five studies [8, 9, 26–28] have investigated and characterised bacterial 16S rRNA sequences in prostate tissue collected from prostate cancer patients. Only

one of these studies [28] found no evidence of 16S rRNA sequences in prostate cancer tissues. Four studies [8, 9, 26, 27] demonstrated the presence of bacterial sequences in 88.9, 85.7, 19.6 and 87% of patients, respectively. The most common organisms identified in these studies were members of the family *Enterobacteriaceae* and specifically species related to *Escherichia coli*. These findings are consistent with the results of the present study. In addition, analysis of the 16S rRNA V4 region sequencing data identified *Actinobacter* spp., *Pseudomonas* spp. and

*Streptococcus* spp. as being present in 95% of all prostate samples therefore members of the 'core' community, in accordance with Sfanos et al. (2008). Analysis of the V2-V3 region also identified *Enterobacteriaceae, Escherichia* spp. as the predominant taxa within this sample of prostate tissues in addition to *Staphylococcus* spp, *Streptococcus* spp, *Moraxella* spp., and *Propionibacterium acnes* as members of the 'core' community.

Distinguishing between contamination of tissue and 'true' prostatic microbial constituents is one of the main challenges of bacterial community studies. Studies [8, 27] have suggested that the presence of bacterial sequences in prostate cancer tissues reflects bacterial contamination of the prostate via transrectal prostate biopsy of prostate which is routinely performed to confirm a diagnosis of prostate cancer. This could explain the presence of bacterial 16S rRNA sequences in prostate tissue samples from prostate cancer patients and the range of organisms detected in our dataset also supports this hypothesis.

Catheterization of patients has also been suggested as a way in which the prostate may be contaminated with bacteria. Hochrieter et al. (2000) detected 16S rRNA sequences in all four prostate tissue samples taken from a benign prostatic hyperplasia (BPH) patient that had an indwelling catheter for several weeks before radical prostatectomy [27]. Gorelick et al. (1988) performed quantitative bacterial culture of prostate tissues from prostatectomy patients to determine the prevalence of prostate bacterial infection or colonization [29]. They reported that 34% of patients with a pre-operative indwelling catheter returned a positive prostatic culture. Organisms were identified as common urinary tract pathogens including *E. coli* and *Streptococcus fecalis*. The pre-operative status with respect to catheterization of patients included in this study is unknown, however, it is a possibility that bacterial sequences identified in our samples could have been introduced in this way.

Sequences representing *Propionibacterium acnes* were detected in the V2-V3 16S rRNA dataset in 95% of samples albeit at low abundance. This study reports a 95% prevalence of *P. acnes* in prostate tissue samples which is consistent with the 100% prevalence of *P. acnes* detected in prostatic intraepithelial neoplasia (PIN) lesions and 78% of prostate cancer tissues reported by Fehri et al. (2011) but approximately two-fold higher than the prevalence of *P. acnes* reported by other studies [1, 2, 9, 30]. The present study could not determine whether the *P. acnes* sequences detected in the V2-V3 dataset represented either urogenital or cutaneous strains. Therefore, it is difficult to ascertain if the *P. acnes* detected in these samples represent contamination through laboratory handling and reagents or if they have biological significance.

The study design and methods employed in this study had several limitations that may have diminished the ability to detect infectious organisms in prostate tissues that were of clinical significance. The study design employed to identify potential infectious agents associated with prostate cancer was limited by study sample collection methods, the sampling of prostate tissue, small sample size and sensitivity of detection (total RNA sequencing). In addition, there were inherent limitations to our study design including the presence of multiple 16S rRNA gene copies, extraction methods, library preparation, experimental controls and bioinformatics approaches.

The 16S rRNA gene occurs in at least one copy of every bacterial genome, however can also occur as multiple and heterogeneous copies with copy number ranging from 1 to 15 [31]. The *E. coli* genome contains seven copies of the 16S rRNA gene and the *P. acnes* genome three copies [32]. Most 16S rRNA gene surveys assume that the relative abundance of 16S sequences are an accurate surrogate measure of the relative abundance of microorganisms in studies of community composition [31]. However, differences in the copy number/heterogeneity of the target 16S rRNA gene may result in overestimation of diversity and abundance [33, 34]. Therefore, inferences made on the basis of relative abundance of 16S rRNA genes may not be an accurate representation of actual community composition [31, 35] and variation in 16S rRNA gene copies can be a source of significant systemic bias within 16S rRNA gene surveys [33]. This study did not normalize for variation in 16S rRNA copy number and therefore it is unlikely that the reported relative abundances of taxa identified reflected *actual* taxa abundance. However, there are software tools [31] and a publicly available curated database (ribosomal RNA operon copy number database or rrnDB [35]) that could be applied to estimate actual organism abundance from 16S rRNA gene abundance data in future work.

There is considerable scope to extend and improve upon the experimental design of this study in investigating a *persistent* infectious aetiology for prostate cancer. Incorporating a prospective study design that collected tissues specifically for PCR- and sequencing-based analyses may reduce the prevalence of contaminating sequences. Inclusion of (a) control group(s) that included samples from lower grade and less aggressive prostate cancer cases and cancer-unaffected prostates such as those from organ donors, cystoprostatectomy and/or BPH cases would allow comparison between the microbial constituents of different prostate pathologies (if any) and normal prostate tissue. In addition, a greater number of cases would ensure that the study is sufficiently powered to detect differences in microbial communities (if any) between groups. Sampling a greater proportion of the prostate gland at several anatomical sites would provide comprehensive coverage of the prostate gland as a whole. With regard to 16S rRNA amplicon sequencing, the inclusion of extraction, PCR and water controls in sequencing runs would also provide a profile of laboratory contaminants so that 'true' microbial constituents (if any) could be distinguished from contaminating sequences. Normalization of 16S rRNA datasets to account for heterogeneity of 16S rRNA gene copies would also provide more accuracy with respect to relative organismal abundance. In terms of RNA sequencing, depletion of host RNA and enrichment of microbial rRNA and mRNA may increase detection sensitivity. If microorganisms of interest were detected, follow-up studies including verification of specific infectious agents in original nucleic acid samples via PCR and tissue localization studies would be warranted.

## Conclusions

An infectious aetiology for prostate cancer has long been conjectured. We evaluated new technology to assess if its use could clarify the inconsistency in evidence related to the nature of possible infection(s) and their relationship to prostate tumour grade. We applied targeted and agnostic approaches both involving MPS. This technology detected endogenous retroviruses providing proof of concept but there was no clear evidence of clinically significant bacterial or viral sequences in prostate cancer tissue. As these investigative methods and protocols become more refined, MPS approaches are anticipated to have significant utility in identifying potential pathogens involved in disease aetiology. Further studies, specifically designed to detect associations between the disease phenotype and aetiological agents, are required.

## Abbreviations

cDNA: complementary DNA; COX-2: Cyclooxygenase-2; DNA: Deoxyribonucleic acid; HERV: Human endogenous retrovirus; MPS: Massively parallel sequencing; mRNA: messenger RNA; OTU: Operational taxonomic unit; PCR: Polymerase chain reaction; RNA: Ribonucleic acid; RNASEL: Ribonuclease L; rRNA: Ribosomal RNA; SD: Standard deviation; TLR4: Toll-like receptor 4

## Acknowledgements

Data analyses of the V2-V3 and V4 16S rRNA datasets were carried out by Gayle Philip, Life Sciences Computation Centre, Victorian Life Sciences Computation Initiative, University of Melbourne. Data analyses of the total RNA sequencing datasets were carried out by Dieter Bulach, Life Sciences Computation Centre, Victorian Life Sciences Computation Initiative, University of Melbourne.
Amplification primers that targeted the V2-V3 hypervariable region of the 16S rRNA gene were adapted/designed by Josef Wagner (JW), Murdoch Children's Research Institute.

The authors would like to express their appreciation to the study participants who kindly donated tissue to the Australian Prostate Cancer BioResource. The Australian Prostate Cancer BioResource is supported by the National Health and Medical Research Council of Australia Enabling Grant (no. 614296) and by a grant from the Prostate Cancer Foundation Australia.

## Funding

This work was supported by the National Health and Medical Research Council (APP504702), the Prostate Cancer Foundation of Australia (projects YIG19 and PG2709) and the Austin Urology Research Foundation supported by the Urologists of the Austin Hospital, Melbourne, Victoria, Australia. The authors would like to express their appreciation to the study participants who kindly donated tissue to the Australian Prostate Cancer BioResource. The Australian Prostate Cancer BioResource is supported by the National Health and Medical Research Council of Australia Enabling Grant (no. 614296) and by a grant from the Prostate Cancer Foundation Australia.

## Authors' contributions

GGG, GS and MS conceived, designed and successfully sought funding for the study. GGG was the principal investigator of the prostate study resources utilized. MS and ST coordinated, designed and supervised the molecular studies. MY carried out the laboratory-based work and drafted the manuscript. JP provided expert pathology review. APCB provided tissue samples. All authors read and approved the manuscript.

## Competing interests

The authors declare that they have no competing interests.

## Author details

[1]Genetic Epidemiology Laboratory, Department of Pathology, Faculty of Medicine, Dentistry and Health Sciences, University of Melbourne, VIC, Australia 3010. [2]Department of Microbiology and Infectious Diseases, Royal Women's Hospital, Parkville, VIC, Australia 3052. [3]Department of Obstetrics and Gynaecology, University of Melbourne, Parkville, VIC, Australia 3010. [4]Murdoch Childrens Research Institute, Parkville, VIC, Australia 3052. [5]Cancer Epidemiology and Intelligence Division, Cancer Epidemiology Centre, Cancer Council Victoria, Level 2, 615 St Kilda Road, Melbourne, VIC, Australia 3004. [6]Centre for Epidemiology and Biostatistics, Melbourne School of Population and Global Health, University of Melbourne, Level 3, 207 Bouverie Street, Carlton, VIC, Australia 3053. [7]Department of Surgery, University of Melbourne, Austin Health, 145 Studley Road, Heidelberg, VIC, Australia 3084. [8]TissuPath, 92-96 Ricketts Road, Mount Waverley, VIC, Australia 3149. [9]Human Genetics Foundation (HuGeF), Via Nizza, 52-10126 Torino, Italy. [10]Australian Prostate Cancer BioResource, the Prostate Cancer Research Program, Department of Anatomy and Developmental Biology, Monash University, Melbourne, VIC, Australia 3800.

## References

1. Cohen RJ, Shannon BA, McNeal JE, Shannon T, Garrett KL. Propionibacterium acnes associated with inflammation in radical prostatectomy specimens: a possible link to cancer evolution? J Urol. 2005; 173:1969–74.

2. Alexeyev OA, Marklund I, Shannon B, Golovleva I, Olsson J, Andersson C, et al. Direct visualization of Propionibacterium acnes in prostate tissue by multicolor fluorescent in situ hybridization assay. J Clin Microbiol. 2007;45:3721–8.

3. Panguluri RCK, Long LO, Chen W, Wang S, Coulibaly A, Ukoli F, et al. COX-2 gene promoter haplotypes and prostate cancer risk. Carcinogenesis. 2004;25:961–6.

4. Casey G, Neville PJ, Plummer SJ, Xiang Y, Krumroy LM, Klein EA, et al. RNASEL Arg462Gln variant is implicated in up to 13% of prostate cancer cases. Nat Genet. 2002;32:581–3. Nature Publishing Group.

5.   Chen Y-C, Giovannucci E, Lazarus R, Kraft P, Ketkar S, Hunter DJ. Sequence variants of Toll-like receptor 4 and susceptibility to prostate cancer. Cancer Res. 2005;65:11771–8.

6.   Riley DE, Berger RE, Miner DC, Krieger JN. Diverse and related 16S rRNA-encoding DNA sequences in prostate tissues of men with chronic prostatitis. J Clin Microbiol. 1998;36:1646–52.

7.   Alexeyev O, Bergh J, Marklund I, Thellenberg-Karlsson C, Wiklund F, Grönberg H, et al. Association between the presence of bacterial 16S RNA in prostate specimens taken during transurethral resection of prostate and subsequent risk of prostate cancer (Sweden). Cancer Causes Control. 2006;17:1127–33.

8.   Krieger JN, Riley DE, Vesella RL, Miner DC, Ross SO, Lange PH. Bacterial dna sequences in prostate tissue from patients with prostate cancer and chronic prostatitis. J Urol. 2000;164:1221–8.

9.   Sfanos KS, Sauvageot J, Fedor HL, Dick JD, De Marzo AM, Isaacs WB. A molecular analysis of prokaryotic and viral DNA sequences in prostate tissue from patients with prostate cancer indicates the presence of multiple and diverse microorganisms. Prostate. 2008;68:306–20.

10.  Australian Prostate Cancer Bioresource [Internet]. apcbioresource.org.au. [cited 2016 Jun 7]. Available from: https://www.apcbioresource.org.au.

11.  Caporaso JG, Lauber CL, Walters WA, Berg-Lyons D, Lozupone CA, Turnbaugh PJ, et al. Colloquium Paper: Global patterns of 16S rRNA diversity at a depth of millions of sequences per sample. Proc Natl Acad Sci. 2011; 108 Suppl 1:4516–22.

12.  Sundquist A, Bigdeli S, Jalili R, Druzin ML, Waller S, Pullen KM, et al. Bacterial flora-typing with targeted, chip-based Pyrosequencing. BMC Microbiol. 2007;7:108.

13.  FastQC v0.10.1 [Internet]. bioinformatics.bbsrc.ac.uk. [cited 2016 Jun 7]. Available from: http://www.bioinformatics.bbsrc.ac.uk/projects/fastqc.

14.  Magoč T, Salzberg SL. FLASH: fast length adjustment of short reads to improve genome assemblies. Bioinformatics. 2011;27:2957–63.

15.  Caporaso JG, Kuczynski J, Stombaugh J, Bittinger K, Bushman FD, Costello EK, et al. QIIME allows analysis of high-throughput community sequencing data. Nat Meth. 2010;7:335–6.

16.  Greengenes [Internet]. greengenes.lbl.gov. [cited 2016 Jun 7]. Available from: http://greengenes.lbl.gov/cgi-bin/nph-index.cgi.

17.  Nesoni [Internet]. https://github.com/Victorian-Bioinformatics-Consortium/nesoni [cited 2016 Oct 19]. Available from: https://github.com/Victorian-Bioinformatics-Consortium/nesoni.

18.  David M, Dzamba M, Lister D, Ilie L, Brudno M. SHRiMP2: sensitive yet practical SHort Read Mapping. Bioinformatics. 2011;27:1011–2.

19.  Li H, Durbin R. Fast and accurate short read alignment with Burrows-Wheeler transform. Bioinformatics. 2009;25:1754–60.

20.  Zerbino DR. Using the Velvet de novo assembler for short-read sequencing technologies. Curr Protoc Bioinformatics. 2010;Chapter 11:Unit11.5.

21.  Easy-Web-BLAST+ [Internet]. github.com. [cited 2016 Jun 7]. Available from: https://github.com/tseemann/easy-web-blast.

22.  NCBI RefSeq [Internet]. ftp.ncbi.nlm.nih.gov. [cited 2016 Jun 7]. Available from: ftp://ftp.ncbi.nlm.nih.gov/refseq/release/viral/.

23.  Sutcliffe S, Viscidi RP, Till C, Goodman PJ, Hoque AM, Hsing AW, et al. Human papillomavirus types 16, 18, and 31 serostatus and prostate cancer risk in the Prostate Cancer Prevention Trial. Cancer Epidemiol Biomarkers Prev. 2010;19:614–8.

24.  Sutcliffe S, Alderete JF, Till C, Goodman PJ, Hsing AW, Zenilman JM, et al. Trichomonosis and subsequent risk of prostate cancer in the Prostate Cancer Prevention Trial. Int J Cancer. 2009;124:2082–7.

25.  Metzker ML. Sequencing technologies — the next generation. Nat Rev Genet. 2010;11:31–46.

26.  Keay S, Zhang CO, Baldwin BR, Alexander RB. Polymerase chain reaction amplification of bacterial 16s rRNA genes in prostate biopsies from men without chronic prostatitis. Urology. 1999;53:487–91.

27.  Hochreiter WW, Duncan JL, Schaeffer AJ. Evaluation of the bacterial flora of the prostate using a 16S rRNA gene based polymerase chain reaction. J Urol. 2000;163:127–30.

28.  Leskinen MJ, Rantakokko-Jalava K, Manninen R, Leppilahti M, Marttila T, Kylmälä T, et al. Negative bacterial polymerase chain reaction (PCR) findings in prostate tissue from patients with symptoms of chronic pelvic pain syndrome (CPPS) and localized prostate cancer. Prostate. 2003;55:105–10.

29.  Gorelick JI, Senterfit LB, Vaughan ED. Quantitative bacterial tissue cultures from 209 prostatectomy specimens: findings and implications. J Urol. 1988;139:57–60.

30.  Mak TN, Fischer N, Laube B, Brinkmann V, Metruccio MME, Sfanos KS, et al. Propionibacterium acnes host cell tropism contributes to vimentin-mediated invasion and induction of inflammation. Cell Microbiol. 2012;14:1720–33.

31.  Kembel SW, Wu M, Eisen JA, Green JL. Incorporating 16S gene copy number information improves estimates of microbial diversity and abundance. PLoS Comput Biol. 2012;8:e1002743.

32.  Shannon BA, Cohen RJ, Garrett KL. Influence of 16S rDNA primer sequence mismatches on the spectrum of bacterial genera detected in prostate tissue by universal eubacterial PCR. Prostate. 2008;68:1487–91.

33.  Acinas SG, Marcelino LA, Klepac-Ceraj V, Polz MF. Divergence and redundancy of 16S rRNA sequences in genomes with multiple rrn operons. J Bacteriol. 2004;186:2629–35.

34.  Jonasson J, Olofsson M, Monstein H-J. Classification, identification and subtyping of bacteria based on pyrosequencing and signature matching of 16S rDNA fragments. APMIS. 2002;110:263–72.

35.  Stoddard SF, Smith BJ, Hein R, Roller BRK, Schmidt TM. rrnDB: improved tools for interpreting rRNA gene abundance in bacteria and archaea and a new foundation for future development. Nucleic Acids Res. 2015;43:D593–8.

# 2

# Frequency and geographic distribution of TERT promoter mutations in primary hepatocellular carcinoma

Francesca Pezzuto, Luigi Buonaguro, Franco M. Buonaguro and Maria Lina Tornesello[*] ⓘ

**Abstract**

Primary hepatocellular carcinoma (HCC) mainly develops in subjects chronically infected with hepatitis B (HBV) and C (HCV) viruses through a multistep process characterized by the accumulation of genetic alterations in the human genome. Nucleotide changes in coding regions (i.e. TP53, CTNNB1, ARID1A and ARID2) as well as in non-coding regions (i.e. TERT promoter) are considered cancer drivers for HCC development with variable frequencies in different geographic regions depending on the etiology and environmental factors. Recurrent hot spot mutations in TERT promoter (G > A at-124 bp; G > A at −146 bp), have shown to be common events in many tumor types including HCC and to up regulate the expression of telomerases. We performed a comprehensive review of the literature evaluating the differential distribution of TERT promoter mutations in 1939 primary HCC from four continents. Mutation rates were found higher in Europe (56.6%) and Africa (53.3%) than America (40%) and Asia (42.5%). In addition, HCV-related HCC were more frequently mutated (44.8% in US and 69.7% in Asia) than HBV-related HCC (21.4% in US and 45.5% in Africa). HCC cases associated to factors other than hepatitis viruses are also frequently mutated in TERT promoter (43.6%, 52.6% and 57.7% in USA, Asia and Europe, respectively). These results support a major role for telomere elongation in HCV-related and non-viral related hepatic carcinogenesis and suggest that TERT promoter mutations could represent a candidate biomarker for the early detection of liver cancer in subjects with HCV infection or with metabolic liver diseases.

**Keywords:** Telomerase, TERT promoter mutations, Hepatocellular carcinoma, Hepatitis B virus, Hepatitis C virus

## Background

Primary liver cancer is one of the commonest and deadliest malignancies in the world accounting for 782,000 new cases and 746,000 deaths in 2012 [1]. The highest incidence has been observed in men from Eastern and South-Eastern Asia (age standardized rates [ASR] 31.9 and 22.2 per 100,000, respectively) and in women from Eastern Asia and Western Africa (ASR 8.1 and 10.2 per 100,000, respectively). On the other hand, liver cancer incidence is intermediate in southern Europe and northern America (ASR 9.5 and 9.3/100,000 men, respectively), and low in western and northern Europe (ASR <7.5/100,000 men and <2.5/100,000 women) [2].

Hepatocellular carcinoma (HCC) and intrahepatic cholangiocarcinoma (ICC) are the most common histotypes of primary liver cancer accounting for about 80%

and 15%, respectively, of all cases worldwide [3–5]. HCC and ICC mainly develops in patients with liver cirrhosis caused by chronic infection with hepatitis B (HBV) and hepatitis C (HCV) or caused by alcohol excess, as well as in patients with non-alcoholic fatty liver disease or other metabolic liver disorders [6]. HBV chronically infects more than 300 million people in the world, mainly in Asia and Africa, while HCV infects approximately 180 million people, mostly in Japan, Europe and United States [6]. Accordingly, HBV-related HCC are more frequent in Asia and Africa (above 50% of all cases), while HCV-related HCC are predominant in Europe and USA (35-50% of all cases) [2, 7, 8].

The complex multistep process of liver carcinogenesis includes inflammation, hepatic damage, cirrhosis, increased liver fibrosis and HCC [9–11]. The molecular mechanisms involved in the malignant transformation of hepatocytes are extremely complex and comprise numerous genetic and epigenetic alterations [12, 13]. Genome instability,

* Correspondence: irccsvir@unina.it; m.tornesello@istitutotumori.na.it
Molecular Biology and Viral Oncology Unit, Istituto Nazionale Tumori IRCCS "Fondazione G Pascale", 80131 Napoli, Italy

mainly involving gains in chromosomes 1q, 5, 6p, 7, 8q, 17q and 20 and losses in chromosomes 1p, 4q, 6q, 8p, 13q, 16, 17p and 21, has been observed in more than 80% of HCC associated to chronic viral hepatitis [14–17].

Several lines of evidence suggest that the pattern of somatic mutations in liver cancer varies in different geographic regions very likely depending on environmental factors or host genetic diversity [18–21]. Indeed, tumor protein 53 (TP53) coding gene mutations in HCC have been observed to occur most commonly in sub-Saharan Africa and Southeast Asia, where the combination of dietary aflatoxin B1 (AFB1) exposure and hepatitis B infection promotes high rate of mutagenesis in the liver [22]. More recently, several new recurrent mutations affecting genes involved in cell cycle regulation and chromatin remodeling have been discovered by whole exome sequencing technology and found differentially distributed in different populations [23–26].

Moreover, the analysis by whole-genome sequencing allowed to discover a substantial fraction of recurrent somatic mutations in non-coding regions of human genome with important regulatory effects on the gene expression in cancer [27]. The most notable example has been the identification of hot spot activating mutations in the promoter region of telomerase reverse transcriptase (TERT) gene in about 85% of human tumors, including liver cancer [28–31]. The newly described mutations at nucleotides 124 (mostly G > A and rarely G > T) or 146 (G > A) before the ATG start site in TERT promoter region have been recognized as frequent and early alterations in the hepatic carcinogenesis [31, 32]. These mutations create a binding site for transcription factors ETS (E-twenty six) and ternary complex factor (TCF), causing TERT over expression and restoring the telomerase activity [33].

Moreover, the single nucleotide polymorphism rs2853669, located at −245 bp upstream of the ATG start codon in TERT promoter, has also shown to deregulate the expression levels of TERT mRNA [34].

We performed a systematic review of published studies to investigate the frequency of TERT promoter mutations in 1939 HCC with diverse etiologies. Moreover, we evaluated the mutational pattern of TERT promoter in tumors from different geographic areas to possibly correlate the type of nucleotide changes with specific environmental or genetic factors in different regions of the world.

### Telomerase and liver diseases

TERT gene encodes for the catalytic subunit of the telomerase reverse transcriptase which is an RNA-dependent DNA polymerase highly expressed in germ cells, in stem cells and in cancer cells [35, 36]. The telomerase synthesizes telomeres which are long stretches of 5'-TTAGGG-3' DNA repeats ending in a single-strand 3' G-rich sequence located at the extremities of human chromosomes. Telomeres protect chromosomes from degradation, end-to-end fusion and recombination and act as an internal clock by regulating the maximal number of cell replication and aging [37–43].

The pathogenesis of liver diseases is strongly dependent on telomeres length and telomerase expression [44]. Several studies have shown a relationship between cirrhosis and telomeres attrition suggesting that this event could be considered a marker of cirrhosis [45–47]. However, telomerase activity and telomere elongation is restored in up to 90% of HCC, compared to the 21% of adjacent non-tumor tissues [8, 48–50]. Moreover, long telomeres and increased telomerase levels have shown to be associated with aggressive HCC phenotype and with poor prognosis [51].

Telomerase is activated by different mechanisms during liver carcinogenesis. In HBV related HCC the telomerase reactivation is frequently caused by the insertion of the HBV DNA within or upstream the TERT gene [52–56]. Sung et al. identified integrated HBV DNA in 86.4% of liver cancers, by whole-genome deep sequencing, and found that genes recurrently affected by HBV integration were TERT (23.7%), myeloid/lymphoid or mixed-lineage leukemia 4 (MLL4) gene (11.8%) and cyclin E1 encoding gene (CCNE1) (5.2%) [57]. Totoki et al. performed a comprehensive transancestry liver cancer genome study on 506 HCC cases from Asia and USA and observed HBV integration in TERT locus in 22% of tumors [31]. Moreover, they observed that TERT promoter mutations were in general mutually exclusive with HBV genome integration in the TERT locus and with TERT focal amplification, suggesting that either event is sufficient to activate telomerases. In addition, Zhao et al. reported that HBV insertional sites are significantly enriched in the proximity of telomeres in HCC DNA but not in non-tumor cell genomes suggesting that the integrated virus in cancer tends to target chromosomal elements critical for the maintenance of chromosome stability [58]. Moreover, Yang et al. analyzed 2199 HBV integration sites and observed that affected genes included 23.1% of protein-coding genes and 24.7% of long noncoding RNAs (lncRNA) [59]. Interestingly, the most frequently lncRNA genes affected by HBV integration were related to telomere maintenance, protein modification processes, and chromosome localization [59].

In HCV-related HCC and non-viral related HCC the telomerase activation is due to TERT promoter mutations in 40% to 75% of HCC cases, however with a considerable variation in different cohorts, as detailed in the next section.

### TERT promoter mutations in different geographical regions

Published data on the analysis of TERT promoter mutations in liver cancer were searched in Medline using the terms ("hepatocellular" OR ("Liver" AND "Cancer")) AND ("TERT" OR "telomerase") AND ("Promoter")

AND ("mutation" OR "variation"), (Fig. 1). For the studies that involved more than one geographic location the data were divided into components for each continent. The search was updated on 31 January 2017.

The frequencies of TERT mutations in HCC have shown to vary by cancer etiology and geographic patient provenance (Table 1). Cevik et al. analyzed TERT promoter mutations in 15 HCC cases from Africa [60]. African patients comprised mainly HBV-positive subjects from Mozambique (n = 6), Transkei (n = 4), Lesotho (n = 2), Swaziland (n = 1) and South Africa (n = 2). The overall frequency of TERT promoter mutation among the HCC African cases was 53.3% and in the subgroup of HBV-related HCC was 45.5%. No other study has analyzed the TERT promoter mutation pattern in African HCC and more cases need to be analyzed to confirm such results.

Two studies evaluated TERT promoter mutations among 150 HCC cases from the United States and the overall mutation rate was 40% [31, 61]. The HCV-related HCC and non viral related cases, mainly associated to alcohol and metabolic syndrome, were more mutated (44.7% and 43.6%, respectively) compared to HBV-related cases (21.4%), Table 1. Both USA cohorts comprised patients with European ancestry (n = 74), Asian ancestry (n = 22) and African-American ancestry (n = 23). Comparable frequencies of TERT promoter mutations were observed between European (43.6%) and African (37.5%) HCV-related HCC. Larger studies are warranted in the USA to analyze the TERT variation frequencies in HBV-related and no-virus

related HCC and to determine whether the genetic background has a role in the accumulation of TERT mutations in HCC in this multiethnic population.

In Asia, a total of 1014 HCC have been analyzed for TERT promoter nucleotide changes comprising 396 cases from Japan, 318 from China, 195 from Taiwan and 105 from South Korea. The overall mutation frequencies in TERT promoter were 28.9% in HBV-positive, 69.7% in HCV-related and 52.6% in non viral related HCC (Table 1). However, there were significant differences between mutation rates observed in HCV-related and no virus related HCC in Japan (74.8% and 62.4%, respectively) and South Korea (83.3% and 61.9%) versus Taiwan (54% and 20.8%). Similarly, variable rates of TERT mutations were observed among HBV positive HCC with high frequency in Japan (37.4%), intermediate in China (30.1%) and South Korea (29.4%) and low in Taiwan (20.6%).

In Europe, among the 760 HCC analyzed in five studies a total of 430 (56.6%) cases were found mutated in TERT promoter. The proportion of hot spot mutations in HCV, no virus and HBV related HCC was 61.5%, 57.7% and 42.7%, respectively. The highest mutation rate was observed in HCV-positive (73.1%) and other etiology HCC (61.7%), mainly related to alcohol, in France. In Italy, lower rates of TERT promoter mutations were observed in HCV-positive HCC, ranging from 40% to 53.6%, and in HBV-positive HCC, ranging from 70% to 41.6%, from northern and southern Italy patients, respectively.

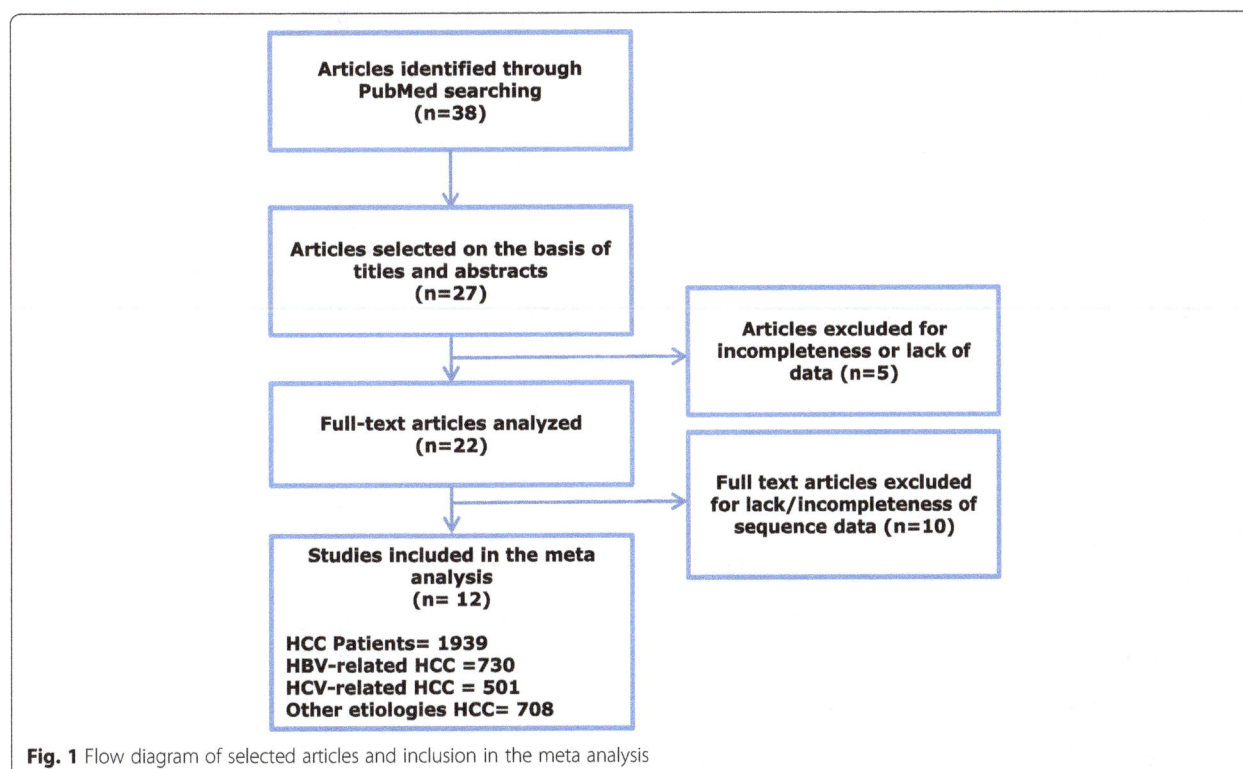

**Fig. 1** Flow diagram of selected articles and inclusion in the meta analysis

**Table 1** Distribution of TERT promoter mutations in HCC, associated to different etiologies, from divers geographic regions

| Patients (n = 1939) | | HBV+ patients (n = 730) | HCV+ patients (n = 501) | Other etiol. (n = 708) | TERTp mut (n = 929) (%) | −124 hotspot (n = 869) (%) | −146 hotspot (n = 43) (%) | HBV+ mut (n = 227) (%) | HCV+ mut (n = 313) (%) | Other etiol. mut^a (n = 389) (%) | Article |
|---|---|---|---|---|---|---|---|---|---|---|---|
| AFRICA | Lesotho (n = 2) | 2 | | | 1 (50) | 1 (100) | 1 (100) | 1 (50) | | 1 (50) | Cevik et al., 2015 [60] |
| | Mozambique (n = 6) | 5 | | 1 | 4 (66.6) | 2 (50) | 2 (50) | 3 (60) | | 1 (100) | Cevik et al., 2015 [60] |
| | South Africa (n = 2) | 2 | | | 1 (50) | 1 (100) | | 1 (50) | | | Cevik et al., 2015 [60] |
| | Swaziland (n = 1) | 1 | | | | | | | | | Cevik et al., 2015 [60] |
| | Transkei (n = 4) | 1 | | 3 | 2 (50) | 2 (100) | | | | 2 (66.6) | Cevik et al., 2015 [60] |
| | **Total cases (n = 15)** | **11** | | **4** | **8 (53.3)** | **5 (62.5)** | **3 (37.5)** | **5 (45.5)** | | **3 (75)** | |
| AMERICA | USA – African Americans (n = 12) | 2 | 7 | 3 | 8 (66.6) | 8 (100) | | 1 (50) | 5 (71.4) | 2 (66.6) | Killela et al., 2013 [61]^b |
| | USA – African Americans (n = 11) | 1 | 9 | 1 | 1 (9.1) | 1 (100) | | | 1 (11.1) | | Totoki et al., 2012 [31] |
| | USA – Asian Ancestry (n = 14) | 8 | 4 | 2 | 5 (35.7) | 4 (80) | 1 (20) | | 4 (100) | 1 (50) | Totoki et al., 2012 [31] |
| | USA – Asian Ancestry (n = 8) | 7 | 7 | 1 | 2 (25) | 2 (100) | | 1 (14.3) | | 1 (100) | Killela et al., 2013 [61]^b |
| | USA – European Ancestry (n = 50) | 3 | 32 | 15 | 21 (42) | 20 (95.2) | 1 (4.8) | 2 (66.6) | 13 (40.6) | 6 (40) | Totoki et al., 2012 [31] |
| | USA – European Ancestry (n = 24) | 1 | 7 | 16 | 12 (50) | 12 (100) | | | 4 (57.1) | 8 (50) | Killela et al., 2013 [61]^b |
| | USA – Unknown Ancestry (n = 17) | 5 | 2 | 10 | 5 (29.4) | 4 (80) | 1 (20) | 2 (40) | 1 (50) | 2 (20) | Killela et al., 2013 [61]^b |
| | USA – Unknown Ancestry (n = 14) | 1 | 6 | 7 | 6 (42.8) | 6 (100) | | | 2 (33.3) | 4 (57.1) | Totoki et al., 2012 [31] |
| | **Total cases (n = 150)** | **28** | **67** | **55** | **60 (40)** | **57 (95)** | **3 (5)** | **6 (21.4)** | **30 (44.8)** | **24 (43.6)** | |
| ASIA | China (n = 275) | 259 | | 16 | 85 (30.9) | 84 (98.8) | 1 (1.2) | 78 (30.1) | | 7 (43.7) | Yang et al., 2016 [74] |
| | China (n = 35) | | | 35 | 11 (31.4) | 9 (81.8) | 2 (18.2) | | | 11 (31.4) | Huang et al., 2015 [74] |
| | China (n = 8) | 8 | | | | | | | | | Cevik et al., 2015 [60] |
| | Japan (n = 374) | 107^e | 139 | 128 | 224^b (59.8) | 208 (92.8) | 9 (4) | 40 (37.4) | 104 (74.8) | 80 (62.5) | Totoki et al., 2014 [31] |

**Table 1** Distribution of TERT promoter mutations in HCC, associated to different etiologies, from divers geographic regions (*Continued*)

| Location | | | | | | | | | | Reference |
|---|---|---|---|---|---|---|---|---|---|---|
| Japan (n = 11) | 11 | | | 9 (81.8) | 9 (100) | | | | 9 (81.8) | Ki et al., 2016 [77] |
| Japan (n = 11) | 10 | 1 | | 4 (36.4) | 3 (75) | 1 (25) | | | 4 (40) | Cevik et al., 2015 [60] |
| South Korea (n = 105) | 78 | 6 | 21 | 41 (39) | 39 (95.1) | 2 (4.9) | 23 (29.4) | 5 (83.3) | 13 (61.9) | Lee et al., 2016 [76] |
| Taiwan (n = 195) | 50 | 12[e] | 133 | 57 (29.2) | 54 (94.7) | 3 (5.3) | 25 (20.6) | 27 (54) | 5 (20.8) | Chen et al., 2014 [73] |
| **Total cases (n = 1014)** | **574** | **245** | **195** | **431 (42.5)** | **406 (94.2)** | **18 (4.2)** | **166 (28.9)** | **136 (69.7)** | **129 (52.6)** | |
| EUROPE France (n = 305) | 67 | 68 | 170 | 179 (58.6) | 168[c] (93.8) | 11 (6.1) | 26 (38.8) | 49 (72.1) | 104 (61.1) | Nault et al., 2013 [69] |
| France (n = 193) | 24[e] | 36 | 133 | 120[d] (62.1) | 106[c] (88.3) | 5 (4.2) | 10 (41.6) | 27 (75) | 83 (62.4) | Schulze et al., 2015 [30] |
| Germany (n = 78) | | | 78 | 37 (47.4) | 37 (100) | | | | 37 (47.4) | Quaas et al., 2014 [78] |
| Germany (n = 7) | 3 | | 4 | 3 (42.8) | 2 (66.6) | 1 (33.3) | 1 (33.3) | | 2 (50) | Cevik et al., 2015 [60] |
| Italy (n = 127) | 12[e] | 110 | 5 | 64 (50.4) | 62 (96.9) | 2 (3.1) | 5 (41.6) | 59 (53.6) | | Pezzuto et al., 2016 [32] |
| Italy (n = 41) | 10 | 20 | 11 | 21[d] (51.2) | 20 (95.2) | | 7 (70) | 8 (40) | 6 (54.5) | Schulze et al., 2015 [30] |
| Spain (n = 9) | 1 | 5 | 3 | 6 (66.6) | 6 (100) | | 1 (100) | 4 (80) | 1 (33.3) | Schulze et al., 2015 [30] |
| **Total cases (n = 760)** | **117** | **239** | **404** | **430 (56.6)** | **401 (93.2)** | **19 (4.4)** | **50 (42.7)** | **147 (61.5)** | **233 (57.7)** | |

[a]This group comprises HCC cases of various etiologies including alcohol intake, metabolic syndrome, NAFLD, NASH, hemochromatosis and cases with unknown etiology (Cevik et al., [60], Huang et al., [74], Killela et al., [61], Quaas et al., [78], Schulze et al., [30])

[b]This group comprises 4 cases of −57 T > G mutations, one case of −64 CG > TC substitution, one case of −69 C > A substitution and one patient showing contemporary −124 G > A substitution and of −116 G > T substitution (Totoki et al., [31])

[c]These groups comprise two (Nault et al., [69]) and one case (Schulze et al., [30]) of −124 G > T mutation, respectively

[d]These groups comprise 4 mutations −57 T > G, one substitution −53 A > G, one substitution g.1271232 A > G, one substitution 1293829 G > T and two cases of deletion (French cohort) and one case of g.1294963 G > A substitution (Italian cohort), respectively (Schulze et al., [30])

[e]These groups comprise twelve cases (Totoki et al., [31]), twenty cases (Chen et al., [73]) four cases (Schulze et al., [30]) and two cases (Pezzuto et al., [32]) of HBV+/HCV+ patients, respectively

In all studies the activating mutation at nucleotide −124 G > A was more frequent than the mutation at position −146 G > A (93.4% versus 4.6%, respectively).

## TERT promoter mutation and rs2853669 polymorphism

Several studies have reported that the single nucleotide polymorphism (SNP) rs2853669 allele G, located at nucleotide −245 from the TERT ATG start site, down regulates the expression of TERT gene caused by hot spot promoter mutations in several types of cancer including bladder, gliomas, and renal cell cancer [62, 63]. In the general population the rs2853669 allele G is less frequent than allele A, except for the south Asia population where it has been observed the reverse [64] (www.ncbi.nlm.nih.gov/projects/SNP/snp_ref.cgi?rs=2853669).

Only two studies evaluated the rs2853669 polymorphism and TERT promoter mutations in liver cancer. The study by Pezzuto et al., analyzed the allele frequency of TERT SNP rs2853669 in HCC from Southern Italy patients and showed allele frequencies of 51% A and 48.9% G among the TERT promoter mutated HCC and 57.6% A and 42.4% G among non-mutated cancer cases [32]. Although G allele appeared more frequent among TERT mutated cases, such difference did not reach statistical significance. Moreover, the Log-rank survival analysis showed no correlation between the presence of TERT promoter mutations, alone or in combination with rs2853669 GG and GA genotypes, and poor prognosis ($p = 0.368$) [32].

Ko et al. analyzed the impact of rs2853669 polymorphism in a cohort of south Korean HCC patients and observed no effect on the overall and recurrence-free survival. However, the combination of rs2853669 G allele and mutation in the TERT promoter was associated with poor survival [65]. Moreover, they showed that the rs2853669 nucleotide G causes increased binding of the transcription factor ETS2 to the TERT promoter and lower activity of the transcription inhibitor E2F1. This condition favors TERT promoter methylation and increased expression of telomerases [65]. Methylation of TERT promoter has been observed in several tumors and transformed cell lines and has been reported to correlate with TERT over expression and poor survival [66, 67].

## Discussion

Telomerase activity has been found strongly up regulated in many human cancers including HCC, highlighting its pivotal role in the neoplastic process [28, 48, 49, 68]. TERT promoter mutations have been recognized as the earliest and most frequent genetic alterations in liver cancer [25, 31, 69]. We have summarized the TERT promoter mutation distribution in HCC cases, associated to different etiologies, from various geographic regions.

In Africa, where HCC cases are mainly related to HBV infection and AFB1 dietary exposure, the frequency of TERT promoter mutations is around 53%. It is not known if there is synergistic effect between AFB1 and HBV on the accumulation of mutations in TERT as observed for the G to T variation at codon 249 in TP53 gene, specifically caused by HBV and AFB1 [70–72]. Interestingly, in USA where patients have no AFB1 exposure, the frequency of TERT promoter mutations

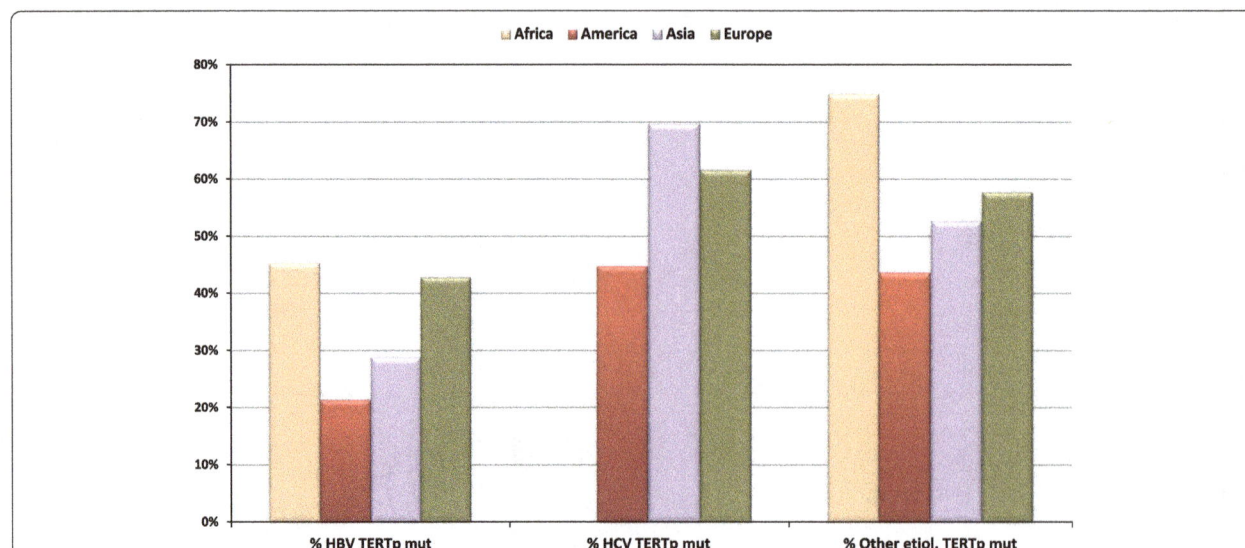

Fig. 2 Frequency of TERT promoter mutations in all HCC from different geographic regions stratified by HBV (% HBV TERTp mut), as percentage of HBV+ HCC cases characterized by TERT promoter mutations, and HCV (% HCV TERTp mut), as percentage of HCV+ HCC cases characterized by TERT promoter mutations. Patients with both HBV and HCV infections have been included in the HBV group. HCC cases of various etiologies including alcohol intake, metabolic syndrome, NAFLD, NASH, hemochromatosis and cases with unknown etiology have been grouped in Other etiologies (% Other etiol. TERTp mut)

among HBV-positive cases is 21.4% [31, 61]. In Asia, the overall rate is 42.5% with lower frequencies in China and Taiwan [31, 60, 73–77]. Higher frequencies of TERT promoter mutations, ranging from 42.8% to 66.6%, have been observed in Europe [30, 32, 60, 69, 78].

As shown in Fig. 2, HCV positive HCC have in general higher TERT promoter mutations rates than HBV positive tumors, in which TERT over expression is frequently caused by HBV integration [31, 32, 60, 73, 74]. HCC caused by non viral factors, such as alcohol consumption, metabolic syndrome, nonalcoholic fatty liver disease (NAFLD), nonalcoholic steatohepatitis (NASH), hemochromatosis, have a striking high frequency of mutation in TERT promoter. In fact, Ki et al. showed that in Japan 81.8% of NAFLD related HCC were mutated in TERT promoter [77]. In Europe, Nault et al. reported TERT promoter mutations in 68% of alcohol related HCC and in 63% of hemochromatosis related HCC cases [69].

Interestingly, TERT promoter mutations were more frequent in older patients [69, 73], and often associated with activating mutations in catenin beta 1 coding gene (CTNNB1) suggesting a cooperation between telomerase activity and β-catenin pathway [69].

## Conclusions

In conclusion, TERT promoter mutations are very frequent in HCC with different etiologies and are tumor specific given their constant absence in non-tumor tissues. There is a substantial heterogeneity in the mutation frequency in HCC from different geographic regions, probably due to environmental factors, such as AFB1, and lifestyle, such as habit of alcohol consumption. The high proportion of HCC mutated cases in different geographic regions and the earliness of occurrence of TERT mutations during hepatocarcinogenesis suggest the use of this reliable biomarker for early HCC diagnosis and as possible target for specific therapies.

## Abbreviations
AFB1: Aflatoxin B1; ARID1A: AT-rich interaction domain 1A coding gene; ARID2: AT-rich interaction domain 2 coding gene; CCNE1: Cyclin E1 coding gene; CTNNB1: catenin beta 1 coding gene; ETS: E-twentysix; HBV: Hepatitis B virus; HCC: Hepatocellular carcinoma; HCV: Hepatitis C virus; ICC: Intrahepatic cholangiocarcinoma; lncRNA: Long noncoding RNAs; MLL4: Myeloid/lymphoid or mixed-lineage leukemia 4; NAFLD: Nonalcoholic fatty liver disease; NASH: Nonalcoholic steatohepatitis; TCF: Ternary complex factor; TERT: Telomerase reverse transcriptase coding gene; TP53: Tumor Protein 53 coding gene

## Acknowledgements
F. Pezzuto is the recipient of a research fellowship awarded by FIRE/AISF ONLUS (Fondazione Italiana per la Ricerca in Epatologia) http://www.fondazionefegato.it/

## Funding
This work was supported by grants from Ministero della Salute Ricerca Corrente 2013–2016 and Ricerca Finalizzata FN 270/RF-2010-2312010.

## Authors' contributions
MLT designed the study and drafted the article; FP conducted the meta analysis and wrote the article; LB contributed to the statistical analyses; FMB supervised the whole project. All authors read and approved the final manuscript.

## Competing interests
The authors declare that they have no competing interests.

## References
1. Ferlay J, Soerjomataram I, Ervik M, Dikshit R, Eser S, Mathers C, Rebelo M, Parkin DM, Forman D, Bray F. GLOBOCAN 2012 v1.0, Cancer Incidence and Mortality Worldwide: IARC CancerBase No. 11. Lyon, France: International Agency for Research on Cancer; 2013.
2. Bosetti C, Turati F, La VC. Hepatocellular carcinoma epidemiology. Best Pract Res Clin Gastroenterol. 2014;28:753–70.
3. Perz JF, Armstrong GL, Farrington LA, Hutin YJ, Bell BP. The contributions of hepatitis B virus and hepatitis C virus infections to cirrhosis and primary liver cancer worldwide. J Hepatol. 2006;45:529–38.
4. Okuda K, Nakanuma Y, Miyazaki M. Cholangiocarcinoma: recent progress, Part 1: epidemiology and etiology. J Gastroenterol Hepatol. 2002;17:1049–55.
5. Petrick JL, Braunlin M, Laversanne M, Valery PC, Bray F, McGlynn KA. International trends in liver cancer incidence, overall and by histologic subtype, 1978–2007. Int J Cancer. 2016;139:1534–45.
6. El-Serag HB. Epidemiology of viral hepatitis and hepatocellular carcinoma. Gastroenterology. 2012;142:1264–73.
7. Raza SA, Clifford GM, Franceschi S. Worldwide variation in the relative importance of hepatitis B and hepatitis C viruses in hepatocellular carcinoma: a systematic review. Br J Cancer. 2007;96:1127–34.
8. Protzer U, Maini MK, Knolle PA. Living in the liver: hepatic infections. Nat Rev Immunol. 2012;12:201–13.
9. Arzumanyan A, Reis HM, Feitelson MA. Pathogenic mechanisms in HBV- and HCV-associated hepatocellular carcinoma. Nat Rev Cancer. 2013;13:123–35.
10. Farazi PA, DePinho RA. Hepatocellular carcinoma pathogenesis: from genes to environment. Nat Rev Cancer. 2006;6:674–87.
11. Tornesello ML, Buonaguro L, Buonaguro FM. An overview of new biomolecular pathways in pathogen-related cancers. Future Oncol. 2015;11:1625–39.
12. Zucman-Rossi J, Villanueva A, Nault JC, Llovet JM. Genetic Landscape and Biomarkers of Hepatocellular Carcinoma. Gastroenterology. 2015;149:1226–39.
13. Tornesello ML, Buonaguro L, Izzo F, Buonaguro FM. Molecular alterations in hepatocellular carcinoma associated with hepatitis B and hepatitis C infections. Oncotarget. 2016;7:25087–102.
14. Guichard C, Amaddeo G, Imbeaud S, Ladeiro Y, Pelletier L, Maad IB, Calderaro J, Bioulac-Sage P, Letexier M, Degos F, Clement B, Balabaud C, Chevet E, Laurent A, Couchy G, Letouze E, Calvo F, Zucman-Rossi J. Integrated analysis of somatic mutations and focal copy-number changes identifies key genes and pathways in hepatocellular carcinoma. Nat Genet. 2012;44:694–8.
15. Thorgeirsson SS, Grisham JW. Molecular pathogenesis of human hepatocellular carcinoma. Nat Genet. 2002;31:339–46.
16. Chochi Y, Kawauchi S, Nakao M, Furuya T, Hashimoto K, Oga A, Oka M, Sasaki K. A copy number gain of the 6p arm is linked with advanced hepatocellular carcinoma: an array-based comparative genomic hybridization study. J Pathol. 2009;217:677–84.
17. Midorikawa Y, Yamamoto S, Tsuji S, Kamimura N, Ishikawa S, Igarashi H, Makuuchi M, Kokudo N, Sugimura H, Aburatani H. Allelic imbalances and homozygous deletion on 8p23.2 for stepwise progression of hepatocarcinogenesis. Hepatology. 2009;49:513–22.

18. Tornesello ML, Buonaguro L, Tatangelo F, Botti G, Izzo F, Buonaguro FM. Mutations in TP53, CTNNB1 and PIK3CA genes in hepatocellular carcinoma associated with hepatitis B and hepatitis C virus infections. Genomics. 2013;102:74–83.

19. Unsal H, Yakicier C, Marcais C, Kew M, Volkmann M, Zentgraf H, Isselbacher KJ, Ozturk M. Genetic heterogeneity of hepatocellular carcinoma. Proc Natl Acad Sci U S A. 1994;91:822–6.

20. De Re V, Caggiari L, De ZM, Repetto O, Zignego AL, Izzo F, Tornesello ML, Buonaguro FM, Mangia A, Sansonno D, Racanelli V, De VS, Pioltelli P, Vaccher E, Berretta M, Mazzaro C, Libra M, Gini A, Zucchetto A, Cannizzaro R, De PP, 10. Genetic diversity of the KIR/HLA system and susceptibility to hepatitis C virus-related diseases. PLoS One. 2015;%20:e0117420.

21. De Re V, De ZM, Caggiari L, Lauletta G, Tornesello ML, Fognani E, Miorin M, Racanelli V, Quartuccio L, Gragnani L, Russi S, Pavone F, Ghersetti M, Costa EG, Casarin P, Bomben R, Mazzaro C, Basaglia G, Berretta M, Vaccher E, Izzo F, Buonaguro FM, De VS, Zignego AL, De PP, Dolcetti R. HCV-related liver and lymphoproliferative diseases: association with polymorphisms of IL28B and TLR2. Oncotarget. 2016;7:37487–97.

22. Gouas D, Shi H, Hainaut P. The aflatoxin-induced TP53 mutation at codon 249 (R249S): biomarker of exposure, early detection and target for therapy. Cancer Lett. 2009;286:29–37.

23. Imbeaud S, Ladeiro Y, Zucman-Rossi J. Identification of novel oncogenes and tumor suppressors in hepatocellular carcinoma. Semin Liver Dis. 2010;30:75–86.

24. Nault JC, Zucman-Rossi J. Genetics of hepatobiliary carcinogenesis. Semin Liver Dis. 2011;31:173–87.

25. Fujimoto A, Totoki Y, Abe T, Boroevich KA, Hosoda F, Nguyen HH, Aoki M, Hosono N, Kubo M, Miya F, Arai Y, Takahashi H, Shirakihara T, Nagasaki M, Shibuya T, Nakano K, Watanabe-Makino K, Tanaka H, Nakamura H, Kusuda J, Ojima H, Shimada K, Okusaka T, Ueno M, Shigekawa Y, Kawakami Y, Arihiro K, Ohdan H, Gotoh K, Ishikawa O, Ariizumi S, Yamamoto M, Yamada T, Chayama K, Kosuge T, Yamaue H, Kamatani N, Miyano S, Nakagama H, Nakamura Y, Tsunoda T, Shibata T, Nakagawa H. Whole-genome sequencing of liver cancers identifies etiological influences on mutation patterns and recurrent mutations in chromatin regulators. Nat Genet. 2012;44:760–4.

26. Huang J, Deng Q, Wang Q, Li KY, Dai JH, Li N, Zhu ZD, Zhou B, Liu XY, Liu RF, Fei QL, Chen H, Cai B, Zhou B, Xiao HS, Qin LX, Han ZG. Exome sequencing of hepatitis B virus-associated hepatocellular carcinoma. Nat Genet. 2012;44:1117–21.

27. Weinhold N, Jacobsen A, Schultz N, Sander C, Lee W. Genome-wide analysis of noncoding regulatory mutations in cancer. Nat Genet. 2014;46:1160–5.

28. Takai H, Smogorzewska A, de LT. DNA damage foci at dysfunctional telomeres. Curr Biol. 2003;13:1549–56.

29. Aubert G, Lansdorp PM. Telomeres and aging. Physiol Rev. 2008;88:557–79.

30. Schulze K, Imbeaud S, Letouze E, Alexandrov LB, Calderaro J, Rebouissou S, Couchy G, Meiller C, Shinde J, Soysouvanh F, Calatayud AL, Pinyol R, Pelletier L, Balabaud C, Laurent A, Blanc JF, Mazzaferro V, Calvo F, Villanueva A, Nault JC, Bioulac-Sage P, Stratton MR, Llovet JM, Zucman-Rossi J. Exome sequencing of hepatocellular carcinomas identifies new mutational signatures and potential therapeutic targets. Nat Genet. 2015;47:505–11.

31. Totoki Y, Tatsuno K, Covington KR, Ueda H, Creighton CJ, Kato M, Tsuji S, Donehower LA, Slagle BL, Nakamura H, Yamamoto S, Shinbrot E, Hama N, Lehmkuhl M, Hosoda F, Arai Y, Walker K, Dahdouli M, Gotoh K, Nagae G, Gingras MC, Muzny DM, Ojima H, Shimada K, Midorikawa Y, Goss JA, Cotton R, Hayashi A, Shibahara J, Ishikawa S, Guiteau J, Tanaka M, Urushidate T, Ohashi S, Okada N, Doddapaneni H, Wang M, Zhu Y, Dinh H, Okusaka T, Kokudo N, Kosuge T, Takayama T, Fukayama M, Gibbs RA, Wheeler DA, Aburatani H, Shibata T. Trans-ancestry mutational landscape of hepatocellular carcinoma genomes. Nat Genet. 2014;46:1267–73.

32. Pezzuto F, Izzo F, Buonaguro L, Annunziata C, Tatangelo F, Botti G, Buonaguro FM, Tornesello ML: Tumor specific mutations in TERT promoter and CTNNB1 gene in hepatitis B and hepatitis C related hepatocellular carcinoma. Oncotarget 2016.

33. Xu D, Dwyer J, Li H, Duan W, Liu JP. Ets2 maintains hTERT gene expression and breast cancer cell proliferation by interacting with c-Myc. J Biol Chem. 2008;283:23567–80.

34. Park CK, Lee SH, Kim JY, Kim JE, Kim TM, Lee ST, Choi SH, Park SH, Kim IH. Expression level of hTERT is regulated by somatic mutation and common single nucleotide polymorphism at promoter region in glioblastoma. Oncotarget. 2014;5:3399–407.

35. Wright WE, Piatyszek MA, Rainey WE, Byrd W, Shay JW. Telomerase activity in human germline and embryonic tissues and cells. Dev Genet. 1996;18:173–9.

36. Levy MZ, Allsopp RC, Futcher AB, Greider CW, Harley CB. Telomere end-replication problem and cell aging. J Mol Biol. 1992;225:951–60.

37. Kim NW, Piatyszek MA, Prowse KR, Harley CB, West MD, Ho PL, Coviello GM, Wright WE, Weinrich SL, Shay JW. Specific association of human telomerase activity with immortal cells and cancer. Science. 1994;266:2011–5.

38. Masutomi K, Yu EY, Khurts S, Ben-Porath I, Currier JL, Metz GB, Brooks MW, Kaneko S, Murakami S, DeCaprio JA, Weinberg RA, Stewart SA, Hahn WC. Telomerase maintains telomere structure in normal human cells. Cell. 2003; 114:241–53.

39. Blackburn EH. Telomere states and cell fates. Nature. 2000;408:53–6.

40. Ramlee MK, Wang J, Toh WX, Li S. Transcription Regulation of the Human Telomerase Reverse Transcriptase (hTERT) Gene. Genes (Basel). 2016;7:50.

41. De LT. How shelterin solves the telomere end-protection problem. Cold Spring Harb Symp Quant Biol. 2010;75:167–77.

42. Makarov VL, Hirose Y, Langmore JP. Long G tails at both ends of human chromosomes suggest a C strand degradation mechanism for telomere shortening. Cell. 1997;88:657–66.

43. Wright WE, Tesmer VM, Huffman KE, Levene SD, Shay JW. Normal human chromosomes have long G-rich telomeric overhangs at one end. Genes Dev. 1997;11:2801–9.

44. Donati B, Valenti L. Telomeres, NAFLD and Chronic Liver Disease. Int J Mol Sci. 2016;17:383.

45. Wiemann SU, Satyanarayana A, Tsahuridu M, Tillmann HL, Zender L, Klempnauer J, Flemming P, Franco S, Blasco MA, Manns MP, Rudolph KL. Hepatocyte telomere shortening and senescence are general markers of human liver cirrhosis. FASEB J. 2002;16:935–42.

46. Kitada T, Seki S, Kawakita N, Kuroki T, Monna T. Telomere shortening in chronic liver diseases. Biochem Biophys Res Commun. 1995;211:33–9.

47. Carulli L, Anzivino C. Telomere and telomerase in chronic liver disease and hepatocarcinoma. World J Gastroenterol. 2014;20:6287–92.

48. Lee CM, Hsu CY, Eng HL, Huang WS, Lu SN, Changchien CS, Chen CL, Cho CL. Telomerase activity and telomerase catalytic subunit in hepatocellular carcinoma. Hepatogastroenterology. 2004;51:796–800.

49. Nakayama J, Tahara H, Tahara E, Saito M, Ito K, Nakamura H, Nakanishi T, Tahara E, Ide T, Ishikawa F. Telomerase activation by hTRT in human normal fibroblasts and hepatocellular carcinomas. Nat Genet. 1998;18:65–8.

50. Nouso K, Urabe Y, Higashi T, Nakatsukasa H, Hino N, Ashida K, Kinugasa N, Yoshida K, Uematsu S, Tsuji T. Telomerase as a tool for the differential diagnosis of human hepatocellular carcinoma. Cancer. 1996;78:232–6.

51. Oh BK, Kim H, Park YN, Yoo JE, Choi J, Kim KS, Lee JJ, Park C. High telomerase activity and long telomeres in advanced hepatocellular carcinomas with poor prognosis. Lab Invest. 2008;88:144–52.

52. Ferber MJ, Montoya DP, Yu C, Aderca I, McGee A, Thorland EC, Nagorney DM, Gostout BS, Burgart LJ, Boix L, Bruix J, McMahon BJ, Cheung TH, Chung TK, Wong YF, Smith DI, Roberts LR. Integrations of the hepatitis B virus (HBV) and human papillomavirus (HPV) into the human telomerase reverse transcriptase (hTERT) gene in liver and cervical cancers. Oncogene. 2003;22:3813–20.

53. Horikawa I, Barrett JC. cis-Activation of the human telomerase gene (hTERT) by the hepatitis B virus genome. J Natl Cancer Inst. 2001;93:1171–3.

54. Levrero M, Zucman-Rossi J. Mechanisms of HBV-induced hepatocellular carcinoma. J Hepatol. 2016;64:S84–101.

55. Brechot C, Pourcel C, Louise A, Rain B, Tiollais P. Presence of integrated hepatitis B virus DNA sequences in cellular DNA of human hepatocellular carcinoma. Nature. 1980;286:533–5.

56. Hai H, Tamori A, Kawada N. Role of hepatitis B virus DNA integration in human hepatocarcinogenesis. World J Gastroenterol. 2014;20:6236–43.

57. Sung WK, Zheng H, Li S, Chen R, Liu X, Li Y, Lee NP, Lee WH, Ariyaratne PN, Tennakoon C, Mulawadi FH, Wong KF, Liu AM, Poon RT, Fan ST, Chan KL, Gong Z, Hu Y, Lin Z, Wang G, Zhang Q, Barber TD, Chou WC, Aggarwal A, Hao K, Zhou W, Zhang C, Hardwick J, Buser C, Xu J, Kan Z, Dai H, Mao M, Reinhard C, Wang J, Luk JM. Genome-wide survey of recurrent HBV integration in hepatocellular carcinoma. Nat Genet. 2012;44:765–9.

58. Zhao LH, Liu X, Yan HX, Li WY, Zeng X, Yang Y, Zhao J, Liu SP, Zhuang XH, Lin C, Qin CJ, Zhao Y, Pan ZY, Huang G, Liu H, Zhang J, Wang RY, Yang Y, Wen W, Lv GS, Zhang HL, Wu H, Huang S, Wang MD, Tang L, Cao HZ, Wang L, Lee TP, Jiang H, Tan YX, Yuan SX, Hou GJ, Tao QF, Xu QG, Zhang XQ, Wu MC, Xu X, Wang J, Yang HM, Zhou WP, Wang HY. Genomic and oncogenic preference of HBV integration in hepatocellular carcinoma. Nat Commun. 2016;7:12992. doi:10.1038/ncomms12992.:12992.

59. Yang X, Wu L, Lin J, Wang A, Wan X, Wu Y, Robson SC, Sang X, Zhao H: Distinct hepatitis B virus integration patterns in hepatocellular carcinoma and adjacent normal liver tissue. Int J Cancer 2016:10.

60. Cevik D, Yildiz G, Ozturk M. Common telomerase reverse transcriptase promoter mutations in hepatocellular carcinomas from different geographical locations. World J Gastroenterol. 2015;21:311–7.

61. Killela PJ, Reitman ZJ, Jiao Y, Bettegowda C, Agrawal N, Diaz Jr LA, Friedman AH, Friedman H, Gallia GL, Giovanella BC, Grollman AP, He TC, He Y, Hruban RH, Jallo GI, Mandahl N, Meeker AK, Mertens F, Netto GJ, Rasheed BA, Riggins GJ, Rosenquist TA, Schiffman M, Shih I, Theodorescu D, Torbenson MS, Velculescu VE, Wang TL, Wentzensen N, Wood LD, Zhang M, McLendon RE, Bigner DD, Kinzler KW, Vogelstein B, Papadopoulos N, Yan H. TERT promoter mutations occur frequently in gliomas and a subset of tumors derived from cells with low rates of self-renewal. Proc Natl Acad Sci U S A. 2013;110:6021–6.

62. Bojesen SE, Pooley KA, Johnatty SE, Beesley J, Michailidou K, Tyrer JP, Edwards SL, Pickett HA, Shen HC, Smart CE, Hillman KM, Mai PL, Lawrenson K, Stutz MD, Lu Y, Karevan R, Woods N, Johnston RL, French JD, Chen X, Weischer M, Nielsen SF, Maranian MJ, Ghoussaini M, Ahmed S, Baynes C, Bolla MK, Wang Q, Dennis J, McGuffog L, Barrowdale D, Lee A, Healey S, Lush M, Tessier DC, Vincent D, Bacot F, Vergote I, Lambrechts S, Despierre E, Risch HA, Gonzalez-Neira A, Rossing MA, Pita G, Doherty JA, Alvarez N, Larson MC, Fridley BL, Schoof N, Chang-Claude J, Cicek MS, Peto J, Kalli KR, Broeks A, Armasu SM, Schmidt MK, Braaf LM, Winterhoff B, Nevanlinna H, Konecny GE, Lambrechts D, Rogmann L, Guenel P, Teoman A, Milne RL, Garcia JJ, Cox A, Shridhar V, Burwinkel B, Marme F, Hein R, Sawyer EJ, Haiman CA, Wang-Gohrke S, Andrulis IL, Moysich KB, Hopper JL, Odunsi K, Lindblom A, Giles GG, Brenner H, Simard J, Lurie G, Fasching PA, Carney ME, Radice P, Wilkens LR, Swerdlow A, Goodman MT, Brauch H, Garcia-Closas M, Hillemanns P, Winqvist R, Durst M, Devilee P, Runnebaum I, Jakubowska A, Lubinski J, Mannermaa A, Butzow R, Bogdanova NV, Dork T, Pelttari LM, Zheng W, Leminen A, Anton-Culver H, Bunker CH, Kristensen V, Ness RB, Muir K, Edwards R, Meindl A, Heitz F, Matsuo K, Du BA, Wu AH, Harter P, Teo SH, Schwaab I, Shu XO, Blot W, Hosono S, Kang D, Nakanishi T, Hartman M, Yatabe Y, Hamann U, Karlan BY, Sangrajrang S, Kjaer SK, Gaborieau V, Jensen A, Eccles D, Hogdall E, Shen CY, Brown J, Woo YL, Shah M, Azmi MA, Luben R, Omar SZ, Czene K, Vierkant RA, Nordestgaard BG, Flyger H, Vachon C, Olson JE, Wang X, Levine DA, Rudolph A, Weber RP, Flesch-Janys D, Iversen E, Nickels S, Schildkraut JM, Silva IS, Cramer DW, Gibson L, Terry KL, Fletcher O, Vitonis AF, van der Schoot CE, Poole EM, Hogervorst FB, Tworoger SS, Liu J, Bandera EV, Li J, Olson SH, Humphreys K, Orlow I, Blomqvist C, Rodriguez-Rodriguez L, Aittomaki K, Salvesen HB, Muranen TA, Wik E, Brouwers B, Krakstad C, Wauters E, Halle MK, Wildiers H, Kiemeney LA, Mulot C, Aben KK, Laurent-Puig P, Altena AM, Truong T, Massuger LF, Benitez J, Pejovic T, Perez JI, Hoatlin M, Zamora MP, Cook LS, Balasubramanian SP, Kelemen LE, Schneeweiss A, Le ND, Sohn C, Brooks-Wilson A, Tomlinson I, Kerin MJ, Miller N, Cybulski C, Henderson BE, Menkiszak J, Schumacher F, Wentzensen N, Le ML, Yang HP, Mulligan AM, Glendon G, Engelholm SA, Knight JA, Hogdall CK, Apicella C, Gore M, Tsimiklis H, Song H, Southey MC, Jager A, den Ouweland AM, Brown R, Martens JW, Flanagan JM, Kriege M, Paul J, Margolin S, Siddiqui N, Severi G, Whittemore AS, Baglietto L, McGuire V, Stegmaier C, Sieh W, Muller H, Arndt V, Labreche F, Gao YT, Goldberg MS, Yang G, Dumont M, McLaughlin JR, Hartmann A, Ekici AB, Beckmann MW, Phelan CM, Lux MP, Permuth-Wey J, Peissel B, Sellers TA, Ficarazzi F, Barile M, Ziogas A. Multiple independent variants at the TERT locus are associated with telomere length and risks of breast and ovarian cancer. Nat Genet. 2013;45:371–2.

63. Zhong R, Liu L, Zou L, Zhu Y, Chen W, Zhu B, Shen N, Rui R, Long L, Ke J, Lu X, Zhang T, Zhang Y, Wang Z, Liu L, Sun Y, Cheng L, Miao X. Genetic variations in TERT-CLPTM1L locus are associated with risk of lung cancer in Chinese population. Mol Carcinog. 2013;52 Suppl 1:E118–26.

64. Abecasis GR, Auton A, Brooks LD, DePristo MA, Durbin RM, Handsaker RE, Kang HM, Marth GT, McVean GA. An integrated map of genetic variation from 1,092 human genomes. Nature. 2012;491:56–65.

65. Ko E, Seo HW, Jung ES, Kim BH, Jung G. The TERT promoter SNP rs2853669 decreases E2F1 transcription factor binding and increases mortality and recurrence risks in liver cancer. Oncotarget. 2016;7:684–99.

66. Castelo-Branco P, Choufani S, Mack S, Gallagher D, Zhang C, Lipman T, Zhukova N, Walker EJ, Martin D, Merino D, Wasserman JD, Elizabeth C, Alon N, Zhang L, Hovestadt V, Kool M, Jones DT, Zadeh G, Croul S, Hawkins C,

Hitzler J, Wang JC, Baruchel S, Dirks PB, Malkin D, Pfister S, Taylor MD, Weksberg R, Tabori U. Methylation of the TERT promoter and risk stratification of childhood brain tumours: an integrative genomic and molecular study. Lancet Oncol. 2013;14:534–42.

67. Dessain SK, Yu H, Reddel RR, Beijersbergen RL, Weinberg RA. Methylation of the human telomerase gene CpG island. Cancer Res. 2000;60:537–41.

68. Kojima H, Yokosuka O, Imazeki F, Saisho H, Omata M. Telomerase activity and telomere length in hepatocellular carcinoma and chronic liver disease. Gastroenterology. 1997;112:493–500.

69. Nault JC, Mallet M, Pilati C, Calderaro J, Bioulac-Sage P, Laurent C, Laurent A, Cherqui D, Balabaud C, Zucman-Rossi J. High frequency of telomerase reverse-transcriptase promoter somatic mutations in hepatocellular carcinoma and preneoplastic lesions. Nat Commun. 2013;4:2218.

70. Hsu IC, Metcalf RA, Sun T, Welsh JA, Wang NJ, Harris CC. Mutational hotspot in the p53 gene in human hepatocellular carcinomas. Nature. 1991;350:427–8.

71. Hussain SP, Schwank J, Staib F, Wang XW, Harris CC. TP53 mutations and hepatocellular carcinoma: insights into the etiology and pathogenesis of liver cancer. Oncogene. 2007;26:2166–76.

72. Gouas DA, Shi H, Hautefeuille AH, Ortiz-Cuaran SL, Legros PC, Szymanska KJ, Galy O, Egevad LA, Bedi-Ardekani B, Wiman KG, Hantz O, de FC C, Chemin IA, Hainaut PL. Effects of the TP53 p.R249S mutant on proliferation and clonogenic properties in human hepatocellular carcinoma cell lines: interaction with hepatitis B virus X protein. Carcinogenesis. 2010;31:1475–82.

73. Chen YL, Jeng YM, Chang CN, Lee HJ, Hsu HC, Lai PL, Yuan RH. TERT promoter mutation in resectable hepatocellular carcinomas: a strong association with hepatitis C infection and absence of hepatitis B infection. Int J Surg. 2014;12:659–65.

74. Yang X, Guo X, Chen Y, Chen G, Ma Y, Huang K, Zhang Y, Zhao Q, Winkler CA, An P, Lyu J. Telomerase reverse transcriptase promoter mutations in hepatitis B virus-associated hepatocellular carcinoma. Oncotarget. 2016;7:27838–47.

75. Huang DS, Wang Z, He XJ, Diplas BH, Yang R, Killela PJ, Meng Q, Ye ZY, Wang W, Jiang XT, Xu L, He XL, Zhao ZS, Xu WJ, Wang HJ, Ma YY, Xia YJ, Li L, Zhang RX, Jin T, Zhao ZK, Xu J, Yu S, Wu F, Liang J, Wang S, Jiao Y, Yan H, Tao HQ. Recurrent TERT promoter mutations identified in a large-scale study of multiple tumour types are associated with increased TERT expression and telomerase activation. Eur J Cancer. 2015;51:969–76.

76. Lee SE, Chang SH, Kim WY, Lim SD, Kim WS, Hwang TS, Han HS: Frequent somatic TERT promoter mutations and CTNNB1 mutations in hepatocellular carcinoma. Oncotarget 2016.

77. Ki Kim S, Ueda Y, Hatano E, Kakiuchi N, Takeda H, Goto T, Shimizu T, Yoshida K, Ikura Y, Shiraishi Y, Chiba K, Tanaka H, Miyano S, Uemoto S, Chiba T, Ogawa S, Marusawa H. TERT promoter mutations and chromosome 8p loss are characteristic of nonalcoholic fatty liver disease-related hepatocellular carcinoma. Int J Cancer. 2016;139:2512–8.

78. Quaas A, Oldopp T, Tharun L, Klingenfeld C, Krech T, Sauter G, Grob TJ. Frequency of TERT promoter mutations in primary tumors of the liver. Virchows Arch. 2014;465:673–7.

# 3

# Review on the role of the human Polyomavirus JC in the development of tumors

Serena Delbue[1*] (iD), Manola Comar[2,3] and Pasquale Ferrante[1,4]

## Abstract

Almost one fifth of human cancers worldwide are associated with infectious agents, either bacteria or viruses, and this makes the possible association between infections and tumors a relevant research issue. We focused our attention on the human Polyomavirus JC (JCPyV), that is a small, naked DNA virus, belonging to the *Polyomaviridae* family. It is the recognized etiological agent of the Progressive Multifocal Leukoencephalopathy (PML), a fatal demyelinating disease, occurring in immunosuppressed individuals.

JCPyV is able to induce cell transformation in vitro when infecting non-permissive cells, that do not support viral replication and JCPyV inoculation into small animal models and non human primates drives to tumor formation. The molecular mechanisms involved in JCPyV oncogenesis have been extensively studied: the main oncogenic viral protein is the large tumor antigen (T-Ag), that is able to bind, among other cellular factors, both Retinoblastoma protein (pRb) and p53 and to dysregulate the cell cycle, but also the early proteins small tumor antigen (t-Ag) and Agnoprotein appear to cooperate in the process of cell transformation.

Consequently, it is not surprising that JCPyV genomic sequences and protein expression have been detected in Central Nervous System (CNS) tumors and colon cancer and an association between this virus and several brain and non CNS-tumors has been proposed. However, the significances of these findings are under debate because there is still insufficient evidence of a casual association between JCPyV and solid cancer development.

In this paper we summarized and critically analyzed the published literature, in order to describe the current knowledge on the possible role of JCPyV in the development of human tumors.

**Keywords:** JC virus, Central nervous system tumors, Colon cancer

## Background

The Human Polyomaviruses (hPyV) are small, naked viruses with icosahedral capsid and circular, double-stranded DNA genome. They belong to the *Polyomaviridae* family and are able to infect and establish latency in the human host. The name "Polyomavirus" derives from the Greek roots poly-, which means "many", and –oma, which means "tumors". To date, at least thirteen human members of the *Polyomaviridae* family have been identified.

The latest demonstration of the oncogenic potential of a polyomavirus in humans, that has been ascribed to Merkel cell PyV (MCPyV), rekindled increasing interest in this viral family. MCPyV was isolated from the skin of a patient affected by Merkel Cell carcinoma (MCC) showing its ability to cause Merkel skin cancers [1]. However, the hypothesis that some among the hPyVs might play an etiological role in malignancies has been formulated more than 40 years ago [2]. Based on experimental models, the human polyomaviruses JC (JCPyV) and BK (BKPyV) have been recently categorized by the International Agency for Research in Cancer as "possible carcinogens", although studies in humans showed inconsistent evidence for an association with cancers at various sites [3].

In this review, the hypothesis that JCPyV could play a role in the development of Central Nervous System (CNS) and colon tumors will be elucidated and in deeply analyzed, based on the results and the reports published in the most recent literature.

* Correspondence: serena.delbue@unimi.it
[1]Department of Biomedical, Surgical and Dental Sciences, University of Milano, Via Pascal, 36-20133 Milan, Italy
Full list of author information is available at the end of the article

## JCPyV: epidemiology, structure, and life cycle

Humans are the natural hosts for JCPyV, that was isolated in 1971 from the brain tissue of a Hodgkin lymphoma patient, with initials J.C., who suffered from Progressive Multifocal Leukoencephalopathy (PML) [4].

JCPyV is ubiquitous and its primary infection, occurring during the childhood, is typically subclinical or linked to a mild respiratory illness. Between the age of 1 and 5 years, up to 50% of children show antibody to JCPyV, and by age of 10 years JCPyV seropositivity can be observed in about 60% of the population [5, 6]. By early adulthood, as many as 70–80% of the population has been infected [7]. Asymptomatic viral shedding in urine has been seen in both healthy and immunocompromised patients [8]. The mode of transmission for JCPyV is not yet well defined, although the presence of JCPyV DNA in B-cells and stromal cells of the tonsils and oropharynx supports the hypothesis of a respiratory route of transmission, with secondary lymphoid tissues serving as the potential site for initial infection [9]. Nevertheless, JCPyV was found also in raw sewage and in a high percentage of normal tissue samples taken from the upper and lower human gastrointestinal tract, suggesting that ingestion of contaminated water or food could be another portal of virus entry [10–13]. Moreover, JCPyV footprints have been reported in other many tissues of asymptomatic individuals, including spleen, lymph node, lung, bone marrow, brain, B lymphocytes and kidney, the last thought as the major site of JCPyV persistence.

The primary infection is followed by a lifelong, subclinical persistence of episomal viral genome in the cells. In the context of profound immunosuppression, the virus can become reactivated, leading to the lytic destruction of the oligodendrocytes, and the consequent development of PML, a fatal demyelinating disease [10]. It is not well assessed whether the immunosuppression of the host promotes the viral spread from the latency sites to the CNS or if JCPyV is already latent in the CNS and reactivates [11, 12].

The structure of the JCPyV virion is characterized by a non-enveloped, icosahedral capsid, measuring 40–45 nm in diameter and comprising 88% proteins and 12% DNA. The capsid is composed of three virus-encoded structural proteins, Viral Protein 1, 2, and 3 (VP1, VP2 and VP3). VP1 is the major component, with 360 molecules per capsid, and VP2 and VP3 contribute with 30–60 molecules each to the capsid. The icosahedron consists of 72 pentamers with no apparent hexamers, each composed of five VP1 molecules and one molecule of VP2 or VP3. Only VP1 is exposed on the surface of the capsid, and this determines the receptor specificity [13, 14].

The capsid surrounds a single, super-coiled, circular, double-stranded DNA molecule of 5130 base pairs (bp), in the case of the prototype JCPyV genome Mad-1 strain.

The viral genome is associated with cellular histones H2A, H2B, H3 and H4 to form the so-called minichromosome, structurally indistinguishable from host cell chromatin; the viral particles do not contain linker histones, but the genome acquires them after entry into the host cell [13–15].

The viral genome of JCPyV is functionally divided into three regions, called the genetically conserved early and late coding regions, of about the same size, which are separated by the hypervariable non-coding control region (NCCR), containing the origin of viral DNA replication (ori), the TATA box, binding sites for cellular transcription factors and bidirectional promoters and enhancers for the transcription of early and late genes. The NCCR of JCPyV is the most variable portion of the viral genome within a single virus. Viral DNA transcription and replication occur bidirectionally starting from the NCCR: the early transcription proceeds in a counterclockwise direction, while the late transcription proceeds clockwise on the opposite strand of DNA [16].

The early coding region spans about 2.4 kb and encodes the alternatively spliced transforming proteins large tumor antigen (T-Ag) and small tumor antigen (t-Ag), which are involved in viral replication, and in promoting transformation of cells in culture and oncogenesis in vivo. Three additional proteins, named $T'_{135}$, $T'_{136}$ and $T'_{165}$, due to the alternative splicing process are also produced at high level in the lytic cycle [17, 18].

T-Ag, a nuclear phosphoprotein of approximately 700 amino acids (aa), is considered the master regulator of the infectious process, because it orchestrates the production of early precursor messenger RNA (pre-mRNA), the initiation of viral DNA replication and the activation of late genes transcription. Moreover, by binding to the hypophosphorylated form of the pRb, T-Ag allows for premature release of the transcription factor E2F, which stimulates resting cells to enter the S-phase of the cell cycle.

T-Ag directly recruits the host cell DNA polymerase complex to the origin in order to initiate bi-directional DNA synthesis. Activation of the late viral promoter by T-Ag and associated cellular transcription factors lead to viral late gene expression [15].

t-Ag is a cysteine-rich protein of 172 aa, the first 80 of which are shared with T-Ag. t-Ag role in the lifecycle of JCPyV is not yet fully understood, though it is believed to serve an ancillary role for T-Ag activity and cell transformation [16, 19].

The late coding region spans 2.3 kb and contains the genetic information for the major structural protein VP1 and the two minor structural proteins VP2 and VP3, that are encoded from a common precursor mRNA by alternative splicing. The late region also encodes the Agnoprotein, a small multifunctional protein, that participates in viral transcriptional regulation, and inhibition of host DNA repair mechanism [20]. Additionally, JCPyV encodes a pre-microRNA (miRNA) that is processed into two unique miRNAs (JCPyV-specific miR-J1-5p and miR-J1-3p) during the late phase of infection. Both miRNAs are capable of downregulating the early phase protein T-Ag [21].

The infection of cell by JCPyV requires the binding between the viral VP1 and an N-linked glycoprotein with sialic acid: JCPyV uses both the α(2,3)- and α(2,6)-linked sialic acids to infect the permissive glial cells [22]. In addition, JCPyV is able to bind the serotonin receptor, 5HT2AR, that is present on cells in the brain and in the kidney, and to the ganglioside GT1b [23, 24]. Once the virus has gained entry into the host cell, by clathrin-dependent endocytosis [25], it travels to the cell nucleus, where it is uncoated and transcription of the early region begins. The early product T-Ag, back into the nucleus, binds to the viral origin of replication and allows the replication of the viral DNA, that depends by the availability of the cell DNA polymerase, replication protein A (RPA) and with host enzymes and cofactors, expressed in the S-phase of the cellular cycle [26]. As JCPyV replication proceeds, the late genes are expressed and the late products, VP1, VP2 and VP3 begin to assemble with the viral DNA, to form the complete virion. The final viral products are released via host cell lysis [27].

There is another possible outcome to infection of a cell by JCPyV: viral entry in nonpermisive cells, that do not support viral replication, can end up with the cell transformation or oncogenesis [28].

## Molecular mechanisms of JCPyV transformation mediated by T-Ag

The JCPyV principal actor, leading to cell transformation and tumor development, is the early protein T-Ag. T-Ag is a multifunctional protein, divided in several domains, defined, from the N-terminal to the C-terminal, as follows: the DNaJ domain, linking to the cellular factor HSc70; the LxCxE motif, that specifically binds and inactivates the Rb family members; the Origin-Binding Domain (OBD) that binds the JCPyV origin of replication; the NLS domain, that is necessary for the nuclear localization of the protein; the Helicase domain (containing the Zn and nucleotide binding domains), and, finally, the p53 binding domain [29, 30]. All these domains cooperate in binding to and inactivating cellular proteins that usually prevent the transition into S-phase; consequently, JCPyV itself, drives the cell cycle from G1 into S-phase. This event promotes viral replication and spread, when JCPyV infects permissive cells, while it drives to cell transformation, when JCPyV infects non permissive cells.

Basically, this progression is mainly the result of the binding between the T-Ag LxCxE motif (aa 103–107) and the members of the Rb tumor suppressor family [31–33]. T-Ag sequestration of the hypophosphorylated form of pRb enables the activation of the transcription factors E2F1, –2, –3a and 3b, that in turn activate the transcription of some genes, needed to enter the S-phase of the cellular cycle, such as *c-fos, c-Myc, cyclins A,D1* and *E, DNA polymerase alpha, thymidine kinas,* and others [29, 34–37]. The disruption of the complex pRb/E2Fs is mediated by the J domain of T-Ag, that binds to the Hsc70, a chaperone, increasing its ATPase activity when associated with T-Ag; the energy produced by the ATP hydrolysis is used to separate the pRb from the E2Fs [38, 39]. In addition, T-Ag can bind other members of the Rb family, that are p130 and p107 [40]. The p130-E2F4/5 association usually anchors a large repressive complex; T-Ag contributes to disrupt the complex p130-E2F4/5 and to release the brakes imposed on cell proliferation [41].

The C-terminal region of T-Ag contains the p53-binding domain [42]. P53 is a tumor suppressor, whose levels are usually kept very low. In conditions of stress, such as DNA damage or presence of oncogenes, p53 rapidly increases its transcription, the p53 protein is accumulated and the DNA repair mechanism or the cell apoptosis or senescence mechanisms are induced. When T-Ag binds and inactivates p53, the growth arrest and the premature cell death are avoided, while the cell cycle progression is favoured also in presence of DNA damage [43, 44].

Additionally, other cellular proteins, such as insulin receptor substrate 1 (IRS-1) [45], β-catenin [46, 47], the neurofibromatosis type 2 gene product [48] and the antiapoptotic protein survivin [49] are implicated in binding to JCPyV T-Ag.

IRS-1 is a membrane associated tyrosine kinase, which mediates both physiological and pathological responses in the cell. Activated IRS-1 triggers cell proliferation, and sends antiapoptotic signals. It has been shown that T-Ag is able to bind directly to the IRS-1 and to cause its translocation into the nucleus and that this event has important consequences in the homologous-recombination-directed DNA repair (HRR) mechanism. In normal conditions, the Insulin Growth Factor-I receptor (IGF-1R)/IRS-1 signaling axis supports HRR: the mechanism involves a direct binding between hypophosphorylated IRS-1 and Rad51 in the cytoplasm. Following IGF-IR stimulation, tyrosine phosphorylated IRS-1 loses the ability to complex Rad51, that translocates to the nucleus, where it participates in homology search and intrastrand invasion to support faithful DNA repair [50, 51]. Following T-Ag-mediated nuclear translocation, IRS-1 binds Rad51 at the site of damaged DNA and attenuates HRR. This indirect inhibition of HRR is associated with an increase number of cells accumulating mutations, that may be the base of the development of a malignant phenotype [45, 50, 52].

β-catenin is part of the Wnt pathway, that is involved in cell proliferation, survival and transcription processes.

Several mutations in the proteins belonging to this pathway have been associated with the development of different tumors [53, 54]. T-Ag binds to β-catenin through the aa 82–628 and induces the stabilization of the cellular protein, whose levels increase [55]. Additionally, following the T-Ag interaction, β-catenin tranlocates into the nucleus and induces the transcription of *c-myc* and cyclin D1 [46].

The interaction between T-Ag and the neurofibromatosis type 2 (NF2) gene product and its translocation to the nucleus were also shown [48], but very few is known about the consequences of this association [56].

Finally, it has been observed that the binding between T-Ag and the antiapoptotic protein survivin leads to a significant decrement of the apoptotic process [49]. Reactivation of Survivin by JCPyV T-Ag can be a critical step in prolonging cell survival, which allows JCPyV to complete its replication cycle. Such a strong reactivation of the normally dormant Survivin has been observed in primary oligodendrocyte and astrocyte cultures infected in vitro, and expressing T-Ag. This can be a critical step in the transformation and proliferation of neural progenitors in vitro and in vivo [57].

T-Ag has also a direct mutagenic effect on the host genome, by inducing spontaneous mutations in the infected cells and cytogenetic alterations, both influencing chromosomal stability and cell kariotype [58]. These damages may precede the morphological transformation [59] (Fig. 1).

The alternative T' early proteins are also able to bind to the Rb family components, with a particular affinity with p107 (T'$_{135}$ and T'$_{136}$); moreover T'$_{135}$ binds Hsc70 [31, 60].

## Molecular mechanisms of JCPyV transformation mediated by t-Ag

The t-Ag is encoded by the same mRNA that encodes the T-Ag, following a mechanism of alternative splicing. Consequently, the N-terminal 82 amino acids are the same as the N-terminus of T-Ag, while the C-terminus

is an unique domain. The t-Ag is not studied as much as T-Ag and the majority of the information regarding its functions derives from what is known about the SV40 t-Ag. SV40 t-Ag cooperates with T-Ag to enhance transformation when T-Ag levels are low [61], it is required for human cells transformation [62], and is needed to keep high level of viral load in persistent infection of human mesothelial cells [63]. It has been demonstrated that, in contrast with SV40 t-Ag, JCPyV plays a relevant role in viral replication, since t-Ag null mutant failed to display detectable DNA replication activity [64].

The unique domain of the JCPyV t-Ag contains the binding site for the Protein Phosphatase 2A (PP2A), a serine/threonine –specific protein phosphatase that is involved in the mitogen-activated protein kinase (MAPK) pathway. The interplay between t-Ag and PP2A is also mediated by the JCPyV Agnoprotein and the result of this binding is an interference with the phosphatase activity of PP2A [65] and the subsequent activation of pathways inducing cell proliferation. Additionally, it has been shown that t-Ag binds to the members of the Rb family pRb, p107 and p130 and these associations are expected to influence cell cycle progression [64] (Fig. 2).

## Molecular mechanisms of JCPyV transformation mediated by Agnoprotein

The JCPyV late genomic region encodes a regulatory protein, known as Agnoprotein. It is a very small protein of 71 aa in length, that was named "agno", because when its encoding ORF was discovered, no protein was associated to it [66]. Agnoprotein is produced late in the infectious cycle, but is not incorporated into the mature virion; additionally, it is phosphorylated and it has been shown that the posphorylation is necessary for the functionality of the protein and the replication of the virus [67]. Over the years, JCPyV Agnoprotein was demonstrated to bind to both viral (T-Ag, t-Ag, VP1) and cellular (YB-1, p53, FEZ1, PP2A, Ku70...) proteins [65, 68–74]. Consequently, it plays a role in the viral transcription, translation, assembly and also in

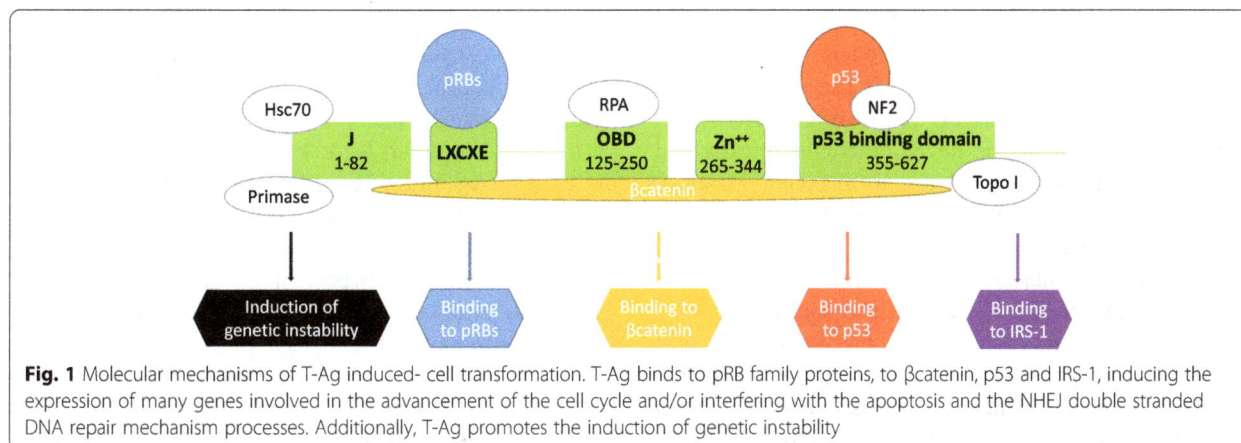

**Fig. 1** Molecular mechanisms of T-Ag induced- cell transformation. T-Ag binds to pRB family proteins, to βcatenin, p53 and IRS-1, inducing the expression of many genes involved in the advancement of the cell cycle and/or interfering with the apoptosis and the NHEJ double stranded DNA repair mechanism processes. Additionally, T-Ag promotes the induction of genetic instability

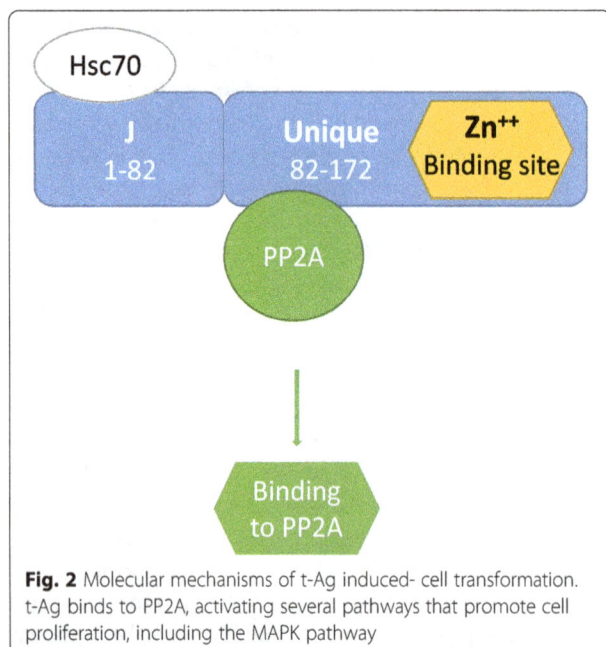

**Fig. 2** Molecular mechanisms of t-Ag induced- cell transformation. t-Ag binds to PP2A, activating several pathways that promote cell proliferation, including the MAPK pathway

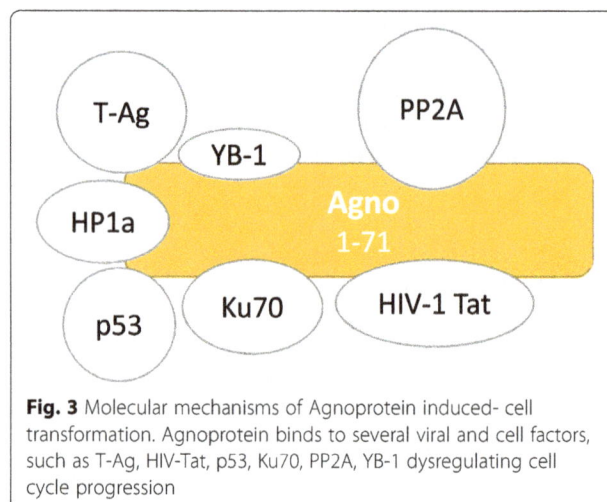

**Fig. 3** Molecular mechanisms of Agnoprotein induced- cell transformation. Agnoprotein binds to several viral and cell factors, such as T-Ag, HIV-Tat, p53, Ku70, PP2A, YB-1 dysregulating cell cycle progression

the cell cycle progression. In particular, Agnoprotein binds directly to p53 causing the arrest of the cell cycle in the G2/M phase due to the activation of p21/WAF-1 promoter [73]. The interaction of the Agnoprotein with Ku70 drives to the inhibition of the non homologous end joining (NHEJ) double stranded DNA repair mechanism, contributing to the genomic instability conferred on cells undergoing JCPyV infection [74]. As already explained before, Agnoprotein is phosphorylated, but the binding with PP2A causes its dephosphorylation; when PP2A is sequestered by t-Ag, it cannot act as a phosphatase on Agnoprotein, and this causes a downregulation of JCPyV replication, but also an activation of the MAPK signaling [65]. All together, the description of the characteristics of the Agnoprotein demonstrated its importance in the cellular transformation process [75] (Fig. 3).

## JCPyV oncogenicity in experimental animals

The highly oncogenic potential of JCPyV has been well established in different animal models, starting from 1973, when it has been shown that the inoculation of the virus into the brain of newborn Golden Syrian hamsters can lead to the development of unexpected tumors, such as medulloblastoma, astrocytoma, glioblastoma multiforme, primitive neuroectodermal tumors and peripheral neuroblastoma [2, 76, 77]. Astrocytoma, glioblastoma and neuroblastoma also developed after intracerebral inoculation of JCPyV into owl and squirrel monkeys [78]. Interestingly, the tumor tissues taken from the hamster and monkeys infected animals showed the presence of the T-Ag protein, but neither the expression of other virion antigens nor evidence of viral replication were found [79].

This is consistent with the fact that the animal cells may not be permissive for the JCPyV replication and leads to the consideration that JCPyV is able to transform the non permissive cells also in the human populations [80].

Other evidences regarding the JCPyV oncogenicity come from studies on transgenic mice, generated to contain the entire T-Ag coding sequence under the control of its own promoter, and without any other viral genes. Adrenal neuroblastoma, pituitary adenoma, malignant peripheral nerve sheat and medulloblastoma were the tumors induced by the expression of the only early protein [81–84].

## JCPyV and human CNS tumors

The ability of JCPyV to transform cells, such as human fetal glial cells and primary hamster brain cells, has been demonstrated in vitro. Furthermore, JCPyV was able to induce different types of brain tumors after injection in hamster, owl and squirrel monkeys [2, 85, 86]. Transgenic mice expressing the JCPyV early region were shown to develop adrenal neuroblastomas, tumors of primitive neuroectodermal origin, tumors arising from the pituitary glan, glioblastoma multiforme, primitive neuroectodernal tumors and malignant peripheral nerve sheath tumors [28, 48, 80], and others.

All the molecular mechanisms previously described in this review appear to be involved in the JCPyV induced - neural oncogenesis, mainly due to the interaction of T-Ag with several cellular factors. Specifically, the binding between T-Ag and pRb promotes the cell cycle progression, while the T-Ag/p53 complex leads to the inhibition of the apoptosis process [28]; the interaction between the JCPyV early protein and IRS-1 or β – catenin is a key factor of the malignant transformation in children medulloblastoma [55, 87].

The first evidence of an association between the presence of JCPyV and a human tumor was reported in 1961, when Richardson [88], who first described PML, diagnosed an oligodendroglioma in a patient with concomitant chronic lymphocytic leukemia and PML. After the identification of JCPyV as the etiologic agent of PML, investigations focused on the possible association with brain tumors were conducted and at least ten cases were published, reporting the concomitant development of CNS neoplasia and PML [89, 90]. These clinical observations represent a strong proof that JCPyV may be involved in the pathogenesis of both the CNS diseases.

Detection of JCPyV sequences and/or protein expression in primary CNS malignancies has been frequently reported also in immunocompetent and/or immunosuppressed patients without PML. These reports regarded a wide variety of CNS neoplasia: gangliocytoma, choroid plexus papilloma, pilocytotic astrocytoma, subependymoma, pleomorphic xanthoastrocytoma, oligodendroglioma, all subtypes of astrocytoma, ependymoma, oligoastrocytoma, glioblastoma multiforme, medulloblastoma, pineoblastoma, gliosarcoma and primitive neuroectodernal tumors, as reported in Table 1.

The percentage of JCPyV positive CNS tumor tissues was highly variable, ranging from 20 to 75%, with regard to the JCPyV genome and from 20 to 68% with regard to the JCPyV protein expression. Interestingly, the studies focusing on the viral protein expression were able to detect the viral early proteins T-Ag in the nuclei and Agnoprotein in the perinuclear area of the cells, but never the late VP1 protein (Table 1). These data are consistent with the fact that most of the CNS cells are non permissive for the JCPyV replication, and that the transforming ability of T-Ag appears limited to neural origin tissue.

Despite the increasing evidence of an association between JCPyV and the CNS tumors, it cannot be omitted that there is a lack of consistency in different studies that failed to detect both viral genome and protein expression in several types of tumors, such as meningioma [91], oligodendroglioma, astrocytoma [92], glioblastoma multiforme [93], glioma, and medulloblatoma [94]. Del Valle and colleagues hypothesized that the wide discrepancy in the viral genome and proteins detection, even within similar tumors, should be ascribed to the different types of collected samples, and to the employment of different techniques. They pointed out the fact that DNA isolated from formalin-fixed paraffin-embedded is usually of inferior quality than those isolated from fresh/frozen tissues and this may cause false negative results. The sensitivity of the routinary used amplification methods (PCR, nested PCR, quantitative-PCR, southern blot hybridization) is another important issue, that should be taken into account, since it can increase the rate of the false negative results [80].

The wide ubiquity of JCPyV, however, was demonstrated by the fact that some studies have underlined the presence of viral genomic sequences, but not DNA expression, also

in brain from healthy immunocompetent subjects, with neither PML nor CNS malignancies [95–99].

This notable observation raises the question of whether the JCPyV found in CNS tumors may have a role in the pathogenesis of the malignancies or whether the brain is a latency site for JCPyV.

The model proposed by Perez-Liz [98] and colleagues and Del Valle and colleagues [80] made an effort in organizing all the puzzle pieces: following the primary infection, JCPyV establishes latency also in the brain and it does not replicate its genome neither express its proteins. In case of profound immunodepression, the virus can infect permissive cells, such as oligodendrocytes and induce a lytic cycle, exiting in the destruction of the infected cells and the subsequent development of PML. On the other hand, transient physiological changes may occur in normal individuals, allowing the expression of the T-Ag, and resulting in the accumulation of this oncogenic protein in brain cells. The result would be the interaction of T-Ag with the host proteins deputized to the cell cycle control, the promotion of uncontrolled cell division and the stimulation of tumor formation [100].

## JCPyV and human colorectal cancer

It is well assessed that JCPyV is commonly excreted in the urine of both immunocompetent and immunodepressed subjects and this is also demonstrated by the findings of JCPyV genome and complete virion in the raw urban sewage from around the world [101, 102] The ingestion of food and/or water contaminated with this virus easily leads to the infection of the gastrointestinal tract by JCPyV, whose structure is particularly resistant at very low pH (up to 1) in raw water [103, 104]. As described here below, an increasing number of studies, conducted worldwide, have reported the presence of JCPyV genomic sequences and the expression of T-Ag in tissues from gastrointestinal tumors, including esophageal carcinoma [105], gastric carcinoma [106–108], sporadic adenomatous polyps [109], and colorectal adenocarcinomas [110–117], but also in normal tissues and in adjacent noncancerous tissue from the gastrointestinal tract [118].

In the context of colorectal cancer, JCPyV seems to be a cofactor for the induction of the chromosomal instability [58, 119, 120], but it also interacts with the β-catenin protein with the consequent enhanced activation of Wnt pathway target genes, such as c-Myc and Cyclin D1. Both c-Myc and Cyclin D1 are involved in cell cycle control and progression and their enhanced activation, mainly due to the intervention of T-Ag, could result in unchecked cell cycle progression, high proliferation rate, and ultimately a more malignant phenotype [46, 47, 121].

**Table 1** Detection of JCPyV in primary central nervous system tumor

| Tumor | Reference | Detected/sampled (%) | | Detection method | |
|---|---|---|---|---|---|
| | | *DNA* | *Proteins* | *DNA* | *Proteins* |
| Adenocarcinoma | [143] | 1/3 (33.3) | - | qPCR | - |
| Anaplastic Astrocytoma | [144] | 6/15 (40.0) | - | qPCR | - |
| | [78, 145] | 3/4 (75.0) | 0/4 (0.0) | PCR, SB | IHC (T-Ag) |
| Anaplastic Ependynoma | [91] | 0/1 (0.0) | - | PCR | - |
| Anaplastic Meningioma | [91] | 0/1 (0.0) | - | PCR | - |
| Anaplastic Oligoastrocytoma | [144] | 0/2 (0.0) | - | qPCR | - |
| Anaplastic Oligodendroglioma | [78, 145] | 2/3 (66.7) | 2/3 (66.7) | PCR, SB | IHC (T-Ag) |
| | [144] | 3/8 (37.5) | - | qPCR | - |
| Astrocytoma | [146] | 4/10 (40.0) | 1/10 (10.0) | nPCR | IHC (T-Ag) |
| | [147] | 1/3 (33.3) | 1/3 (33.3) | nPCR, PCR | IHC (T-Ag) |
| | [78, 145] | 10/16 (62.5) | 7/16 (43.8) | PCR, SB | IHC (T-Ag) |
| | [148] | 1/5 (20.0) | - | nPCR | - |
| | [144] | 31/78 (39.7) | - | qPCR | - |
| | [144] | 5/12 (41.7) | - | qPCR | - |
| | [143] | 1/3 (33.3) | - | qPCR | - |
| | [149] | 6/19 (31.6) | - | qPCR | - |
| | [150] | 0/23 (0.0) | - | PCR | - |
| Chroid plexus papilloma | [151] | 1/5 (20.0) | 1/5 (20.0) | PCR, SB | IHC(T-Ag,Agno) |
| | [150] | 0/14 (0.0) | - | PCR | - |
| Ependyomomas | [145] | 5/6 (83.3) | 4/6 (66.7) | PCR, SB | IHC (T-Ag) |
| | [151] | 5/18 (27.8) | 4/18 (22.2) 3/18 (16.7) | PCR, SB | IHC(T-Ag,Agno) |
| | [147] | 0/2 (0.0) | 0/2 (0.0) | nPCR, PCR | IHC (T-Ag) |
| | [146] | 1/5 (20.0) | 0/5 (0.0) | nPCR | IHC (T-Ag) |
| | [150] | 1/34 (2.9) | - | PCR | - |
| | [148] | 0/2 (0.0) | - | nPCR | - |
| | [143] | 0/1 (0.0) | - | qPCR | - |
| | [149] | 0/5 (0.0) | - | qPCR | - |
| Gangliocytoma | [147] | 0/1 (0.0) | 0/1 (0.0) | nPCR, PCR | IHC (T-Ag) |
| | [148] | 0/1 (0.0) | - | nPCR | - |
| Gangliogioma | [149] | 2/5 (40.0) | - | qPCR | - |
| Glioblastoma | [144] | 20/51 (39.2) | - | qPCR | - |
| | [150] | 2/102 (2.0) | - | PCR | - |
| | [148] | 11/21 (52.4) | - | nPCR | - |
| | [149] | 19/39 (48.7) | - | qPCR | - |
| Glioblastoma Multiforme | [78, 145] | 12/21 (57.1) | 5/21 (23.8) | PCR, SB | IHC (T-Ag) |
| | [152] | 1/100 (1.0) | 1/100 (1.0) | PCR, SB | IHC (T-Ag) |
| | [147] | 7/13 (53.8) | 7/13 (53.8) | nPCR, PCR | IHC (T-Ag) |
| | [153] | 1/100 (1.0) | 1/100 (1.0) 1/100 (1.0) | PCR | IHC(T-Ag,Agno) |
| | [143] | 0/7 (0.0) | - | qPCR | - |
| Glioblastosis celebri | [78, 145] | 1/100 (1.0) | 1/100 (1.0) | PCR, SB | IHC (T-Ag) |
| Gliosarcoma | [149] | 2/5 (40.0) | - | qPCR | - |
| Lymphoma | [149] | 1/7 (14.3) | - | qPCR | - |

**Table 1** Detection of JCPyV in primary central nervous system tumor *(Continued)*

| | | | | | |
|---|---|---|---|---|---|
| Medulloblastoma | [154] | 11/16 (68.8) | 9/16 (56.3) 11/16(68.8) | PCR, SB | IHC (T-Ag) |
| | [155] | 0/8 (0.0) | 0/8 (0.0) | PCR, SB | IHC (T-Ag) |
| | [156] | 11/23 (47.8) | 4/23 (17.4) | PCR, SB | IHC (T-Ag) |
| | [157] | 0/15 (0.0) | 0/15 (0.0) | PCR, SB | IHC (T-Ag) |
| | [158] | - | 0/22 | - | IHC (T-Ag,Agno) |
| | [151] | 0/32 (0.0) | 0/32 (0.0) | PCR, SB | IHC (T-Ag) |
| | [143] | 0/1 (0.0) | - | qPCR | - |
| | [149] | 2/5 (40.0) | - | qPCR | - |
| | [150] | 0/21 (0.0) | - | PCR | - |
| | [91] | 0/2 (0.0) | - | PCR | - |
| Meningioma | [150] | 0/15 (0.0) | - | PCR | - |
| | [148] | 3/8 (37.5) | - | nPCR | - |
| | [91] | 1/1 (100.0) | - | PCR | - |
| | [143] | 6/12 (50.0) | - | qPCR | - |
| Oligoastrocytoma | [78, 145] | 5/8 (62.5) | 2/8 (25.0) | PCR, SB | IHC (T-Ag) |
| | [159] | 1/100 (1.0) | 1/100 (1.0) | PCR | IPPt (T-Ag) |
| | [143] | 0/1 (0.0) | - | qPCR | - |
| | [149] | 2/3 (66.7) | - | qPCR | - |
| | [144] | 2/6 (33.3) | - | qPCR | - |
| Oligodendroglioma | [148] | 1/2 (50.0) | - | nPCR | - |
| | [149] | 4/12 (33.3) | - | qPCR | - |
| | [143] | 0/2 (0.0) | - | qPCR | - |
| | [78, 145] | 4/7 (57.1) | - | PCR, SB | - |
| | [160] | 13/15 (86.7) | 8/18 (44.4) 10/18(55.6) | PCR, SB | IHC (T-Ag,Agno) |
| | [147] | 1/2 (50.0) | 1/2 (50.0) | nPCR, PCR | IHC (T-Ag) |
| | [146] | 1/5 (20.0) | 0/5 (0.0) | nPCR | IHC (T-Ag) |
| | [144] | 5/17 (29.4) | - | qPCR | - |
| Pilocytic Astrocytoma | [78, 145] | 4/5 (80.0) | 1/5 (20.0) | PCR, SB | IHC (T-Ag) |
| | [151] | 0/7 (0.0) | 0/7 (0.0) | PCR, SB | IHC (T-Ag,Agno) |
| Pineocytoma | [147] | 0/1 (0.0) | 0/1 (0.0) | nPCR, PCR | IHC (T-Ag) |
| | [143] | 0/2 (0.0) | - | qPCR | - |
| | [149]. | 1/3 (33.3) | - | qPCR | - |
| | [148] | 0/1 (0.0) | - | nPCR | - |
| Pituitary adenoma | [143] | 0/3 (0.0) | - | qPCR | - |
| Pleomorphic xanthoastrocytoma | [161] | 1/1 (100.0) | - | nPCR | - |
| Rare brain tumors | [149] | 0/6 (0.0) | - | qPCR | - |
| Schwannoma | [143] | 5/14 (35.7) | - | qPCR | - |
| sPNET | [157] | 0/5 (0.0) | 0/5 (0.0) | PCR, SB | IHC (T-Ag) |
| Subependymoma | [91] | 0/1 (0.0) | - | PCR | - |
| | [78, 145] | 1/1 (100.0) | 1/1 (100.0) | PCR, SB | IHC (T-Ag) |
| Xanthoatrocytoma | [143] | 0/1 (0.0) | - | qPCR | - |

Legend: *qPCR* quantitative PCR, *nPCR* nested PCR, *IHC* immunohistochemistry, *SB* Southern Blot, *IPPt* immunoprecipitation, *sPNET* supratentorial primary neuroectodermal tumor

Overall, 18 different studies evaluated the presence of JCPyV in colorectal cancer, including studies that were aimed to identify only the viral genomic sequences or both viral genomic sequences and viral protein expression.

The first paper was published in 1999 by Laghi and colleagues and reported the presence of the T-Ag genomic sequence in 12 tissues samples out of 46 analyzed tissues (23 pairs of normal colorectal epithelium and adjacent cancers). The authors also showed that larger number of viral copies was present in cancer cells than in non-neoplastic colon cells [110]. The same research group also demonstrated some years later that 81.2% of normal colonic tissues and 70.6% of normal tissues from the upper gastrointestinal tract contained the T-Ag DNA sequences [104]. The presence of the JCPyV genome was confirmed by Enam and colleagues, who found 22 out of 27 tissues of malignant tumors of the large intestine positive for the presence of the T-Ag DNA; the expression of the oncogenic proteins T-Ag and Agnoprotein was observed only in 14 of these samples [46]. In adenomatous polyps of the colon, that are premalignant lesions, JCPyV T-Ag DNA sequences were found to be frequently present (82%), and T-Ag was found to be expressed specifically in the nuclei of 16% of these samples [109].

The remaining 14 studies evaluated the presence of JCPyV in colorectal cancer cases and controls. Eleven of them were extensively reviewed by Chen and colleagues in 2015 [118]. Additionally, a new case–control study was published in 2015, regarding JCPyV DNA in immunocompetent colorectal patients from Tunisia [117]. The remaining two studies focused on immunosuppressed patients and will be analyzed later [122, 123].

Taken together, ten papers reported the data obtained by the employment of Polymerase Chain Reaction (PCR), nested-PCR or quantitative PCR for the search of viral genomic sequences in a total of 746 colorectal cancer tissues and of 828 normal tissues (both adjacent noncancerous or tissues from healthy controls). Overall, 256/746 (34.3%) colorectal cancer tissues and 120/828(14.5%) were positive for the presence of the JCPyV genome [112, 115, 124–129]. Additionally 240 adenoma tissues were analyzed and compared with 257 normal tissues from healthy controls: JCPyV DNA was found in 77 adenoma (32.1%) and 48 normal (18.7%) tissues, respectively (Table 2) [115, 127, 128]. The expression of the JCPyV proteins was analyzed only in 4 studies [126, 130–132] and it has been observed that the early T-Ag protein was present in 9 out of 172 (5.2%) colorectal cancer or adenoma tissues and in 7 out of 38 (18.4%) adjacent noncancerous tissues or normal tissues from healthy controls (Table 3). Rollison and colleagues and Lundstig and colleagues collected blood samples from colorectal patients, and healthy controls and found a total of 210 (41.3%), and 179 (38.4%) seropositive subjects out

of 509 colorectal patients, and 466 and healthy subjects (Table 3) [130, 131].

Interestingly, Selgrad and colleagues [122] and Boltin and colleagues [133] highlighted the important issue of JCPyV infection in the gastrointestinal tract in immunosuppressed patients. In particular, Selgrad and colleagues focused their attention on liver transplant patients who developed colorectal neoplasia and they showed that both the viral genome and early protein were present in higher percentage in colorectal mucosa and adenoma tissues from transplant patients than in non transplant patients. The hypothesis that has been formulated based on this finding was that the use of immunosuppressive agents may contribute in the reactivation of the virus and that the expression of T-Ag may represent a risk for the developing of neoplasia in immunosuppression conditions [122]. Similarly, Boltin and colleagues reported that JCPyV T-Ag DNA was more prevalent in the upper and lower gastrointestinal mucosa of 38 immunosuppressed patients than in the gastrointestinal mucosa of 48 immunocompetent subjects, possibly indicating that the virus resides in these patients. This may account for the higher prevalence of gastrointestinal carcinomas in immunosuppressed patients.

A very innovative starting point for the next research studies on the association between JCPyV and colorectal cancer comes from a recent publication, reporting that JCPyV specific miR-J1-5p miRNA could be used as a potential biomarker for viral infection in colorectal patients, since JCPyV miRNA lower expression was showed in the stools from patients with colorectal cancer, compared to healthy subjects [134]. However, the role of JCPyV miRNA in the development of the neoplasia remains to be elucidated.

Taken together, these reports demonstrated the presence of both JCPyV genome and proteins in tumor tissues, but also in the normal adjacent part or in normal colorectal mucosa and only in two studies the JCPyV prevalence was significantly higher in patients than in controls [112, 124]. Consequently, it is not possible yet to affirm whether JCPyV should be considered as an etiological cofactor, a risk factor or a simple bystander in the development of colorectal cancer. To this regard, Coelho and colleagues hypothesized that JCPyV might participate in different steps of the colorectal carcinogenesis: its latency might favor a transient inflammatory reaction, generating a microenvironment rich in cytokines, which can promote the expansion of transformed cells; the binding between T-Ag, Agnoprotein and several cell proteins might induce genetic instability, that can drive to irreversible genetic damages. The mechanism employed by JCPyV for inducing tumorigenesis might be the "hit and run", where PyV infection is associated with the early stages of tumorigenesis, but is not needed for the progression of

**Table 2** Studies comparing JCPyV DNA prevalence between cases and controls

| Reference | Positive cases/total cases (%) Type of Sample | Positive controls/total controls (%) Type of Sample |
|---|---|---|
| [125] | 0/233 (0%) CRC tumor tissue | 1/233 (0.4%) Adjacent noncancerous tissue |
| [128] | 49/80 (61.3%) CRC tumor tissue | 6/20 (30.0%) Healthy tissue |
| | 15/25 (60.0%) Adenoma tissue | |
| [115] | 6/23 (26.1%) CRC tumor tissue | 0/20 (0%) Healthy tissue |
| | 1/21 (4.8%) Adenoma tissue | |
| [126] | 15/18 (8.3%) CRC tumor tissue | 13/16 (81.2%) Adjacent noncancerous tissue |
| [112] | 19/22 (86.4%) CRC tumor tissue | 0/22 (0.0%) Adjacent noncancerous tissue |
| [129] | 0/94 (0.0%) Adenoma tissue | 0/91 (0.0%) Healthy tissue |
| [124] | 56/137 (40.9%) CRC tumor tissue | 34/137 (24.8%) Adjacent noncancerous tissue |
| | | 11/80 (13.8%) Healthy tissue |
| [127] | 12/14 (85.7%) CRC tumor tissue | 40/100 (40.0%) Healthy tissue |
| | 55/60 (91.7%) Adenoma tissue | |
| [132] | 38/114 (33.3%) CRC glandular/stromal tissue | 2/20 (10%) Healthy glandular/stromal tissue |
| | 6/40 (15.0%) Adenoma glandular/stromal tissue | |
| [117] | 61/105 (58.1%) CRC tumor tissue | 13/89 (14.6%) Adjacent noncancerous tissue |

**Table 3** Studies comparing JCPyV protein prevalence between cases and controls

| Reference | Positive cases/total cases (%) Type of Sample | Positive controls/total controls (%) Type of Sample |
|---|---|---|
| [126] | 9/18 (50.0%) CRC tumor tissue | 7/18 (38.9%) Adjacent noncancerous tissue |
| [132] | 0/114 (0.0%) CRC glandular/stromal tissue | 0/20 (0.0%) Healthy glandular/stromal tissue |
| | 0/40 (0.0%) Adenoma glandular/stromal tissue | |
| [131] | 152/386 (39.4%) CRC patient's blood | 168/386 (43.5%) Healthy subject's blood |
| [130] | 58/123 (47.2%) CRC patient's blood | 11/80 (13.8%) Healthy subject's blood |

the disease, and this could explain why JCPyV genome/proteins were not always detected in the tumor tissues [135].

## Conclusions

Almost one fifth of human cancers worldwide are associated with infectious agents, either bacteria or viruses, and this makes the potential association between infections and tumors a relevant research issue. It is well assessed that the exposure to some viruses, such as Human Papillomavirus [136], Hepatitis B Virus [137], Human T leukemia virus [138] and MCPyV [1], can trigger the development of cervical carcinoma, liver carcinoma, leukemia and MCC, respectively. In this article, we have reviewed data concerning the possible link between JCPyV with CNS tumors and colorectal cancer.

Some of the biological features of JCPyV makes it a fully compatible candidate as risk factor of human tumors, because (a) it is usually acquired early in life; (b) it establishes a persistent infection in the host; (c) it encodes oncoproteins that interfere with tumor suppressors pathways, thus altering the normal progression of cell cycle; (d) it causes cancer in laboratory animals, and (e) viral sequences are often detected in human tumors. However, some other characteristics are not consistent with the known pattern of viral oncogenesis: it is ubiquitous in the human population and its genome/proteins can be easily detected in biological samples from healthy individuals; the length of infection is not determinable, since the primary infection is asymptomatic. In addition, it is well known that environmental and/or host cofactors could modulate the tumor pathogenesis, where viral infections could play a trigger role in the first step of transformation mechanism.

Some guidelines have been provided in order to prove cancer causation by a viral infection. JCPyV should have all the following requirements for being definitely associated to the development of CNS tumors and colon cancer: (a) the presence of its genome/proteins should be higher in cases than in controls; (b) the infection should always precede the disease symptoms; (c) the virus should have a highest prevalence in the geographical area where there is a highest prevalence of the tumor; (d) the virus should be able to transform human cell in vitro and to induce cancer in animal models [139, 140]. While JCPyV fulfills the second and the last criteria, it is difficult to apply the other two criteria to JCPyV: in fact it is ubiquitous in nature, but only a limited fraction of infected subjects develops disease; in addition, a variable time occurs between infection and the development of a cancer, making markers of exposure difficult to evaluate along the carcinogenic process [141]. Moreover, these criteria do not consider that some viruses, such as, probably, JCPyV may employ an "hit and run" oncogenic mechanism, where the virus induces cell transformation and, subsequently, is silenced or even lost during tumor progression [142].

At the light of all these observations, a causative role of JCPyV in human cancers is still to be defined, but, despite the "inadequate evidence of carcinogenicity in humans", the WHO International Agency for Cancer Research Monograph Working Group decided to classify JCPyV as "possibly carcinogenic to humans", belonging to group 2B, on the basis of the "sufficient evidence in experimental animals" [3]. Since the presence of JCPyV has been demonstrated in multiple human tumor tissues, it is reasonable to hypothesize that it could play a role as relevant cofactor in human tumorigenesis.

Therefore, only further solid, clear-cut epidemiologic, histopathologic and DNA evidence will ultimately settle this urgent issue and will help to answer the still unsolved question: "Does JCPyV cause tumors in the human population?" When a complete understanding is reached, a vaccination approach for the prevention of JCPyV infection may be proposed, based to the fact that JCPyV infection is acquired early in life and that, besides its possible transforming ability, this virus causes PML, a disease with no available and specific treatment.

## Abbreviations
aa: Amino acids; BKPyV: Human Polyomavirus BK; CNS: Central nervous system; hPyVs: Human polyomaviruses; HRR: Homologous-recombination-directed DNA repair; IGF-1R: Insulin Growth Factor-I receptor; IRS-1: Insulin receptor substrate 1; JCPyV: Human Polyomavirus JC; MAPK: Mitogen-activated protein kinase; MCC: Merkel cell carcinoma; MCPyV: Merkel cell PyV; miRNA: microRNA; mRNA: messenger RNA; NCCR: Non-coding control region; NF2: Neurofibromatosis type 2; NHEJ: Nonhomologous endjoining; OBD: Origin-Binding Domain; ori: Origin of replication; PCR: Polymerase chain reaction; PML: Progressive Multifocal Leukoencephalopathy; T-Ag: Large tumor antigen; t-Ag: Small tumor antigen; VP1, VP2, VP3: Viral Protein 1, 2, and 3

## Acknowledgements
We would like to thank Dr. Sonia Villani and Mrs. Rosalia Ticozzi for the technical support.

## Funding
The Authors declare no study sponsors involvement in the study design, in the collection, analysis and interpretation of data, in the writing of the manuscript and in the decision to submit the manuscript for publication.

## Authors' contributions
SD acquired the data; SD drafted the article and contributed to conception and design; MC and PF contributed to critical revision for important intellectual content; all authors approved the final version to be published.

## Competing interests
The authors declare that they have no competing interests.

## Author details
[1]Department of Biomedical, Surgical and Dental Sciences, University of Milano, Via Pascal, 36-20133 Milan, Italy. [2]Department of Medical Sciences, University of Trieste, Trieste, Italy. [3]Institute for Maternal and Child Health-IRCCS "Burlo Garofolo", 34137 Trieste, Italy. [4]Istituto Clinico Città Studi, Milan, Italy.

## References
1. Feng H, Shuda M, Chang Y, Moore PS. Clonal integration of a polyomavirus in human Merkel cell carcinoma. Science. 2008;319:1096–100.
2. Walker DL, Padgett BL, ZuRhein GM, Albert AE, Marsh RF. Human papovavirus (JC): induction of brain tumors in hamsters. Science. 1973;181:674–6.
3. Bouvard V, Baan RA, Grosse Y, Lauby-Secretan B, El Ghissassi F, Benbrahim-Tallaa L, Guha N, Straif K. Carcinogenicity of malaria and of some polyomaviruses. Lancet Oncol. 2012;13:339–40.
4. Padgett BL, Walker DL, ZuRhein GM, Eckroade RJ, Dessel BH. Cultivation of papova-like virus from human brain with progressive multifocal leucoencephalopathy. Lancet. 1971;1:1257–60.
5. Elia F, Villani S, Ambrogi F, Signorini L, Dallari S, Binda S, Primache V, Pellegrinelli L, Ferrante P, Delbue S. JC virus infection is acquired very early in life: evidence from a longitudinal serological study. J Neurovirol. 2016. [Epub ahead of print] PubMed PMID: 27538993.
6. White MK, Gordon J, Khalili K. The rapidly expanding family of human polyomaviruses: recent developments in understanding their life cycle and role in human pathology. PLoS Pathog. 2013;9:e1003206.
7. Kean JM, Rao S, Wang M, Garcea RL. Seroepidemiology of human polyomaviruses. PLoS Pathog. 2009;5:e1000363.
8. Arthur RR, Shah KV. Occurrence and significance of papovaviruses BK and JC in the urine. Prog Med Virol. 1989;36:42–61.
9. Monaco MC, Jensen PN, Hou J, Durham LC, Major EO. Detection of JC virus DNA in human tonsil tissue: evidence for site of initial viral infection. J Virol. 1998;72:9918–23.
10. Doerries K. Human polyomavirus JC and BK persistent infection. Adv Exp Med Biol. 2006;577:102–16.
11. Dorries K, Sbiera S, Drews K, Arendt G, Eggers C, Dorries R. Association of human polyomavirus JC with peripheral blood of immunoimpaired and healthy individuals. J Neurovirol. 2003;9 Suppl 1:81–7.
12. White MK, Khalili K. Pathogenesis of progressive multifocal leukoencephalopathy–revisited. J Infect Dis. 2011;203:578–86.
13. Imperiale MJ. Oncogenic transformation by the human polyomaviruses. Oncogene. 2001;20:7917–23.
14. Ferenczy MW, Marshall LJ, Nelson CD, Atwood WJ, Nath A, Khalili K, Major EO. Molecular biology, epidemiology, and pathogenesis of progressive multifocal leukoencephalopathy, the JC virus-induced demyelinating disease of the human brain. Clin Microbiol Rev. 2012;25:471–506.
15. Eash S, Manley K, Gasparovic M, Querbes W, Atwood WJ. The human polyomaviruses. Cell Mol Life Sci. 2006;63:865–76.
16. Khalili K, White MK. Human demyelinating disease and the polyomavirus JCV. Mult Scler. 2006;12:133–42.
17. Trowbridge PW, Frisque RJ. Identification of three new JC virus proteins generated by alternative splicing of the early viral mRNA. J Neurovirol. 1995; 1:195–206.
18. Frisque RJ. Structure and function of JC virus T' proteins. J Neurovirol. 2001; 7:293–7.
19. Lee W, Langhoff E. Polyomavirus in human cancer development. Adv Exp Med Biol. 2006;577:310–8.
20. Khalili K, White MK, Sawa H, Nagashima K, Safak M. The agnoprotein of polyomaviruses: a multifunctional auxiliary protein. J Cell Physiol. 2005;204:1–7.
21. Seo GJ, Fink LH, O'Hara B, Atwood WJ, Sullivan CS. Evolutionarily conserved function of a viral microRNA. J Virol. 2008;82:9823–8.

22. Liu CK, Wei G, Atwood WJ. Infection of glial cells by the human polyomavirus JC is mediated by an N-linked glycoprotein containing terminal alpha(2–6)-linked sialic acids. J Virol. 1998;72:4643–9.

23. Elphick GF, Querbes W, Jordan JA, Gee GV, Eash S, Manley K, Dugan A, Stanifer M, Bhatnagar A, Kroeze WK, et al. The human polyomavirus, JCV, uses serotonin receptors to infect cells. Science. 2004;306:1380–3.

24. Maginnis MS, Haley SA, Gee GV, Atwood WJ. Role of N-linked glycosylation of the 5-HT2A receptor in JC virus infection. J Virol. 2010;84:9677–84.

25. Querbes W, Benmerah A, Tosoni D, Di Fiore PP, Atwood WJ. A JC virus-induced signal is required for infection of glial cells by a clathrin- and eps15-dependent pathway. J Virol. 2004;78:250–6.

26. Melendy T, Stillman B. An interaction between replication protein A and SV40 T antigen appears essential for primosome assembly during SV40 DNA replication. J Biol Chem. 1993;268:3389–95.

27. Boothpur R, Brennan DC. Human polyoma viruses and disease with emphasis on clinical BK and JC. J Clin Virol. 2010;47:306–12.

28. White MK, Khalili K. Polyomaviruses and human cancer: molecular mechanisms underlying patterns of tumorigenesis. Virology. 2004;324:1–16.

29. Moens U, Van Ghelue M, Johannessen M. Oncogenic potentials of the human polyomavirus regulatory proteins. Cell Mol Life Sci. 2007;64:1656–78.

30. Moens U, Van Ghelue M, Ehlers B. Are human polyomaviruses co-factors for cancers induced by other oncoviruses? Rev Med Virol. 2014;24:343–60.

31. Bollag B, Prins C, Snyder EL, Frisque RJ. Purified JC virus T and T' proteins differentially interact with the retinoblastoma family of tumor suppressor proteins. Virology. 2000;274:165–78.

32. DeCaprio JA, Ludlow JW, Figge J, Shew JY, Huang CM, Lee WH, Marsilio E, Paucha E, Livingston DM. SV40 large tumor antigen forms a specific complex with the product of the retinoblastoma susceptibility gene. Cell. 1988;54:275–83.

33. Felsani A, Mileo AM, Paggi MG. Retinoblastoma family proteins as key targets of the small DNA virus oncoproteins. Oncogene. 2006;25:5277–85.

34. Dyson N, Bernards R, Friend SH, Gooding LR, Hassell JA, Major EO, Pipas JM, Vandyke T, Harlow E. Large T antigens of many polyomaviruses are able to form complexes with the retinoblastoma protein. J Virol. 1990;64:1353–6.

35. Ludlow JW, Skuse GR. Viral oncoprotein binding to pRB, p107, p130, and p300. Virus Res. 1995;35:113–21.

36. Harris KF, Christensen JB, Radany EH, Imperiale MJ. Novel mechanisms of E2F induction by BK virus large-T antigen: requirement of both the pRb-binding and the J domains. Mol Cell Biol. 1998;18:1746–56.

37. White MK, Khalili K. Interaction of retinoblastoma protein family members with large T-antigen of primate polyomaviruses. Oncogene. 2006;25:5286–93.

38. Sullivan CS, Pipas JM. T antigens of simian virus 40: molecular chaperones for viral replication and tumorigenesis. Microbiol Mol Biol Rev. 2002;66:179–202.

39. Craig EA, Huang P, Aron R, Andrew A. The diverse roles of J-proteins, the obligate Hsp70 co-chaperone. Rev Physiol Biochem Pharmacol. 2006;156:1–21.

40. Dyson N, Buchkovich K, Whyte P, Harlow E. The cellular 107 K protein that binds to adenovirus E1A also associates with the large T antigens of SV40 and JC virus. Cell. 1989;58:249–55.

41. An P, Saenz Robles MT, Pipas JM. Large T antigens of polyomaviruses: amazing molecular machines. Annu Rev Microbiol. 2012;66:213–36.

42. Sharma AK, Kumar G. A 53 kDa protein binds to the negative regulatory region of JC virus early promoter. FEBS Lett. 1991;281:272–4.

43. Bollag B, Chuke WF, Frisque RJ. Hybrid genomes of the polyomaviruses JC virus, BK virus, and simian virus 40: identification of sequences important for efficient transformation. J Virol. 1989;63:863–72.

44. Vogelstein B, Lane D, Levine AJ. Surfing the p53 network. Nature. 2000;408:307–10.

45. Lassak A, Del Valle L, Peruzzi F, Wang JY, Enam S, Croul S, Khalili K, Reiss K. Insulin receptor substrate 1 translocation to the nucleus by the human JC virus T-antigen. J Biol Chem. 2002;277:17231–8.

46. Enam S, Del Valle L, Lara C, Gan DD, Ortiz-Hidalgo C, Palazzo JP, Khalili K. Association of human polyomavirus JCV with colon cancer: evidence for interaction of viral T-antigen and beta-catenin. Cancer Res. 2002;62:7093–101.

47. Gan DD, Khalili K. Interaction between JCV large T-antigen and beta-catenin. Oncogene. 2004;23:483–90.

48. Shollar D, Del Valle L, Khalili K, Otte J, Gordon J. JCV T-antigen interacts with the neurofibromatosis type 2 gene product in a transgenic mouse model of malignant peripheral nerve sheath tumors. Oncogene. 2004;23:5459–67.

49. Piña-Oviedo S, Urbanska K, Radhakrishnan S, Sweet T, Reiss K, Khalili K, Del Valle L. Effects of JC virus infection on anti-apoptotic protein survivin in progressive multifocal leukoencephalopathy. Am J Pathol. 2007;170:1291–304.

50. Trojanek J, Croul S, Ho T, Wang JY, Darbinyan A, Nowicki M, Del Valle L, Skorski T, Khalili K, Reiss K. T-antigen of the human polyomavirus JC attenuates faithful DNA repair by forcing nuclear interaction between IRS-1 and Rad51. J Cell Physiol. 2006;206:35–46.

51. Davies AA, Masson JY, McIlwraith MJ, Stasiak AZ, Stasiak A, Venkitaraman AR, West SC. Role of BRCA2 in control of the RAD51 recombination and DNA repair protein. Mol Cell. 2001;7:273–82.

52. Reiss K, Del Valle L, Lassak A, Trojanek J. Nuclear IRS-1 and cancer. J Cell Physiol. 2012;227:2992–3000.

53. Reya T, Clevers H. Wnt signalling in stem cells and cancer. Nature. 2005;434:843–50.

54. Moon RT, Gough NR. Beyond canonical: the Wnt and β-catenin story. Sci Signal. 2016;9(422):eg5.

55. Gan DD, Reiss K, Carrill T, Del Valle L, Croul S, Giordano A, Fishman P, Khalili K. Involvement of Wnt signaling pathway in murine medulloblastoma induced by human neurotropic JC virus. Oncogene. 2001;20:4864–70.

56. Beltrami S, Branchetti E, Sariyer IK, Otte J, Weaver M, Gordon J. Neurofibromatosis type 2 tumor suppressor protein, NF2, induces proteasome-mediated degradation of JC virus T-antigen in human glioblastoma. PLoS One. 2013;8:e53447.

57. Gualco E, Urbanska K, Perez-Liz G, Sweet T, Peruzzi F, Reiss K, Del Valle L. IGF-IR-dependent expression of Survivin is required for T-antigen-mediated protection from apoptosis and proliferation of neural progenitors. Cell Death Differ. 2010;17:439–51.

58. Ricciardiello L, Baglioni M, Giovannini C, Pariali M, Cenacchi G, Ripalti A, Landini MP, Sawa H, Nagashima K, Frisque RJ, et al. Induction of chromosomal instability in colonic cells by the human polyomavirus JC virus. Cancer Res. 2003;63:7256–62.

59. Trabanelli C, Corallini A, Gruppioni R, Sensi A, Bonfatti A, Campioni D, Merlin M, Calza N, Possati L, Barbanti-Brodano G. Chromosomal aberrations induced by BK virus T antigen in human fibroblasts. Virology. 1998;243:492–6.

60. Bollag B, Kilpatrick LH, Tyagarajan SK, Tevethia MJ, Frisque RJ. JC virus T'135, T'136 and T'165 proteins interact with cellular p107 and p130 in vivo and influence viral transformation potential. J Neurovirol. 2006;12:428–42.

61. Sáenz-Robles MT, Sullivan CS, Pipas JM. Transforming functions of Simian Virus 40. Oncogene. 2001;20:7899–907.

62. Chang LS, Pan S, Pater MM, Di Mayorca G. Differential requirement for SV40 early genes in immortalization and transformation of primary rat and human embryonic cells. Virology. 1985;146:246–61.

63. Fahrbach KM, Katzman RB, Rundell K. Role of SV40 ST antigen in the persistent infection of mesothelial cells. Virology. 2008;370:255–63.

64. Bollag B, Hofstetter CA, Reviriego-Mendoza MM, Frisque RJ. JC virus small T antigen binds phosphatase PP2A and Rb family proteins and is required for efficient viral DNA replication activity. PLoS One. 2010;5:e10606.

65. Sariyer IK, Khalili K, Safak M. Dephosphorylation of JC virus agnoprotein by protein phosphatase 2A: inhibition by small t antigen. Virology. 2008;375:464–79.

66. Fiers W, Contreras R, Haegemann G, Rogiers R, Van de Voorde A, Van Heuverswyn H, Van Herreweghe J, Volckaert G, Ysebaert M. Complete nucleotide sequence of SV40 DNA. Nature. 1978;273:113–20.

67. Sariyer IK, Akan I, Palermo V, Gordon J, Khalili K, Safak M. Phosphorylation mutants of JC virus agnoprotein are unable to sustain the viral infection cycle. J Virol. 2006;80:3893–903.

68. Safak M, Barrucco R, Darbinyan A, Okada Y, Nagashima K, Khalili K. Interaction of JC virus agno protein with T antigen modulates transcription and replication of the viral genome in glial cells. J Virol. 2001;75:1476–86.

69. Safak M, Sadowska B, Barrucco R, Khalili K. Functional interaction between JC virus late regulatory agnoprotein and cellular Y-box binding transcription factor, YB-1. J Virol. 2002;76:3828–38.

70. Suzuki T, Okada Y, Semba S, Orba Y, Yamanouchi S, Endo S, Tanaka S, Fujita T, Kuroda S, Nagashima K, Sawa H. Identification of FEZ1 as a protein that interacts with JC virus agnoprotein and microtubules: role of agnoprotein-induced dissociation of FEZ1 from microtubules in viral propagation. J Biol Chem. 2005;280:24948–56.

71. Suzuki T, Semba S, Sunden Y, Orba Y, Kobayashi S, Nagashima K, Kimura T, Hasegawa H, Sawa H. Role of JC virus agnoprotein in virion formation. Microbiol Immunol. 2012;56:639–46.

72. Suzuki T, Orba Y, Makino Y, Okada Y, Sunden Y, Hasegawa H, Hall WW, Sawa H. Viroporin activity of the JC polyomavirus is regulated by interactions with the adaptor protein complex 3. Proc Natl Acad Sci U S A. 2013;110:18668–73.

73. Darbinyan A, Darbinian N, Safak M, Radhakrishnan S, Giordano A, Khalili K. Evidence for dysregulation of cell cycle by human polyomavirus, JCV, late auxiliary protein. Oncogene. 2002;21:5574–81.

74. Darbinyan A, Siddiqui KM, Slonina D, Darbinian N, Amini S, White MK, Khalili K. Role of JC virus agnoprotein in DNA repair. J Virol. 2004;78:8593–600.

75. Saribas AS, Coric P, Hamazaspyan A, Davis W, Axman R, White MK, Abou-Gharbia M, Childers W, Condra JH, Bouaziz S, Safak M. Emerging from the unknown: structural and functional features of agnoprotein of polyomaviruses. J Cell Physiol. 2016;231:2115–27.

76. Zu Rhein GM. Studies of JC virus-induced nervous system tumors in the Syrian hamster: a review. Prog Clin Biol Res. 1983;105:205–21.

77. Zu Rhein GM, Varakis JN. Perinatal induction of medulloblastomas in Syrian golden hamsters by a human polyoma virus (JC). Natl Cancer Inst Monogr. 1979;(51):205–8.

78. Del Valle L, Baehring J, Lorenzana C, Giordano A, Khalili K, Croul S. Expression of a human polyomavirus oncoprotein and tumour suppressor proteins in medulloblastomas. Mol Pathol. 2001;54:331–7.

79. Major EO, Amemiya K, Tornatore CS, Houff SA, Berger JR. Pathogenesis and molecular biology of progressive multifocal leukoencephalopathy, the JC virus-induced demyelinating disease of the human brain. Clin Microbiol Rev. 1992;5:49–73.

80. Del Valle L, White MK, Khalili K. Potential mechanisms of the human polyomavirus JC in neural oncogenesis. J Neuropathol Exp Neurol. 2008;67: 729–40.

81. Small JA, Khoury G, Jay G, Howley PM, Scangos GA. Early regions of JC virus and BK virus induce distinct and tissue-specific tumors in transgenic mice. Proc Natl Acad Sci U S A. 1986;83:8288–92.

82. Franks RR, Rencic A, Gordon J, Zoltick PW, Curtis M, Knobler RL, Khalili K. Formation of undifferentiated mesenteric tumors in transgenic mice expressing human neurotropic polymavirus early protein. Oncogene. 1996; 12:2573–8.

83. Krynska B, Otte J, Franks R, Khalili K, Croul S. Human ubiquitous JCV(CY) T-antigen gene induces brain tumors in experimental animals. Oncogene. 1999;18:39–46.

84. Gordon J, Del Valle L, Otte J, Khalili K. Pituitary neoplasia induced by expression of human neurotropic polyomavirus, JCV, early genome in transgenic mice. Oncogene. 2000;19:4840–6.

85. London WT, Houff SA, Madden DL, Fuccillo DA, Gravell M, Wallen WC, Palmer AE, Sever JL, Padgett BL, Walker DL, et al. Brain tumors in owl monkeys inoculated with a human polyomavirus (JC virus). Science. 1978; 201:1246–9.

86. London WT, Houff SA, McKeever PE, Wallen WC, Sever JL, Padgett BL, Walker DL. Viral-induced astrocytomas in squirrel monkeys. Prog Clin Biol Res. 1983;105:227–37.

87. Khalili K, Del Valle L, Wang JY, Darbinian N, Lassak A, Safak M, Reiss K. T-antigen of human polyomavirus JC cooperates withIGF-IR signaling system in cerebellar tumors of the childhood-medulloblastomas. Anticancer Res. 2003;23:2035–41.

88. Richardson Jr EP. Progressive multifocal leukoencephalopathy. N Engl J Med. 1961;265:815–23.

89. White MK, Khalili K. Expression of JC virus regulatory proteins in human cancer: potential mechanisms for tumourigenesis. Eur J Cancer. 2005;41: 2537–48.

90. Brassesco MS, Darrigo Jr LG, Valera ET, Oliveira RS, Yamamoto YA, de Castro Barros MV, Tone LG. Giant-cell glioblastoma of childhood associated with HIV-1 and JC virus coinfection. Childs Nerv Syst. 2013;29:1387–90.

91. Weggen S, Bayer TA, von Deimling A, Reifenberger G, von Schweinitz D, Wiestler OD, Pietsch T. Low frequency of SV40, JC and BK polyomavirus sequences in human medulloblastomas, meningiomas and ependymomas. Brain Pathol. 2000;10:85–92.

92. Herbarth B, Meissner H, Westphal M, Wegner M. Absence of polyomavirus JC in glial brain tumors and glioma-derived cell lines. Glia. 1998;22:415–20.

93. Arthur RR, Grossman SA, Ronnett BM, Bigner SH, Vogelstein B, Shah KV. Lack of association of human polyomaviruses with human brain tumors. J Neurooncol. 1994;20:55–8.

94. Munoz-Marmol AM, Mola G, Ruiz-Larroya T, Fernandez-Vasalo A, Vela E, Mate JL, Ariza A. Rarity of JC virus DNA sequences and early proteins in human gliomas and medulloblastomas: the controversial role of JC virus in human neurooncogenesis. Neuropathol Appl Neurobiol. 2006;32:131–40.

95. Elsner C, Dorries K. Evidence of human polyomavirus BK and JC infection in normal brain tissue. Virology. 1992;191:72–80.

96. Mori M, Aoki N, Shimada H, Tajima M, Kato K. Detection of JC virus in the brains of aged patients without progressive multifocal leukoencephalopathy by the polymerase chain reaction and Southern hybridization analysis. Neurosci Lett. 1992;141:151–5.

97. White 3rd FA, Ishaq M, Stoner GL, Frisque RJ. JC virus DNA is present in many human brain samples from patients without progressive multifocal leukoencephalopathy. J Virol. 1992;66:5726–34.

98. Perez-Liz G, Del Valle L, Gentilella A, Croul S, Khalili K. Detection of JC virus DNA fragments but not proteins in normal brain tissue. Ann Neurol. 2008; 64:379–87.

99. Delbue S, Branchetti E, Boldorini R, Vago L, Zerbi P, Veggiani C, Tremolada S, Ferrante P. Presence and expression of JCV early gene large T Antigen in the brains of immunocompromised and immunocompetent individuals. J Med Virol. 2008;80:2147–52.

100. Khalili K, Stoner G, editors. Human polyomaviruses: molecular and clinical perspectives. New York: Wiley-Liss. 2001.

101. Rossi A, Delbue S, Mazziotti R, Valli M, Borghi E, Mancuso R, Calvo MG, Ferrante P. Presence, quantitation and characterization of JC virus in the urine of Italian immunocompetent subjects. J Med Virol. 2007;79:408–12.

102. Bofill-Mas S, Rodriguez-Manzano J, Calgua B, Carratala A, Girones R. Newly described human polyomaviruses Merkel cell, KI and WU are present in urban sewage and may represent potential environmental contaminants. Virol J. 2010;7:141.

103. Bofill-Mas S, Formiga-Cruz M, Clemente-Casares P, Calafell F, Girones R. Potential transmission of human polyomaviruses through the gastrointestinal tract after exposure to virions or viral DNA. J Virol. 2001;75:10290–9.

104. Ricciardiello L, Laghi L, Ramamirtham P, Chang CL, Chang DK, Randolph AE, Boland CR. JC virus DNA sequences are frequently present in the human upper and lower gastrointestinal tract. Gastroenterology. 2000;119:1228–35.

105. Del Valle L, White MK, Enam S, Pina Oviedo S, Bromer MQ, Thomas RM, Parkman HP, Khalili K. Detection of JC virus DNA sequences and expression of viral T antigen and agnoprotein in esophageal carcinoma. Cancer. 2005;103:516–27.

106. Murai Y, Zheng HC, Abdel Aziz HO, Mei H, Kutsuna T, Nakanishi Y, Tsuneyama K, Takano Y. High JC virus load in gastric cancer and adjacent non-cancerous mucosa. Cancer Sci. 2007;98:25–31.

107. Ksiaa F, Ziadi S, Mokni M, Korbi S, Trimeche M. The presence of JC virus in gastric carcinomas correlates with patient's age, intestinal histological type and aberrant methylation of tumor suppressor genes. Mod Pathol. 2010;23:522–30.

108. Shin SK, Li MS, Fuerst F, Hotchkiss E, Meyer R, Kim IT, Goel A, Boland CR. Oncogenic T-antigen of JC virus is present frequently in human gastric cancers. Cancer. 2006;107:481–8.

109. Jung WT, Li MS, Goel A, Boland CR. JC virus T-antigen expression in sporadic adenomatous polyps of the colon. Cancer. 2008;112:1028–36.

110. Laghi L, Randolph AE, Chauhan DP, Marra G, Major EO, Neel JV, Boland CR. JC virus DNA is present in the mucosa of the human colon and in colorectal cancers. Proc Natl Acad Sci U S A. 1999;96:7484–9.

111. Ricciardiello L, Chang DK, Laghi L, Goel A, Chang CL, Boland CR. Mad-1 is the exclusive JC virus strain present in the human colon, and its transcriptional control region has a deleted 98-base-pair sequence in colon cancer tissues. J Virol. 2001;75:1996–2001.

112. Lin PY, Fung CY, Chang FP, Huang WS, Chen WC, Wang JY, Chang D. Prevalence and genotype identification of human JC virus in colon cancer in Taiwan. J Med Virol. 2008;80:1828–34.

113. Link A, Shin SK, Nagasaka T, Balaguer F, Koi M, Jung B, Boland CR, Goel A. JC virus mediates invasion and migration in colorectal metastasis. PLoS One. 2009;4:e8146.

114. Vilkin A, Ronen Z, Levi Z, Morgenstern S, Halpern M, Niv Y. Presence of JC virus DNA in the tumor tissue and normal mucosa of patients with sporadic colorectal cancer (CRC) or with positive family history and Bethesda criteria. Dig Dis Sci. 2012;57:79–84.

115. Hori R, Murai Y, Tsuneyama K, Abdel-Aziz HO, Nomoto K, Takahashi H, Cheng CM, Kuchina T, Harman BV, Takano Y. Detection of JC virus DNA sequences in colorectal cancers in Japan. Virchows Arch. 2005;447:723–30.

116. Wang JP, Wang ZZ, Zheng YS, Xia P, Yang XH, Liu YP, Takano Y, Zheng HC. JC virus existence in Chinese gastrointestinal carcinomas. Oncol Lett. 2012;3:1073–8.

117. Ksiaa F, Allous A, Ziadi S, Mokni M, Trimeche M. Assessment and biological significance of JC polyomavirus in colorectal cancer in Tunisia. J buon. 2015; 20:762–9.

118. Chen H, Chen XZ, Waterboer T, Castro FA, Brenner H. Viral infections and colorectal cancer: a systematic review of epidemiological studies. Int J Cancer. 2015;137:12–24.

119. Niv Y, Goel A, Boland CR. JC virus and colorectal cancer: a possible trigger in the chromosomal instability pathways. Curr Opin Gastroenterol. 2005;21:85–9.

120. Goel A, Li MS, Nagasaka T, Shin SK, Fuerst F, Ricciardiello L, Wasserman L, Boland CR. Association of JC virus T-antigen expression with the methylator phenotype in sporadic colorectal cancers. Gastroenterology. 2006;130:1950–61.

121. Ripple MJ, Parker Struckhoff A, Trillo-Tinoco J, Li L, Margolin DA, McGoey R, Del Valle L. Activation of c-Myc and Cyclin D1 by JCV T-Antigen and beta-catenin in colon cancer. PLoS One. 2014;9:e106257.

122. Selgrad M, Koornstra JJ, Fini L, Blom M, Huang R, Devol EB, Boersma-van Ek W, Dijkstra G, Verdonk RC, de Jong S, et al. JC virus infection in colorectal neoplasia that develops after liver transplantation. Clin Cancer Res. 2008;14:6717–21.

123. Burnett-Hartman AN, Newcomb PA, Potter JD. Infectious agents and colorectal cancer: a review of Helicobacter pylori, Streptococcus bovis, JC virus, and human papillomavirus. Cancer Epidemiol Biomarkers Prev. 2008;17:2970–9.

124. Mou X, Chen L, Liu F, Lin J, Diao P, Wang H, Li Y, Teng L, Xiang C. Prevalence of JC virus in Chinese patients with colorectal cancer. PLoS One. 2012;7:e35900.

125. Newcomb PA, Bush AC, Stoner GL, Lampe JW, Potter JD, Bigler J. No evidence of an association of JC virus and colon neoplasia. Cancer Epidemiol Biomarkers Prev. 2004;13:662–6.

126. Casini B, Borgese L, Del Nonno F, Galati G, Izzo L, Caputo M, Perrone Donnorso R, Castelli M, Risuleo G, Visca P. Presence and incidence of DNA sequences of human polyomaviruses BKV and JCV in colorectal tumor tissues. Anticancer Res. 2005;25:1079–85.

127. Coelho TR, Gaspar R, Figueiredo P, Mendonca C, Lazo PA, Almeida L. Human JC polyomavirus in normal colorectal mucosa, hyperplastic polyps, sporadic adenomas, and adenocarcinomas in Portugal. J Med Virol. 2013;85:2119–27.

128. Theodoropoulos G, Panoussopoulos D, Papaconstantinou I, Gazouli M, Perdiki M, Bramis J, Lazaris A. Assessment of JC polyoma virus in colon neoplasms. Dis Colon Rectum. 2005;48:86–91.

129. Campello C, Comar M, Zanotta N, Minicozzi A, Rodella L, Poli A. Detection of SV40 in colon cancer: a molecular case–control study from northeast Italy. J Med Virol. 2010;82:1197–200.

130. Rollison DE, Helzlsouer KJ, Lee JH, Fulp W, Clipp S, Hoffman-Bolton JA, Giuliano AR, Platz EA, Viscidi RP. Prospective study of JC virus seroreactivity and the development of colorectal cancers and adenomas. Cancer Epidemiol Biomarkers Prev. 2009;18:1515–23.

131. Lundstig A, Stattin P, Persson K, Sasnauskas K, Viscidi RP, Gislefoss RE, Dillner J. No excess risk for colorectal cancer among subjects seropositive for the JC polyomavirus. Int J Cancer. 2007;121:1098–102.

132. Samaka RM, Abd El-Wahed MM, Aiad HA, Kandil MA, Al-Sharaky DR. Does JC virus have a role in the etiology and prognosis of Egyptian colorectal carcinoma? Apmis. 2013;121:316–26.

133. Boltin D, Vilkin A, Levi Z, Elkayam O, Niv Y. JC virus T-Antigen DNA in gastrointestinal mucosa of immunosuppressed patients: a prospective, controlled study. Dig Dis Sci. 2010;55:1975–81.

134. Link A, Balaguer F, Nagasaka T, Boland CR, Goel A. MicroRNA miR-J1-5p as a potential biomarker for JC virus infection in the gastrointestinal tract. PLoS One. 2014;9:e100036.

135. Coelho TR, Almeida L, Lazo PA. JC virus in the pathogenesis of colorectal cancer, an etiological agent or another component in a multistep process? Virol J. 2010;7:42.

136. zur Hausen H. Papillomaviruses and cancer: from basic studies to clinical application. Nat Rev Cancer. 2002;2:342–50.

137. Blumberg BS, London WT. Hepatitis B virus and the prevention of primary cancer of the liver. J Natl Cancer Inst. 1985;74:267–73.

138. Matsuoka M, Jeang KT. Human T-cell leukaemia virus type 1 (HTLV-1) infectivity and cellular transformation. Nat Rev Cancer. 2007;7:270–80.

139. Pagano JS, Blaser M, Buendia MA, Damania B, Khalili K, Raab-Traub N, Roizman B. Infectious agents and cancer: criteria for a causal relation. Semin Cancer Biol. 2004;14:453–71.

140. Zur Hausen H. The search for infectious causes of human cancers: where and why. Virology. 2009;392:1–10.

141. De Paoli P, Carbone A. Carcinogenic viruses and solid cancers without sufficient evidence of causal association. Int J Cancer. 2013;133:1517–29.

142. Ambinder RF. Gammaherpesviruses and "Hit-and-Run" oncogenesis. Am J Pathol. 2000;156:1–3.

143. Sadeghi F, Salehi-Vaziri M, Ghodsi SM, Alizadeh A, Bokharaei-Salim F, Saroukalaei ST, Mirbolouk M, Monavari SH, Keyvani H. Prevalence of JC polyomavirus large T antigen sequences among Iranian patients with central nervous system tumors. Arch Virol. 2015;160:61–8.

144. Eftimov T, Enchev Y, Tsekov I, Simeonov P, Kalvatchev Z, Encheva E. JC polyomavirus in the aetiology and pathophysiology of glial tumours. Neurosurg Rev. 2016;39:47–53.

145. Del Valle L, Gordon J, Assimakopoulou M, Enam S, Geddes JF, Varakis JN, Katsetos CD, Croul S, Khalili K. Detection of JC virus DNA sequences and expression of the viral regulatory protein T-antigen in tumors of the central nervous system. Cancer Res. 2001;61:4287–93.

146. Caldarelli-Stefano R, Boldorini R, Monga G, Meraviglia E, Zorini EO, Ferrante P. JC virus in human glial-derived tumors. Hum Pathol. 2000;31:394–5.

147. Boldorini R, Pagani E, Car PG, Omodeo-Zorini E, Borghi E, Tarantini L, Bellotti C, Ferrante P, Monga G. Molecular characterisation of JC virus strains detected in human brain tumours. Pathology. 2003;35:248–53.

148. Delbue S, Pagani E, Guerini FR, Agliardi C, Mancuso R, Borghi E, Rossi F, Boldorini R, Veggiani C, Car PG, Ferrante P. Distribution, characterization and significance of polyomavirus genomic sequences in tumors of the brain and its covering. J Med Virol. 2005;77:447–54.

149. Tsekov I, Ferdinandov D, Bussarsky V, Hristova S, Kalvatchev Z. Prevalence of JC polyomavirus genomic sequences from the large T-antigen and non-coding control regions among Bulgarian patients with primary brain tumors. J Med Virol. 2011;83:1608–13.

150. Rollison DE, Utaipat U, Ryschkewitsch C, Hou J, Goldthwaite P, Daniel R, Helzlsouer KJ, Burger PC, Shah KV, Major EO. Investigation of human brain tumors for the presence of polyomavirus genome sequences by two independent laboratories. Int J Cancer. 2005;113:769–74.

151. Okamoto H, Mineta T, Ueda S, Nakahara Y, Shiraishi T, Tamiya T, Tabuchi K. Detection of JC virus DNA sequences in brain tumors in pediatric patients. J Neurosurg. 2005;102:294–8.

152. Del Valle L, Azizi SA, Krynska B, Enam S, Croul SE, Khalili K. Reactivation of human neurotropic JC virus expressing oncogenic protein in a recurrent glioblastoma multiforme. Ann Neurol. 2000;48:932–6.

153. Pina-Oviedo S, De Leon-Bojorge B, Cuesta-Mejias T, White MK, Ortiz-Hidalgo C, Khalili K, Del Valle L. Glioblastoma multiforme with small cell neuronal-like component: association with human neurotropic JC virus. Acta Neuropathol. 2006;111:388–96.

154. Del Valle L, Wang JY, Lassak A, Peruzzi F, Croul S, Khalili K, Reiss K. Insulin-like growth factor I receptor signaling system in JC virus T antigen-induced primitive neuroectodermal tumors–medulloblastomas. J Neurovirol. 2002;8 Suppl 2:138–47.

155. Hayashi H, Endo S, Suzuki S, Tanaka S, Sawa H, Ozaki Y, Sawamura Y, Nagashima K. JC virus large T protein transforms rodent cells but is not involved in human medulloblastoma. Neuropathology. 2001;21:129–37.

156. Krynska B, Del Valle L, Croul S, Gordon J, Katsetos CD, Carbone M, Giordano A, Khalili K. Detection of human neurotropic JC virus DNA sequence and expression of the viral oncogenic protein in pediatric medulloblastomas. Proc Natl Acad Sci U S A. 1999;96:11519–24.

157. Kim JY, Koralnik IJ, LeFave M, Segal RA, Pfister LA, Pomeroy SL. Medulloblastomas and primitive neuroectodermal tumors rarely contain polyomavirus DNA sequences. Neuro Oncol. 2002;4:165–70.

158. Vasishta RK, Pasricha N, Nath A, Sehgal S. The absence of JC virus antigens in Indian children with medulloblastomas. Indian J Pathol Microbiol. 2009;52:42–5.

159. Rencic A, Gordon J, Otte J, Curtis M, Kovatich A, Zoltick P, Khalili K, Andrews D. Detection of JC virus DNA sequence and expression of the viral oncoprotein, tumor antigen, in brain of immunocompetent patient with oligoastrocytoma. Proc Natl Acad Sci U S A. 1996;93:7352–7.

160. Del Valle L, Enam S, Lara C, Ortiz-Hidalgo C, Katsetos CD, Khalili K. Detection of JC polyomavirus DNA sequences and cellular localization of T-antigen and agnoprotein in oligodendrogliomas. Clin Cancer Res. 2002;8:3332–40.

161. Boldorini R, Caldarelli-Stefano R, Monga G, Zocchi M, Mediati M, Tosoni A, Ferrante P. PCR detection of JC virus DNA in the brain tissue of a 9-year-old child with pleomorphic xanthoastrocytoma. J Neurovirol. 1998;4:242–5.

# 4

# The effects of antiviral treatment on breast cancer cell line

Madina Shaimerdenova[1], Orynbassar Karapina[2], Damel Mektepbayeva[1], Kenneth Alibek[3] and Dana Akilbekova[1*]

## Abstract

**Background:** Recent studies have revealed the positive antiproliferative and cytotoxic effects of antiviral agents in cancer treatment. The real effect of adjuvant antiviral therapy is still controversial due to the lack of studies in biochemical mechanisms. Here, we studied the effect of the antiviral agent acyclovir on morphometric and migratory features of the MCF7 breast cancer cell line. Molecular levels of various proteins have also been examined.

**Methods:** To evaluate and assess the effect of antiviral treatment on morphometric, migratory and other cellular characteristics of MCF7 breast cancer cells, the following experiments were performed: (i) MTT assay to measure the viability of MCF7 cells; (ii) Colony formation ability by soft agar assay; (iii) Morphometric characterization by immunofluorescent analysis using confocal microscopy; (iv) wound healing and transwell membrane assays to evaluate migration and invasion capacity of the cells; (v) ELISA colorimetric assays to assess expression levels of caspase-3, E-cadherin and enzymatic activity of aldehyde dehydrogenase (ALDH).

**Results:** We demonstrate the suppressive effect of acyclovir on breast cancer cells. Acyclovir treatment decreases the growth and the proliferation rate of cells and correlates with the upregulated levels of apoptosis associated cytokine Caspase-3. Moreover, acyclovir inhibits colony formation ability and cell invasion capacity of the cancer cells while enhancing the expression of E-cadherin protein in MCF7 cells. Breast cancer cells are characterized by high ALDH activity and associated with upregulated proliferation and invasion. According to this study, acyclovir downregulates ALDH activity in MCF7 cells.

**Conclusions:** These results are encouraging and demonstrate the possibility of partial suppression of cancer cell proliferation using an antiviral agent. Acyclovir antiviral agents have a great potential as an adjuvant therapy in the cancer treatment. However, more research is necessary to identify relevant biochemical mechanisms by which acyclovir induces a potent anti-cancer effect.

**Keywords:** MCF7 breast cancer cell line, Acyclovir, Antiproliferative effect, ALDH activity

## Background

Current cancer therapy includes the use of chemotherapeutic agents, surgery and radiation therapy. It is estimated that four types of viruses alone could cause 12% of cancer cases worldwide. These are human papillomavirus (HPV), hepatitis B (HBV), hepatitis C (HCV), and Epstein–Barr virus (EBV) [1]. Investigation of the virus-associated cancer serves as a unique platform for the development of novel strategies to prevent the development of infection that can predispose tumorigenesis. Studies on antiviral drug treatments demonstrate promising results on the prognosis through the prevention of carcinogenesis. Administration of the antiviral agents in combination with the anticancer drugs is known for positively influencing the effectiveness of the treatment [2]. This combined therapy is termed as an adjuvant antiviral therapy [3]. Complex combinations of the chemotherapeutic agents together with the antiviral drugs are used to treat a number of infection-associated malignancies such as Kaposi sarcoma, hepatocellular carcinoma (HCC) and nasopharyngeal carcinoma [4, 5]. A study based on the electronic health records of 2671 adult participants diagnosed with chronic HBV infection from 1992 to 2011 also indicates that an antiviral treatment against chronic HBV

* Correspondence: dana.akilbekova@nu.edu.kz
[1]National Laboratory Astana, Nazarbayev University, Qabanbay Batyr Avenue 53, Astana 010000, Kazakhstan
Full list of author information is available at the end of the article

infection markedly decreases the incidence of HCC in the treated patients [5].

Adjuvant antiviral therapy also has a reported antiproliferative effect in some types of cancer [2]. Treatment of breast cancer cells with ribavirin decreases the level of one of the biomarkers of this malignancy, eukaryotic translation initiation factor (eIF4E), which is usually elevated in more than 25% of cancer cases [6]. Ribavirin disrupts the structure of eIF4E, leading to the inhibition of cyclin D1 and expression of NBS1 oncogene [7, 8].

Namba et al. demonstrated the use of zidovudine, an antiviral drug, in combination with gemcitabine, a chemotherapeutic agent - in an attempt to overcome a gemcitabine resistance for the pancreatic cancer treatment. In this type of malignancy, the gemcitabine resistance is associated with a decreased level of human equilibrative nucleoside transporter 1 (hENT1) and acquisition of epithelial-to-mesenchymal transition (EMT) - like phenotype. The zidovudine adjunct therapy was shown to reverse both events in this study [9]. Furthermore, authors demonstrated that activation of Akt-GSK3β-Snail mechanism, one of the major signaling pathways during gemcitabine resistance, is inhibited by zidovudine so that gemcitabine-resistant cancer cells were resensitized.

Although there is a plethora of evidence suggesting the beneficial effect of the antiviral agents in cancer treatment, the therapeutic benefit of their use in cancer treatment remains a grey area due to the lack of studies of the biochemical mechanisms. Antiviral agents such as acyclovir and ribavirin have been reported to have a suppressive effect on the proliferation and ability to increase an apoptosis in various cancers [7, 8]. Acyclovir was discovered 40 years ago and remains one of the main existing therapies for herpes simplex virus (HSV) infections. This drug is a highly potent inhibitor of this virus and commonly used for the treatment of the infections caused by the herpes viruses, CMV and EBV. It also has a low toxicity for the normal cells [10].

In the present study, we propose to investigate how cancer cells respond to the antiviral agent as acyclovir in vitro and whether this treatment can affect the metastatic phenotype of cancer cells. We report results on the potential effect of acyclovir treatment on the cell proliferation, invasion capacity, cytotoxicity, and the expression of tumor suppressing genes.

## Methods
### Cell culture
Breast cancer cell line MCF7 (American Type Cell Collection, ATCC® HTB 22™) and human breast epithelial primary cells (Celprogen, Benelux, Netherlands) were cultured in a complete media (CM) (Dulbecco's modified Eagle's medium (DMEM) (D6421, Sigma-Aldrich, St Louis, MO, USA) supplemented with 10% fetal bovine serum (12103C-500 ml, Sigma-Aldrich, Buchs, Switzerland), 100 U/mL penicillin, 100 µg/mL streptomycin and 25 ug/mL Amphotericin B (SV30079.01, HyClone, Thermo Scientific, South Logan, Utah, USA) at 37 °C in 5% $CO_2$. Cells were subcultured every three days using 0.25% trypsin-EDTA (25-052-CI, Cellgro, Mediatech Inc, Manassas, VA, USA) for detachment.

### Treatment with Acyclovir
Antiviral agent – acyclovir (ACV) in powder form was purchased from Sigma-Aldrich (PHR1254-1G, St Louis, MO, USA). A 10 mM (stock) solution was prepared in phosphate buffered saline (PBS) and sterilized through filtering (0.45 µM PVDF 25 mm filters, (094.01.003, Isolab, Wertheim, Germany). Stock solution was stored at -20 °C. MCF7 cells were cultured in 12-well plate at 26,000 cells/cm$^2$ (92412, TPP, Switzerland) in the presence of 5 uM acyclovir solution and incubated for 72 h at 37 °C in 5% $CO_2$. In a positive control experiment, cells were cultured in the absence of acyclovir. A control of acyclovir without cells was also conducted. All experiments were performed in triplicate.

### Viability assay
Cell viability after the acyclovir treatment was evaluated with MTT (3-(4,5-dimethylthiazol-2- yl)-2,5-diphenyltetrazolium bromide (M5655-1G, Sigma Aldrich, St Louis, MO, USA) assay. Concentration of 5 mg/ml was achieved by reconstituting MTT in DI water. After removal of the supernatant from the wells, 500 µl of warm culture media and 50 µl of MTT solution were added in each well for two hours at 37 °C in 5% $CO_2$. Then 400 µl of media was removed and crystals of formazan were diluted with 500 µl of dimethyl sulfoxide (DMSO) (D4540-100 ml, Sigma Aldrich, St Louis, MO, USA). Absorbance of cells was measured at 570 nm (BioTek ELx800 plate reader, Winooski, Vermont, USA).

### Proliferation assay
Proliferation in MCF7 cells was determined by plating 6500 cells/cm$^2$ into 12-well plate and cultured in a medium with and without ACV. After overnight incubation cells were detached with trypsin and counted using automated cell counter (TC20™, 1450102, Bio-rad Laboratories, Berkeley, California) at 24, 48, 72 and 96 h.

### Soft agar assay
The ability of cancer cells to form colonies was characterized using a soft agar assay. This assay required 21 days of growth on the soft agar medium. At the end of 3 weeks, a number of colonies formed per petri dish were counted using a crystal violet stain. Briefly, 1% sterile agar solution was warmed in a microwave and place to 37 °C water bath to cool down. 500 µg of agarose

powder (BP165-25, Thermo Fisher Scientific, Fair Lawn, New Jersey, USA) was dissolved in 50 mL distilled water. The bottom of the petri dish (502014-07P, Sterilin petri dishes 9.6 cm$^2$, Dynalon Labware, Rochester, NY, USA) was coated with 0.7% agar and 0.3% CM by adding 3 ml/dish at room temperature for 30 min. following this, the upper layer of 3 mL of agar solution with 0.3% agar and 0.7% cell suspension (3125 cells/cm$^2$) was plated. The top agar layer was allowed to solidify and then incubated for 3 weeks at 37 °C in 5% CO$_2$. CM was refreshed 2 times a week. In 21 days crystal violet was used as a staining for colonies (C3886, Sigma-Aldrich, Munich, Germany) and counting was performed using Leica DMI3000 B light microscope.

### Cell staining for fluorescent imaging
#### Morphological analysis
Glass coverslips were cleaned for 2 h in 200 mL ethanol, 50 g NaOH, and 300 mL DI water and finally rinsed with PBS. Cells were seeded on glass coverslips at 10,500 cells/cm$^2$, placed in petri dishes (Sterilin petri dishes 9.6 cm$^2$) and incubated at 37 °C in 5% CO$_2$ overnight before the treatment. After the 72 h incubation with acyclovir, coverslips with cells were rinsed briefly with PBS for thrice for 5 min each time. 4% paraformaldehyde was used as a fixative for 10 min at room temperature. The samples were blocked with 1% BSA and 0.3% Tween-20 (P2287-500 ml, Sigma-Aldrich, St Louis, MO, USA) in PBS and incubated at room temperature for 1 h. Following 1 h incubation, α-tubulin rabbit mAb Alexa Fluor® 488 conjugate (322588, Invitrogen, Life Technologies, Rockford, IL, USA) diluted as 1:200 was used for staining and incubation at 4 °C overnight in the dark. After 24 h, the coverslips were washed 3 times for 5 min with PBS and then incubated with 0.1 μg/mL DAPI for 2 min. After rinsing again with PBS, aqueous mounting medium (ab128982, Abcam, Cambridge, MA) was used for mounting coverslips on microscope slides. Finally, coverslips were sealed with a clear nail polish. Images were acquired using EVOS® FLoid® Cell Imaging Station (4471136, Life Technologies, Carlsbad, California, USA). Cellprofiler software was used to evaluate morphometric features of treated MCF7 cells (Broad Institute, www.cellprofiler.org). The equation used for the quantitative measurement of the shape of the cell is given below. This equation uses form factor, FF:

$$FF = 4 * \pi * area/perimeter^2 \tag{1}$$

The pipeline for this analysis included four modules: Identify Primary Objects, Identify Secondary Objects, Identify Tertiary Objects and Measure Object Size Shape [11].

Area ratio was calculated by dividing area of nucleus over area of cytoplasm.

### Immunofluorescence staining for the presence of E-cadherin
4% paraformaldehyde in PBS was used as a fixative for 10 min at room temperature and 0.1% Triton was used as a permeabilization solution for 10 min on ice. Following this, cells were washed 3 times with ice cold PBS and blocked with 1% BSA in PBST at room temperature for 1 h. Blocked cells were stained with 1 mg/ml of Ms mAb to E-cadherin (ab1416, Abcam, Cambridge, MA, USA) in 1% BSA in PBST in a humidified chamber for 24 h at 4 °C. The stained samples were then washed 3x5 min with PBS and incubated overnight with a 2 mg/ml of secondary antibody goat pAb to Ms IgG Alexa fluor 488 (ab150113, Abcam, Cambridge, MA, USA) in 1% BSA in PBST. Coverslips were washed 3x5 min with PBS in the dark and incubated with DAPI for 2 min, and mounted on the microscope slides using glycerol. Images were acquired using EVOS® FLoid® Cell Imaging Station (4471136, Life Technologies, Carlsbad, California, USA).

### Aldehyde dehydrogenase activity colorimetric assay (ALDH)
NAD-dependent ALDH activity was measured using colorimetric assay kit (MAK082-1KT, Sigma Aldrich, Saint Louis, MO, USA) and performed as described in the manufacturer's instructions. The absorbance was measured at 450 nm on BioTek *ELx*800 plate reader. Measurements were recorded every 3 min until the value of the control sample exceeded the value of the most active standard (10 nmole/well). The following equation was used to calculate the activity of the enzyme:

$$ALDH\ Activity = \frac{NADH\ Amount\ (nmole)\ x\ Sample\ Dilution\ Factor}{(Reaction\ time)\ x\ Sample\ volume\ (mL)} \tag{2}$$

### Transwell migration assay
Cells were cultured for 72 h with and without acyclovir at 37 °C in 5% CO2, and then in serum-free medium for another 24 h at 37 °C in 5% CO$_2$. After detachment with 0.05% trypsin- EDTA the cells were re-suspended in a serum-free medium. Upper insert was filled with 100 μl of the cell suspension ($\sim$9x10$^4$-1x10$^6$ cells per well) while reservoir chamber was filled with 600 μl of culture medium. Migration of cells was monitored at 3, 6, and 12 h at 37 °C in 5% CO$_2$. Crystal violet was used as the staining solution to distinguish between migrated and non-migrated cells. A cotton swab was used to remove the cells that were left in the upper chamber of the membrane. Those cells that migrated through the insert were examined and counted with bright-field microscope (LEICA DMI3000 B, Wetzlar, Germany).

## Wound healing

Cell culture was performed at a concentration of 260,000 cells/cm$^2$ in 12-well plates incubated overnight at 37 °C in 5% $CO_2$. The medium was then substituted with $CO_2$ free media with and without ACV. A scratch using sharpened toothpick was made on the surface of the well to simulate a wound in vitro. Four randomly areas in a well were selected and imaged in 10 min intervals for 12 h using time-lapse microscopy system (AMAFD1000, EVOS FL Auto imaging system, Life Technologies, Thermo Fisher Scientific, Carlsbad, CA, USA). The images obtained were processed using ImageJ (image processing software). The sequence of images was analyzed and the open wound area was measured for each image at every hour. A scatter plot of wound area measurements (units) vs. time (in hours) was generated as seen in Additional data 5. A line-of-best fit was used to calculate the slope, which corresponded to the rate of migrated cells.

## E-cadherin, C-Myc, NF-kB p65 and caspase-3 levels colorimetric assays

Secretion levels of E-cadherin in a cell culture were measured using a human E-cadherin ELISA colorimetric assay kit (99-1700, Invitrogen, Novex by Life Technologies, Frederick, MD, USA) and performed as described in the manufacturer's instructions. Cellular levels of C-Myc, NF-kB p65 and caspase-3 in cell lysates were measured using a human C-Myc ELISA colorimetric assay kit (KHO 2041, Novex by Life Technologies, Frederick, MD, USA); a human NF-kB p65 Total ELISA colorimetric assay kit (KHO 0371, Novex by Life Technologies, Frederick, MD, USA) and a human caspase-3 ELISA Kit (KHO 1091, Novex by Life Technologies, Frederick, MD, USA).

Cell lysates were prepared using a 1 mM phenylmethylsulfonyl fluoride (PMSF) cell extraction buffer, a protease inhibitor cocktail (78439, Thermo Scientific, Rockford, IL, USA) and RIPA buffer (89900, Thermo Scientific, Rockford, IL, USA). Lysis was performed by adding 500 µl extraction buffer to the cell pellet for 30 min on ice while vortexing every 10 min. Then the cells were placed in the microcentrifuge tubes at 13,000 rpm for 10 min at 4 °C. Lysates were stored at -80 °C. All experiments were performed in triplicate. Results were expressed as mean concentration ± standard deviation and normalized to the number of live cells.

## Apoptosis assay

Programmed cell death was studied using annexin V-FITC apoptosis detection kit (331200, Invitrogen, Camarillo, CA, USA). Treated and control cells were harvested and re-suspended in CM to obtain a target concentration of 1×10$^6$/ml in 1.5 ml Eppendorf tubes. Cells were centrifuged for 1 min at 3000 rpm, washed with ice cold PBS and centrifuged again. Cell pellets were re-suspended in 190 ul of 1x binding buffer with 10 ul Annexin V-FITC and 10 ul of 20ug/ml propidium iodide for 15 min at room temperature in the dark. Apoptosis of the cells was analyzed by flow cytometry (SORP FACSAria -II with 6 lasers, BD Biosciences, San Jose, USA).

## Statistics

All reported results below are presented as mean values ± standard error values. To calculate differences between means, one-way analysis of variance (ANOVA) was implemented, where a null hypothesis was accepted when all means were equal. Population differences were calculated only for a treatment and a control within the cell line. If at least one mean was different, a follow-up Tukey's HSD test to compare between groups and calculate p-values of each sample ($\alpha = 0.05$).

## Results

Viability of MCF7 cells and breast epithelial cells after the treatment with 5 µM ACV were measured and normalized to the untreated culture cells [Additional file 1]. MCF7 cells and breast epithelial cells demonstrated 80,687 and 97,194% of viable cells after the ACV treatment, respectively.

First, we sought to evaluate the influence of ACV on the proliferation ability and apoptosis of MCF7 cells. Regulated interplay between apoptosis and cell proliferation is essential for the processes like tissue development and deregulation mechanisms [12]. Deregulated mechanism of apoptosis that correlates with an uncontrolled cell proliferation eventually leads to the carcinogenesis [13]. Several antiviral agents demonstrated the ability to inhibit proliferation and increase proapoptotic activity of the cancer cells [2]. Here, the rate of proliferation decreased during 96 h treatment with ACV (Fig. 1a). ACV significantly increased a population doubling time compared to the control cells ∞1.4 fold [Additional file 2]. Caspase-3 level in MCF7 cells was estimated to evaluate the apoptotic activity of cancer cells in response to ACV treatment. ACV upregulated caspase-3 expression in the treated cells ∞1.7 compared to the control cells ($p < 0.05$) (Fig. 1b). Annexin V staining and flow cytometry analysis demonstrated a slight increase of the number of the apoptotic cells in response to ACV treatment ($p > 0.05$ for the late and early apoptosis) (Fig. 1c, Additional file 3).

When examining normal cells and cancerous cells under the microscope, we observed distinctive external characteristic features. Results of the IF staining indicate that cancer cells underwent changes in their morphological characteristics in response to ACV treatment (Fig. 1d). FF shape descriptor was used quantitative

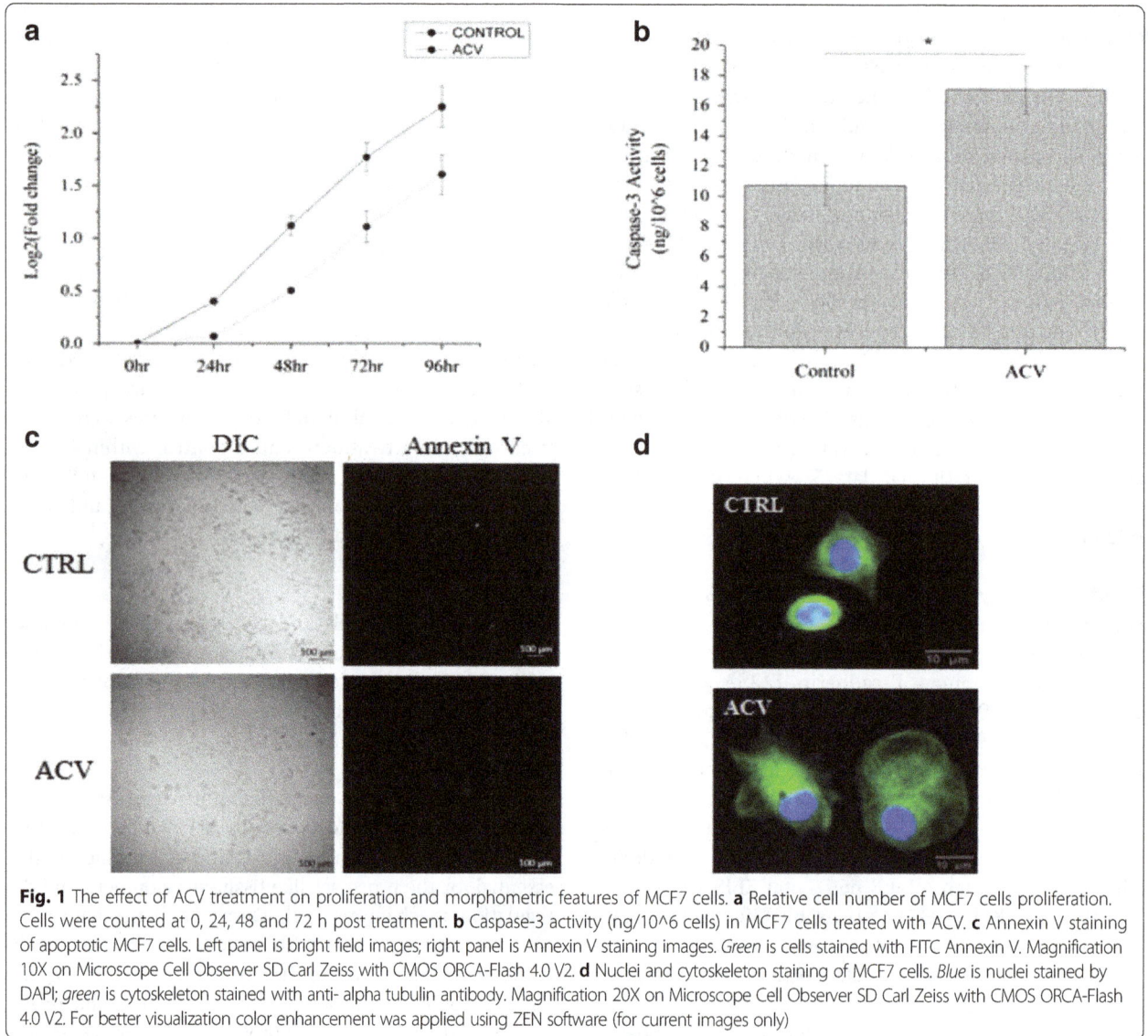

**Fig. 1** The effect of ACV treatment on proliferation and morphometric features of MCF7 cells. **a** Relative cell number of MCF7 cells proliferation. Cells were counted at 0, 24, 48 and 72 h post treatment. **b** Caspase-3 activity (ng/10^6 cells) in MCF7 cells treated with ACV. **c** Annexin V staining of apoptotic MCF7 cells. Left panel is bright field images; right panel is Annexin V staining images. Green is cells stained with FITC Annexin V. Magnification 10X on Microscope Cell Observer SD Carl Zeiss with CMOS ORCA-Flash 4.0 V2. **d** Nuclei and cytoskeleton staining of MCF7 cells. Blue is nuclei stained by DAPI; green is cytoskeleton stained with anti- alpha tubulin antibody. Magnification 20X on Microscope Cell Observer SD Carl Zeiss with CMOS ORCA-Flash 4.0 V2. For better visualization color enhancement was applied using ZEN software (for current images only)

characterization of these changes, where FF value of 1 served as a detector of a circular shape and 0 indicated linear or star shaped object [Additional file 4]. ACV treated cancer cells displayed a decrease of FF compared to the control cells from $0.828 \pm 0.014$ to $0.659 \pm 0.012$, indicating that ACV treated cells were more spread out with a non-uniform shape ($\infty 1.25$ fold). Furthermore, ACV treated cancer cells had a larger cytoplasmic volume compared to the control cells.

The effect of ACV treatment on the migratory and invasive capacities of the breast cancer cells was also tested. Various environmental factors can modulate the motility of cancer cells and affect invasion capacity of these cells. Teng et al. showed that antiviral drug ribavirin causes a considerable suppression of the migration of renal cell carcinoma cell lines [14]. Boyden chamber migration assay was performed to assess whether ACV

affects MCF7 chemopolarised migration. As seen in Fig. 2a, ACV treatment reduces the number of cells migrating towards the chemoattractants as compared to the control cells. The cell invasion capacity of the treated cancer cells dropped $\infty 15$ times compared to the untreated cells ($p < 0.05$). Fig. 2b shows the effect of ACV on the collective motility and rates of migration of both normal and cancer cells. The rate of the wound closure of ACV treated cancer cells decreased significantly compared to the control cells with $\infty 1.34$ fold and was comparable to the rate of normal breast epithelial cells (24.74 μm/h and 21.95 μm/h for ACV treated and normal cells, respectively) ($p < 0.05$) [Additional file 5].

E-cadherin is secreted in most of the epithelial tissues and normal expression of E-cadherin has been reported to inhibit metastasis and invasion by suppressing epithelial-mesenchymal transition as well as stimulating cell-cell

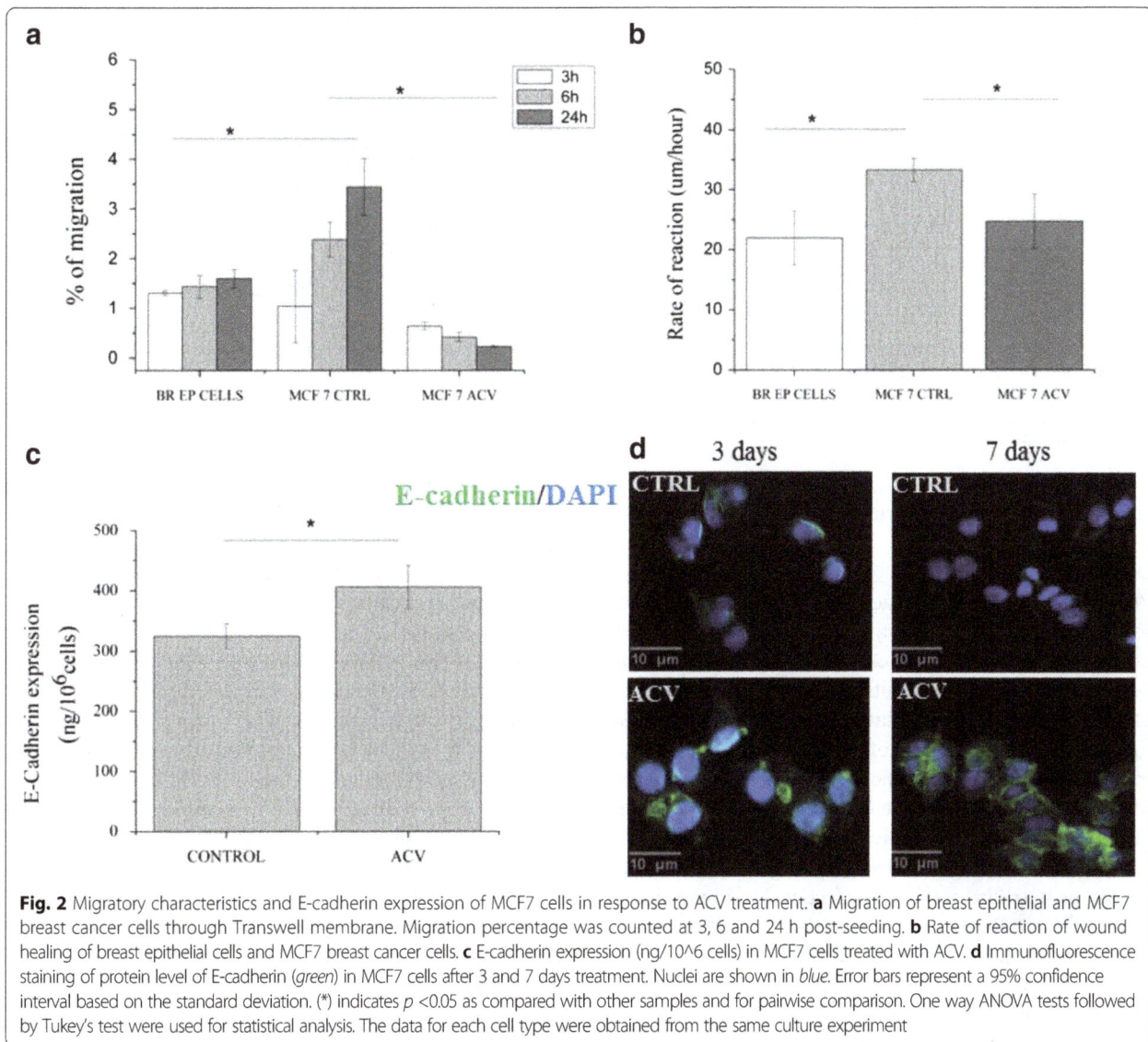

**Fig. 2** Migratory characteristics and E-cadherin expression of MCF7 cells in response to ACV treatment. **a** Migration of breast epithelial and MCF7 breast cancer cells through Transwell membrane. Migration percentage was counted at 3, 6 and 24 h post-seeding. **b** Rate of reaction of wound healing of breast epithelial cells and MCF7 breast cancer cells. **c** E-cadherin expression (ng/10^6 cells) in MCF7 cells treated with ACV. **d** Immunofluorescence staining of protein level of E-cadherin (*green*) in MCF7 cells after 3 and 7 days treatment. Nuclei are shown in *blue*. Error bars represent a 95% confidence interval based on the standard deviation. (*) indicates $p < 0.05$ as compared with other samples and for pairwise comparison. One way ANOVA tests followed by Tukey's test were used for statistical analysis. The data for each cell type were obtained from the same culture experiment

adhesions [15, 16]. We observed a significant increase of E-cadherin secretion in ACV treated cells compared to the control ∞1,25 ($p < 0.05$) as shown in Fig. 2c, d.

Next, we evaluated the action of ACV on the ability of MCF7 cells to form colonies. This distinguishing feature of the cell transformation and its deregulated growth served as a marker to distinguish between cancer and normal cells, since normal cells do not have the ability to grow in semisolid matrices [17]. ACV treatment effectively decreased (∞ 2 fold) the number of colonies formed by cancer cells compared to the untreated cells as seen in Fig. 3a. Also the differences in external features are clearly observable in rough scabrous surface of control cells (R - shape) versus smoother surface of ACV treated cells (S -shape). (Fig. 3b).

The concentration changes of C-Myc protein secreted by MCF7 cells were determined in response to ACV treatment. C-Myc oncogene regulates cellular growth and metabolic mechanisms as well as their interconnection [18]. Our results demonstrate a non-significant effect of ACV on the level of secretion of C-Myc in MCF7 cells. The concentration of C-Myc protein was similar to the control (Fig. 4a). Additional examinations of the viral protein NF-kB p65 demonstrated an elevated level after treatment with ACV [Additional file 6].

ALDH activity is one of the detectors of cancer progression [19]. Upregulated expression of ALDH1, one of the isoforms of ALDH family, has been reported as a crucial event in the breast cancer prognosis correlated with a poor clinical outcome [20, 21]. Moreover, studies show that ALDH activity is linked to the differentiation and expansion. It is also associated with a self-protective ability [22]. Our assessment of the effect of ACV treatment on ALDH activity of breast cancer cells shows a

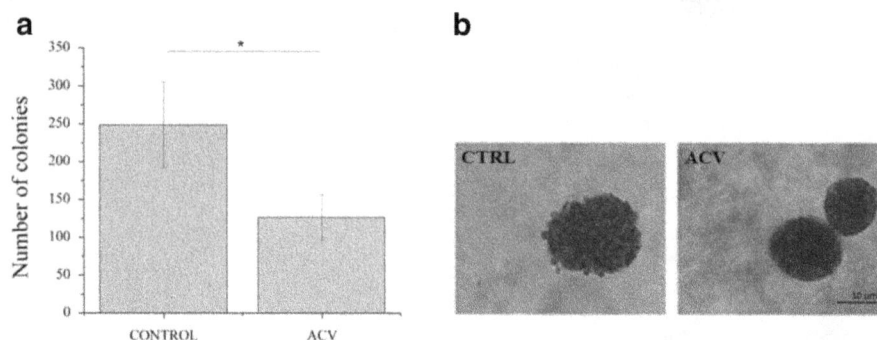

**Fig. 3** ACV altered ability to form colonies of MCF7 breast cancer cells (**a**) Number of colonies of MCF7 cells in response to ACV treatment. **b** Representative images of colonies formed. Duration of growing on a soft agar was 21 days. Error bars represent a 95% confidence interval based on the standard deviation. (*) indicates $p < 0.05$ compared with control and other samples. One way ANOVA followed by Tukey's test were used for statistical analysis. The data for each cell type were taken from the same culture experiment

significant decrease (~3 fold) of ALDH activity in MCF7 cells compared to the control cells (Fig. 4b).

## Discussion

Recently, several antiviral agents have been found to possess the ability to decrease the rate of the cells' proliferation and to promote apoptosis in cancer cells. However, despite the compelling results supporting the clinical use of antiviral agents as an adjuvant therapy in cancer treatment, there is still a lack of studies of the biochemical mechanisms of their anticancer effects [23, 24]. There are several factors that might be involved in a therapeutic approach of the antiviral adjuvant therapy in cancer treatment: an antiviral agent selectively targets cancer related viruses or post-chemotherapy infections and may also result in the cytotoxic and antiproliferative effects on the cancer cells, causing apoptosis [2]. Our implementation of ACV as an antiviral strategy demonstrated a positive effect on the prevention as well as successful predictive capability in the treatment of various types of malignancies.

In this study, we used acyclovir (ACV) to examine the potential of the antiviral treatment on MCF7 breast cancer cell line. Acyclovir is an antiviral drug used in treating infections of *Herpesviridae* family [25]. In several studies antiviral agents similar to ACV were used as an adjuvant therapy along with the chemotherapy [26, 27]. Records of the patients diagnosed with nasopharyngeal carcinoma demonstrate a suppression of the tumor growth for several months where injection of antiviral was used in tandem with the chemotherapy [26]. Moreover, *in situ* hybridization shows that the tumor cell populations were reduced in EBV-encoded RNAs [26]. In another study, the effect of acyclic nucleoside phosphonate against HPV-associated cancer was examined. The results indicate that the adjunct therapy using a cytotoxic drug and acyclic nucleoside phosphonates is more effective than one therapy alone. The authors also report an inhibited rate of the virus replication that led to a decreased expression of the viral oncoproteins and upregulation of the tumor-suppressor genes [27].

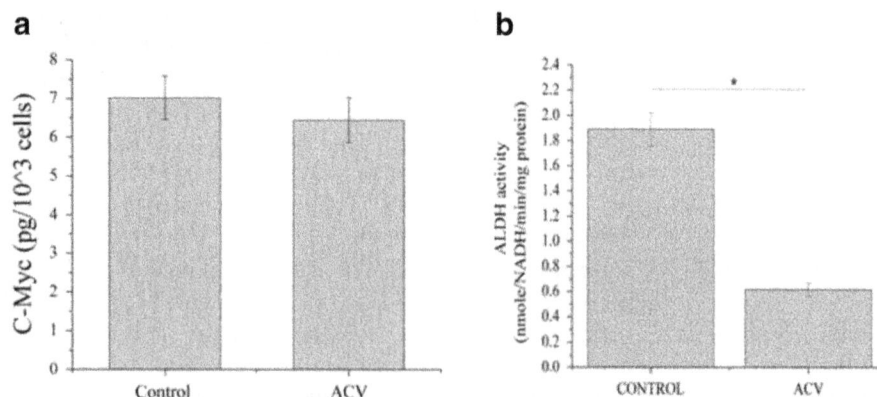

**Fig. 4 a** C-Myc (pg/10^3 cells) and (**b**) ALDH activity (nmol NADH/min/mg protein) expressions of MCF7 cells in response to ACV treatment. Error bars represent 95% confidence interval based on the standard deviation. (*) indicate $p < 0.05$ as compared with other samples and for pairwise comparison. One way ANOVA tests followed by Tukey's test were used for statistical analysis. The data for each cell type were obtained from the same culture experiment

Based on our results, we conclude that ACV as an antiviral agent has a potential suppressive effect on MCF7 breast cancer cells. ACV does not affect viability of non-cancerous breast epithelial cells, while showing a decrease of the viability of MCF7 breast cancer cells. Observed morphological changes and apoptosis analysis demonstrated the ability of ACV to affect the process of programmed cell death of MCF7 cells. The mechanism of apoptosis requires a number of proteins that regulate a proper cell death. One of these proteins is caspase-3 which is included in a family of cysteine proteases [28]. An upregulated level of the apoptosis associated cytokine Caspase-3 was detected in ACV treated cells, correlating with the higher number of apoptotic cells and decreased rate of the cancer cell proliferation. Previously, it was reported that zidovudine treatment combined with a chemotherapeutic agent cisplatin has increased the apoptosis level of head and neck cancer cells [29]. This synergistic strategy of zidovudine and cisplatin was shown to trigger abnormal regulation of the mitochondria, increase of oxidative stress response and cause a significant cytotoxic effect on the cancer cells through the inhibition of a thiol metabolism [29]. Quantitative analysis revealed a moderate effect of acyclovir with a slight increase of the apoptotic cells.

ACV was also able to decrease the rate of the growth, colony formation ability, and cell invasion capacity of MCF7 breast cancer cells. These observations correlate with an upregulated secretion of E-cadherin in ACV treated cells. As previously mentioned, E-cadherin is an essential marker in the building of cell-to-cell adhesion and downregulation of this protein leads to the stimulation of invasion and metastasis [30].

Previous studies also report that antiviral agents can affect the secretion of the specific translation initiation factors, oncogenes, and angiogenic genes [8, 31, 32]. Borden et al. showed the ability of ribavirin to decrease the oncogenic potential of eukaryotic translation initiation factor (eIF4E) in the case of acute myeloid leukemia with a poor prognosis. Ribavirin binds eIF4E around the m7G cap-binding site leading to the reduction of affinity of this translation initiator factor [32]. While, we observed that ACV did not affect the expression levels of C-Myc oncogene, suggesting that antiviral agents might have a selective impact on the secretion of specific proteins.

Moreover, our study showed that acyclovir was able to influence ALDH activity in the breast cancer cells. The ALDH superfamily consists of 19 isoenzymes with various cellular localizations, tissue/organ distributions and functions. ALDH enzymes catalyze highly reactive aldehydes and some isoenzymes play structural roles related to the osmoregulation and possess antioxidant functions [30]. Following cancer stem cell theories, where cancer is suggested to have a stem origin, ALDH was found to be a common marker for both normal and cancer stem cells [22, 33, 34]. Increased level of ALDH enzyme is an indicator of a high tumorigenic potential of the cancer cell and ability to self-renew and initiate tumor progression [21]. In the breast cancer cells upregulated expression of ALDH is associated with a poor clinical outcome [19, 20]. Our results suggest that ACV affects multiple aspects of cellular life related to the carcinogenesis and ALDH fulfills the role of a marker for these changes.

A study by Curiel et al. reported that ACV had an inhibitory effect on one of the immune system components as T-regulatory cells (Treg) in glioblastomas through the suppression of indoleamine 2, 3-dioxygenase activity [35]. Another antiviral agent - ribavirin was also reported as an immune response inducer in the renal cell carcinoma lines through the downregulation of IL-10 expression and the upregulation of TGF-β expression [14]. The mechanisms by which ACV enables its anticancer effects might involve an enhanced immune response of the cancer cells and further study is required in this area.

There are several limitations in this study. All experiments were performed in vitro only on one cell line. Future research should focus on an adjuvant strategy of different antiviral agents to determine whether a combinatorial effect exists, and if so, which pathways are affected during the mechanism. Additionally, an examination of epigenetic modifications might serve as a platform for understanding the molecular mechanism underlying the antiviral therapy.

## Conclusion

In summary, we present evidence that ACV has an anticancer effect on breast cancer cell line. Our study shows that ACV was able to inhibit cancer cells proliferation, colony formation ability and cell invasion capacity, while having no effect on the secretion of certain tumor suppressor genes. Treatment with ACV induced downregulation of ALDH activity, suggesting a decrease of the tumorigenic potential of the treated cancer cells. These results provide new insights on the effect of antiviral agents on the tumorigenesis and metastasis. However, more research is necessary to identify the primary target of ACV and maximize its potential.

## Additional files

**Additional file 1:** Viability of MCF7 breast cancer and normal breast epithelial cells in response to acyclovir. Error bars represent 95% confidence interval based on the standard deviation. (*) indicates $p < 0.05$ as compared with other samples and for pairwise comparison. One way ANOVA followed by Tukey's test were used for statistical analysis. The data for each cell type were taken from same culture experiment.

**Additional file 2:** Population doubling time (hours) of proliferation of MCF7 cells treated with ACV. Error bars represent 95% confidence interval based on the standard deviation. (*) indicates *p* <0.05 as compared with other samples and for pairwise comparison. One way ANOVA followed by Tukey's test were used for statistical analysis. The data for each cell type were taken from same culture experiment.

**Additional file 3:** Annexin V staining of apoptotic MCF7 cells after treatment with acyclovir. Left panel is early apoptosis, right panel is late apoptosis. Error bars represent 95% confidence interval based on the standard deviation. One way ANOVA followed by Tukey's test were used for statistical analysis. Means are not significant, *p* > 0.05. *P*-value for early apoptosis = 1.31579; for late apoptosis = 0.91371. The data for each cell type were taken from same culture experiment.

**Additional file 4:** Quantitative analysis of nucleus and cytoplasm of MCF7 breast cancer cells without and with acyclovir treatment.

**Additional file 5:** A scatter plot of measurements where best fit line and a slope indicate rate of migrating cells.

**Additional file 6:** NF-kB p65 (pg/10^3 cells) expression of MCF7 cells in response to ACV treatment. Error bars represent 95% confidence interval based on the standard deviation. (*) indicates *p* <0.05 as compared with other samples and for pairwise comparison. One way ANOVA followed by Tukey's test were used for statistical analysis. The data for each cell type were taken from the same culture experiment.

## Abbreviations

ACV: Acyclovir; ALDH: aldehyde dehydrogenase; BCS: Bovine calf serum; BSA: Bovine serum albumin; CMV: Cytomegalovirus; DMEM: Dulbecco's modified eagle's medium; DMSO: Dimethyl sulfoxide; EBV: Epstein–barr virus; eIF4E: Eukaryotic translation initiation factor 4E; ELISA: Enzyme-linked immunosorbent assay; EMT: Epithelial-to-mesenchymal transition; FF: Form factor; HBV: Hepatitis B; HCC: Hepatocellular carcinoma; HCV: Hepatitis C; hENT1: Human equilibrative nucleoside transporter 1; HPV: Human papillomavirus; HSV: Herpes simplex virus; IF: Immunofluorescence; MTT: 3-(4,5-dimethylthiazol-2-yl)-2,5-diphenyltetrazolium bromide; NAD: Nicotinamide adenine dinucleotide; NF-kB: Nuclear factor kappa-light-chain-enhancer of activated B cells; PBS: Phosphate buffered saline; PMSF: Phenylmethylsulfonyl fluoride; RIPA buffer: Radioimmunoprecipitation assay buffer; Treg: T-regulatory cells

## Acknowledgment
Authors would like to thank Samal Zhussupbekova, Sabina Murzakhmetova and Tomiris Atazhanova for their help with the collection of colony formation, cell migration and IF staining data.

## Funding
This work was supported by №0121-1 Program-oriented funding-13 by the Ministry of Education and Science of the Republic of Kazakhstan.

## Authors' contributions
MS, KA, and DA. designed the study. MS, OK and DM performed experiments. MS, OK, KA and DA. analyzed data. MS and DA wrote the manuscript. All authors read and approved the final manuscript.

## Competing interests
Authors declare that they have no competing interests.

## Author details
[1]National Laboratory Astana, Nazarbayev University, Qabanbay Batyr Avenue 53, Astana 010000, Kazakhstan. [2]Nazarbayev University Research and Innovation System, Nazarbayev University, Astana, Kazakhstan. [3]Locus Solutions LLC, Solon, OH, USA.

## References
1. Shih WL, Fang CT, Chen PJ. Anti-viral treatment and cancer control. Recent Results Cancer Res. 2014;193:269–90.
2. Alibek K, Bekmurzayeva A, Mussabekova A, Sultankulov B. Using antimicrobial adjuvant therapy in cancer treatment: a review. Infect Agent Cancer. 2012;7(1):33.
3. Alibek K, Kakpenova A, Baiken Y. Role of infectious agents in the carcinogenesis of brain and head and neck cancers. Infect Agent Cancer. 2013;8(1):7.
4. Cathomas G. Kaposi's sarcoma-associated herpesvirus (KSHV)/human herpesvirus 8 (HHV-8) as a tumour virus. Herpes. 2003;10(3):72–7.
5. Gordon SC, et al. Antiviral therapy for chronic hepatitis B virus infection and development of hepatocellular carcinoma in a US population. Clin Gastroenterol Hepatol. 2013;12(5):885–93.
6. Pettersson F, et al. Ribavirin treatment effects on breast cancers overexpressing eIF4E, a biomarker with prognostic specificity for luminal B-type breast cancer. Clin Cancer Res. 2011;17(9):2874–84.
7. Assouline S, et al. Molecular targeting of the oncogene eIF4E in acute myeloid leukemia (AML): A proof-of-principle clinical trial with ribavirin. Blood. 2009;114(2):257–60.
8. Kentsis A, Topisirovic I, Culjkovic B, Shao L, Borden KLB. Ribavirin suppresses eIF4E-mediated oncogenic transformation by physical mimicry of the 7-methyl guanosine mRNA cap. Proc Natl Acad Sci U S A. 2004;101(52):18105–10.
9. Namba T, Kodama R, Moritomo S, Hoshino T, Mizushima T. Zidovudine, an anti-viral drug, resensitizes gemcitabine-resistant pancreatic cancer cells to gemcitabine by inhibition of the Akt-GSK3β-Snail pathway. Cell Death Dis. 2015;6:e1795.
10. Elion GB. Mechanism of action and selectivity of acyclovir. Am J Med. 1982; 73(1 PART 1):7–13.
11. Bygd HC, Akilbekova D, Muñoz A, Forsmark KD, Bratlie KM. Poly-l-arginine based materials as instructive substrates for fibroblast synthesis of collagen. Biomaterials. 2015;63:47–57.
12. Alenzi FQB. Links between apoptosis, proliferation and the cell cycle. Br J Biomed Sci. 2004;61(2):99–102.
13. Evan GI, Vousden KH. Proliferation, cell cycle and apoptosis in cancer. Nature. 2001;411(6835):342–8.
14. Teng L, et al. Anti-tumor effect of ribavirin in combination with interferon-α on renal cell carcinoma cell lines in vitro. Cancer Cell Int. 2014;14:63.
15. Singhai R, Patil VW, Jaiswal SR, Patil SD, Tayade MB, Patil AV. E-Cadherin as a diagnostic biomarker in breast cancer. N Am J Med Sci. 2011;3(5):227–33.
16. Kowalski PJ, Rubin M a, Kleer CG. E-cadherin expression in primary carcinomas of the breast and its distant metastases. Breast Cancer Res. 2003;5(6):R217–22.
17. Borowicz S, et al. The soft agar colony formation assay. J Vis Exp. 2014;92: e51998.
18. Miller DM, Thomas SD, Islam A, Muench D, Sedoris K. c-Myc and cancer metabolism. Clin Cancer Res. 2012;18(20):5546–53.
19. Marcato P, Dean CA, Giacomantonio CA, Lee PWK. Aldehyde dehydrogenase its role as a cancer stem cell marker comes down to the specific isoform. Cell Cycle. 2011;10(9):1378–84.
20. Chaterjee M, van Golen KL. Breast cancer stem cells survive periods of farnesyl-transferase inhibitor-induced dormancy by undergoing autophagy. Bone Marrow Res. 2011;2011:362938.
21. Ginestier C, et al. ALDH1 is a marker of normal and malignant human mammary stem cells and a predictor of poor clinical outcome. Cell Stem Cell. 2007;1(5):555–67.
22. Ma I, Allan AL. The role of human aldehyde dehydrogenase in normal and cancer stem cells. Stem Cell Rev. 2011;7(2):292–306.
23. Söderlund J, Erhardt S, Kast RE. Acyclovir inhibition of IDO to decrease Tregs as a glioblastoma treatment adjunct. J Neuroinflammation. 2010;7:44.
24. Zhou FX, et al. Radiosensitization effect of zidovudine on human malignant glioma cells. Biochem Biophys Res Commun. 2007;354(2):351–6.
25. Spruance SL, Nett R, Marbury T, Wolff R, Johnson J, Spaulding T. Acyclovir cream for treatment of herpes simplex labialis: Results of two randomized,

double-blind, vehicle-controlled, multicenter clinical trials. Antimicrob Agents Chemother. 2002;46(7):2238–43.

26. Yoshizaki T, et al. Treatment of locally recurrent Epstein-Barr virus-associated nasopharyngeal carcinoma using the anti-viral agent cidofovir. J Med Virol. 2008;80(5):879–82.

27. Abdulkarim B, Bourhis J. Antiviral approaches for cancers related to Epstein-Barr virus and human papillomavirus. Lancet Oncol. 2001;2(10):622–30.

28. Devarajan E, et al. Down-regulation of caspase 3 in breast cancer: a possible mechanism for chemoresistance. Oncogene. 2002;21(57):8843–51.

29. Mattson DM, et al. Cisplatin combined with zidovudine enhances cytotoxicity and oxidative stress in human head and neck cancer cells via a thiol-dependent mechanism. Free Radic Biol Med. 2009;46(2):232–7.

30. Hanahan D, Weinberg RA. Hallmarks of cancer: the next generation. Cell. 2011;144(5):646–74.

31. Flore O, Rafii S, Ely S, O'Leary JJ, Hyjek EM, Cesarman E. Transformation of primary human endothelial cells by Kaposi's sarcoma-associated herpesvirus. Nature. 1998;394(6693):588–92.

32. Borden KLB, Culjkovic-Kraljacic B. Ribavirin as an anti-cancer therapy: acute myeloid leukemia and beyond? Leuk Lymphoma. 2010;51(10):1805–15.

33. Sell S. Stem cell origin of cancer and differentiation therapy. Crit Rev Oncol Hematol. 2004;51(1):1–28.

34. Reya T, Morrison SJ, Clarke MF, Weissman IL. Stem cells, cancer, and cancer stem cells. Nature. 2001;414(6859):105–11.

35. Curiel TJ. Tregs and rethinking cancer immunotherapy. J Clin Investig. 2007; 117(5):1167–74.

# 5

# Differences in age-specific HPV prevalence between self-collected and health personnel collected specimen

Adolf K. Awua[1,2*], Richard M. K. Adanu[3], Edwin K. Wiredu[4], Edwin A. Afari[1] and Alberto Severini[5,6]

## Abstract

**Background:** HPV infections are ubiquitous and particularly common among sexually active young women. However, there are regional and national variations in age-specific HPV prevalence, which have implications for cervical cancer control. Data on age-specific HPV prevalences for Ghana and most sub-Saharan countries are scanty. Therefore, this study primarily sought to determine the age-specific HPV prevalence among women in a Ghanaian community and to determine whether these prevalences determined with health-personnel and self-collected specimens were comparable.

**Methods:** In this cross-sectional study, conducted between March 2012 and March 2013, cervical specimens were collected by self- and health-personnel collection from 251 women who were between the ages of 15 and 65 years. HPV present in these specimens were genotyped by a nested-multiplex PCR and Luminex fluoro-microspheres based method. Information on the demographic, sexual and reproductive characteristics of the women were also obtained. A Chi-square test of association was employed to determine the association of the distribution of age groups with each categorised sexual and reproductive characteristic and HPV risk type's status.

**Results:** The age group distribution of the participants was significantly associated with overall ($x^2 = 36.1$; $p = 0.001$), high risk ($x^2 = 26.09$; $p = 0.002$) and low risk ($x^2 = 21.49$; $p = 0.011$) HPV prevalences. The age-specific HPV prevalence pattern for each of the HPV risk types, determined with self-collected specimen, showed three peaks (at 20–24 years; 40–44 years and ≥ 55 years), while those determined with health-personnel collected specimen, showed two peaks (at 20–24 years and ≥ 55 years) for each HPV risk type's prevalence pattern. The high risk HPV prevalences determined with self-collected specimen were often higher than those determined with health-personnel specimen for the age groups between 25 and 45 years, who are mostly targeted for screening by HPV testing. Additionally, there were interesting variations in patterns of age-specific HPV genotype-specific prevalence between the two specimen collection methods.

**Conclusions:** The usefulness of self-collected specimen for high risk HPV burden determination and the existence of a two peaked and three peaked age-specific HPV prevalences in Ghana have been clearly indicated.

**Keywords:** Human Papillomavirus, Age-specific, Cervical cancer, Self-sample collection, Screening, Ghana

* Correspondence: a_awua@yahoo.com
[1]Department of Epidemiology and Disease Control, School of Public Health, College of Health Sciences, University of Ghana, Accra, Ghana
[2]Cellular and Clinical Research Centre, Radiological and Medical Sciences Research Institute, GAEC, Accra, Ghana
Full list of author information is available at the end of the article

## Background

Human Papillomaviruses are small, single coated, double stranded DNA virus that have been classified to belong to 30 species and about 200 distinct genotypes [1–3]. Of these, about 50 types infect the mucosal epithelia of most parts of the human body, including the cervix, vagina, vulva, penis, anus and the oropharynx [1, 3]. They are transmitted by almost all forms of sexual contacts, including penetrative intercourse, oral sex, genital contacts and genital skin to skin contact as well as by self-inoculation [4, 5]. These ubiquitous viruses are particularly common among young sexually active women; however, variations in the age specific cervical HPV prevalence, within and between countries and the WHO world regions have been well documented [6]. Similar variations have been reported for other genital tissues, oral, head and neck malignancies [7].

Based on a meta-analysis of 78 studies, which used health personnel collected specimen reported and data of women with normal cytology [6], and also on a few research studies (which used self-collected specimen [8]) and other articles, which did not indicate specimen collection [9, 10], it was clear that women who were younger than 25 years were the most infected by HPV (with a peak between 20 and 22 years). This peak was followed by a progressive decrease in prevalence as age increased until a small increase was observed among women 45–54 years from Africa and Europe, and between 34 and 45 years for those from the North, Central and South America regions. Data from the Asia region did not show a second increase in prevalence as observed for the other regions [6]. Further to these, pooled analysis of country specific multi-centre study HPV data, obtained with health personnel collected specimen from women with normal cytology, showed only a single peak at 25–34 years [11], although data from the individual countries showed different prevalence trends. For instance, data from the Nigerian study in this pooled data showed two peaks, at 25–34 years and 45–54 years; while data form Italy and Netherlands showed one peak, at 55–64 years and 45–54 years respectively; data from Thailand and Vietnam showed two peaks. at 25–34 years and 55–64 years; data form Columbia, Argentina and Chile all showed one peak, but at 25–34 years, 35–44 years and 35–44 years respectively [11]. Similarly a Canadian study, which tested for only high risk HPV types using health-personnel collected specimen, showed a single peak at 20–24 years [12], while as reported by Bosch et. al., [13] a study in Spain, that used health personnel collected specimen, showed two peaks at 20–24 years and 45–54 among the general population of women.

For reasons not clearly understood, the variation in age-specific HPV prevalence trends for African countries seems to have both one peak (unimodal) and two peaks

(bimodal) but not three peaks (trimodal) prevalence. That is, in rural Nigeria, South Africa and Senegal an initial high peak among younger women was followed by a second small prevalence peak among mid-age women (bimodal prevalence) [14–17]. In other studies conducted in South Africa, Nigeria and Mozambique, it was determined that HPV prevalence reduced with increase in age, showing a peak (unimodal) among younger women [14, 18–20]. In the Gambia, the age-specific HPV prevalence was seemingly consistent with increase in age [21]. It is worth noting that these and most age-specific prevalence studies had been based on the analysis of specimen collected by health personnel (HPC), particularly for Pap testing [6].

An effective cervical cancer screening strategy, referred to as self-collection has gained a lot research attention in recent times [22–24]. This strategy involves women themselves collecting cervicovaginal swabs in the privacy of their home for HPV testing, and has been compared with cytology and HPC-HPV testing for the reduction of cervical intraepithelial neoplasia (CIN) and the determination of overall HPV prevalence. Such studies reported a variety of Kappa estimates (ranging between 0.24 and 0.96) and concordances (ranging between 70 and > 90%) for the overall HPV prevalence agreement between self-collected (SC) and HPC specimen [22, 23, 25–29]. Most of these studies have suggested that the difference in overall HPV prevalence between these methods may be due to LR HPV preferentially infecting the vagina than the cervix and therefore they become more detectable with SC than HPC, since the time-to-clearance were similar for both LR HPV and HR HPV detected by both methods [22, 23, 25–28].

Among these studies, only the studies from South Africa [26] and Uganda [27] presented a limited comparison of the age-specific HPV prevalences obtained with the two collection methods, and these showed a non-significant difference. Therefore, the aim of our study was to determine the differences, if any, between the age-specific HPV prevalences determined with SC specimen and those determined with HPC specimen in Ghana and compare the age-specific HPV detection concordance between the two methods. We present the first age-specific HPV prevalence for a Ghanaian population and an assessment of the distribution of related participant characteristics stratified by age.

## Methods

### Study population

In this cross-sectional study of the multi-ethnic population of the Akuse sub-district, women were recruited between March 2012 and March 2013 by a house survey and invited for specimen collection either at the Akuse Government Hospital or at a specified location within the individual communities. In each of 17 communities, the major roads/paths through it were identified by the use of Google Map computer application and grouped in order of direction, from one end of the community to the other. Based on the crude estimate of the average number of houses and the population of women in each of the communities, it was assessed that visiting every 5th house or less will ensure a wide coverage of the communities. Therefore, starting from the first randomly selected road/path, every third house to the right and left of the road/path was visited. Not more than three women in each house, who met the inclusion criteria were invited to participate in the study, after explaining the study, the consent form and the options available to them as participants as well as giving them basic information about cervical cancer.

Women between the ages of 15 and 65 years who had ever been sexually active and were willing to provide specimen by at least one of the two specimen collection methods (data not shown) were included in this study. Women having their menses were asked to come back 1 week after their menstrual period. Women who were pregnant (self-report), had undergone hysterectomy or cervical conisation were excluded from the study. Two trained Public Health Nurses assisted the study participants, by a one-on-one interview, to complete a study questionnaire that obtained information on the socio-demographic characteristics, sexual behaviour, sexual and reproductive history, menstrual factors, use of oral contraception and history of sexually transmitted infections and cervical cancer screening history.

### Compliance with ethical standards

The study was conducted in accordance with the ethical standards as laid down in the 1964 Declaration of Helsinki and its later amendments and comparable ethical standards. The participants either read and signed an informed consent form (in English) or it was translated to a local language and explained to them with the assistance of a witness; the explanation in each of the four local languages (Hausa, Ewe, Ga-Adangbe and Twi) was performed by one particular person throughout the study. The informed consent included the main research goals, sample collection procedures, potential benefits and harms and privacy and confidentiality. The name and mobile phone number (s) (personal or that of another family member) of the women were obtained and each was recorded at separate places alongside a unique identification code, after informed consent had been obtained. The study was approved as a part of a bigger study by the Ethics Review Committee of the Ghana Health Service (ID No GHS-ERC: 06/11/10).

### Specimen collection and smear preparation

Each participant was instructed on how to use the Rover® Viba-Brush vaginal sampler, (Rovers Medical Devices, The Netherlands). The instructions were given verbally and in the language the participant understood (the option of four local languages was available) with demonstrations, using an illustrations on the packaging of the brush, that showed the steps and positioning of the body. The participants were asked to describe the process they going to following to the investigator, before they allowed to go to the private room to perform the specimen collection. The collected specimen was transferred into a sterile 15 mL screw-capped tube containing 5 mL PBS with 5 mM ethylene diamine tetraacetic acid (EDTA), pH 8.0. These specimens were designated as self-collected (SC) for HPV testing.

The health personnel then performed a standardized pelvic examination and with the aid of a sterile plastic disposable speculum, a wooden spatula and a cytobrush collected cervical specimen according to the manufacturer's instructions. The cytobrush was then rinsed in 50 µL of DNAgard®Tissue (Biomatrica, Inc., San Diego) and head of the wooden spatula was rinsed in the same 50 µL of DNAgard®Tissue. The specimen was designated as Health Personnel Collected (HPC). Both collected specimens were transported at 4 °C and thereafter store at −20 °C until used for HPV testing.

### DNA extraction

The volume of specimen obtained by HPC was made-up to 1 mL with PBS and vortexed thoroughly. DNA was extracted from 200 µL of each specimen (SC and HPC) on the MagNA Pure LC automated system (Roche Molecular Systems, Inc, Pleasanton, USA) using the MagNA Pure DNA Extraction Kit (Roche Molecular Systems, Inc, Pleasanton, USA) according to the manufactures specification and a modification by adding 15 µL of RNase to the lysis buffer for each specimen. The negative controls included for each set of extraction were PBS, DNase/RNase free water and DNAGard while the positive control was a suspension of SiHa cells with an integrated HPV 16 genome. The specimen DNA quality was assessed by a real-time PCR amplification of the house keeping gene, RNase H in 10 µL of DNA extract and analysed with Light Cycler 480 and related software (Roche Molecular Systems, Inc, Pleasanton, USA).

### Nested-multiplex PCR based detection of HPV genotype

The extracted DNA was amplified by a nested PCR reaction using PGMY09/PGMY11 and GP5+/GP6+ primers as previously described [30].

The typing of 46 mucosal HPV types was carried out by a multiplex system based on the xMAP® technology as previously described by Zubach et al., [30]. Briefly, 46 fluorescence sortable microspheres (Luminex Corporation, Austin, TX) were coupled to the 46 specific probes for HPV types 6, 11, 13, 16, 18, 26, 30, 31, 32, 33, 34, 35, 39, 40, 42, 43, 44, 45, 51, 52, 53, 54, 56, 58, 59, 61, 62, 66, 67, 68, 69, 70, 71, 72, 73, 74, 81, 82, 83, 84, 85, 86, 87, 89, 90 and 91.. The double stranded second round PCR products, labelled with biotin, were made single-stranded by digestion with 2 µL of bacteriophage T7 gene6 exonuclease (New England BioLabs, Pickering, ON, Canada) that removed the non-labelled strand after 40 min incubation at room temperature. The single stranded HPV DNA was incubated for hybridization at 60 °C for 10 min and streptavidin-phycoerythrin (PE) (Invitrogen) in 1-tetramethyl ammonium chloride (TMAC) (Sigma), was added and incubated for 5 min at 60 °C. Genotype specific hybridization was detected on a Luminex Liquid Chip 200 flow cytometer (Qiagen) using the Luminex IS software (Luminex).

## Statistical analysis

All the participants' sexual and reproductive characteristics were categorised into the known groups widely reported for HPV risk factors analysis. The age of the participants were also categorised into groups of 5 year intervals. Frequencies and proportions were used to describe the distributions and summarize data of demographic characteristics and the categorized sexual and reproductive characteristics stratified by age groups (5 year intervals). Chi-square test of association (at 95% confidence level) was used for the determination of the univariate association between the categorised participants' characteristics and grouped age, and between grouped age and the HPV prevalence for each of the HPV risk types and for overall HPV. A bivariate and multivariate Chi-square association were subsequently determined for each of the HPV risk types and for overall HPV For the Chi-square analysis of the age at first sexual intercourse (AFSI) stratified by age group, the analysis was conducted, first, excluding women 20 years and younger and secondly, grouping the women within the age groups 15–19 and 20–24 to a new group labelled as < 25 years. For both analyses the association was significant by Chi-square test at 95% confidence level. The Cohen's Kappa analysis was used to determine the extent of agreement between the two methods for the detection of the following; overall/any HPV type, high risk types and low risk types, using data of only 226 women who provided both specimen. For overall HPV type, agreement was defined as Individuals positive for any HPV genotypes in both samples. For high risk HPV, agreement was defined as Individuals positive for any of the high risk HPV genotypes in both. For the Low risk HPV, agreement was defined as Individuals positive for any of

the Low risk HPV types in both samples. For of the three criteria it was not necessarily the same genotype in both samples.

## Results

### Specimens

Of the 415 women contacted during the study, 258 women provided specimens. Of this number 4 self-collected (SC) and 3 health personnel collected (HPC) specimens were excluded because their labels were destroyed during handling of the samples. The quality of the specimens of the remaining 251 women was found to be appropriate for further analysis; although 17 of the 244 SC and 6 of the 233 HPC specimen were not consistently positive with triplicate analyses for the RNase H gene (2 of 3 were positive); these specimen were included in the HPV analysis. Overall 226 women provided both SC and HPC specimen. The distribution of the demographic characteristics of the 415 women and those of them who were HPV positive are shown in Table 1.

### Age specific distribution of characteristics

Following the stratification of the distribution of the sexual and reproductive characteristics by age (Table 2), it was determined that a significant generational difference in age at first sexual intercourse (AFSI) existed for this population ($\chi^2 = 42.8$, $p = 0.0001$). Also, the distributions of lifetime number of male sexual partners ($\chi^2 = 34.6$, $p = 0.01$), the contraction of a sexually transmitted infection (STI) ($\chi^2 = 44.4$, $p = 0.0001$), use of condoms ($\chi^2 = 52.0$, $p = 0.0001$), current number of male sexual partners ($\chi^2 = 72.3$, 0.0001), number of pregnancies ($\chi^2 = 146.8$, $p = 0.001$) and ever had an abortion ($\chi^2 = 29.1$, $p = 0.001$) were all significantly associated with age. However, the use of OC was not significantly associated with age ($\chi^2 = 9.0$, $p = 0.437$).

### Age specific HPV prevalences

Age was determined to be significantly associated with the following, overall/any HPV positivity ($\chi^2 = 36.1$; $p = 0.001$), HR HPV positivity ($\chi^2 = 26.09$; $p = 0.002$) and LR HPV positivity ($\chi^2 = 21.49$; $p = 0.011$) detected with both self and health personnel collected specimen. The bivariate association controlling for each of the following potential confounders; Age at first sexual intercourse, Lifetime number of sexual partners, Current number of male sexual partners, Contracted a sexually transmitted infection in the past 10 years and Use of condom during sexual intercourses remained significant for each risk type and overall HPV prevalence obtained with self-collected specimen (Additional file 1: Table S1). However, for the health-personnel collected specimen, the association remained significant for overall HPV and HR HPV but become non-significant for LR HPV (Additional file 1: Table S1). With

**Table 1** Distribution of the demographic data of the participants who were positive for HPV by at least one of the specimen collected

| Demographic characteristics | Sub-categories | Frequency (%) | |
|---|---|---|---|
| | | All Women | Women HPV positive by any specimen |
| Grouped Age | 15–19 | 26 (6.3) | 8 (6.5) |
| | 20–24 | 65 (15.8) | 28 (22.6) |
| | 25–29 | 97 (23.5) | 34 (27.4) |
| | 30–34 | 46 (11.2) | 8 (6.5) |
| | 35–39 | 52 (12.6) | 13 (10.5) |
| | 40–44 | 51 (12.4) | 15 (12.1) |
| | 45–49 | 30 (7.3) | 3 (2.4) |
| | 50–54 | 22 (5.3) | 6 (4.8) |
| | 55–59 | 13 (3.2) | 8 (6.5) |
| | 60 Or Older | 10 (2.4) | 1 (.8) |
| | Total | 412 (100.0) | 124 (100.0) |
| Religion | Christian | 373 (90.5) | 121 (97.6) |
| | Muslim | 35 (8.5) | 3 (2.4) |
| | Other | 4 (1.0) | 0.0 (0.0) |
| | Total | 412 (100.0) | 124 (100.0) |
| Marital Status | Unmarried | 150 (36.9) | 47 (37.9) |
| | Married | 257 (63.1) | 74 (59.7) |
| | Total | 407 (100.0) | 124 (100.0) |
| Educational Status | No Formal | 68 (16.6) | 19 (15.3) |
| | Primary | 77 (18.8) | 25 (20.2) |
| | Junior Secondary | 194 (47.4) | 56 (45.2) |
| | Senior Secondary | 48 (11.7) | 11 (8.9) |
| | Post-Secondary | 22 (5.4) | 13 (10.5) |
| | Total | 409 (100.0) | 124 (100.0) |
| Occupation | Unemployed | 25 (6.2) | 9 (7.3) |
| | Formally employed | 66 (16.4) | 25 (20.2) |
| | Skilled Worker | 93 (23.1) | 34 (27.4) |
| | Trader | 172 (42.8) | 43 (34.7) |
| | Agro-worker | 46 (11.4) | 8 (6.5) |
| | Total | 402 (100.0) | 124 (100.0) |

respect to the multivariate association, age remained significant for self-collected specimen determine overall HPV ($x^2 = 36.44$; $p = 0.0001$), HR HPV ($x^2 = 26.25$; $p = 0.002$) and LR HPV ($x^2 = 20.69$; $p = 0.014$). However, for health-personnel collected specimen, the association was significant for both overall HPV prevalence ($x^2 = 17.76$; $p = 0.038$) and HR HPV prevalence ($x^2 = 17.73$; 0.038) but non-significant for LR HPV prevalence ($x^2 = 8.82$; 0.365). The trend of this distribution are as shown in the prevalence curves (Figs. 1, 2 and 3). In respect of the overall HPV infection by both SC and HPC specimen (Fig. 1), a major peak among women of the age group of 20–24 years was followed by a rapid reduction until the age group

of 30–34 years. Thereafter, for the SC specimen, a steady rise in prevalence resulted in a second peak at the age group of 40–44 years and sharp drop at age 45–49 years. On the other hand, for the HPC specimen, the prevalence plateaued between the age group 30–34 years and 45–49 years. Then for both SC and HPC specimen, the prevalence increased until among the age group of 55 years or older.

The prevalence curve for high risk HPVs (Fig. 2) was very similar to that of the overall HPV prevalence described above. That is, an initial peak at age group (20–24 years) for both SC and HPC specimen, was followed by a second peak at the age group of 40–44 years for the SC specimen but a plateaued between the

**Table 2** Distribution and association of sexual and reproductive characteristics stratified by age

| Risk factors | Category | Age group (years), n (%) | | | | | | | | | $\chi^2$ (p-value) |
|---|---|---|---|---|---|---|---|---|---|---|---|
| | | 15–19[e] (n = 26) | 20–24[e] (n = 64) | 25–29 (n = 97) | 30–34 (n = 47) | 35–39 (n = 52) | 40–44 (n = 51) | 45–49 (n = 31) | 50–54 (n = 24) | ≥55 (n = 23) | |
| Age at first sexual intercourse | <20 | 16 (100) | 56 (87.5) | 53 (55.2) | 25 (54.3) | 30 (57.7) | 34 (69.4) | 16 (53.3) | 9 (42.9) | 11 (50.0) | 42.8[e] (0.0001)[a] |
| | ≥20 | 0 (0.0) | 8 (12.5) | 43 (44.8) | 21 (45.7) | 22 (42.3) | 15 (30.6) | 14 (46.7) | 12 (57.1) | 11 (50.9) | |
| Lifetime number of sexual partners | 1 | 8 (53.3) | 19 (29.7) | 22 (22.9) | 5 (10.9) | 9 (17.6) | 11 (22.4) | 7 (23.3) | 4 (18.2) | 6 (26.1) | 34.6 (0.010)[a] |
| | 2 | 5 (33.3) | 21 (32.8) | 30 (31.3) | 16 (34.8) | 12 (23.5) | 13 (26.5) | 6 (20.0) | 4 (18.2) | 4 (17.4) | |
| | ≥3 | 2 (13.3) | 24 (37.5) | 44 (45.8) | 25 (54.3) | 30 (58.8) | 25 (51.0) | 17 (56.7) | 14 (63.6) | 13 (56.5) | |
| [c]Current number of male sexual partners | 0 | 16 (61.5) | 6 (9.4) | 6 (6.2) | 5 (10.9) | 4 (7.7) | 6 (12.0) | 4 (13.3) | 6 (27.3) | 8 (36.4) | 72.3 (0.0001)[a] |
| | 1 | 10 (38.5) | 58 (90.6) | 89 (91.8) | 41 (89.1) | 48 (92.3) | 44 (88.0) | 26 (86.7) | 16 (72.7) | 14 (63.6) | |
| Contracted a sexually transmitted infection in the past 10 years | No | 10 (38.5) | 18 (28.6) | 36 (37.1) | 18 (40.0) | 22 (43.1) | 34 (68.0) | 15 (51.7) | 16 (72.7) | 20 (86.9) | 44.4 (0.0001)[a] |
| | Yes | 16 (61.5) | 45 (71.4) | 61 (62.9) | 27 (60.0) | 29 (56.9) | 16 (32.0) | 14 (48.3) | 6 (27.3) | 3 (13.0) | |
| [b]Use of condom during sexual intercourse | No | 12 (48.0) | 28 (44.4) | 38 (39.2) | 24 (52.2) | 36 (70.6) | 40 (78.4) | 22 (73.3) | 19 (86.4) | 20 (76.9) | 52.0 (0.0001)[a] |
| | Yes | 13 (52.0) | 35 (55.6) | 59 (60.8) | 22 (47.8) | 15 (29.4) | 11 (21.6) | 8 (26.7) | 3 (13.6) | 3 (23.1) | |
| Number of pregnancies | 1 | 4 (80.0) | 23 (43.4) | 17 (21.5) | 6 (13.3) | 2 (4.1) | 3 (6.0) | 1 (3.4) | 0 (0.0) | 1 (4.5) | 146.8 (0.0001)[a] |
| | 2–4 | 1 (20.0) | 27 (50.9) | 54 (68.4) | 27 (60.0) | 17 (34.7) | 17 (34.0) | 10 (34.5) | 4 (18.2) | 5 (22.7) | |
| | ≥5 | 0 (0.0) | 3 (5.7) | 8 (10.1) | 12 (26.7) | 30 (61.2) | 30 (60.0) | 18 (62.1) | 18 (81.8) | 16 (72.7) | |
| [d]Have you ever had any abortion | No | 24 (92.3) | 43 (68.3) | 59 (60.8) | 21 (45.7) | 24 (46.2) | 24 (47.1) | 17 (56.7) | 9 (40.9) | 17 (73.9) | 29.1 (0.001)[a] |
| | Yes | 2 (7.7) | 20 (31.7) | 38 (39.2) | 25 (54.3) | 28 (53.8) | 27 (52.9) | 13 (43.3) | 13 (59.1) | 6 (26.1) | |
| Number of abortion | 1 | 2 (100) | 15 (75.0) | 24 (63.2) | 14 (56.0) | 12 (42.9) | 13 (48.1) | 8 (61.5) | 8 (61.5) | 4 (66.7) | 11.0 (0.272) |
| | ≥2 | 0 (0.0) | 5 (25.0) | 14 (36.8) | 11 (44.0) | 16 (57.1) | 14 (51.9) | 5 (38.5) | 5 (38.5) | 2 (33.3) | |
| Use of oral contraceptive in the past 10 years | No | 24 (96.0) | 49 (77.8) | 74 (77.1) | 30 (65.2) | 37 (75.5) | 39 (78.0) | 22 (75.9) | 16 (72.7) | 18 (78.3) | 9.0 (0.437) |
| | Yes | 1 (4.0) | 14 (22.2) | 22 (22.9) | 16 (34.8) | 12 (24.5) | 11 (22.0) | 7 (24.1) | 6 (27.3) | 5 (21.7) | |

[a]Significant differences within age groups
[b]condom used was not consistent among all the participants
[c]only 2 women in age group 25–29 years had more than 1 current male sexual partner
[d]both spontaneous and induced abortion
[e]For the Chi-square analysis of AFSI stratified by age group, the analysis was conducted, first, excluding women 20 years and younger (the p value is reported) and secondly, grouping the women within the age group 15–19 and 20–24 to a new group labelled as < 25 years. For both analyses the association was significant by Chi-square test at 95% confidence level

age group of 35–39 and 45–49 years for HPC specimen. Interestingly, the subsequent increase in HR HPV prevalence for both the SC and HPC specimen (between 45 and 55 or older years) were almost the same (Fig. 2). Conversely, the low risk (LR) HPV prevalence curve of the SC specimen showed a peak at the age group of 20–24 years followed by a sharp reduction until the age group of 30–34 years. This was followed by a marginal increase at 30 – 34 years and a plateauing until the age group of 45–49 years. The prevalence then increased until the

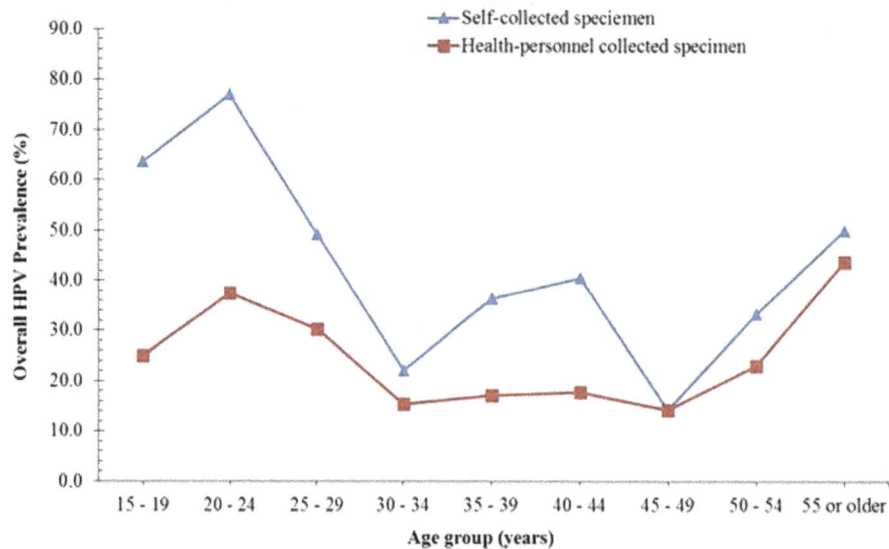

**Fig. 1** Overall HPV prevalence curves obtained with self and health personnel collected specimen

age group 55 or older years. On the other hand, the LR HPV prevalence curve determined with the HPC specimen showed a gradual decreased from a high prevalence among the age of 15–19 years until the age of 30–34 years and then plateaued until the age 50–54 years, then an increase in prevalence was observed at the age group of 55 or older years (Fig. 3).

The age-specific HPV genotype-specific prevalence for each of the detected HPVs are shown as a heat-map (Fig. 4). Clear differences in pattern were obtained with SC specimen as compared to the HPC specimen. A close look at the heat-map for SC specimen showed that the a few HPV genotypes contributed to the mid-age peak

(40–45 years) in HPV prevalence curves (Figs. 1, 2 and 3). These were for high risk genotypes, HPV16, 18, 31, 45, 52 and 59; for probable high risk HPV genotypes, HPV 30 and 53 and for low risk HPV genotypes HPV 40, 41 and 81.

### Age-specific concordance between SC and HPC HPV positivity

The concordance between SC and HPC in respect of the *overall HPV positivity* ranged between 53.1 and 60.0% among the aged 15–29 years (Table 3). This range increased among the women in their thirties to between 75.0 and 76.9%. The concordance reduced to 60.7% for women in the age group 40–44 years. Among women

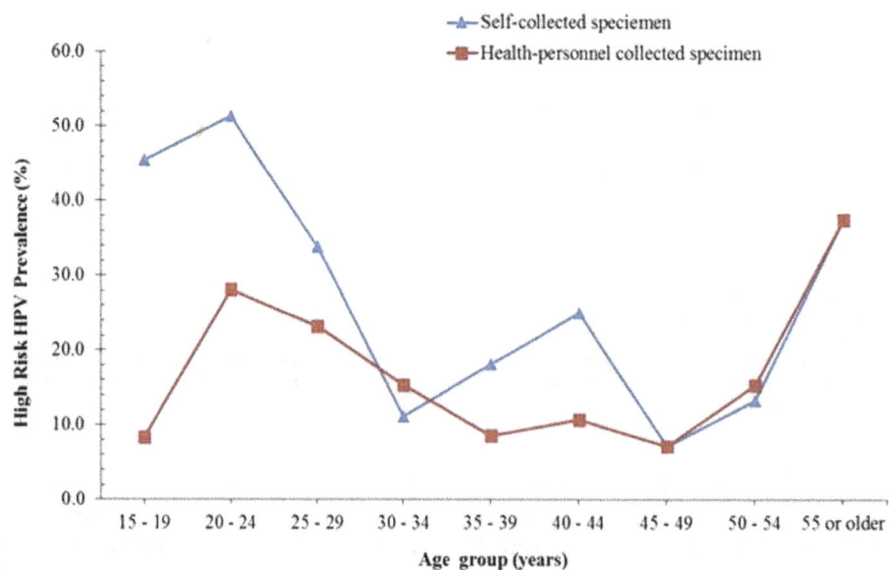

**Fig. 2** High risk (HR) HPV prevalence curves obtained with self and health personnel collected specimen

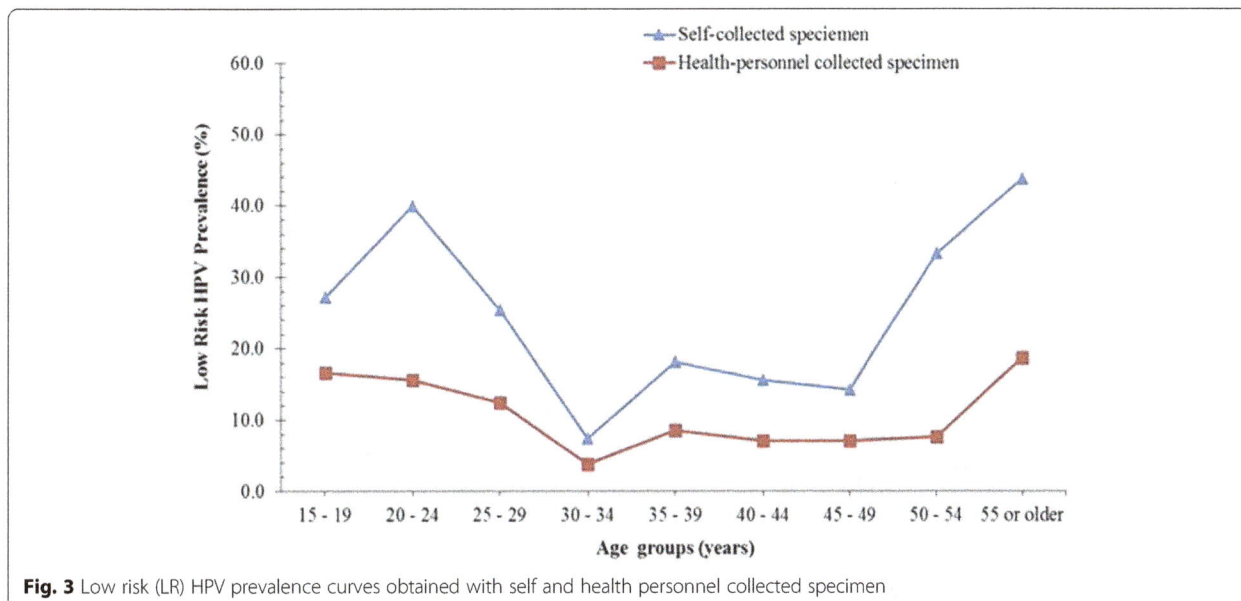

**Fig. 3** Low risk (LR) HPV prevalence curves obtained with self and health personnel collected specimen

45 years or older, the concordance ranged between 81.3 and 85.7% (Table 3).

Similarly, the concordance between the two methods in respect of the detection of HR HPVs ranged between 62.5 and 63.6% for women aged 15–24 years. However, it increased to 76.8% among the women aged 25–29 years and then even higher among women in their 30s, ranging between 84.4 and 88.5%. It then reduced to 78.6% among women 40–44 years and increased to 85.7% among women 45–49 years and 91.7% among women 50–54 years. Among women 55 years or older, the concordance for HR HPV was 75.0%. However, the concordance between the two methods in respect of LR HPV positivity remained consistently high with age except among women 50–54 years old (Table 3). Despite these variation, the observed differences within the concordance for overall, high risk and low risk HPV detection were not significant.

## Discussion

Overall, our study adds to the evidence of bimodal and trimodal trends in the age-specific HPV prevalence in West Africa and how different this is to those reported for other world regions and countries. For example, a unimodal prevalence curve (20–25 years) in South African [14], Denmark, Spain, Italy, Canada and the Netherlands [12, 31–33]; a bimodal prevalence curve in Hong Kong (26–30 years and 46–50 years) [34], Chine (<25 years and 40–44 years) [35] and in Japan (15–20 years and 50 years) [36]. Additionally, our study provides a more convincing evidence, by using a wider age range, that there was a clear difference in the age-specific HPV prevalences between SC and HPC specimen, which was contrary to those reported by Wright et al., in South

Africa [26] and Safaeian et al., in Uganda [27], the only two studies in Africa to have reported similar investigation but within a narrower age range.

The generally higher HR HPV prevalence with SC specimen as well as the additional peak (among the age group 40–44 years) of this curve (Fig. 2), strongly suggest that the use of SC specimens for cervical screening in Ghana will result in additional information on the extent of within-country HPV prevalence variation, which is not likely to be obtained with the use of health personnel-collected specimen. Additionally, the occurrence of a major prevalence peak at the age group of 20–24 years, for both SC and HPC on both the overall and HR HPV prevalence curves, suggests that the use of SC specimen for determining the age-group with a high HPV burden will most likely not be different from that of HPC, rather, it is more likely to give a better indication of the HR HPV infection prevalence at each specific age group in the population. By extension, this potential of SC as a better predictor of the age group at higher risk of developing lower genital tract lesions in future needs to be confirmed by a fellow-up (Figs. 1 and 2).

Comparing the prevalence curves, it is also clear that the mid-age (40–44 years) peak observed in the overall HPV curve for SC was due to the high prevalence of HR HPV for SC among the mid-age group, but not the prevalence of LR HPV. However, other studies have indicated that a higher overall HPV prevalence obtained with SC specimen are often due to a higher LR HPV detection [22, 25]. These studies explained that HR HPV preferentially infects the cervix than the vagina, therefore it was expected that an effectively collected SC specimen should record HPV prevalence at best, similar to that with HPC specimen, but not consistently higher as

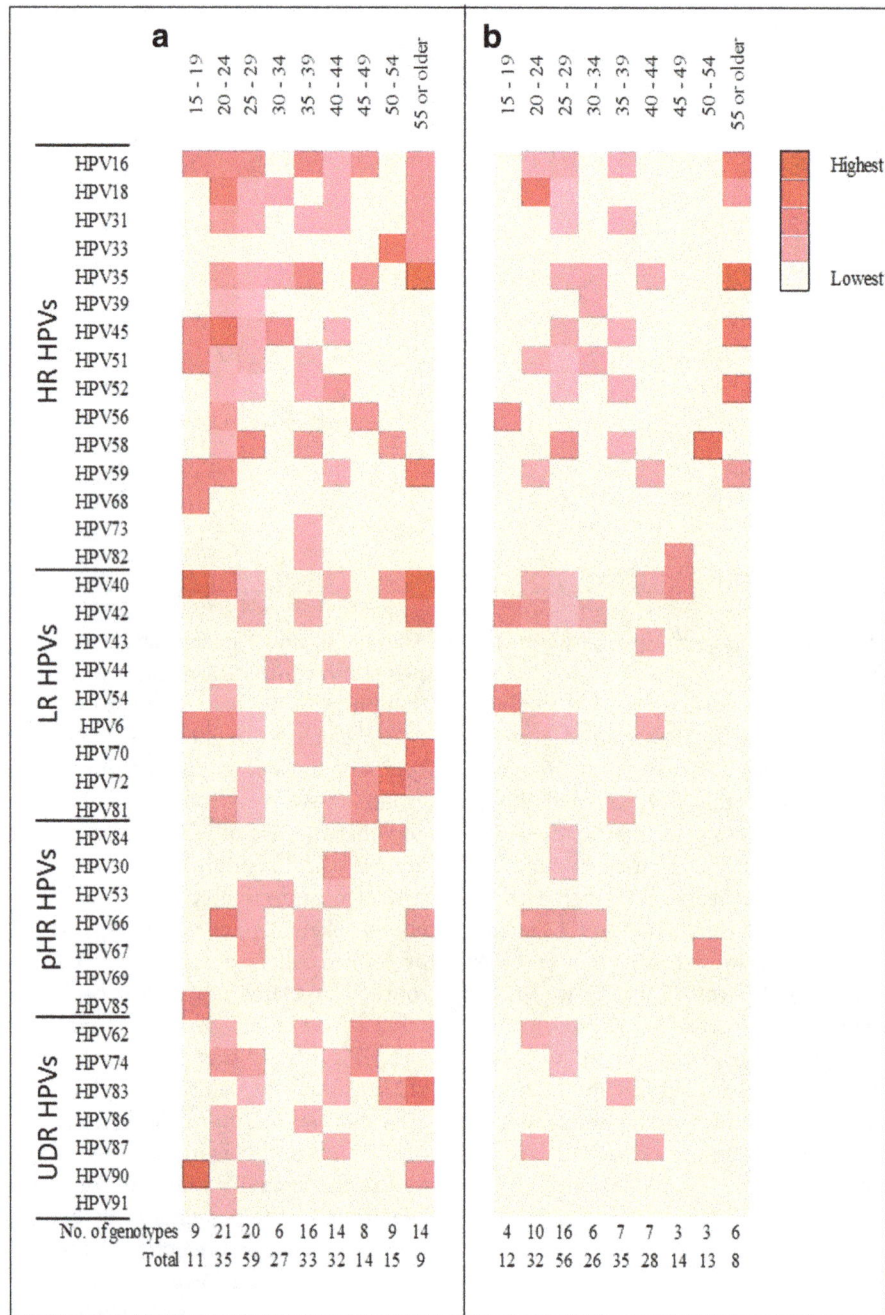

**Fig. 4** Heat map of the genotype specific prevalence as determined with **a** self-collected specimen and **b** health personnel-collected specimen. HR = high risk; LR = low risk; pHR = probable high risk; UDR = undetermined risk. No. = Number

obtained in our study. Therefore, what remains unclear, in light of the facts that the cytology analysis of the HPC specimen indicated it was well performed (data not shown), is, do these imply that for this population/cohort the vagina harbours more HR HPV infections than the cervix? Furthermore, does the HR HPV prevalence peak at mid-age observed for the SC specimen identify a high risk of cervical lesion that may be missed by using HPC

specimen? It is however not clear from these data, whether these additional HR HPV infections detected with SC are infections that may be transient or persist and whether they may lead to the development of lesions. However, the age group showing this additional HR HPV peak prevalence is the age group (30–49) recommended for primary HPV testing, based on the thoughts that this age group mostly harbour persistent HPV infection [37–40].

**Table 3** Age-specific concordance of HPV positivity determined with SC and HPC specimen

| Grouped age | Both specimens positive for | | | | | | | | |
| --- | --- | --- | --- | --- | --- | --- | --- | --- | --- |
| | Overall/Any HPV Type | | | Low Risk HPV Types | | | High Risk HPV Types | | |
| | Concordance | 95% CI | | Concordance | 95% CI | | Concordance | 95% CI | |
| 15–19 | 54.5 | 48.69 | 97.43 | 81.8 | 52.30 | 94.86 | 63.6 | 35.38 | 84.83 |
| 20–24 | 53.1 | 48.41 | 82.79 | 75.0 | 57.89 | 86.75 | 62.5 | 45.26 | 77.07 |
| 25–29 | 60.0 | 46.81 | 71.88 | 71.4 | 58.53 | 81.58 | 76.8 | 64.23 | 85.90 |
| 30–34 | 76.9 | 57.95 | 88.97 | 88.5 | 71.03 | 96.00 | 88.5 | 71.03 | 96.00 |
| 35–39 | 75.0 | 57.89 | 86.75 | 90.6 | 75.78 | 96.76 | 84.4 | 68.25 | 93.14 |
| 40–44 | 60.7 | 24.1 | 76.43 | 82.1 | 64.41 | 92.12 | 78.6 | 60.46 | 89.79 |
| 45–49 | 85.7 | 60.06 | 95.99 | 92.9 | 68.53 | 98.73 | 85.7 | 60.06 | 95.99 |
| 50–54 | 83.3 | 55.20 | 95.30 | 66.7 | 39.06 | 86.19 | 91.7 | 64.61 | 98.51 |
| 55 or older | 81.3 | 47.6 | 93.2 | 74.1 | 44.80 | 95.14 | 75.0 | 64.57 | 89.24 |
| All ages | 67.3 | 60.89 | 73.04 | 79.7 | 74.03 | 84.45 | 78.0 | 72.14 | 82.87 |

Comparatively, the middle-age peak of overall HPV and HR HPV prevalences has been shown in some cohort studies with the suggestion that in addition to the persistence of previously acquired HPV infection, the acquisition of new HPV infection by these women accounted for such peaks in prevalence [41, 42]. However in this study, the persistence of the HPV infection were not determined. The only indication that suggest a likelihood of a higher prevalence among this age group is the data on the age at first sexual intercourse, which shows that 70.0% of women within this age group (40–44 years) reported a an AFSI of less than 20 years, which was higher compared to those of the flanking age groups, 25–39 years and 45–59 years (Table 2).

Generally, the high prevalence among younger women (particularly those aged between 20 and 29 years) as has been widely accepted, is related to sexual behaviour, particular those associated with the initiation (AFSI) and conducts of sexual activities [14, 16, 34, 36, 42, 43]. This association was evident in this study since slightly more than 90.0% of the women within the age groups of 20–24 and 25–29 years had at least one current male sexual partner and that only women in the age group of 25–29 years reported 2 and 3 current male sexual partners (Table 2). Also, between 61.5 and 71.4% of the women between 15 and 29 years had contracted an STI in the past 5–10 years prior to the study, compared to the lower proportion in the older age groups. Furthermore, 100 and 87.5% of the women within the age groups of 15–19 years and 20–24 years respectively reported an age at first sexual intercourse of less than 20 years (which is a very significant risk factor for HPV acquisition), while most of the older age groups reported an age at first sexual intercourse of 20 years or more (Table 2).

The high HR HPV prevalence peak among women aged 55 years or older determined with both SC and HPC specimen has been shown only in selected

geographical regions. For instance, a very similar age-specific overall HPV and HR HPV prevalence distribution has been reported in a community based study in China, where an initial major peak was observed among women aged 20–24 years, small increase among women aged 34–39 years, a second major peak among women aged 50–54 years [44]. A study in Nigeria showed a first peak and a second high prevalence among women aged between 20 and 24 years and 55–64 years respectively [16, 42]. Another study in Nigeria showed two peaks for women 24–29 years and 55–64 years [16, 42]. Similar high prevalence peak among older women (50 years or older) have also been shown by a meta-analysis for the Central America and West Africa WHO regions [43]. Although the high prevalence among the older women is still not clearly understood, in the larger Nigerian study, no risk factor was identified to have had any significant association (by a logistic regression analysis) with the high prevalence among the age group of 55–64 years [16]. Some studies have suggested that this could have been due to changes in sexual behaviour of both the women and their male sexual partners at that age while other studies have stated that this could be a population specific cohort effect [4, 14, 16, 42, 43]. These population specific cohort effect may include, the lack, low coverage or poor follow-ups of screening and treatment, and some unidentified population characteristic relating to sexual and reproductive behaviour in one population compared to another. For instance, it is common some populations in Ghana for older women to insert all kind of herbal preparations into their vagina with the intension of restoring its elasticity or improving the lubrication thereof. This high prevalence may also result from an increased HPV infection due to the reduced protection (local immunity) and increased dryness of the female reproductive organ as a result of menopausal changes [45, 46]. For instance, during or after menopause, there is a reduction in the secretions of the female reproductive organ, which are known to protect against infections and provide lubrication that reduce/prevent the occurrence micro-abrasion and subsequent HPV infection [46–48]. However, it was not possible in this study to comment extensively on these due to the small number of participants in sub-group analysis. However, for a population with a relatively lower life-expectance (<80 years), and given the natural history of HPV and cervical cancer, which indicates that a period of 10–15 years passes before a few of the HR HPV infection may progress to cervical lesion [10], most of the women may not be alive to develop the disease and therefore HPV based screening among women of this age group may have very little value, if any, particularly in developing countries.

It was important to determine whether the observed difference between SC and HPC specimen prevalence curves, for both the overall and HR HPV prevalence curves, (Figs. 1 and 2) resulted in significant difference in the age-specific concordance between the two collection methods. This will show if the overall concordance between SC and HPC vary significantly with age and if for all ages SC specimen may be used in place of HPC specimen. Considering the age-specific overall HPV prevalence concordances, it was observed that for the age group that SC overall HPV prevalence was much higher than that of HPC (15–19 years and 20–24 years), the concordance were lower (Fig. 1 and Table 3), and where the difference between their prevalence was lowest (30–34 years; 45–49, 50–54 and ≥ 55 years), the concordances were highest. These were also evident with the HR HPV and LR HPV prevalence curves and concordances. Do these suggest that the variation in the concordance between SC and HPC reported by most studies may be related to the HPV types (LR HPV) that preferential infection of the vagina and possibly more among younger women as well as with how high the overall HPV prevalence is for that study? That is, for a population with a high HPV prevalence, there is a high likelihood of a lower concordance between SC and HPC HPV prevalence and vise versa. A close look at the mini review by Gravitt et al. shows a similar trend between the SC HR HPV prevalence and the measure of agreement (Kappa values) between SC and HPC methods [22]. Furthermore, it was interesting to note that the highest concordances in our study were among women between 30 years and 54 years, an age range recommended for HPV testing (in co-testing) [38]. Therefore, the use of SC based HPV testing instead of HPC based HPV testing is further strengthened, since the best concordances were within these age group that need to be screened for persistent HPV.

The results and subsequent conclusions of our study must be viewed in the light of the fact that the number of participants was not even distributed the across age groups and was limited in some of the older age groups, as such resulted in wider 95% confidence intervals and in some cases did not allow for the further more rigours statistical analyses.

## Conclusions

Based on these findings, the existence of a bimodal and or a trimodal HPV prevalence in some Ghanaian population is to be expected in future investigations and also that the use of SC specimen is mostly likely going to provide more information in respect of the HR HPV burden. In respect of the difference between age-specific HR HPV prevalence curve, and concordance between SC and HPC, further investigations are needed to throw more light on the question, does the overall HPV prevalence (particularly determined with SC) and/or age of women influence the level of concordance between HR HPV test by SC and HPC specimen? Further investigation will shed light on the possible utility of HR HPV testing with SC or HPC in determining screening recommendations for this and other similar populations in low income countries..

## Abbreviations

CI: Confidence interval; EDTA: Ethylene diamine tetraacetic acid; ERC: Ethical Review Committee; GHS: Ghana Health Service; HPC: Health personnel collected; HPV: Human Papillomavirus; OR: Odds ratio; PE: Streptavidin-phycoerythrin; SC: Self-collected; TMAC: 1-tetramethyl ammonium chloride

## Acknowledgements

The authors are grateful to the Ghanaian-German Centre for Health Research Ph.D programme and its counterparts (Prof. Fred Binka, Prof. Thomas Junghanss, Prof. Oliver Razum), coordinators (Prof. Richard Adanu, Dr. Micheal Kaeser and Dr. Fenna Veeltmann) and the support staff of this programme. Also, we are grateful to the German Academic Exchange Services (DAAD) for its funding and sponsorship of this programme and to the staff of Department of Epidemiology and Disease Control, School of Public Health, University of Ghana. We are very thankful to the Hospital Administration and Staff of the Public Health Unit and the Reproductive and Child Health Unit of the Akuse Government Hospital, particularly Nurses Yaaba Essien and Gifty Tekushie and also, to the community and religious leaders within the Akuse sub-district. We are also thankful to Mr. Meindert Dzwart, CEO of Rovers Medical Devices for supporting this study with a donation of the Rover® Viba-Brush vaginal sampler, the self-collection devises used in this study. We are grateful to all the staff of the National Microbiology Laboratory of the Public Health Agency of Canada for all their support during the laboratory analyses.

## Funding

German Academic Exchange Services (DAAD) through the Ghanaian-German Centre for Health Research Ph.D programme provided scholarship and support funding for the field work as well as funding for travel, accommodation and living expense in Canada. Additionally, the National Microbiology Laboratory of the Public Health Agency of Canada, Winnipeg, hosted, provided technical support and all the inputs for the laboratory analyses (the molecular genotyping of HPV) of the collected samples.

## Authors' contributions

Conception of the study and the drafting of proposal: AKA. Supervision, Review of and contribution to draft proposal and progress of study: RMA, EKW, EAA, AS. Conduct of the field work/specimen collection: AKA, RMA. Conduct laboratory analyses: AKA, VAZ, AS. Draft of manuscript: AKA. Review of and contribution to the manuscript: All the authors. All authors read and approved the final manuscript.

## Competing interests

The authors declare that they have no competing interests.

## Author details

[1]Department of Epidemiology and Disease Control, School of Public Health, College of Health Sciences, University of Ghana, Accra, Ghana. [2]Cellular and Clinical Research Centre, Radiological and Medical Sciences Research Institute, GAEC, Accra, Ghana. [3]Population, Family and Reproductive Health, School of Public Health, College of Health Sciences, University of Ghana, Accra, Ghana. [4]Department of Pathology, School of Biomedical and Allied Health Science, College of Health Sciences, University of Ghana, Korle-Bu, Accra, Ghana. [5]National Microbiology Laboratory, Public Health Agency of Canada, Winnipeg, MB, Canada. [6]University of Manitoba, Winnipeg, MB, Canada.

## References

1. Bernard H-U, Burk RD, Chen Z, van Doorslaer K, zur Hausen H, de Villiers E-M. Classification of papillomaviruses (PVs) based on 189 PV types and proposal of taxonomic amendments. Virology. 2010;401:70–9.
2. Chen Z, Schiffman M, Herrero R, DeSalle R, Anastos K, Segondy M, Sahasrabuddhe VV, Gravitt PE, Hsing AW, Burk RD. Evolution and taxonomic classification of alphapapillomavirus 7 complete genomes: HPV18, HPV39, HPV45, HPV59, HPV68 and HPV70. PLoS ONE (Zheng, Z-M, ed). 2013;8:e72565.
3. de Villiers E-M, Fauquet C, Broker TR, Bernard H-U, zur Hausen H. Classification of papillomaviruses. Virology. 2004;324:17–27.
4. Moscicki A-B, Schiffman M, Kjaer S, Villa LL. Chapter 5: Updating the natural history of HPV and anogenital cancer. Vaccine. 2006;24(Supplement 3):S42–51.
5. Schiffman M, Kjaer SK. Chapter 2: natural history of anogenital human papillomavirus infection and neoplasia. J Natl Cancer Inst Monogr. 2003;2003:14–9.
6. de Sanjosé S, Diaz M, Castellsagué X, Clifford G, Bruni L, Muñoz N, Bosch FX. Worldwide prevalence and genotype distribution of cervical human papillomavirus DNA in women with normal cytology: a meta-analysis. Lancet Infect Dis. 2007;7:453–9.
7. Muñoz N, Castellsagué X, de González AB, Gissmann L. Chapter 1: HPV in the etiology of human cancer. Vaccine. 2006;24(Supplement 3):S1–S10.
8. Lenselink CH, Melchers WJG, Quint WGV, Hoebers AMJ, Hendriks JCM, Massuger LFAG, Bekkers RLM. Sexual behaviour and HPV infections in 18 to 29 year old women in the pre-vaccine era in the Netherlands. PLoS ONE (Ramqvist, T, ed). 2008;3:e3743.
9. Burchell AN, Winer RL, de Sanjosé S, Franco EL. Chapter 6: epidemiology and transmission dynamics of genital HPV infection. Vaccine. 2006;24(Supplement 3):S52–61.
10. Schiffman M, Castle PE. The promise of global cervical-cancer prevention. N Engl J Med. 2005;353:2101–4.
11. Clifford GM, Gallus S, Herrero R, Muñoz N, Snijders PJF, Vaccarella S, Anh PTH, Ferreccio C, Hieu NT, Matos E, et al. Worldwide distribution of human papillomavirus types in cytologically normal women in the International Agency for Research on Cancer HPV prevalence surveys: a pooled analysis. Lancet. 2005;366:991–8.
12. Ogilvie GS, Cook DA, Taylor DL, Rank C, Kan L, Yu A, Mei W, van Niekerk DJ, Coldman AJ, Krajden M. Population-based evaluation of type-specific HPV prevalence among women in British Columbia, Canada. Vaccine. 2013;31:1129–33.
13. Bosch FX, Qiao Y-L, Castellsagué X. CHAPTER 2 The epidemiology of human papillomavirus infection and its association with cervical cancer. Int J Gynecol Obstet. 2006;94:S8–S21.
14. Richter K, Becker P, Horton A, Dreyer G. Age-specific prevalence of cervical human papillomavirus infection and cytological abnormalities in women in Gauteng Province. S Afr Med J. 2013;103:313.
15. Gage JC, Ajenifuja KO, Wentzensen NA, Adepiti AC, Eklund C, Reilly M, Hutchinson M, Wacholder S, Harford J, Soliman AS, et al. The age-specific prevalence of human papillomavirus and risk of cytologic abnormalities in rural Nigeria: implications for screen-and-treat strategies. Int J Cancer. 2012;130:2111–7.
16. Clarke MA, Gage JC, Ajenifuja KO, Wentzensen NA, Adepiti AC, Wacholder S, Burk RD, Schiffman M. A population-based cross-sectional study of age-specific risk factors for high risk human papillomavirus prevalence in rural Nigeria. Infect Agent Cancer. 2011;6:12.
17. Xi LF, Touré P, Critchlow CW, Hawes SE, Dembele B, Sow PS, Kiviat NB. Prevalence of specific types of human papillomavirus and cervical squamous intraepithelial lesions in consecutive, previously unscreened, West-African women over 35 years of age. Int J Cancer. 2003;103:803–9.
18. Akarolo-Anthony SN, Famooto AO, Dareng EO, Olaniyan OB, Offiong R, Wheeler CM, Adebamowo CA. Age-specific prevalence of human papilloma virus infection among Nigerian women. BMC Public Health. 2014;14:656.
19. Thomas JO, Herrero R, Omigbodun AA, Ojemakinde K, Ajayi IO, Fawole A, Oladepo O, Smith JS, Arslan A, Muñoz N, et al. Prevalence of papillomavirus infection in women in Ibadan, Nigeria: a population-based study. Br J Cancer. 2004;90:638–45.
20. Castellsagué X, Menéndez C, Loscertales M-P, Kornegay JR, dos Santos F, Gómez-Olivé FX, Lloveras B, Abarca N, Vaz N, Barreto A, et al. Human papillomavirus genotypes in rural Mozambique. Lancet. 2001;358:1429–30.
21. Wall SR, Scherf CF, Morison L, Hart KW, West B, Ekpo G, Fiander AN, Man S, Gelder CM, Walraven G, et al. Cervical human papillomavirus infection and squamous intraepithelial lesions in rural Gambia, West Africa: viral sequence analysis and epidemiology. Br J Cancer. 2005;93:1068–76.
22. Gravitt PE, Belinson JL, Salmeron J, Shah KV. Looking ahead: a case for human papillomavirus testing of self-sampled vaginal specimens as a cervical cancer screening strategy. Int J Cancer. 2011;129:517–27.
23. Moscicki A-B, Widdice L, Ma Y, Farhat S, Miller-Benningfield S, Jonte J, Jay J, Godwin de Medina C, Hanson E, Clayton L, et al. Comparison of natural histories of human papillomavirus detected by clinician- and self-sampling. Int J Cancer. 2010;127:1882–92.
24. Catarino R, Vassilakos P, Stadali-Ullrich H, Royannez-Drevard I, Guillot C, Petignat P. Feasibility of at-home self-sampling for HPV testing as an appropriate screening strategy for nonparticipants in Switzerland: preliminary results of the DEPIST study. J Low Genit Tract Dis. 2015;19:27–34.
25. Petignat P, Faltin DL, Bruchim I, Tramèr MR, Franco EL, Coutlée F. Are self-collected samples comparable to physician-collected cervical specimens for human papillomavirus DNA testing? A systematic review and meta-analysis. Gynecol Oncol. 2007;105:530–5.
26. Wright Jr TC, Denny L, Kuhn L, Pollack A, Lorincz A. HPV DNA testing of self-collected vaginal samples compared with cytologic screening to detect cervical cancer. JAMA. 2000;283:81.
27. Safaeian M, Kiddugavu M, Gravitt PE, Ssekasanvu J, Murokora D, Sklar M, Serwadda D, Wawer MJ, Shah KV, Gray R. Comparability of self-collected vaginal swabs and physician-collected cervical swabs for detection of human papillomavirus infections in Rakai, Uganda. Sex Transm Dis. 2007;34:429–36.
28. Jones HE, Allan BR, van de Wijgert JHHM, Altini L, Taylor SM, de Kock A, Coetzee N, Williamson A-L. Agreement between self- and clinician-collected specimen results for detection and typing of high risk human palliomavirus in specimen from women in Gugulethu, South Africa. J Clin Microbiol. 2007;45:1679–83.
29. Lack N, West B, Jeffries D, Ekpo G, Morison L, Soutter WP, Walraven G, Boryseiwicz L. comparison of non-invasive sampling methods for detection of HPV in rural African women. Sex Transm Infect. 2005;81:239–41.

30. Zubach V, Smart G, Ratnam S, Severini A. Novel microsphere-based method for detection and typing of 46 mucosal human papillomavirus types. J Clin Microbiol. 2011;50:460–4.

31. Jiang Y, Brassard P, Severini A, Mao Y, Li Y, Laroche J, Chatwood S, Corriveau A, Kandola K, Hanley B, et al. The prevalence of human papillomavirus and its impact on cervical dysplasia in Northern Canada. Infect Agent Cancer. 2013;8:25.

32. Kjaer SK, Breugelmans G, Munk C, Junge J, Watson M, Iftner T. Population-based prevalence, type- and age-specific distribution of HPV in women before introduction of an HPV-vaccination program in Denmark. Int J Cancer. 2008;123:1864–70.

33. Franceschi S, Herrero R, Clifford GM, Snijders PJF, Arslan A, Anh PTH, Bosch FX, Ferreccio C, Hieu NT, Lazcano-Ponce E, et al. Variations in the age-specific curves of human papillomavirus prevalence in women worldwide. Int J Cancer. 2006;119:2677–84.

34. Chan PKS, Chang AR, Yu MY, Li W-H, Chan MYM, Yeung ACM, Cheung T-H, Yau T-N, Wong S-M, Yau C-W, et al. Age distribution of human papillomavirus infection and cervical neoplasia reflects caveats of cervical screening policies. Int J Cancer. 2010;126:297–301.

35. Wu E-Q, Liu B, Cui J-F, Chen W, Wang J-B, Lu L, Niyazi M, Zhao C, Ren S-D, Li C-Q, et al. Prevalence of type-specific human papillomavirus and pap results in Chinese women: a multi-center, population-based cross-sectional study. Cancer Causes Control. 2013;24:795–803.

36. Onuki M, Matsumoto K, Satoh T, Oki A, Okada S, Minaguchi T, Ochi H, Nakao S, Someya K, Yamada N, et al. Human papillomavirus infections among Japanese women: age-related prevalence and type-specific risk for cervical cancer. Cancer Sci. 2009;100:1312–6.

37. WHO; Guideline Development Group. Comprehensive cervical cancer control: a guide to essential practice. 2nd ed. Geneva: World Health Organization; 2014.

38. Saslow D, Solomon D, Lawson HW, Killackey M, Kulasingam SL, Cain J, Garcia FAR, Moriarty AT, Waxman AG, Wilbur DC, et al. American cancer society, American society for colposcopy and cervical pathology, and American society for clinical pathology screening guidelines for the prevention and early detection of cervical cancer. CA Cancer J Clin. 2012;62:147–72.

39. Arbyn M, European Commission. Directorate-General Health & Consumer Protection. European guidelines for quality assurance in cervical cancer screening, office for official publications of the European communities, Luxembourg. 2008.

40. Money DM, Roy M, Scrivener J, Allen L, Brewer M, Bryson P, Evans G, Frappier J-Y, Jamieson MA, Lynde C, et al. Canadian consensus guidelines on human papillomavirus. J Obstet Gynaecol Can. 2007;29:S1.

41. Baussano I, Franceschi S, Gillio-Tos A, Carozzi F, Confortini M, Palma P, De Lillo M, Del Mistro A, De Marco L, Naldoni C, et al. Difference in overall and age-specific prevalence of high-risk human papillomavirus infection in Italy: evidence from NTCC trial. BMC Infect Dis. 2013;13:238.

42. Gage JC, Partridge EE, Rausa A, Gravitt PE, Wacholder S, Schiffman M, Scarinci I, Castle PE. Comparative performance of human papillomavirus DNA testing using novel sample collection methods. J Clin Microbiol. 2011;49:4185–9.

43. Bruni L, Diaz M, Castellsagué X, Ferrer E, Bosch FX, de Sanjosé S. Cervical human papillomavirus prevalence in 5 continents: meta-analysis of 1 million women with normal cytological findings. J Infect Dis. 2010;202:1789–99.

44. Ye J, Cheng X, Chen X, Ye F, Lu W, Xie X. Prevalence and risk profile of cervical human papillomavirus infection in Zhejiang Province, southeast China: a population-based study. Virol J. 2010;7:66.

45. Sivro A, Lajoie J, Kimani J, Jaoko W, Plummer FA, Fowke K, Ball T. Age and menopause affect the expression of specific cytokines/chemokines in plasma and cervical lavage samples from female sex workers in Nairobi, Kenya. Immun Ageing. 2013;10:42.

46. Hale GE, Burger HG. Hormonal changes and biomarkers in late reproductive age, menopausal transition and menopause. Best Pract Res Clin Obstet Gynaecol. 2009;23:7–23.

47. Ribeiro AA, Costa MC, Alves RRF, Villa LL, Saddi VA, Carneiro MA, Zeferino LC, Rabelo-Santos SH. HPV infection and cervical neoplasia: associated risk factors. Infect Agent Cancer. 2015;10:16.

48. Hwang LY, Scott ME, Ma Y, Moscicki A-B. Higher levels of cervicovaginal inflammatory and regulatory cytokines and chemokines in healthy young women with immature cervical epithelium. J Reprod Immunol. 2011;88:66–71.

# 6

# Multiple HPV infections in female sex workers in Western Kenya: implications for prophylactic vaccines within this sub population

Sonia Menon[1,5*], Davy van den Broeck[1,4], Rodolfo Rossi[3], Emilomo Ogbe[1] and Hillary Mabeya[1,2]

## Abstract

**Background:** Whilst the imputed role of High Risk (HR) HPV infection in the development of cervical lesions and cancer has been established, the high number of HPV genotypes that Female Sex workers (FSW) harbour warrants that the synergistic effects of potential HR (pHR) and HR HPV genotypes be elucidated to assess the potential impact of prophylactic vaccines. This population in Kenya also harbours a number of other vaginal infections and STIs, including bacterial vaginosis (BV), trichomonas vaginalis (TV) and *candida spp.*
The aims of this cross-sectional analysis in Kenya are to explore the epidemiology of abnormal cytology and the pairing of pHR/HPV genotypes in HIV-negative and HIV-infected FSW.

**Methods:** A cross-sectional study design of 616 FSW from Western Kenya aged between 18 and 61 years during 2009–2015 using a peer recruitment sampling strategy.

**Results:** Of the 599 FSW who underwent cytological examination, 87 had abnormal cytology (14.5%; 95% CI: 12.0–17.6%). A combined prevalence of HPV16 and 18 (29.6%; 95% CI: 22.2–37.8%) was observed in abnormal cytology. HPV 53 and 51 were the most observed pairing in FSW with abnormal cytology. Significant adjusted associations were found between abnormal cytology and TV (aOR: 30; 95% CI: 14.1–62.9), multiple HR HPV (aOR: 3.7; 95% CI: 1.9–7.3), HPV 51 (aOR 3.7; 95% CI 1.6–8.6) and HPV 52 (aOR 6.1; 95% CI: 2.8–13.3).

**Conclusion:** HPV 51 and 52 were independently associated with abnormal cervical cytology in both HIV negative/positive FSW. The strong association between TV and cervical dysplasia and the high percentage of FSW harbouring more than one STI underscore the need for enhanced STI management within the framework of cervical cancer prevention.

**Keywords:** FSW, HIV, High risk HPV, Potential high risk HPV, Multiple pHR/HR coinfections, Vaccine efficacy

## Background

Human Papilloma Viruses (HPV) are double-stranded DNA viruses which are now deemed to be the chief etiological agents in cervical intraepithelial neoplasias and cancers [1]. High risk (HR) genotypes, which are associated with cervical cancer include HPV genotypes 16, 18, 31, 33, 35, 39, 45, 51, 52, 56, 58, 59, 66, 68 while HPV types 26, 53, 67, 70, 73 and 82 are now classified as possible carcinogenic, and low risk (LR) HPV genotypes considered benign include 6, 11, 42, 43, and 44 [2]. The 15 HR oncological viral strains, which have been identified can be broken down into different species: the HPV 16 group (alpha-9) of the alpha-papillomavirus genus (HPV 31, HPV33, HPV 35, HPV 52, and HPV 58) and the HPV 18 group (alpha-7) (HPV39, HPV 45, HPV 59, and HPV 68).

Cervical intraepithelial neoplasia (CIN) can be histologically graded into mild dysplasia (CIN 1), moderate dysplasia (CIN 2), and severe dysplasia to carcinoma in situ (CIN 3). Several studies have reported a robust

* Correspondence: soniasimonemenon@gmail.com
[1]International Centre for Reproductive health, Department of Obstetrics and Gynaecology, Ghent University, De Pintelaan 185 P3, 9000 Ghent, Belgium
[5]CDC Foundation Atlanta, Atlanta, USA
Full list of author information is available at the end of the article

association between HIV and HPV co-infection and therefore the development of CIN and genital cancer, [3, 4] along with a persistence and recurrence of pre-invasive cervical lesions, CIN 2 or CIN 3 [5].

It is well recognized that among the 14 HR HPV geno-types, HPV 16 and 18 are associated with approximately two thirds of all invasive cervical carcinomas [6]. After HPV16/18, data confirm HPV31/33/35/45/52/58 as the most frequently detected genotypes in Invasive Cervical Cancer (ICC) worldwide [7, 8].

Prophylactic vaccines against HPV 16 and 18 are currently being rolled out across the globe for the prevention of cervical cancer, which is likely to yield a significant impact on the future burden of cervical cancer, particularly in sub Saharan Africa, where screening is scarce. Although the bivalent/quadrivalent vaccines, including the LR HPV 6 and 11 consti-tute a crucial milestone in cervical cancer prevention in HIV-negative women, epidemiological data available suggest that in HIV positive populations, HPV 16 has shown to be frequent, but not as predominant as seen in most HIV negative popula-tions [9, 10]. Moreover, HIV immunosuppression has been linked to multiple HPV infection [11, 12]. Concomitant infection with multiple HPV genotypes has been found to be attributable to the inability to clear HPV infections as well as to the reactivation of latent HPV infections; both occurring as a consequence of immune suppression [13, 14].

Also, epidemiological knowledge of pHR HPV types is highly limited, mainly because commercial molecular as-says focus on HR HPV genotypes. There is a paucity of data on these genotypes in HIV positive women with ab-normal cytology, notwithstanding their potential enhanced role in cervical dysplasia development in HIV positive patients [15, 16].

In Kenya, the Ministry of Public Health and Sanitation has developed a comprehensive cervical cancer preven-tion strategy, entailing plans for administrating quadriva-lent vaccine to preteen girls in the near future. Currently they are running the pilot programme Kituwi in Eastern Kenya and awaiting approval for nationwide rollout and successful global funding [17]. The not yet commercialized nonavalent vaccine in Kenya, containing additional HPV types HPV 6, 11, 16, 18, 31, 33, 45, 52, and 58 antigens may have the ability to prevent 90% of ICC cases worldwide.

In Kenya, as in many parts of sub-Saharan Africa, where the penal code specifically penalizes prostitution [18], FSW bear the greatest burden of HIV and STI infections. Concomitant STIs and vaginal infections may lead to pro-longed HPV infection, which may in turn increase the risk of CIN [19, 20]. Bacterial vaginosis (BV) and *Trichomonas vaginalis* (TV), have been associated with an increased risk of squamous intraepithelial lesions and/or CIN based on biopsy results [21, 22].

As early as 1985, a study reported that HIV prevalence was as high as 61% among a group of FSW in Nairobi [23]. A recent study reported that in Kenya, 5% of the urban female population of reproductive age could be sex workers [24].

The objectives of this analysis were primarily to assess genotype-specific distribution of pHR/HR HPVs in FSW with abnormal cytology, as well as the pairing prevalence of certain pHR/HR HPV genotypes found in HIV nega-tive and HIV infected women with abnormal cytology; secondly, to investigate which HPV genotypes and other variables were associated with abnormal cytology.

## Methods
### Study design
A cross-sectional design was used to explore associa-tions between abnormal cytology and pHR/HR HPV ge-notypes. This cross-sectional study based on record reviews adhered to the methodological guidelines rec-ommended in the STROBE document on observational studies [25].

Women were excluded if they were pregnant, <18 years of age, had a history of cervical dysplasia or cancer, had current abnormal bleeding or bloody discharge, and/or had a hysterectomy. Snowball sampling was undertaken instead of randomized sampling, which is an often used strategy for locating difficult-to-reach and stigmatized populations [26]. This involved a sample of women en-gaged in sex work being recruited through informational gatherings, snowball sampling and neighborhood out-reach. Inclusion criteria for the study entailed being fe-male, giving consent after being explained the objectives of the study, and having engaged in sex in exchange for money, goods, services, or drugs in the last three months. In order to reduce friendship bias, a limit of referral of 10 FSW was established. This activity was undertaken by means of an extensive community outreach program by Gynocare Women and Fistula Hospital, two non-governmental organizations specializing in reproductive health, to identify women with obstetric fistula, STI screening and cervical screening in Western Kenya. The screening was supported by Gent University, Belgium.

### Sample size
The sample size was calculated to allow for a prevalence of at least 15% for abnormal cytology, [27] with a confi-dence interval of 95% and a power of 80%.

### Data collection
#### Structured questionnaire
A structured paper questionnaire was privately adminis-tered by trained interviewers covering socio-demographic characteristics, and sexual behavior. Participants were of-fered testing for HIV and HPV. HIV results were disclosed to participants and women infected with HIV received counseling and treatment.

## Specimen collection and laboratory testing

A gynaecological examination was performed using a swab. Candida colonization was diagnosed by Gram stain; bacterial vaginosis was scored according to Nugent's criteria. Infection with *Trichomonas vaginalis* was diagnosed by PCR, using a validated method which was part of the HPV genotyping essay.

A HIV diagnosis was performed using rapid immunoassays: Uni-Gold™ Recombigen® HIV (Trinity Biotech plc, Bray, Ireland) and Determine® HIV-1/2 (Abbott Japan co Ltd, Minato-Ku, Tokyo, Japan). In the case of indeterminate results, an enzyme-linked immunosorbent assay was used to confirm HIV status.

## Biologic specimens

Cervical samples were collected using a cervix brush (Cervex-brush®, Rovers®, Oss, The Netherlands), and cervical cytology was assessed with conventional Papanicolaou (Pap) smears. Slides were read by a cytologist with master level training, supervised by a pathologist. An external cytopathologist provided quality control. The Bethesda Reporting System was used for cytological classification [28].

The cervix brush tips were preserved in a liquid-based cytology collection medium (SurePath®, Tripath Imaging Inc., Burlington, North Carolina, USA) and stored at 4 °C until further processing.

## Ethical approval

Ethical approval for the study was obtained from the Institutional Research and Ethics Committee at the MOI University in Kenya (No 000187) on August 11th, 2011.

## Statistics and data analysis

Data analysis was done using STATA version 12 (StataCorp LP, College Station, TX). Due to incomplete information about the study samples, we checked whether the missing data (10%) were randomly distributed by performing the Little's MCAR test. Continuous variables were then converted into categorical. Age was dichotomized into ≥30 years and <30 years; this categorization was used to reflect the WHO 2014 guideline concerning cervical screening. The number of pHR/HR HPV co-infections was also dichotomized as a categorical variable with 1 and ≥2 genotypes.

We first described the distribution of pHR/HR HPV types observed among women with both normal cytology and abnormal cytology, for which the overall prevalence and 95% confidence intervals (95% CI) based upon normal distributions were calculated.

To examine patterns of clustering of high-risk HPV types, the prevalence of pHR/HR HPV genotypes in presence of another pHR/HR HPV genotypes by abnormal cytology was calculated, which was defined as the proportion of women with abnormal cytology who were positive for the pHR/HR HPV genotypes. The prevalence of pairings detected in women with HSIL was also calculated.

The variables were explored by means of tabulation and cross-tabulation. The $\chi^2$ test was used to assess whether there was an association between CIN 2+ and various risk factors. In building the regression models, age, STIs and multiple pHR/HR HPV genotypes tested were entered. A multivariable logistic regression analysis was performed to assess the association between pHR/HR HPV genotypes and abnormal cytology, ASC-US or higher, the main outcome of interest and to simultaneously control for potential confounders. The Likelihood Ratio Test (LRT) was used to measure the association of each variable with the outcome.

To assess for a possible interaction due to age, logistic regression models were fitted with and without the interaction term; significance for interaction was then checked through visual inspection of the OR and LRT. Statistical significance was considered at $p \leq 0.05$.

## Results

Out of the 616 participants, data from only 599 participants could be analysed because of the quality of the specimen. Missing values were observed for BV (61), TV (7) and *candida spp* (7). The Little's MCAR test revealed that the missing values were randomly distributed among the participants ($p = 0.4$), therefore unlikely to have introduced information bias.

The mean age of study participants was 28 years and median parity was 2 (range: 0–7 children). Regular condom use, which was defined as always or almost always was reported in 21.7% of 369 women. (95% CI = 17.6–26.2%). The median number of partners in the past week was 4 (IQR: 2–7). Table 1 depicts the prevalence of categories for age and sexual behavior.

Of the 616 FSW who underwent cytological examination, 512 (85.5%: 95% CI: 82.4–88.2) had normal cytology, 87 had abnormal cytology (14.5%; 95% CI: 12.0–17.6%) and 17 were excluded due to poor quality of the sample, leaving 599 participants on whom we could perform the analysis. Of the FSW population, 192 FSW were HIV positive, of

**Table 1** Reports the prevalence of categories for age and sexual behaviour

| Socio demographic variables | Percentage (95% CI) |
|---|---|
| >30 years | 40.1% (95% CI: 36.2–44.1) |
| ≤30 years | 59.9% (95% CI: 55.9–63.8) |
| Sexual behavior: | |
| > 4 sexual partners the past week | 1.9% (95% CI:1.0–3.3) |
| ≤ 4 sexual partners | 98.1% (95% CI: 96.7–99.0) |
| Regular use of condom | 21.7% (95% CI 17.6–26.2) |
| No regular use of condom | 78.3% (95% CI: 73.8–92.3) |

which 27.1% (95% CI: 20.9–34.0%) had abnormal cytology. Table 2 in annex reports the prevalence of cervical abnormalities observed in the sample ($N = 616$).

The prevalence of pHR/HR HPV and multiple pHR/HR co-infections in the 616 FSW was 57.7 and 32.8% respectively. In HPV infected FSW, HIV-infected FSW had a significantly higher number of co-infections (2.0) than HIV negative FSW (0.9), $p < 0.001$.

The prevalence of BV in this population was 48.3%, followed by TV 31.4%, and *candida spp* 19.9%. FSW with BV had the highest prevalence of multiple pHR/HR co-infections with 53.4%, followed by TV, and *candida spp*, 38.8and 23.9% respectively. Table 3 reports the prevalence of each HPV genotypes and vaginal infections/TV.

### Normal and abnormal cytology and each HPV genotypes

The combined prevalence of HPV 16 and HPV 18 was 27.1%, and of the two pHR HPV genotypes tested, HPV 53 and 66, 20.8% (95% CI: 17.6–24.2%). In women with abnormal cytology, we observed a multiple pHR/HR HPV genotype prevalence of 65.5%. See Table 4 in annex, which reports the prevalence of each HPV genotypes.

### Potential HR HPV in abnormal cytology

HPV 53 and HPV 66 were found as a stand-alone pHR HPV genotype in two LSIL cases.

### Pairings of pHR/HR HPV genotypes in abnormal cytology

A higher prevalence of pairings in abnormal cytology were observed in HIV infected FSW than HIV negative FSW. The most frequently observed pairings in HIV- negative FSW were HPV 18 and 31 ($n = 3$) occurrences, and HPV 31 and 52 ($n = 2$), involving genotypes phylogenetically related to the HPV 16.

In HIV-infected women, HPV 53 and HPV 51 are observed in 5 of the most prevalent pairings, followed by HPV 16, observed in 4 of the most prevalent pairings. Whilst in HIV negative FSW, the most prevalent co-infection pairings exhibited a mixed alpha 9-alpha 7 combination or a homogenous alpha 9 pattern, in HIV infected women, the non-alpha 9/7 pHR HPV genotypes, HPV 53 (alpha 6) and HPV 51 (alpha 5) figure prominently. See Table 5 in annex which depicts the most prevalent pairing occurrences in women with abnormal cytology and HSIL.

**Table 2** Reports the prevalence of cervical abnormalities observed in the sample ($N = 616$)

| Cytological status | n | % of FSW (95% CI) |
|---|---|---|
| Normal cytology | 512 | 85.5% (82.4–88.2) |
| ASC-US | 10 | 1.7% (0.8–3.04) |
| LSIL | 63 | 10.5% (8.2–13.3) |
| HSIL | 14 | 2.3% (12.8–3.9) |
| Excluded samples due to poor quality | 17 | 2.8% |

**Table 3** Reports the prevalence of each HPV genotypes and vaginal infections/TV

| pHR/HR HPV Genotype | Frequency (n) | Percentage ($N = 616$) | 95% CI |
|---|---|---|---|
| HPV 16 ($N = 616$) | 99 | 16.10% | 13.3%–19.2% |
| HPV 18 ($N = 616$) | 68 | 11.04% | 08.7%–13.8% |
| HPV 31 ($N = 616$) | 49 | 8.00% | 5.9%–10.4% |
| HPV 33 ($N = 616$) | 2 | 0.30% | 0.04%–1.2% |
| HPV 35 ($N = 616$) | 70 | 11.40% | 9.0%–14.1% |
| HPV 39 ($N = 616$) | 48 | 7.80% | 5.8%–10.2% |
| HPV 51 ($N = 615$) | 52 | 8.50% | 3.7%–7.4% |
| HPV 53 ($N = 616$) | 68 | 11.04% | 8.7%–13.8% |
| HPV 56 ($N = 616$) | 45 | 7.30% | 5.4%–9.7% |
| HPV 58 ($N = 616$) | 30 | 4.90% | 3.3%–6.9% |
| HPV 59 ($N = 616$) | 75 | 12.20% | 9.7%–15.02% |
| HPV 66 ($N = 616$) | 60 | 9.70% | 7.5%–12.4% |
| HPV 68 ($N = 616$) | 9 | 4.90% | 3.3%–6.9% |
| Vaginal infections and TV | | | |
| BV ($N = 555$) | 268 | 48.30% | 44.06%–52.5% |
| TV ($N = 609$) | 191 | 31.4% | 27.6%–35.2% |
| Candida ($N = 609$) | 121 | 19.90% | 16.8%–23.3% |

### Risk factors for abnormal cytology

In the univariate analysis, age did not appear to be associated with abnormal cytology: women under 30 years of age have a crude OR 1.1 (95% CI: 0.7–1.8 $p = 0.6$) of having abnormal cytology compared to older women.

**Table 4** Reports the prevalence of each HPV genotype in women with abnormal cytology

| HPV genotype | Abnormal cytology | % ($N = 87$) | 95% CI |
|---|---|---|---|
| HPV 16 | 24 | 28.6% | 19.2–39.5 |
| HPV 18 | 15 | 17.9% | 10.0–27.0 |
| HPV 31 | 13 | 15.5% | 8.5–25.0 |
| HPV 33 | 1 | 1.2% | 0.03–6.5 |
| HPV 35 | 18 | 21.4% | 13.2–31.7 |
| HPV 39 | 13 | 15.5% | 8.5–25.0 |
| HPV 45 | 9 | 10.7% | 5.0–19.4 |
| HPV 51 | 18 | 21.4% | 13.2–31.7 |
| HPV 52 | 26 | 31.0% | 21.3–42.0 |
| HPV 53 | 21 | 25.0% | 16.2–35.6 |
| HPV 56 | 13 | 15.5% | 8.5–25.0 |
| HPV 58 | 4 | 13.3% | 3.8–30.7 |
| HPV 59 | 17 | 23.6% | 14.4–35.1 |
| HPV 66 | 9 | 10.7% | 5.0–19.4 |
| HPV 67 | | | |
| HPV 68 | 4 | 4.8% | 1.3–11.7 |

**Table 5** Most prevalent pairing occurrences in women with abnormal cytology and HSIL

| Prevalent pairings in abnormal cytology in HIV-negative women | Occurrences (n) | % in abnormal cytology |
|---|---|---|
| HPV 18 and 31 | 2 | 3 |
| HPV 31 and 52 | 7 | 2 |
| Prevalent pairings in HIV infected women with abnormal cytology | | |
| HPV 16 and 39 | 2 | 6 |
| HPV 16 and 52 | 9 | 7 |
| HPV 16 and 51 | 4 | 5 |
| HPV 16 and 53 | 10 | 7 |
| HPV 18 and 52 | 12 | 5 |
| HPV 18 and 53 | 8 | 5 |
| HPV 31 and 51 | 2 | 5 |
| HPV 35 and 51 | 2 | 5 |
| HPV 35 and 53 | 4 | 7 |
| HPV 45 and 53 | 0 | 6 |
| HPV 45 and 59 | 2 | 5 |
| HPV 51 and 53 | 2 | 7 |
| HPV 51 and 56 | 1 | 6 |
| HPV 52 and 56 | 3 | 6 |
| HPV 53 and 56 | 1 | 5 |

A very strong significant association was found between TV and abnormal cytology OR: 30.0 (95% CI: 14.1–62.9) adjusting for age and pHR/HR HPV genotypes, BV and *candida spp* and HIV.

A statistically significant OR, adjusted for age was found for multiple HPV and abnormal cytology compared to single HPV genotype infection. This association decreased but remained significant (OR; 3.9; $p < 0.001$; 95%CI: 1.9–7.8) when adjusted for HIV.

Whilst all pHR/HR HPV genotypes were significant predictors of abnormal cytology, when adjusted for age pHR/HR HPV genotypes co-infections, HIV, BV, TV, and *candida spp* these associations became statistically insignificant, except for HPV 51 and 52. Table 6 in annex depicts the age, BV, TV and *candida spp* adjusted association between specific pHR/HR HPV genotypes and abnormal cytology.

As no interaction terms were significant, no result reflecting the differential impact for that particular outcome was presented.

## Discussion
### Summary of results
In the present study, we observed a high prevalence of women harbouring more than two pHR/HR HPV genotypes, which was significantly higher in HIV-1–infected women, consistent with results of several studies illustrating that HIV-1–infected women not only have a greater prevalence of HR-HPV infection but multiple coinfections [29, 30].

Our observations are in agreement with those of a large study on multiple HPV infections in Costa Rica in which young healthy women with multiple infections were at significantly increased risk of CIN 2+, Although our findings of an association between TV and abnormal cytology are congruent with other observations [31] demonstrating an association between TV and abnormal cytology, [32, 33] our study suggest an unprecedented strong association.

After adjusting for age and multiple pHR/HR HPV co-infections, BV, TV and *candida spp*, no significant association was observed between any single pHR/HR HPV and abnormal cytology, except for HPV 51 and 52 in both HIV negative and positive women. This is incongruent with our previous findings in an exclusively HIV-infected study population in Belgium, [34] in which only the association between HPV 39 and abnormal cytology became statistically significant.

In contrast to HPV 31 and 58 being the most observed frequent pairing in Brazil in HIV infected women, and HPV 31 and 66 and HPV 39 and 52 in our Belgian study population, in this FSW study population, HPV 31, 52 and 66 do not figure prominently within pairings observed in HIV-infected women despite a higher prevalence of HPV 52 than HPV 53.

Also, our high prevalence of women with abnormal cytology without any detected HPV genotypes can be attributed to our testing of only 18 genotypes out of the over 200 HPV types described. Whilst some types may be inducing low grade lesions, they may also lack a cancer-initiating capacity.

### Strengths and limitations
Our major strength was that all cervical smears were histologically confirmed and the high sensitivity of the HPV DNA diagnostics employed. However, whilst our sample was large, the number of FSW with abnormal cytology was small, which precluded us from exploring particular co-infection patterns as a risk factor. Moreover, due to our lack of behavioral and clinico-epidemiological data, including smoking, CD4 count, HAART use or the presence of other co-infections, we have not been able to adjust for these potential confounders, nor assess whether these factors were associated with cervical abnormalities. Also, there may be potential for selection bias as FSW with similar characteristics may have been sampled, as a result of the convenience sampling method used. However, a convenience sampling strategy may have inadvertently excluded those FSW operating in a more clandestine fashion and thereby not benefitting from a social network.

A limitation related to a cross sectional study design may be the lack of data concerning age of acquisition of

**Table 6** Association between vaginal infections, TV, specific pHR/HR HPV genotypes and abnormal cytology; OR from Logistic regression; p-value from LRT

| Vaginal infections and STIs | OR Model 1 (95% CI) | p-value | OR Model 2 (95% CI) | p-value |
|---|---|---|---|---|
| BV | 0.9 (0.6–1.5) | 0.8 | 0.8 (0.5–1.4) | 0.5 |
| TV | 24.8 (12.7–48.3) | <0.001 | 30.0 (14.1–62.9) | <0.001 |
| Candida spp | 1.0 (0.5–1.7) | 1.0 | 0.9 (0.5–1.7) | 0.7 |
| Multiple HPV infection | 5.3 (2.9–9.7) | <0.001 | 3.7 (1.9–7.3) | <0.001 |
| HPV 16 | 1.9 (0.8–4.5) | 0.1 | 1.2 (0.5–3.2) | 0.5 |
| HPV 18 | 0.8 (0.3–2.1) | 0.7 | 1.04 (0.4–2.8) | 0.9 |
| HPV 31 | 0.5 (0.2–1.5) | 0.2 | 0.6 (0.2–1.7) | 0.3 |
| HPV 33 | 3.9 (0.05–293.9) | 0.5 | 2.8 (0.03–254.6) | 0.6 |
| HPV 35 | 1.3 (0.6–3.0) | 0.5 | 1.1 (0.5–2.7) | 0.9 |
| HPV 39 | 3.3 (1.3–8.7) | 0.03 | 2.5 (0.9–7.1) | 0.09 |
| HPV 51 | 3.7 (1.6–8.6) | 0.002 | 3.7 (1.5–9.0) | 0.004 |
| HPV 52 | 6.1 (2.8–13.3) | <0.001 | 4.0 (1.6–8.2) | 0.002 |
| HPV 53 | 2.0 (0.8–4.9) | 0.1 | 1.4; (0.5–3.8) | 0.5 |
| HPV 56 | 2.5 (1.0–6.6) | 0.06 | 2.0 (0.7–5.7) | 0.2 |
| HPV 58 | 0.9 (0.2–3.6) | 0.9 | 1.1 (0.3–5.2) | 0.9 |
| HPV 66 | 1.2 (0.5–3.0) | 0.7 | 1.0 (0.4–3.0) | 0.9 |
| HPV 68 | 1.7 (0.2–17.0) | 0.7 | 0.8 (0.1–7.4) | 0.8 |

Model 1: OR adjusting for age, pHR/HR HPV genotypes, vaginal infections/TV
Model 2: OR adjusting for age and pHR/HR genotypes, vaginal infections/TV and HIV

HIV infection since it is possible this may have occurred too late in life for some of the women in our study to influence abnormal cytology. Similarly, an analysis of a cross sectional study for exploring associations between multiple HPV genotypes and abnormal cytology may have inherent limitations as infections may have been acquired concurrently or sequentially, therefore, resulting in the criterion of temporality for causation not being met. This may have an impact as immunologic responses may differ following concurrent acquisition of multiple HPV genotypes from infections that are acquired sequentially.

### Implications for vaccination programs

The only significant association observed between abnormal cytology and HPV 51 and HPV 52 underscore the need for post quadrivalent and nonavalent vaccine surveillance in both HIV negative and HIV infected FSW.

In light of a high prevalence of multiple HR HPV infections in this FSW HIV-negative and infected population, it will need to be elucidated whether cross protection may be hampered by the additional burden due to other synergistic relationships among HR HPV genotypes present. A recent systematic review and meta-analysis [35] found that bivalent Cervarix© vaccine from GlaxoSmithKline had better cross protection against HPV 31 in persistent infection, but that efficacy against persistent infections with types 31 appeared to decrease with longer follow-up, suggesting a waning of cross-protection. It still remains to be determined whether a cross protection can be extrapolated to HIV-infected women and in presence of multiple HR HPV genotypes.

Moreover, with a high prevalence of the pHR HPV 53 in pairings with the vaccine preventable HPV 16 and HPV 18 in HIV infected women, it will need to be determined how HPV 53 will fare within the vacuum that ensues the quadrivalent vaccine [36]. In addition, given the high median number of pHR/HR HPV genotypes harboured by this population, the synergies between not only two pHR/HR HPV genotypes need to be determined but within a context of other prevalent genotypes, capable of inducing cervical cancer genesis. Whether Gardasil and Cervarix can attain a 70% reduction of cervical cancer may be contingent upon the natural history of the imputed pHR/HR HPV genotypes in cancer genesis along with their synergistic effects.

Our very high association between TV and cervical dysplasia underscores the need for STI management to be integrated within cervical cancer prevention program. Furthermore, the biological interaction between TV and HPV and its subsequent capacity to induce progression of cervical dysplasia should be further explored. Moreover, the impact of immune modulating infections, such as tuberculosis, malaria and helminthic infections on cervical disease progression should be elucidated in HIV triple co-infected women with HPV and TV.

## Conclusion

Co-infection with pHR/HR HPV genotypes was more strongly associated with abnormal cytology than any single high-risk HPV. In light of the high prevalence of multiple pHR/HR HPV genotypes harboured by FSW and especially HIV infected women, its micro epidemiology in cervical carcinoma in HIV positive women needs to be explored in order for the vaccine efficacy to be assessed.

Whilst the quadrivalent vaccine may be effective in reducing the prevalence of abnormal cytology in HIV negative and HIV infected FSW, the high presence of multiple infections with HPV 16 requires that the micro epidemiology of concurrent be elucidated. In particular, the high prevalence of the non alpha 9 and 7 genotypes, HPV 51 and HPV 53 observed in pairings with HPV 16 and HPV 18 in HIV infected FSW requires further characterization.

These current gaps in epidemiology underscore the need for FSW, HIV negative or positive to be regularly monitored in the post quadrivalent/nonavalent vaccine era.

The strong association observed between TV and cervical dysplasia as well as the high percentage of FSW harbouring more than one vaginal infection/STI begs for the elucidation of synergistic interactions between multiple STIs to be better assessed as factor(s) for cervical dysplasia and for a wider encompassing cervical cancer prevention framework.

## Abbreviations

ASC-H: Typical squamous cells-cannot exclude high-grade squamous intraepithelial lesion; ASC-U: Atypical cells of undetermined significance; FSW: Female sex workers; HIV: Human immunodeficiency virus; HPV: Human Papilloma virus; HSIL: High grade squamous intraepithelial lesion; LR HPV: Low risk HPV; LSIL: Low grade squamous intraepithelial lesion; pHR HPV: Potential high risk

## Acknowledgement

Dr Stacy Harmon and Dr Mbabazi Kariisa for their editing, critical feedback of the intellectual content. This research received no specific grant. HM is supported by VLIR-UOS.

## Funding

Our research was funded by the VLIR IUC Moi University.

## Authors' contributions

SM lead author conceived and drafted the manuscript, performed the statistical analysis, and interpreted the findings. DB participated in the conception of the paper, revision and validation of the article. RR participated in the data analysis, interpretation of findings, and in the revision of the article. EO: participated in the data analysis, interpretation of findings, and in the revision of the article. HM: participated in designing the study, interpretation of findings and in the revision of the article. All authors read and approved the final manuscript.

## Competing interests

The authors declare that they have no competing financial, political, personal, religious, ideological, academic, intellectual, commercial or any other interests.

## Author details

[1]International Centre for Reproductive health, Department of Obstetrics and Gynaecology, Ghent University, De Pintelaan 185 P3, 9000 Ghent, Belgium. [2]Moi University/Gynocare Fistula Centre, Eldoret, Kenya. [3]AMBIOR (Applied Molecular Biology Research Group), Antwerpen, Belgium. [4]Faculty of Medicine and Health Sciences, Laboratory of Cell Biology & Histology, University of Antwerp, Antwerp, Belgium. [5]CDC Foundation Atlanta, Atlanta, USA.

## References

1. Ng'andwe C, Lowe JJ, Richards PJ, Hause L, Wood C, Angeletti PC. The distribution of sexually-transmitted Human Papillomaviruses in HIV positive and negative patients in Zambia, Africa. BMC Infect Dis. 2007;7:77. doi:10.1186/1471-2334-7-77.
2. Bouvard V, Baan R, Straif K, Grosse Y, Secretan B, El Ghissassi F, Benbrahim-Tallaa L, Guha N, Freeman C, Galichet L, Cogliano V, WHO International Agency for Research on Cancer Monograph Working Group. A review of human carcinogens—Part B: biological agents. Lancet Oncol. 2009;10:321–2.
3. Hawes SE, et al. Increased risk of high-grade cervical squamous intraepithelial lesions and invasive cervical cancer among African women with human immunodeficiency virus type 1 and 2 infections. J Infect Dis. 2003;188(4):555–63.
4. De Sanjose S, Diaz M, Castellsague X, et al. Worldwide prevalence and genotype distribution of cervical human papilloman DNA in women with normal cytology: a meta-analysis. Lancet Infect Dis. 2007;7:453–9.
5. Russomano F, Paz BR, Camargo MJ, Grinstejn BG, Friedman RK, Tristao MA, Oliveira CA. Recurrence of cervical intraepithelial neoplasia in human immunodeficiency virus-infected women treated by means of electrosurgical excision of the transformation zone (LLETZ) in Rio de Janeiro, Brazil. Sao Paulo Med J. 2013;131(6):405–10. doi:10.1590/1516-3180.2013.1316578.
6. Bosch FX, de Sanjose S. Chapter 1: Human papillomavirus and cervical cancer: burden and assessment of causality. J Natl Cancer Inst Monogr. 2003;31:3–13.
7. Li N, Franceschi S, Howell-Jones R, Snijders PJ, Clifford GM. Human papillomavirus type distribution in 30,848 invasive cervical cancers worldwide: Variation by geographical region, histological type and year of publication. Int J Cancer. 2011;128(4):927–35.
8. Rahman M, Sasagawa T, Yamada R, Kingoro A, Ichimura H, Makinoda S. High prevalence of intermediate-risk human papillomavirus infection in uterine cervices of kenyan women infected with human immunodeficiency virus. J Med Virol. 2011;83:1988–96.
9. Didelot-Rousseau MN, Nagot N, Costes-Martineau V, Valles X, Ouedraogo A, Konate I, Weiss HA, Van de Perre P, Mayaud P, Segondy M, Yerelon Study Group. Human papillomavirus genotype distribution and cervical squamous intraepithelial lesions among high-risk women with and without HIV-1 infection in Burkina Faso. Br J Cancer. 2006;95:355–62.
10. Ahdieh L, Klein RS, Burk R, et al. Prevalence, incidence, and type-specific persistence of human papillomavirus in Human Immunodeficiency Virus (HIV)-positive and HIV-negative women. J Infect Dis. 2001;184:682–90.
11. Levi JE, Kleter B, Quint WG, Fink MC, Canto CL, Matsubara R, et al. High prevalence of human papillomavirus (HPV) infections and high frequency of multiple HPV genotypes in human immunodeficiency virus-infected women in Brazil. J Clin Microbiol. 2002;40:3341–5.
12. Moscicki AB, Ellenberg JH, Farhat S, Xu J. Persistence of human papillomavirus infection in HIV-infected and -uninfected adolescent girls: risk factors and differences, by phylogenetic type. J Infect Dis. 2004;190:37–45.
13. Strickler HD, Burk RD, Fazzari M, Anastos K, Minkoff H, Massad LS, Hall C, Bacon M, Levine AM, Watts DH, Silverberg MJ, Xue X, Schlecht NF, Melnick S, Palefsky JM. Natural history and possible reactivation of human papillomavirus in human immunodeficiency virus-positive women. J Natl Cancer Inst. 2005;97:577–86.
14. Palefsky JM, Minkoff H, Kalish LA, Levine A, Sacks HS, Garcia P, Young M, Melnick S, Miotti P, Burk R. Cervicovaginal human papillomavirus infection in

human immunodeficiency virus-1 (HIV)-positive and high-risk HIV-negative women. J Natl Cancer Inst. 1999;91:226–36.

15. Schopp B, Holz B, Zago M, Stubenrauch F, Petry KU, Kjaer SK, et al. Evaluation of the performance of the novel PapilloCheck HPV genotyping test by comparison with two other genotyping systems and the HC2 test. J Med Virol. 2010;82:605–15.

16. Barcellos RB, Almeida SE, Sperhacke RD, Verza M, Rosso F, Medeiros RM, et al. Evaluation of a novel microplate colorimetric hybridization genotyping assay for human papillomavirus. J Virol Methods. 2011;77:38–43.

17. Friedman AL, Oruko KO, et al. Preparing for human papillomavirus vaccine introduction in Kenya: implications from focus-group and interview discussions with caregivers and opinion leaders in Western Kenya. BMC Public Health. 2014;14:855.

18. International Models project on women's right. Current Legal Framework: Prostitution in Kenya. 2011. http://www.impowr.org/content/current-legal-framework-prostitution-kenya. Accessed 8 May 2016.

19. Finan RR, Tamim H, Almawi WY. Identification of Chlamydia trachomatis DNA in human papillomavirus (HPV) positive women with normal and abnormal cytology. Arch Gynecol Obstet. 2002;266(3):168–71.

20. Syrjanen K, Mantyjarvi R, Vayrynen M, et al. Chlamydial cervicitis in women followed-up for human papillomavirus (HPV) lesions of the uterine cervix. Acta Obstet Gynecol Scand. 1985;64:467–71.

21. Platz-Christensen JJ, Sundstrom E, Larsson PG. Bacterial vaginosis and cervical intraepithelial neoplasia. Acta Obstet Gynecol Scand. 1994;73:586–8.

22. Noel JC, Fayt I, Romero Munoz MR, et al. High prevalence of high-risk human papillomavirus infection among women with Trichomonas vaginalis infection on monolayer cytology. Arch Gynecol Obstet. 2010;282:503–5.

23. Ngugi EN, Plummer FA, Simonsen JA, Cameron DW, Bosire M, et al. Prevention of transmission of human immunodeficiency virus in Africa: effectiveness of condom promotion and health education among prostitutes. Lancet. 1988; 2(8616):887–90. doi:10.1016/s0140-6736(88)92480-4.

24. Odek WO, Githuka GN, Avery L, Njoroge PK, Kasonde L, Gorgens M, et al. Estimating the size of the female sex worker population in Kenya to inform HIV prevention programming. PLoS One. 2014;9(3):e89180. doi:10.1371/journal.pone.0089180.

25. von Elm E, Altman DG, Egger M, Pocock SJ, Gotzsche PC, Vandenbroucke JP, the STROBE initiative. The Strengthening the Reporting of Observational Studies in Epidemiology (STROBE) statement: guidelines for reporting observational studies. Lancet. 2007;370:1453–7.

26. Ulin PR, Robinson ET, Tolley EE. Qualitative methods in public health: A field guide for applied research. San Francisco: APA (6th ed.) Jossey-Bass; 2005.

27. Musa J, Achenbach C, Taiwo B, et al. High-risk human papilloma virus and cervical abnormalities in HIV-infected women with normal cervical cytology. Infect Agents Cancer. 2014;9:36.

28. Davey DD. Cervical cytology classification and the Bethesda System. Cancer J. 2003;9(5):327–34.

29. Grinsztejn B, Veloso VG, Levi JE, Velasque L, Luz PM, et al. Factors associated with increased prevalence of human papillomavirus infection in a cohort of HIV-1-infected Brazilian women. Int J Infect Dis. 2008;13(1):72–80.

30. Temmerman M, Tyndall MW, Kidula N, Claeys P, Muchiri L, et al. Risk factors for human papillomavirus and cervical precancerous lesions, and the role of concurrent HIV-1 infection. Int J Gynaecol Obstet. 1999;65(2):171–81.

31. Yap EH, Ho TH, Chan YC, et al. Serum antibodies to Trichomonas vaginalis in invasive cervical cancer patients. Genitourin Med. 1995;71:402–4.

32. Donders GGG, Depuydt CE, Bogers J-P, Vereecken AJ. Association of Trichomonas vaginalis and Cytological Abnormalities of the Cervix in Low Risk Women. Kaul R, ed. PLoS ONE. 2013;8(12):e86266. doi:10.1371/journal.pone.0086266.

33. Viikki M, Pukkala E, Nieminen P, Hakama M. Gynaecological infections as risk determinants of subsequent cervical neoplasia. Acta Oncol. 2000;39:71–5.

34. Menon S, Rossi R, Benoy I, Bogers JP, van den Broeck D. Human papilloma virus infection in HIV-infected women in Belgium: implications for prophylactic vaccines within this subpopulation. Eur J Cancer Prev. 2016. [Epub ahead of print].

35. Malagón T, Drolet M, Boily MC, Franco EL, Jit M, Brisson J, Brisson M. Cross-protective efficacy of two human papillomavirus vaccines: a systematic review and meta-analysis. Lancet Infect Dis. 2012;12(10):781–9. doi:10.1016/S1473-3099(12)70187-1.

36. Padalko E, Ali-Risasi C, Van Renterghem L, Bamelis M, De Mey A, Sturtewagen Y, Vastenavond H, Vanden Broeck D, Weyers S, Praet M. Evaluation of the clinical significance of human papillomavirus (HPV) 53. Eur J Obstet Gynecol Reprod Biol. 2015;191:7–9. doi:10.1016/j.ejogrb.2015.04.004.

# 7

# Serum EBV antibodies and LMP-1 in Polish patients with oropharyngeal and laryngeal cancer

Sylwia Fołtyn[1], Małgorzata Strycharz-Dudziak[2*], Bartłomiej Drop[3], Anastazja Boguszewska[1] and Małgorzata Polz-Dacewicz[1]

## Abstract

**Background:** The association between Epstein-Barr virus (EBV) and the development of head and neck cancer was reported by many researchers. The aim of the present study was to detect EBV DNA and EBV antibodies in 110 Polish patients with oropharyngeal and laryngeal cancer compared to 40 healthy individuals.

**Methods:** Frozen tumor tissue fragments were tested using nested PCR assay for EBV DNA detection. Sera from all individuals were investigated using ELISA tests to detect the presence of VCA IgM and IgG, EBNA IgG, EA IgG.

**Results:** EBV DNA was detected in 52.7% of the patients (25% in controls). EBVCA were detected in 94.5%, EBNA in 96.4% and EA in 94.5% of patients. The significantly higher level of EA in the patients suggests EBV reactivation. The majority of patients (83%) were infected with wild-type EBV.

**Conclusion:** Our study showed that this variant seems to be associated with oropharyngeal and laryngeal cancer in the Polish population.

**Keywords:** EBV antibodies, LMP1, Oropharyngeal cancer, Laryngeal cancer

## Background

The Epstein-Barr virus (EBV) is a ubiquitous gammaherpesvirus that infects more than 90% of the global adult human population [1–3]. For the past two decades, increasing interest has been focused on the EBV-associated cancers including Burkitt's lymphoma (BL), Hodgkin lymphoma (HL), nasopharyngeal carcinoma and gastric cancer [4–8].

The global burden of mortality from EBV-related cancers accounts for 1.8% of all cancer deaths in 2010 [9]. The trends indicate that both this burden and life-expectancy in the world population will increase. About 92% of all EBV-associated cancer deaths are caused by nasopharyngeal cancer and gastric cancer. After primary infection, EBV establishes latent infection in B lymphocytes with periodic reactivation and viral transmission in the oropharyngeal epithelium. Chronic viral infection is an important risk factor, particularly for tongue cancer and oropharyngeal cancer [1, 7, 8, 10–14]. The association between the latent EBV infection and the development of head and neck cancer (HNC) was reported by several investigators [11, 12, 14, 15].

The present study analysed the serum level of EBV antibodies (VCA IgM and IgG, EBNA IgG, EA IgG) and determined LMP1 variant in patients with oropharyngeal and laryngeal cancers in the Polish population.

## Methods

### Patients

The present study comprised of a group of 110 patients with a diagnosed cancer of the pharynx or larynx who were hospitalized in Otolaryngology Division of the Hospital in Radom, Poland. The results were compared to the control group, involving 40 persons hospitalized at the Otolaryngology Ward due to diseases other than cancer. There were no statistically significant differences between the patients and the control group (age, sex, tobacco and alcohol consumption (Table 1)). The socio-

* Correspondence: malgorzata.strycharz-dudziak@umlub.pl
[2]Chair and Department of Conservative Dentistry with Endodontics, Medical University of Lublin, Lublin, Poland
Full list of author information is available at the end of the article

**Table 1** Epidemiological characteristics of patients and control group

|  |  | Patients ($n = 110$) | | Controls ($n = 40$) | | p |
|---|---|---|---|---|---|---|
|  |  | n | % | n | % |  |
| Sex | female | 8 | 7.3 | 2 | 5.0 | >0.05 |
|  | male | 102 | 92.7 | 38 | 95.0 |  |
| Age | <49 | 12 | 10.9 | 6 | 15.0 | >0.05 |
|  | 50–59 | 46 | 41.8 | 16 | 40.0 |  |
|  | >60 | 52 | 47.3 | 18 | 45.0 |  |
| Place of residence | urban | 72 | 65.5 | 28 | 70.0 | >0.05 |
|  | rural | 38 | 34.5 | 12 | 30.0 |  |
| Smoking | yes | 94 | 85.5 | 36 | 90.0 | >0.05 |
|  | no | 16 | 14.5 | 4 | 10.0 |  |
| Alcohol abuse | yes | 50 | 45.5 | 14 | 35.0 | >0.05 |
|  | no | 60 | 54.5 | 13 | 65.0 |  |
| EBV DNA | positive | 58 | 52.7 | 10 | 25.0 | <0.001 |
|  | negative | 52 | 47.3 | 30 | 75.0 |  |

demographic and clinicopathological characteristics of the study group are shown in Table 2 in relation to EBV DNA. The research material consisted of the sera and frozen tumor tissue fragments. This research was approved by the Ethics Committee and is in accordance with the GCP regulations (no. KE-0254/133/2013).

**DNA extraction from fresh frozen tumour tissue**

Fragments of the fresh frozen tumour tissue (20 mg), both from the patients with OSCC and from the control subjects (biopsies), were cut and homogenized in a manual homogenizer Omni TH/Omni International/Kennesewa/Georgia/USA. DNA was extracted using a protocol as described in the DNeasy Tissue Kit Handbook (QiagenGmBH, Hilden, Germany). Purified DNA was quantified by spectrophoto-metery (Epoch Microplate Spectrophotometer, BioTek Instruments Inc., Vinooski, Vermont, USA). The isolates were kept at −20 °C until the test was conducted. To verify the quality of the obtained DNA (presence of inhibitors of Polymerase Chain Reaction), a β-globinassay was performed.

**Detection of viruses**

EBV DNA detection: All PCR reactions were carried out in the final volume of 25 μl using HotStartTaq DNA Polymerase (Qiagen, Germany). Concentrations of PCR reaction components were prepared as follows: 2.0 mM $MgCl_2$, 0.2 mM dNTPs, 0.5 μM of each forward and reverse primers and 0.5 U of HotStartTaq polymerase. During each run the samples were tested together with one negative (nuclease-free water) and positive control (EBV-positive cell line, Namalwa, ATCC-CRL-1432).

**Table 2** Epidemiological and clinical characteristics of patients in relation to EBV DNA

|  |  | EBV DNA+ | | EBV DNA- | | p |
|---|---|---|---|---|---|---|
|  |  | n | % | n | % |  |
| Sex | female | 0 | 0 | 8 | 100 | 0.0282* |
|  | male | 58 | 56.9 | 44 | 43.1 |  |
| Age | <49 | 8 | 50.0 | 4 | 50.0 | 0.8969 |
|  | 50–59 | 22 | 47.8 | 24 | 52.2 |  |
|  | >60 | 28 | 50.0 | 24 | 50.0 |  |
| Place of residence | urban | 40 | 55.6 | 32 | 44.4 | 0.5630 |
|  | rural | 18 | 47.4 | 20 | 52.6 |  |
| Smoking | yes | 50 | 53.2 | 44 | 46.8 | 0.8672 |
|  | no | 8 | 50.0 | 8 | 50.0 |  |
| Alcohol abuse | yes | 28 | 56.0 | 22 | 44.0 | 0.6571 |
|  | no | 30 | 50.0 | 30 | 50.0 |  |
| Histological grading | G1 | 22 | 61.1 | 14 | 38.9 | 0.6852 |
|  | G2 | 34 | 48.57 | 36 | 51.43 |  |
|  | G3 | 2 | 50.0 | 2 | 50.0 |  |
| T stage | T1 | 6 | 42.9 | 8 | 57.1 | 0.1826 |
|  | T2 | 28 | 58.3 | 20 | 41.7 |  |
|  | T3 | 16 | 72.7 | 6 | 27.3 |  |
|  | T4 | 8 | 30.8 | 18 | 69.2 |  |
| N stage | N0 | 30 | 51.7 | 28 | 48.3 | 0.9768 |
|  | N1 | 10 | 50.0 | 10 | 50.0 |  |
|  | N2 | 14 | 58.3 | 10 | 41.7 |  |
|  | N3 | 4 | 50.0 | 4 | 50.0 |  |
| M stage | M0 | 58 | 52.7 | 52 | 47.3 |  |
|  | M1 | 0 | 0 | 0 | 0 |  |
| Location of cancer | pharynx | 23 | 50.0 | 23 | 50.0 | 0.6452 |
|  | larynx | 35 | 54.7 | 29 | 45.3 |  |
| EBV type | wild | 48 | 82.8 | - | - | - |
|  | del-LMP1 | 10 | 17.2 | - | - |  |

*statistically significant

**Amplification of EBNA-2 gene**

The nested PCR was carried out for amplification of EBNA-2. The sequence of primers used for PCR was as follows: outer pair 5′ – TTT CAC CAA TAC ATG ACC C – 3′, 5′ – TGG CAA AGT GCT GAG AGC AA – 3′ and inner pair 5′ – CAA TAC ATG AAC CRG AGT CC – 3′, 5′ – AAG TGC TGA GAG CAA GGC MC – 3′. 2 μl of extracted DNA was subjected to the PCR mixture with the concentration as described above. The first-round amplification consisted of the activation of polymerase 95 °C for 15 min, 35 cycles of 94 °C for 1 min, 55 °C for 1 min, 72 °C for 2 min and the final extension at 72 °C for 5 min. The second-round amplification was performed with 1 μl of first round PCR product in 30 cycles with an annealing temperature at 60 °C. The amplicons 368 bp, 473 bp in length (depending on the EBV type EBV-1 and EBV-2, respectively) were separated on 2% agarose gel and purified using a Gel-Out kit (A&A Biotechnology, Poland) for further analysis. Purified PCR products were sent to Genomed Warsaw company for sequencing.

## Genotyping of LMP1

PCR screening for the EBV LMP1 subtype based on exon 3, defined as wild-type (wtLMP1) or del-LMP1, was done using specific primers: forward 5′-AGC GAC TCT GCT GGA AAT GAT- 3′; revers 5′-TGA TTA GCT AAG GCA TTC CCA- 3′. Concentrations of PCR reaction components were prepared as follows: 2.0 mM $MgCl_2$, 0.2 mM dNTPs, 0.5 μM of each forward and revers primers and 0.5 U Hot Start DNA polymerase and 5 μl of extracted DNA. The reaction mixture (25 μl) was incubated at 95 °C for 15 min., followed by 45 cycles at 94 °C for 1 min., 57 °C for 1 min., 72 °C for 1 min., a final extension at 72 °C for 10 mins. The PCR products were analyzed by gel electrophoresis in a 3% agarose gel and visualized under UV light.

## Serological tests

To detect antibody levels serological tests were used with ELISA method. Designed antibodies: anti-VCA IgM (Nova-Lisa Epstein-Barr Virus VCA IgM/Nova Tec Immunodiagnostica GmbH/Germany/catalog number: EBVM0150), anti-VCA IgG (NovaLisa Epstein-Barr Virus VCA IgG/Nova Tec Immunodiagnostica GmbH/Germany/catalog number: EBVG0150), and anti-EBNA IgG (NovaLisa Epstein-Barr Virus EBNA IgG/Nova Tec Immunodiagnostica GmbH/Germany/catalog number: EBVG0580), antibodies anti-EA IgG (ELISA-VIDITEST anti-EA (D) EBV IgG/Vidia/Czech Republic/catalog number: ODZ-006). All tests were performed according to the manufacturer's instructions.

The NovaTec Epstein-Barr Virus (EBV) IgG-ELISA is intended for the qualitative determination of IgG class antibodies against Epstein-Barr virus. Samples are considered positive if the absorbance value is higher than 10% over the cut-off. The level of antibodies is expressed as NovaTec-Units = NTU.

ELISA-VIDITEST anti-EA is semiquantitative test. Samples with absorbances higher than 110% of the cut-off value are considered positive.

## Statistical analysis

Descriptive statistics were used to characterize patient baseline characteristics. The Mann-Whitney $U$-test and Kruskal-Wallis test were used to compare antibody levels. Pearson's chi-square test was used to investigate the relationship between EBNA2 subtypes and LMP1 subtype and clinical and demographical parameters. Statistical significance was defined as $p < 0.05$.

## Results

EBV DNA was detected in 52.70% of the patients with pharyngeal and laryngeal cancer and in 25.0% of controls ($p < 0.001$). In all patients with EBV DNA type 1 of the virus was detected. Epidemiological and demographical characteristics of the patients and controls are shown in Table 1.

The prevalence of EBV in patients group was significantly higher in males than in females ($p < 0.05$). No statistically significant differences were found between EBV infection and other demographical features, smoking and alcohol consumption (Table 2). The majority of patients (82.8%) were infected with wild type of EBV.

All the patients and controls were EBVCA IgM antibodies negative. IgG EBVCA antibodies were detected in 94.5% of patients, EBNA in 96.4% (Table 3). A statistically significant difference was observed in the prevalence of IgG EA antibodies in patients and controls (94.5% vs 22.5%). High level of EA was stated in 70% of cancer cases and in 0% of controls ($p < 0.05$). The level of IgG EBVCA and IgG EBNA antibodies was higher in the patients than in control group; however, the difference was not statistically significant.

Patients with an advanced stage of tumour development (T3-T4 stage) had a significantly higher level of EBNA antibodies than patients with T1-T2 stage ($p < 0.05$), while the level of EBVCA antibodies was the highest in patients with N1 stage. The level of EBVCA antibodies decreased with more advanced nodal stage ($p < 0.05$) (Table 4).

In patients infected with the wild-type of EBV, the level of anti-EBVCA was significantly higher than in cases with EBV type with deletion ($p < 0.05$). There was no relationship between EBV type on the basis of the

**Table 3** EBVCA, EBNA and EA level in serum of patients and control group

| Antibodies level (IgG) | | Patients | | Controls | | p |
|---|---|---|---|---|---|---|
| | | n | % | n | % | |
| EBVCA | negative | 6 | 5.5 | 0 | 0 | >0.05 |
| | low | 24 | 21.8 | 14 | 35.0 | |
| | high | 80 | 72.7 | 26 | 65.0 | |
| EBNA | negative | 4 | 3.6 | 0 | 0 | >0.05 |
| | low | 23 | 20.9 | 12 | 30.0 | |
| | high | 83 | 75.5 | 28 | 70.0 | |
| EA | negative | 6 | 5.5 | 31 | 77.5 | <0.05* |
| | low | 27 | 24.5 | 9 | 22.5 | |
| | high | 77 | 70.0 | 0 | 0 | |

*statistically significant

**Table 4** Association between EBVCA, EBNA, EA antibodies level in patients serum and selected features (p value)

| Histological grading TN classification | EBVCA IgG | EBNA IgG | EA IgG |
|---|---|---|---|
| Histological grade G | 0.9139 | 0.2222 | 0.5587 |
| T stage | 0.6359 | 0.0174[a] | 0.1759 |
| N stage | 0.0126[a] | 0.5920 | 0.4201 |
| EBV type LMP1 vs del-LMP1 | 0.0379[a] | 0.4479 | 0.3622 |
| Location of cancer | 0.8875 | 0.9363 | 0.9485 |

[a]statistically significant

sequence in LMP1 gene, histological grading, and TN stage (Table 5).

## Discussion

Two major types of EBV (EBV-1 and EBV-2) have been identified (a classification based on the EBNA2 gene sequence) and according to the researchers they differ in geographic distribution [6, 16]. According to some investigators, these genetic differences in EBV DNA sequence may be responsible for varied interactions with host cells, immunological response and cancer transformation, but the role of specific EBV types in the etiology of different cancers is not fully understood [17, 18]. EBV type 1 has a greater potential to transform B lymphocytes than EBV type 2 and is more common in Western and Asian countries, while EBV-2 is more frequently detected in Africa [16]. The results of our present and previous studies are consistent with the existing reports as type 1 EBV was detected in all examined patients [19]. Similar results were presented by Neves et al. [18], who demonstrated that 96.3% of the examined Portuguese individuals carried EBV type 1.

**Table 5** Relationship between EBV type according to the LMP1 gene sequence and histological grading, TN stage

| Histological grading TN classification | EBV LMP1 | | EBV del-LMP1 | | p |
|---|---|---|---|---|---|
| | n | % | n | % | |
| G1 | 16 | 72.7 | 6 | 27.3 | 0.05113 |
| G2 | 30 | 88.2 | 4 | 11.8 | |
| G3 | 2 | 100.0 | 0 | 0 | |
| T1 | 6 | 100.0 | 0 | 0 | 0.2786 |
| T2 | 24 | 85.7 | 4 | 14.3 | |
| T3 | 14 | 87.5 | 2 | 12.5 | |
| T4 | 4 | 50.0 | 2 | 50.0 | |
| N0 | 26 | 86.7 | 4 | 13.3 | 0.6293 |
| N1 | 8 | 80.0 | 2 | 20.0 | |
| N2 | 12 | 85.7 | 2 | 14.3 | |
| N3 | 2 | 50.0 | 2 | 50.0 | |

As the disease progresses, EBV is activated into the replicative stage, in which major viral proteins are expressed [20, 21]. Patients with nasopharyngeal carcinoma show an elevated level of antibodies to several EBV antigens, including the viral capsid antigen (VCA), early antigen (EA) and EB nuclear antigen (EBNA) [22–25]. Traditional assays of EBV antibodies have been very useful in clinical diagnosis of nasopharyngeal cancer (NPC) [26].

Our study revealed that more than half of the patients were EBV positive but also the level of IgG EBV antibodies was higher in patients than in controls and it increased with the tumour development stage. Moreover, the difference in EBV DNA prevalence between patients and controls was statistically significant.

Serological testing was performed both in the patients and in the controls to clarify whether there is a relationship between pharyngeal and laryngeal cancer development and past EBV infection. Various studies revealed that IgG EBV antibodies were detected in a greater part of the examined patients and their level was higher in the patients with pharyngeal and laryngeal cancers than in controls [24, 27, 28]. Other researchers report IgG EBVCA antibodies detection in more than 60% of patients with laryngeal and pharyngeal cancers [29].

Our study did not reveal any significant difference between the presence and the level of EBV antibodies and demographical features of the patients, cancer location and histological grading of malignant lesions. However, patients with an advanced stage of tumour development (T3-T4 stage) had a significantly higher level of EBNA antibodies than patients with T1-T2 stage, while the level of EBVCA antibodies was the highest in patients with N1 stage. The more advanced nodal stage was, the more the level of these antibodies decreased.

The level of EA antibodies among our patients was higher than in control group. Our results are similar to other researchers' findings and may indicate a reactivation of latent EBV infection, because a high titer of EA antibodies can be seen in cases of reactivation of latent infection [25].

Statistically significant differences were observed by Chen et al. [30] in the scores/levels of six markers (EVB-IgG, VCA-IgG, EA-D p43-IgG, EA-IgG, EA-IgG + EBNA1-IgG, and EA-D p45-IgG) between NPC patients and healthy subjects. The lytic cycle of EBV is important and plays more active roles in oncogenesis [31].

Many authors show that EBV DNA load and IgA antibodies are more effective and useful in the clinical diagnosis and screening of NPC [32–34]. In our study only IgG antibodies were analysed. Immunoglobulins against viral proteins, including EA-IgG, VCA-IgA, and Rta-IgG, may be used as molecular biomarkers for predicting the prognosis of nasopharyngeal cancer. According to Tay et al. [24], EBV DNA load correlated with EA IgA serology titers may be useful in detecting early NPC in screening studies.

EBV is transmitted via oral route and primary infection establishes a lifelong virus latent infection. The establishment of latent EBV infection in premalignant nasopharyngeal epithelial cells and the expression of latent viral genes are crucial features of NPC [14, 35].

Latent infection was divided into different subgroups due to specific viral proteins expression [12, 31, 34]. Nasopharyngeal carcinoma can display both latency type I and II EBV infections [36]. During type I latency EBNA1, EBER1 and 2, BamHI-A rightward transcripts (BART) are expressed, but type II latency can also express latent membrane protein 1 (LMP1). The oncogenic role of LMP1 is well established. In nasopharyngeal carcinoma LMP1 expression is associated with TNM stage and lymph node metastasis [37]. The EBV variant with a 30 bp deletion ((amino acids 346–355) includes part of C terminal activating region 2) isolated from an NPC tumor had a greater transforming activity than the reference LMP1 [38]. The 30 bp deletion variant (del-LMP1) was first detected in EBV isolated from cell lines derived from NPC patients from Southern China [39]. Molecular studies demonstrated that a higher frequency of nasopharyngeal cancer detected in Asian population contains a variant of EBV LMP1 gene with a 30-bp deletion (del-LMP1) [16, 34].

According to some researchers, EBV del-LMP1 plays a key role in nasopharyngeal cancer development and might be detected at higher frequencies in NPC patients than in the general population. Other investigators, however, suggest that del-LMP1 is only a geographic variation – it is more common in the Chinese population but not involved in the pathogenesis of NPC, as no association was found between the del-LMP1 and NPC. Hadhri et al. [40] found that del-LMP1 variant was significantly more frequent in NPC (71.42%) than in control biopsies (52%) in Tunisia. Tiwawech et al. [16] also reported that a significant association between the del-LMP1 variant and NPC susceptibility was found in the Thai. Moreover, the frequency of del-LMP1 in NPC patients was associated with the clinical stage of NPC [39].

Our study demonstrated that in the Polish population with oropharyngeal and laryngeal cancer wild-type LMP1 was more frequent (83%). A limitation of our research is, however, small size of del-LMP1 group, which makes statistical data comparing relationship between EBV type on the basis of the sequence in LMP1 gene and histological grading or TN stage not sufficiently strong. Neves et al. [18] demonstrated that EBV-2 and wt-LMP1 were associated with NPC in the Portuguese population. Their research performed in a similar ethnic group – Portuguese individuals – revealed no predominance of a specific LPM1 variant as not only both variants

but also co-infection was common in this population. However, contrary to the Chinese population these authors found that the majority of NPC patients were wt-LMP1, which pointed to a differential geographic association of EBV-strains with NPC development.

Although the association between EBV infection and head and neck cancer was reported in various studies, the mechanism of malignancy development is still not clear. Understanding the role of the EBV latent genes expressed in pharyngeal and laryngeal cancers is crucial in determining the role of viral infection in the development and progression of cancer in this area.

## Conclusions

Our results reveal that EBV DNA and a high level of antibodies, particularly EA, are most frequent and the wild type EBV is predominant in Polish patients with both pharyngeal and laryngeal carcinoma. However, further studies are necessary to clarify the role of Epstein-Barr virus in cancer development because genetic and epigenetic changes occur after EBV infection.

**Abbreviations**
BL: Burkitt's lymphoma; del-LMP1: deletion variant of latent membrane protein 1; EA: Early antigen; EBNA: Epstein-Barr nuclear antigen; EBV: Epstein-Barr virus; EBVCA: Epstein-Barr viral capsid antigen; HL: Hodgkin lymphoma; HNC: Head and neck cancer; LMP1: Latent membrane protein 1; NPC: Nasopharyngeal cancer; TN: Tumour, node; VCA: Viral capsid antigen; wt-LMP1: wild type latent membrane protein 1

**Acknowledgements**
Not applicable.

**Funding**
This study was supported by a Research Grant from the Medical University of Lublin, Lublin, Poland (DS 233).

**Authors' contributions**
SF: Conceived the study, its design, data and clinical samples collection. MS-D: data analysis, manuscript preparation. BD: Statistical and data analysis. AB: carried out serological and molecular identification. MP-D: conceived the study, data analysis, coordination and help in drafting the manuscript. All authors read and approved the final manuscript.

**Competing interests**
The authors declare that they have no competing interests.

**Author details**
[1]Department of Virology, Medical University of Lublin, Lublin, Poland. [2]Chair and Department of Conservative Dentistry with Endodontics, Medical University of Lublin, Lublin, Poland. [3]Chair and Department of Public Health, Medical University of Lublin, Lublin, Poland.

## References

1. Hillbertz NS, Hirsch JM, Jalouli J, Jalouli MM, Sand L. Viral and molecular aspects of oral cancer. Anticancer Res. 2012;32(10):4201–12.

2. Young LS, Rickinson AB. Epstein-Barr virus: 40 years on. Nat Rev Cancer. 2004;4(10):757–68.

3. Macsween KF, Higgins CD, McAulay KA, Williams H, Harrison N, Swerdlow AJ, et al. Infectious mononucleosis in university students in the United Kingdom: evaluation of the clinical features and consequences of the disease. Clin Infect Dis. 2010;50(5):699–706.

4. Tsang CM, Tsao SW. The role of Epstein-Barr virus infection in the pathogenesis of nasopharyngeal carcinoma. Virol Sin. 2015;30(2):107–21.

5. Raab-Traub N. Nasopharyngeal carcinoma: an evolving role for the Epstein-Barr virus. Curr Top Microbiol Immunol. 2015;390:339–63.

6. Deng Z, Uehara T, Maeda H, Hasegawa M, Matayoshi S, Kiyuna A, et al. Epstein-Barr virus and human papillomavirus infections and genotype distribution in head and neck cancers. PLoS One. 2014;9(11), e113702.

7. Jalouli J, Jalouli MM, Sapkota D, Ibrahim SO, Larsson PA, Sand L. Human Papilloma virus, Herpes Simplex virus and Epstein Barr virus in oral squamous cell carcinoma from eight different countries. Anticancer Res. 2012;32:571–80.

8. Alibek K, Kakpenova A, Baiken Y. Role of infectious agents in the carcinogenesis of brain and head and neck cancers. Infect Agent Cancer. 2013;8(1):7.

9. Khan G, Hashim MJ. Global burden of deaths from Epstein-Barr virus attributable malignancies 1990–2010. Infect Agent Cancer. 2014;9(1):38.

10. Gandini S, Negri E, Boffetta P, La Vecchia C, Boyle P. Mouthwash and oral cancer risk quantitative meta-analysis of epidemiologic studies. Ann Agric Environ Med. 2012;19(2):173–80.

11. Sand L, Jalouli J. Viruses and oral cancer. Is there a link? Microbes Infect. 2014;16(5):371–8.

12. Bornkamm GW. Epstein-Barr virus and the pathogenesis of Burkitt's lymphoma: more questions than answers. Int J Cancer. 2009;124(8):1745–55.

13. Shield KD, Ferlay J, Jemal A, Sankaranarayanan R, Chaturvedi AK, Bray F, et al. The global incidence of lip, oral cavity, and pharyngeal cancers by subsite in 2012. CA Cancer J Clin. 2017;67(1):51–64.

14. Young LS, Dawson CW. Epstein-Barr virus and nasopharyngeal carcinoma. Chin J Cancer. 2014;33(12):581–90.

15. Kis A, Fehér E, Gáll T, Tar I, Boda R, Tóth ED, et al. Epstein-Barr virus prevalence in oral squamous cell cancer and in potentially malignant oral disorders in an eastern Hungarian population. Eur J OralSci. 2009;117(5):536–40.

16. Tiwawech D, Srivatanakul P, Karalak A, Ishida T. Association between EBNA2 and LMP1 subtypes of Epstein-Barr virus and nasopharyngeal carcinoma in Thais. J Clin Virol. 2008;42(1):1–6.

17. IARC monographs on the evaluation of carcinogenic risks to humans. A review of human carcinogens. Biological agents. Lyon: World Health Organization; 2012. p. 255.

18. Neves M, Marinho-Dias J, Ribeiro J, Esteves M, Maltez E, Baldaque I, et al. Characterization of Epstein-Barr virus strains and LMP1-deletion variants in Portugal. J Med Virol. 2015;87(8):1382–8.

19. Polz D, Podsiadło Ł, Stec A, Polz-Dacewicz M. Prevalence of EBV genotypes in Polish, Taiwanese and Arabic healthy students and association between genotypes and 30-bp deletion in the LMP-1 gene phylogenetic analysis. Pol J Microbiol. 2014;63(1):105–9.

20. Makielski KR, Lee D, Lorenz LD, Nawandar DM, Chiu YF, Kenney SC, et al. Human papillomavirus promotes Epstein-Barr virus maintenance and lytic reactivation in immortalized oral keratinocytes. Virology. 2016;495:52–62.

21. Ji MF, Huang QH, Yu X, Liu Z, Li X, Zhang LF, et al. Evaluation of plasma Epstein-Barr virus DNA load to distinguish nasopharyngeal carcinoma patients from healthy high-risk populations in Southern China. Cancer. 2014;120(9):1353–60.

22. Abdulamir AS, Hafidh RR, Abu Bakar F, Abbas K. Novel Epstein-Barr virus immunoglobulin G-based approach for the specific detection of nasopharyngeal carcinoma. Am J Otolaryngol. 2010;31(6):410–7.

23. Linde A. Diagnosis of Epstein-Barr virus-related diseases. Scand J Infect Dis Suppl. 1996;100:83–8.

24. Tay JK, Chan SH, Lim CM, Siow CH, Goh HL, Loh KS. The role of Epstein-Barr Virus DNA load and serology as screening tools for nasopharyngeal carcinoma. Otolaryngol Head Neck Surg. 2016;155(2):274–80.

25. De Paschale M, Clerici P. Serological diagnosis of Epstein-Barr virus infection: problems and solutions. World J Virol. 2012;1(1):31–43.

26. Chang KP, Hsu CL, Chang YL, Tsang NM, Chen CK, Lee TJ, et al. Complementary serum test of antibodies to Epstein-Barr virus nuclear antigen-1 and early antigen: a possible alternative for primary screening of nasopharyngeal carcinoma. Oral Oncol. 2008;44(8):784–92.

27. Chien YC, Chen JY, Liu MY, Yang HI, Hsu MM, Chen CJ, et al. Serologic markers of Epstein-Barr virus infection and nasopharyngeal carcinoma in Taiwanese men. N Engl J Med. 2001;345(26):1877–82.

28. Coghill AE, Hsu WL, Pfeiffer RM, Juwana H, Yu KJ, Lou PJ, et al. Epstein-Barr virus serology as a potential screening marker for nasopharyngeal carcinoma among high-risk individuals from multiplex families in Taiwan. Cancer Epidemiol Biomarkers Prev. 2014;23(7):1213–9.

29. Roy A, Dey S, Chatterjee R. Prevalence of serum IgG and IgM antibodies against Epstein-Barr virus capsid antigen in Indian patients with respiratory tract carcinomas. Neoplasma. 1994;41(1):29–33.

30. Chen H, Luo YL, Zhang L, Tian LZ, Feng ZT, Liu WL. EA-D p45-IgG as a potential biomarker for nasopharyngeal carcinoma diagnosis. Asian Pac J Cancer Prev. 2013;14(12):7433–8.

31. Murata T. Regulation of Epstein–Barr virus reactivation from latency. Microbiol Immunol. 2014;58(6):307–17.

32. Li Y, Wang K, Yin SK, Zheng HL, Min DL. Expression of Epstein-Barr virus antibodies EA-IgG, Rta-IgG, and VCA-IgA in nasopharyngeal carcinoma and their use in a combined diagnostic assay. Genet Mol Res. 2016;15(1).

33. Peng YH, Xu YW, Huang LS, Zhai TT, Dai LH, Qiu SQ, et al. Autoantibody signatures combined with Epstein-Barr virus capsid antigen-IgA as a biomarker panel for the detection of nasopharyngeal carcinoma. Cancer Prev Res (Phila). 2015;8(8):729–36.

34. Kikuchi K, Noguchi Y, de Rivera MW, Hoshino M, Sakashita H, Yamada T, et al. Detection of Epstein-Barr virus genome and latent infection gene expression in normal epithelia, epithelial dysplasia, and squamous cell carcinoma of the oral cavity. Tumour Biol. 2016;37(3):3389–404.

35. Kang MS, Kieff E. Epstein-Barr virus latent genes. Exp Mol Med. 2015;47:e131.

36. Frappier L. Role of EBNA1 in NPC tumourigenesis. Semin Cancer Biol. 2012;22(2):154–61.

37. Wang A, Zhang W, Jin M, Zhang J, Li S, Tong F, Zhou Y. Differential expression of EBV proteins LMP1 and BHFR1 in EBV-associated gastric and nasopharyngeal cancer tissues. Mol Med Rep. 2016;13(5):4151–8.

38. Tzellos S, Farrell PJ. Epstein-Barr virus sequence variation ⁻ biology and disease. Pathogens. 2012;1(2):156–74.

39. Ai J, Xie Z, Liu C, Huang Z, Xu J. Analysis of EBNA-1 and LMP-1 variants in diseases associated with EBV infection in Chinese children. Virol J. 2012;9:13.

40. Hadhri-Guiga B, Khabir AM, Mokdad-Gargouri R, Ghorbel AM, Drira M, Daoud J, Frikha M, et al. Various 30 and 69 bp deletion variants of the Epstein-Barr virus LMP1 may arise by homologous recombination in nasopharyngeal carcinoma of Tunisian patients. Virus Res. 2006;115(1):24–30.

# 8

# Low prevalence of human mammary tumor virus (HMTV) in breast cancer patients from Myanmar

Thar Htet San[1], Masayoshi Fujisawa[1], Soichiro Fushimi[1,2], Teizo Yoshimura[1], Toshiaki Ohara[1], Lamin Soe[3], Ngu Wah Min[4], Ohnmar Kyaw[5], Xu Yang[1] and Akihiro Matsukawa[1*]

## Abstract

**Background:** Human mammary tumor virus (HMTV) is 90–95% homologous to mouse mammary tumor virus (MMTV), one of the causal agents of murine mammary tumors. HMTV (MMTV-like) sequences were reported to be present in human breast cancers from several populations with a prevalence range of 0–78%; however, the prevalence of HMTV in breast cancers from Myanmar remains unknown.

**Methods:** Fifty-eight breast cancer samples from Myanmar women were examined in this study. DNA was isolated from formalin-fixed paraffin-embedded specimens, and HMTV envelope sequences were detected by semi-nested PCR. The sequence of the PCR products was also confirmed.

**Results:** Only 1.7% (1 of 58) of the breast cancers were positive for HMTV, and the sequence of PCR products was 98.9% identical to the reference HMTV sequence (GenBank accession No. AF243039). The tumor with HMTV was grade III invasive ductal carcinoma, 7.0 cm in size with lymph node metastasis (T3, N1, M0).

**Conclusions:** We, for the first time, investigated the presence of HMTV in Myanmar breast cancer patients. In accordance with other Asian studies, the prevalence of HMTV in Myanmar was quite low, supporting the hypothesis that Asian breast cancers have different etiologies than in Western countries, where HMTV is more prevalent.

**Keywords:** Human mammary tumor virus, Mouse mammary tumor virus, Breast cancer

## Background

Worldwide, breast cancer is the most frequently diagnosed cancer affecting women, with an estimated 1.7 million cases and 521,900 deaths in 2012 [1, 2]. The incidence of breast cancer is higher in developed countries, while the mortality is higher in developing countries. These discrepancies in incidence and mortality are attributed to early detection as well as risk factors including geographic variation, racial/ethnic background, genetic variation, lifestyle, and reproductive patterns associated with urbanization and economic development [3, 4].

The etiology of human breast cancer can be significantly affected by environmental factors, including viruses [5, 6]. Among them, mouse mammary tumor virus (MMTV) is a non-acute transforming type B retrovirus that causes the majority of mammary tumors in mice. MMTV induces premalignant lesions and malignant tumors of the breast by acting as an insertional mutagen or activating the transcription of nearby oncogenes [7, 8]. In 1995, retroviral sequences 90–95% homologous to MMTV were detected in 39% of human breast cancers in the United States [9]. Subsequently, a 9.9-kb proviral structure, which was 95% homologous to MMTV, was successfully amplified from two distinct human breast cancers. The retrovirus with MMTV-like sequence was subsequently designated human mammary tumor virus (HMTV) [10]. Very recently, MMTV-like sequences were found in breast tissues prior to the development of virus-positive breast cancer, indicating a

* Correspondence: amatsu@md.okayama-u.ac.jp
[1]Department of Pathology and Experimental Medicine, Graduate School of Medicine, Dentistry and Pharmaceutical Sciences, Okayama University, 2-5-1 Shikata, Okayama 700-8558, Japan
Full list of author information is available at the end of the article

possible causal role in the development of breast cancer [11]. To understand the involvement of HMTV/MMTV-like sequence in the carcinogenesis of breast cancer, it is important to obtain more clinical and epidemiological data in breast cancer worldwide.

As with other countries, breast cancer is a leading cause of morbidity and mortality in Myanmar women [12]. The purpose of this study was to investigate the prevalence of HMTV in breast cancers in Myanmar.

## Methods

### Study subjects

In this study, we employed 58 breast cancer cases diagnosed in 2015 at Myeik General Hospital (Myeik City, Myanmar) and Sakura Specialist Hospital (Yangon City, Myanmar). All hematoxylin and eosin-stained sections were reviewed by two independent pathologists. The criteria defined by the World Health Organization (2012) were used for the histopathological diagnosis and classification of breast carcinoma [13]. Nottingham combined histological grading system [14] was used for tumor grading. American Joint Committee on Cancer staging system 8th edition was applied for tumor staging. The experimental protocol employed in this study was approved by the Ethics Committee of Okayama University and the Ethics Review Committee of Department of Medical Research of Yangon City (Myanmar).

### DNA extraction

Two to four 10-μm-thick sections were cut from each paraffin block, and genomic DNA was extracted using the Nucleospin DNA FFPE XS kit (Macherey-Nagel, Düren, Germany) according to the manufacturer's instructions. The amount of extracted DNA was measured on a Nanodrop 1000 spectrophotometer (Thermo Fisher Scientific, Waltham, MA, USA). The A260:A280 ratio was used to measure the purity of DNA (~1.80). DNA quality was also confirmed by PCR amplification of the 268 bp β-globin gene using GH20 and PC04 primers

(Table 1). All samples employed in this study were qualified for HMTV detection.

### Detection of HMTV sequence by PCR

The detection of HMTV DNA sequences was performed using a semi-nested PCR approach. Primers were carefully selected from those stated to successfully amplify HMTV sequences in previous literature [15–18]. In the first-round of PCR, primers 5 F and MR1 were used to amplify a 246-bp segment. In the second-round of PCR, the same forward primer (5 F) and a different reverse primer (2NR) were used to amplify a 189-bp HMTV sequence. PCR reactions were performed in a 20 μl volume and contained 0.02 μM and 0.2 μM of primers, together with reagents from the Pyromark PCR kit (QIAGEN, Hilden, Germany) according to the manufacturer's instructions. Approximately 250 ng of extracted DNA was used as template for first-round PCR and 2 μl of first-round PCR product was used as template for second-round PCR. PCR products were electrophoresed on 2% agarose gels containing ethidium bromide and visualized with ultraviolet light. RCB0526:Jyg-MC(A) cells (Riken Bioresource Center, Tsukuba, Japan), a murine mammary tumor cell line expressing high MMTV levels, were cultivated, harvested and the extracted DNA was used as a positive control.

To exclude murine DNA contamination in the HMTV-positive sample, mouse-specific mitochondrial (mt) DNA was amplified by semi-nested PCR using the primers mt15982F and mt16267R for the first-round PCR and mt16115F and mt16267R for the second-round PCR, which yielded a final PCR product of 153-bp. DNA extracted from the 4 T1 murine breast cancer cell line was used as positive control.

The list of all primers used and their positions in the genome are shown in Table 1. PCR conditions were as follows: β-globin: 95 °C for 15 min, 40 cycles of 95 °C for 30 s, 55 °C for 30 s, and 72 °C for 1 min, and then 72 °C for 7 min; HMTV: first-round PCR: 95 °C for

**Table 1** List of primers, their sequences and positions in the genome

| gene | primer | sequence (5′–3′) | nucleotide position |
|---|---|---|---|
| β-globin | GH20 | GAAGAGCCAAGGACAGGTAC | 1417-1436[a] |
| | PC04 | CAACTTCATCCACGTTCACC | 1684-1665[a] |
| HMTV | 5 F | GTATGAAGCAGGATGGGTAGA | 235-255[b] |
| | MR1 | CCTCTTTTCTCTATATCTATTAGCTGAGGTAATC | 480-446[b] |
| | 2NR | GTAACACAGGCAGATGTAGG | 423-404[b] |
| mt DNA | mt15982F | AGACGCACCTACGGTGAAGA | 15982-16001[c] |
| | mt16115F | TGCCAAACCCCAAAAACACT | 16115-16134[c] |
| | mt16267R | AGAGTTTTGGTTCACGGAACATGA | 16267-16244[c] |

[a]Refers to *Homo sapiens* β-globin gene, complete cds (Genbank AH001475)
[b]Refers to human mammary tumor virus SAG pseudogene, complete sequence (Genbank AF243039)
[c]Refers to *Mus musculus* complete mitochondrial genome, strain Balb/cJ (Genbank AJ512208)

15 min and 40 cycles of 30 s at 95 °C, 30 s at 58 °C and 1 min at 72 °C, and then 72 °C for 7 min; second-round PCR: 95 °C for 15 min and 35 cycles of 30 s at 95 °C, 30 s at 60 °C and 1 min at 72 °C, and then 72 °C for 7 min; mt DNA: first-round PCR: 95 °C for 15 min and 40 cycles of 30 s at 95 °C, 30 s at 55 °C and 1 min at 72 °C, and then 72 °C for 7 min; second-round PCR: 95 °C for 15 min and 35 cycles of 30 s at 95 °C, 30 s at 55 °C and 1 min at 72 °C, and then 72 °C for 7 min.

## DNA sequencing

Sequencing was performed using an ABI3130*xl* Genetic Analyzer (Applied Biosystems, Waltham, MA, USA) at the Central Research Laboratory of Okayama University. PCR products were isolated from gels, sequenced and aligned by a BLAST search (NCBI).

## Results

### Patient characteristics

Clinical data for the 58 breast cancer patients are shown in Table 2. Ages ranged from 30 to 81 years with a mean age of 50.3 years. Tumor sizes ranged from 1.5 cm to 7.2 cm with an average size of 4.0 cm. Most of the cancers (97%) were invasive ductal carcinoma with high histological grade (grade II and III). No grade I malignancies were found. There were lymph nodes metastases in 57% of the cases.

**Table 2** Clinical data for the enrolled breast cancer patients

|  | categories | number of cases (%) |
|---|---|---|
| Age (years) | <35 | 4 (6.9) |
|  | 35–50 | 24 (41.4) |
|  | >50 | 30 (51.7) |
| Tumor size (cm) | ≦2.0 | 4 (6.9) |
|  | 2.1–5.0 | 39 (67.2) |
|  | >5.0 | 15 (25.9) |
| Pathological diagnosis | Invasive ductal carcinoma | 56 (96.6) |
|  | Mucinous carcinoma | 1 (1.7) |
|  | Carcinoma with neuroendocrine differentiation | 1 (1.7) |
| Histological grade | Grade I | 0 (0.0) |
|  | Grade II | 26 (44.8) |
|  | Grade III | 32 (55.2) |
| Lymph node metastasis | Absent | 25 (43.1) |
|  | Present | 33 (56.9) |
| Stage | Stage I | 4 (6.9) |
|  | Stage II | 30 (51.7) |
|  | Stage III | 22 (37.9) |
|  | Stage IV | 2 (3.4) |

## Detection of HMTV

Experiments were conducted to analyze the prevalence of HMTV. Genomic DNA was extracted from each paraffin block and its quality was measured using the A260:A280 ratio (>1.80) and a distinct β-globin PCR product. HMTV sequence was investigated in all 58 samples using semi-nested PCR, which revealed one case (MB14) was positive for HMTV (Fig. 1). The PCR reaction was confirmed by repeating the semi-nested PCR using newly extracted DNA from the paraffin block (not shown). The positive band was cut from the gel, and the PCR product was sequenced. The complete 189-bp PCR product sequence was aligned to two published HMTV sequences, and the reference sequence of the positive control (Fig. 2). The sequence was 98.9% identical to the original proviral HMTV sequence (GenBank AF243039) and HMTV sequence from Vietnam (GenBank AY161347). Although MB14-sequence showed 92% homology with control MMTV (GenBank AK145002), we attempted to exclude murine DNA contamination in MB14-DNA. For this, MB14-DNA (250 ng) was amplified using primers for mouse mitochondrial DNA. 4 T1-DNA was used as a positive control murine DNA. The data in Fig. 3 demonstrated that there was no contamination of murine DNA in MB14-DNA. The detection limit of this assay was more than 0.8 pg DNA (Fig. 3). The HMTV-positive case was invasive carcinoma, 7.0 cm in size, histological grade III, with lymph node metastasis.

## Discussion

HMTV has been detected at different frequencies in different countries. We, for the first time in this study, investigated the prevalence of HMTV in breast cancers in Myanmar. Semi-nested PCR and sequencing data showed that the prevalence of HMTV was very low (1.7%, 1 of 58 cases). To the best of our knowledge, the prevalence of HMTV (MMTV-like) sequences in breast cancers has been reported for 17 countries, including the present study. Figure 4 shows the prevalence of HMTV on the world-map from these reports.

The prevalence of HMTV shows geographic heterogeneity. A high prevalence of HMTV was detected in North and South America, Australia and Mediterranean countries, where the range is from 12 to 78% (average 49.4%) [18–25]. Conversely, HMTV was not detected in Central and Northern Europe [26–29]. In Asia, no or few cases are positive for HMTV in Japan [30], Iran [31], Vietnam [15] and Myanmar (this study). The prevalence of HMTV in Myanmar breast cancers (1.7%) is comparable to that of a Vietnamese study (0.8%) [15]. More intriguingly, the sequence of HMTV reported in the Vietnamese study (GenBank AY161347) was 98.9%

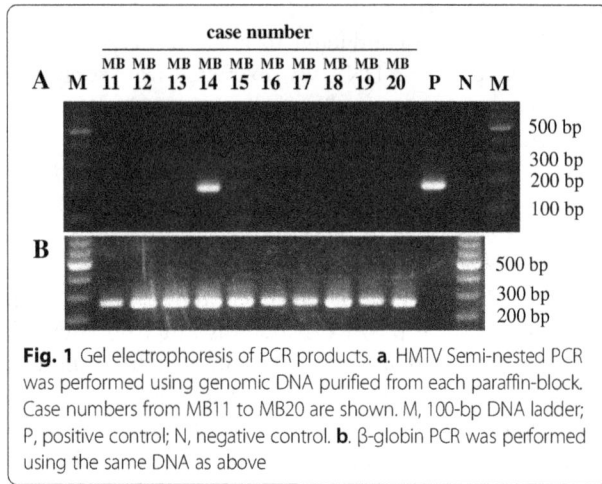

**Fig. 1** Gel electrophoresis of PCR products. **a.** HMTV Semi-nested PCR was performed using genomic DNA purified from each paraffin-block. Case numbers from MB11 to MB20 are shown. M, 100-bp DNA ladder; P, positive control; N, negative control. **b.** β-globin PCR was performed using the same DNA as above

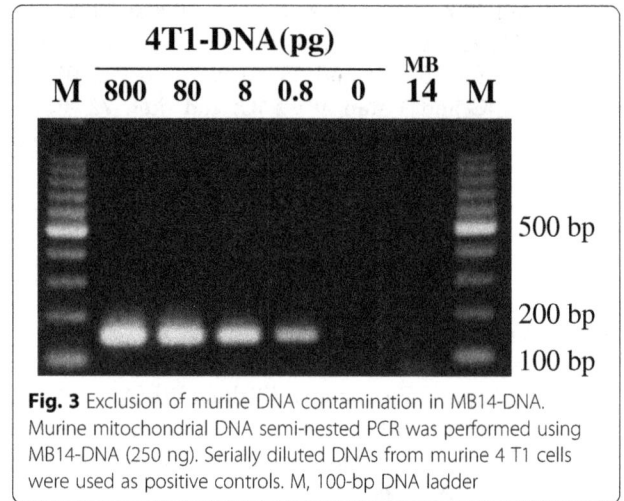

**Fig. 3** Exclusion of murine DNA contamination in MB14-DNA. Murine mitochondrial DNA semi-nested PCR was performed using MB14-DNA (250 ng). Serially diluted DNAs from murine 4 T1 cells were used as positive controls. M, 100-bp DNA ladder

identical to that seen in this Myanmar case, suggesting there may be a close etiological relationship between the two countries. Although the prevalence in China and Pakistan was high (16.8 and 20.0%, respectively) [32, 33], no sequence was confirmed in the Chinese study, and only 2 of 16 positive cases were confirmed in the Pakistani study. A recent study in Iran showed that 12% of cases were positive, but none of the sequences were confirmed [34]. These data appear to be contingent and necessitate further study.

Interestingly, Asian countries with zero or low HMTV prevalence such as Japan, Vietnam and Myanmar have low breast cancer incidence (51.5, 23.0 and 22.1 per 100,000 women, respectively) compared with countries with high HMTV prevalence like the United States, Italy and Australia (92.9, 91.3 and 86.0 per 100,000 women, respectively) (http://globocan.iarc.fr.). Breast cancer develops at earlier ages in Asia (peak incidence between 40 and 50 years) than in Western countries (peak incidence

between 60 and 70 years) [35]. These differences may reflect distinct characteristics and etiological backgrounds. There is an interesting report hypothesizing that human breast cancer could be correlated with the natural ranges of different species of wild mice [36]. *Mus domesticus,* having the highest numbers of endogenous MMTV proviral loci, inhabits the United States, Italy and Australia, where the prevalence of HMTV in breast cancers is high. On the other hand, *M. musculus* and *M. castaneus,* having the fewest MMTV proviral loci, ranges from central Europe east to China and Japan and from southern China to central Iran, respectively.

A question arises about the sensitivity of the detection system. False negatives may be present in zero or low prevalence reports as primers and/or reaction conditions are critical in the detection system [37, 38]; however, this is unlikely in this study. We employed a highly sensitive methodology (semi-nested PCR) together with a proper positive control, a murine mammary tumor

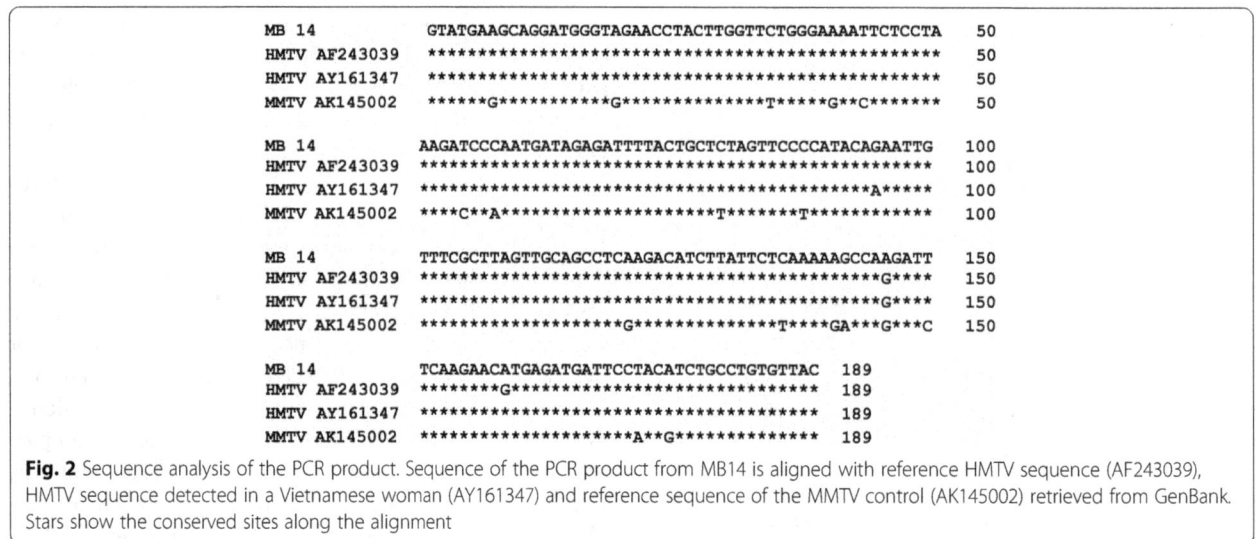

**Fig. 2** Sequence analysis of the PCR product. Sequence of the PCR product from MB14 is aligned with reference HMTV sequence (AF243039), HMTV sequence detected in a Vietnamese woman (AY161347) and reference sequence of the MMTV control (AK145002) retrieved from GenBank. Stars show the conserved sites along the alignment

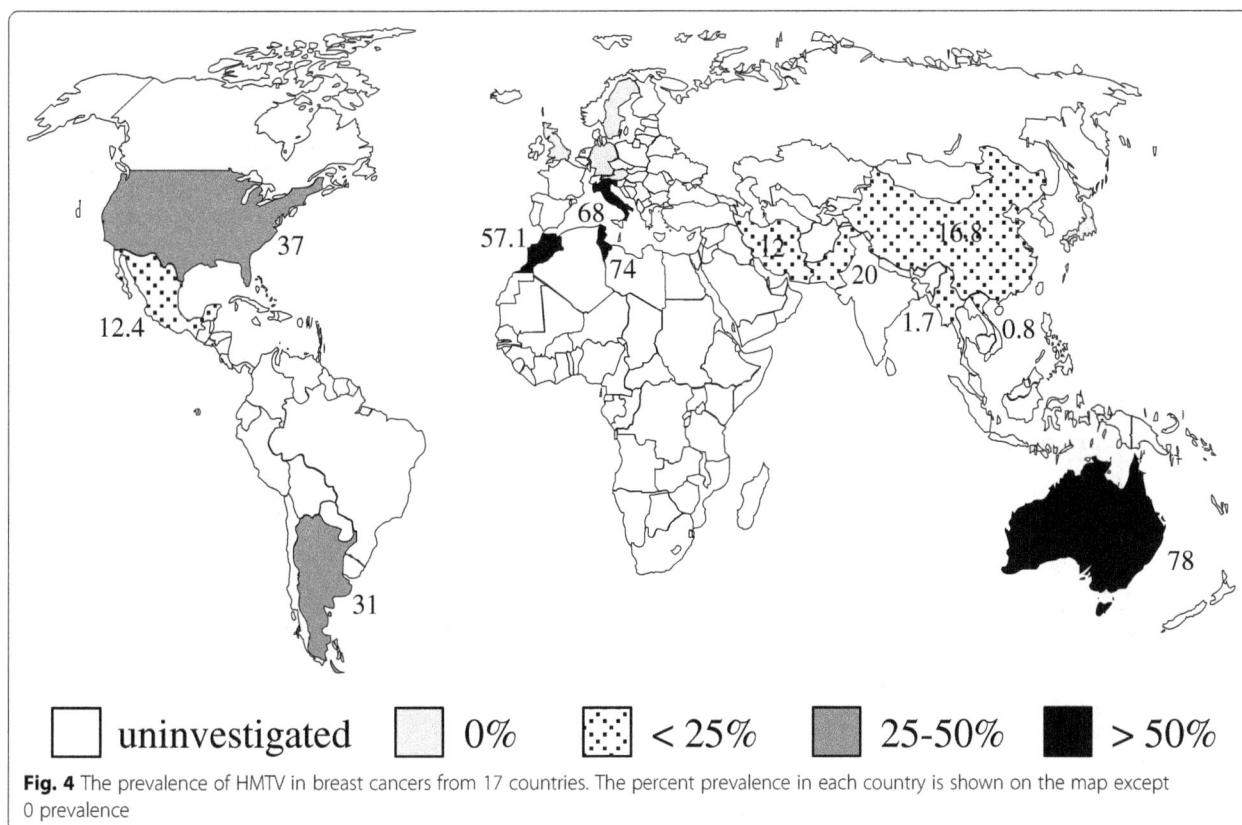

**Fig. 4** The prevalence of HMTV in breast cancers from 17 countries. The percent prevalence in each country is shown on the map except 0 prevalence

cell line expressing high level MMTV. We estimated the detection limit of this semi-nested PCR method using serially diluted positive control DNA, which was highly sensitive (as little as 80 pg of DNA, not shown). In addition, the primers and PCR conditions used in this study are same as those in previous studies [15–18].

It would be interesting if there was a correlation between HMTV status and clinicopathological parameters. Although several reports demonstrated causal association between these [16, 17, 24, 39], no strong correlation could be found after comprehensive meta-analysis [40]. The HMTV-positive case in this study showed histological grade III with lymph node metastasis. Further studies may reveal some unexplored or unnoticed characteristics of HMTV-associated breast cancers.

## Conclusions

This is the first study to report the prevalence of HMTV in breast cancers in Myanmar. The prevalence of HMTV in Myanmar was consistent with other Asian countries with low or zero prevalence. The frequency of infection and HMTV sequence closely resembled that from Vietnam. It appears that HMTV does not play an important role in breast cancer carcinogenesis in most Asian populations.

**Abbreviations**
HMTV: Human mammary tumor virus; MMTV: Mouse mammary tumor virus; PCR: Polymerase chain reaction.

**Acknowledgements**
The authors would like to thank Mr. Yasuharu Arashima and Mr. Haruyuki Watanabe for their technical assistance.

**Funding**
Not applicable.

**Authors' contributions**
THS carried out data collection and wrote the draft. MF and SF reviewed HE sections and the original draft. TY and TO co-supervised molecular experiments. LS, NWM and OK carried out the initial screening of breast cancer samples. XY supported the preparation of the draft. AM coordinated the study and reviewed the manuscript. All authors have approved the final manuscript for publication.

**Competing interests**
The authors declare that they have no competing interests.

**Author details**
[1]Department of Pathology and Experimental Medicine, Graduate School of Medicine, Dentistry and Pharmaceutical Sciences, Okayama University, 2-5-1 Shikata, Okayama 700-8558, Japan. [2]Department of Pathology, Himeji Red Cross Hospital, Himeji, Japan. [3]Department of Pathology, Myeik General Hospital, Myeik, Myanmar. [4]Department of Pathology, Sakura Specialist

Hospital, Yangon, Myanmar. [5]Immunology Research Division, Department of Medical Research, Yangon, Myanmar.

## References

1. Ferlay J, Soerjomataram I, Dikshit R, Eser S, Mathers C, Rebelo M, Parkin DM, Forman D, Bray F. Cancer incidence and mortality worldwide: sources, methods and major patterns in GLOBOCAN 2012. Int J Cancer. 2015; 136(5):E359–86.

2. Torre LA, Bray F, Siegel RL, Ferlay J, Lortet-Tieulent J, Jemal A. Global cancer statistics, 2012. CA Cancer J Clin. 2015;65(2):87–108.

3. Hortobagyi GN, de la Garza SJ, Pritchard K, Amadori D, Haidinger R, Hudis CA, Khaled H, Liu MC, Martin M, Namer M, O'haughnessy JA, Shen ZZ, Albain KS, ABREAST I. The global breast cancer burden: variations in epidemiology and survival. Clin Breast Cancer. 2005;6(5):391–401.

4. Jemal A, Center MM, DeSantis C, Ward EM. Global patterns of cancer incidence and mortality rates and trends. Cancer Epidemiol Biomarkers Prev. 2010;19(8):1893–907.

5. Amarante MK, Watanabe MA. The possible involvement of virus in breast cancer. J Cancer Res Clin Oncol. 2009;135(3):329–37.

6. Lawson JS. Do Viruses Cause Breast Cancer? In: Verma M, editor. Cancer Epidemiology. Totowa: Humana Press; 2009. p. 421–38.

7. Callahan R, Smith GH. MMTV-induced mammary tumorigenesis: gene discovery, progression to malignancy and cellular pathways. Oncogene. 2000;19(8):992–1001.

8. Callahan R, Smith GH. Common integration sites for MMTV in viral induced mouse mammary tumors. J Mammary Gland Biol Neoplasia. 2008;13(3):309–21.

9. Wang Y, Holland JF, Bleiweiss IJ, Melana S, Liu X, Pelisson I, Cantarella A, Stellrecht K, Mani S, Pogo BG. Detection of mammary tumor virus env gene-like sequences in human breast cancer. Cancer Res. 1995;55(22):5173–9.

10. Liu B, Wang Y, Melana SM, Pelisson I, Najfeld V, Holland JF, Pogo BG. Identification of a proviral structure in human breast cancer. Cancer Res. 2001;61(4):1754–9.

11. Nartey T, Mazzanti CM, Melana S, Glenn WK, Bevilacqua G, Holland JF, Whitaker NJ, Lawson JS, Pogo BG. Mouse mammary tumor-like virus (MMTV) is present in human breast tissue before development of virally associated breast cancer. Infect Agent Cancer. 2017;12:1.

12. Moore MA. Cancer control programs in East Asia: evidence from the international literature. J Prev Med Public Health. 2014;47(4):183–200.

13. Lakhani SR, Ellis IO, Schnitt SJ, Tan PH, van de Vijver MJ, editors. WHO Classification of Tumours of the Breast. Lyon: IARC; 2012.

14. Elston CW, Ellis IO. Pathological prognostic factors in breast cancer. I. The value of histological grade in breast cancer: experience from a large study with long-term follow-up. Histopathology. 1991;19(5):403–10.

15. Ford CE, Tran D, Deng Y, Ta VT, Rawlinson WD, Lawson JS. Mouse mammary tumor virus-like gene sequences in breast tumors of Australian and Vietnamese women. Clin Cancer Res. 2003;9(3):1118–20.

16. Ford CE, Faedo M, Crouch R, Lawson JS, Rawlinson WD. Progression from normal breast pathology to breast cancer is associated with increasing prevalence of mouse mammary tumor virus-like sequences in men and women. Cancer Res. 2004;64(14):4755–9.

17. Hachana M, Trimeche M, Ziadi S, Amara K, Gaddas N, Mokni M, Korbi S. Prevalence and characteristics of the MMTV-like associated breast carcinomas in Tunisia. Cancer Lett. 2008;271(2):222–30.

18. Mazzanti CM, Al Hamad M, Fanelli G, Scatena C, Zammarchi F, Zavaglia K, Lessi F, Pistello M, Naccarato AG, Bevilacqua G. A mouse mammary tumor virus env-like exogenous sequence is strictly related to progression of human sporadic breast carcinoma. Am J Pathol. 2011; 179(4):2083–90.

19. Cedro-Tanda A, Códova-Solis A, Juáez-Cedillo T, Pina-Jiméez E, Hernádez-Caballero ME, Moctezuma-Meza C, Castelazo-Rico G, Góez-Delgado A, Monsalvo-Reyes AC, Salamanca-Góez FA, Arenas-Aranda DJ, Garcí-Hernádez N. Prevalence of HMTV in breast carcinomas and unaffected tissue from Mexican women. BMC Cancer. 2014;14:942.

20. Etkind P, Du J, Khan A, Pillitteri J, Wiernik PH. Mouse mammary tumor virus-like ENV gene sequences in human breast tumors and in a lymphoma of a breast cancer patient. Clin Cancer Res. 2000;6(4):1273–8.

21. Glenn WK, Heng B, Delprado W, Iacopetta B, Whitaker NJ, Lawson JS. Epstein-Barr virus, human papillomavirus and mouse mammary tumour virus as multiple viruses in breast cancer. PLoS One. 2012;7(11):e48788.

22. Levine PH, Pogo BG, Klouj A, Coronel S, Woodson K, Melana SM, Mourali N, Holland JF. Increasing evidence for a human breast carcinoma virus with geographic differences. Cancer. 2004;101(4):721–6.

23. Melana SM, Picconi MA, Rossi C, Mural J, Alonio LV, Teyssie A, Holland JF, Pogo BG. [Detection of murine mammary tumor virus (MMTV) env gene-like sequences in breast cancer from Argentine patients]. Medicina (B Aires). 2002;62(4):323–7.

24. Pogo BG, Melana SM, Holland JF, Mandeli JF, Pilotti S, Casalini P, Menard S. Sequences homologous to the mouse mammary tumor virus env gene in human breast carcinoma correlate with overexpression of laminin receptor. Clin Cancer Res. 1999;5(8):2108–11.

25. Slaoui M, El Mzibri M, Razine R, Qmichou Z, Attaleb M, Amrani M. Detection of MMTV-Like sequences in Moroccan breast cancer cases. Infect Agent Cancer. 2014;9:37.

26. Bindra A, Muradrasoli S, Kisekka R, Nordgren H, Warnberg F, Blomberg J. Search for DNA of exogenous mouse mammary tumor virus-related virus in human breast cancer samples. J Gen Virol. 2007;88(Pt 6):1806–9.

27. Frank O, Verbeke C, Schwarz N, Mayer J, Fabarius A, Hehlmann R, Leib-Mosch C, Seifarth W. Variable transcriptional activity of endogenous retroviruses in human breast cancer. J Virol. 2008;82(4):1808–18.

28. Mant C, Gillett C, D'rrigo C, Cason J. Human murine mammary tumour virus-like agents are genetically distinct from endogenous retroviruses and are not detectable in breast cancer cell lines or biopsies. Virology. 2004;318(1):393–404.

29. Witt A, Hartmann B, Marton E, Zeillinger R, Schreiber M, Kubista E. The mouse mammary tumor virus-like env gene sequence is not detectable in breast cancer tissue of Austrian patients. Oncol Rep. 2003;10(4):1025–9.

30. Fukuoka H, Moriuchi M, Yano H, Nagayasu T, Moriuchi H. No association of mouse mammary tumor virus-related retrovirus with Japanese cases of breast cancer. J Med Virol. 2008;80(8):1447–51.

31. Ahangar Oskouee M, Shahmahmoodi S, Jalilvand S, Mahmoodi M, Ziaee AA, Esmaeili HA, Mokhtari-Azad T, Yousefi M, Mollaei-Kandelous Y, Nategh R. No evidence of mammary tumor virus env gene-like sequences among Iranian women with breast cancer. Intervirology. 2014;57(6):353–6.

32. Luo T, Wu XT, Zhang MM, Qian K. [Study of mouse mammary tumor virus-like gene sequences expressing in breast tumors of Chinese women]. Sichuan Da Xue Xue Bao Yi Xue Ban. 2006;37(6):844–6. 851.

33. Naushad W, Bin Rahat T, Gomez MK, Ashiq MT, Younas M, Sadia H. Detection and identification of mouse mammary tumor virus-like DNA sequences in blood and breast tissues of breast cancer patients. Tumour Biol. 2014;35(8):8077–86.

34. Reza MA, Reza MH, Mahdiyeh L, Mehdi F, Hamid ZN. Evaluation Frequency of Merkel Cell Polyoma, Epstein-Barr and Mouse Mammary Tumor Viruses in Patients with Breast Cancer in Kerman, Southeast of Iran. Asian Pac J Cancer Prev. 2015;16:7351–7.

35. Leong SP, Shen ZZ, Liu TJ, Agarwal G, Tajima T, Paik NS, Sandelin K, Derossis A, Cody H, Foulkes WD. Is breast cancer the same disease in Asian and Western countries. World J Surg. 2010;34(10):2308–24.

36. Stewart TH, Sage RD, Stewart AF, Cameron DW. Breast cancer incidence highest in the range of one species of house mouse, Mus domesticus. Br J Cancer. 2000;82(2):446–51.

37. Glenn WK, Salmons B, Lawson JS, Whitaker NJ. Mouse mammary tumor-like virus and human breast cancer. Breast Cancer Res Treat. 2010;123(3):907–9.

38. Holland JF, Pogo BG. Comment on the review by Joshi and Buehring. Breast Cancer Res Treat. 2012;136(1):303–7.

39. Faedo M, Ford CE, Mehta R, Blazek K, Rawlinson WD. Mouse mammary tumor-like virus is associated with p53 nuclear accumulation and progesterone receptor positivity but not estrogen positivity in human female breast cancer. Clin Cancer Res. 2004;10(13):4417–9.

40. Wang F, Hou J, Shen Q, Yue Y, Xie F, Wang X, Jin H. Mouse mammary tumor virus-like virus infection and the risk of human breast cancer. Am J Transl Res. 2014;6(3):248–66.

# 9

# The efficacy of Epigallocatechin-3-gallate (green tea) in the treatment of Alzheimer's disease: an overview of pre-clinical studies and translational perspectives in clinical practice

Marco Cascella[1†], Sabrina Bimonte[1*†] (ID), Maria Rosaria Muzio[2], Vincenzo Schiavone[3] and Arturo Cuomo[1]

## Abstract

Alzheimer's disease (AD) is a neurodegenerative disorder and the most common form of dementia characterized by cognitive and memory impairment. One of the mechanism involved in the pathogenesis of AD, is the oxidative stress being involved in AD's development and progression. In addition, several studies proved that chronic viral infections, mainly induced by Human herpesvirus 1 (HHV-1), Cytomegalovirus (CMV), Human herpesvirus 2 (HHV-2), and Hepatitis C virus (HCV) could be responsible for AD's neuropathology. Despite the large amount of data regarding the pathogenesis of Alzheimer's disease (AD), a very limited number of therapeutic drugs and/or pharmacological approaches, have been developed so far. It is important to underline that, in recent years, natural compounds, due their antioxidants and anti-inflammatory properties have been largely studied and identified as promising agents for the prevention and treatment of neurodegenerative diseases, including AD. The ester of epigallocatechin and gallic acid, (−)-Epigallocatechin-3-Gallate (EGCG), is the main and most significantly bioactive polyphenol found in solid green tea extract. Several studies showed that this compound has important anti-inflammatory and antiatherogenic properties as well as protective effects against neuronal damage and brain edema. To date, many studies regarding the potential effects of EGCG in AD's treatment have been reported in literature. The purpose of this review is to summarize the in vitro and in vivo pre-clinical studies on the use of EGCG in the prevention and the treatment of AD as well as to offer new insights for translational perspectives into clinical practice.

**Keywords:** (−) - Epigallocatechin-3-O-gallate (EGCG), Natural compound, Inflammation, Oxidative stress, Alzheimer's disease

## Background

The term dementia covers a large range of heterogeneous diseases at clinical and histopathological levels. Loss of memory and progressive dysfunctions of neuronal materials are features commonly present in patients with dementia and severely impairing theirs quality of life. Classically, dementia is defined as "syndrome caused by neurodegeneration" whereas Alzheimer's disease (AD), is the most common type of dementia, accounting for an estimated 60 to 80% of cases. Although the exact pathophysiology of AD is still unclear, emerging evidence suggests that microglia-mediated neuroinflammatory responses play an important role in AD's pathogenesis [1, 2]. In addition, several studies proved that chronic viral infections, mainly induced by Human herpesvirus 1 (HHV-1), Cytomegalovirus (CMV), Human herpesvirus 2 (HHV-2), and Hepatitis C virus (HCV) could be responsible for AD's neuropathology. It is of note that microglia, resident immune cells of the central nervous system (CNS), are

* Correspondence: s.bimonte@istitutotumori.na.it
†Equal contributors
[1]Division of Anesthesia and Pain Medicine, Istituto Nazionale Tumori – IRCCS - "Fondazione G. Pascale", Via Mariano Semmola, 80131 Naples, Italy
Full list of author information is available at the end of the article

significantly involved in the neuroinflammation process. Current evidences on AD's mechanism showed that the principal pathological features of AD are represented by the accumulation of soluble amyloid β peptide (Aβ) in the brain and the neurofibrillary tangles [3]. Aβ is considered an important neuroinflammatory stimulus for microglia. Moreover, it is of note that Aβ-dependent microglial activation induces neuronal injury due to the secretion of various pro-inflammatory molecules such as tumour necrosis factor-α (TNFα), interleukin (I) L-6, IL-1β, reactive oxygen species (ROS), and reactive nitrogen species (NOS) [4]. Neuroinflammation and oxidative stress processes are responsible for the impairments of neurovascular unit's functions, leading to axonal demyelination, local hypoxia–ischemia, and reduced repair of white matter damages [5].

Despite the large amount of data published on the AD's pathogenesis, a limited number of therapeutic drugs have been developed so far. Natural compounds have been identified as promising agents for the prevention and treatment of neurological disorders [6] and AD due their antioxidants and anti-inflammatory properties [7]. As a consequence, many investigations have been performed, with the aim of to evaluate the neuroprotective effects of nutraceuticals, such as resveratrol [8], curcumin [9], pinocembrin [10], caffeine [11], the combination of *Panax ginseng*, *Ginkgo biloba*, and *Crocus sativus* [12], and salvia triloba associated to *Piper nigrum* [13].

Catechins flavonoids are contained in Green tea extract (GTE) and are defined as the active components of green tea, accounting for its therapeutic properties. The ester of epigallocatechin and gallic acid, (−)-Epigallocatechin-3-Gallate [EGCG; (2R,3R)-5,7-dihydroxy-2-(3,4,5-trihydroxyphenyl)-3,4-dihydro-2H-1-benzopyran-3-yl 3,4,5-trihydroxybenzoate] (Pubchem CID: 65,064), represents the principal bioactive polyphenol in the solid GTE (65% catechin content). Several studies showed that EGCG has important anti-atherogenic and anti-inflammatory properties [14, 15] with potential neuroprotective effects against cerebrovascular diseases. For examples, *Ahn* et al. showed that EGCG was able to inhibit the production of TNFα-induced monocyte chemotactic protein-1 from vascular endothelial cells [16], whereas *Lee* et al. studied the protective effects of EGCG against brain edema and neuronal damage after unilateral cerebral ischemia in gerbils [17]. In addition, it has been proved that EGCG bypassed the blood–brain barrier (BBB) and to reach the functional parts of the brain [18]. Moreover, EGCG appears to be safe even when administered at relatively high dose. Indeed, as *Lee* et al. showed, an amount up to 6 mg/kg of EGCG can be used without any side effects [19].

As regards to the role of EGCG in the treatment of AD's disorder, a large amount of in vitro and in vivo studies, have been reported so far [19–37], indicating that EGCG

plays a neuroprotective role and be potentially used as therapeutic agent for AD's treatment (Fig. 1).

On the other side, studies have been also performed by using computational methods. For example, Ali et al., in order to demonstrate a potential role of cholinesterase inhibitors for AD's treatment, performed an in silico analysis by using green tea polyphenols. Data emerged from this study, suggested that the cholinergic neurotransmission was enhanced by these synthetically compounds through the inhibition of acetylcholinesterase (AChE) and butyrylcholinesterase (BChE) enzymes [38].

The aim of this article is to highlight the potential use of EGCG for the prevention and/or treatment of AD, by summarize the pre-clinical studies reported in literature. Insights for translational perspectives into clinical practice are also given.

## Anti-neuroinflammatory properties of EGCG in the prevention and the treatment of Alzheimer's disease

a) **In vitro** *studies: an update*

In vitro studies on the anti-neuroinflammatory effects of EGCG have been performed on different cells lines including *MC65, EOC 13.31, SweAPP N2a, N2a/APP695, DIV8, CHO, and M146 L* cells (Table 1). Results from these studies showed that the anti-neuroinflammatory capacity of EGCG is mainly associated to the inhibition of microglia-induced cytotoxicity.

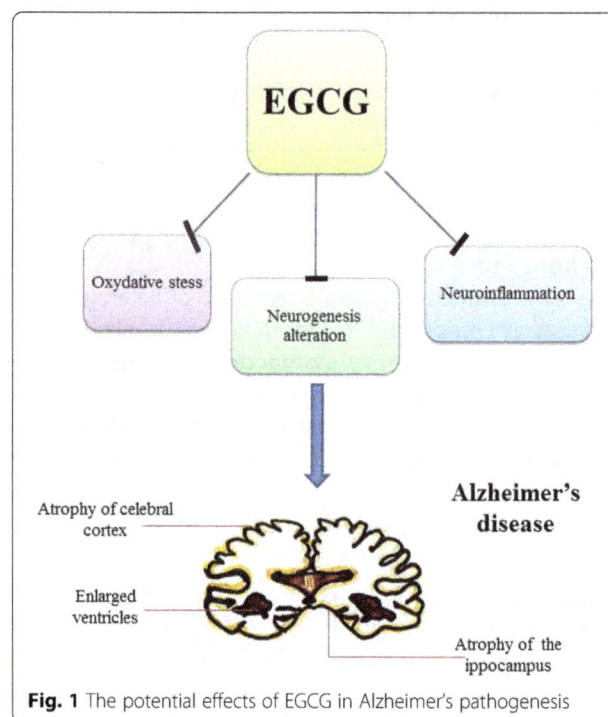

**Fig. 1** The potential effects of EGCG in Alzheimer's pathogenesis

**Table 1** A summary of in vitro studies on the role of EGCG on AD prevention

| Cell lines | Drug and dosage | Results | References |
|---|---|---|---|
| MC65 | EGCG 20 μM | EGCG reduced the Aβ levels by enhancing endogenous APP proteolysis and decreased nuclear translocation of c-Abl. | [20] |
| EOC 13.31 | EGCG 5 to 20 μM | EGCG suppressed the expression of Aβ-induced TNFα, IL-1β, IL-6, and iNOS, and restored the levels of intracellular antioxidants Nrf2 and HO-1. | [23] |
| SweAPP N2a | GTE | EGCG reduced the Aβ generation and activated nonamyloidogenic processing of APP by promoting its α-secretase cleavage. | [24] |
| Div8 | EGCG 12.5–50 μM | EGCG induced an increase in the key autophagy adaptor proteins NDP52 and p62. | [27] |
| M146 L, CHO | EGCG 16–32 μmol/L | EGCG reduced the accumulation of β-amyloid (Aβ). | [28] |
| N2a/APP695 | EGCG (5–100 μM) | EGCG suppressed the production of Aβ and reduced inflammation, oxidative stress and cell apoptosis. | [29] |

*Lin* et al. demonstrated that EGCG was able to suppress the neurotoxicity induced by Aβ, through the activation of the glycogen synthase kinase-3β (GSK-3β) and the inhibition of c-Abl/FE65 nuclear translocation [20]. This was a relevant finding, since it is of note that c-Abl is a cytoplasmic nonreceptor tyrosine kinase involved in the development of the nervous system and implicated in the regulation of cell apoptosis, whereas the β-isoform of GSK3 is a proline-directed serine-threonine kinase involved in neuronal cell development and energy metabolism [21]. These data suggest that c-Abl/GSK-3β signaling is involved in neuronal loss, neuroinflammation and gliosis. It is of note that, related to AD's pathogenesis, the proteolytic processing of a transmembrane glycoprotein, known as amyloid precursor protein (APP), is responsible for the Aβ's origin [22]. Other investigations have been conducted to evaluate the effect of EGCG on Aβ-induced inflammatory responses in microglia. To this regard, *Wei* et al., investigated on the inhibitory effects of EGCG on microglial activation induced by Aβ and on neurotoxicity in Aβ-stimulated EOC 13.31 microglia. Results revealed that that EGCG was able to suppress the expression of TNFα, IL-1β, IL-6, and inducible nitric oxide synthase (iNOS) and to restore the levels of intracellular antioxidants against free radical-induced pro-inflammatory effects in microglia, the nuclear erythroid-2 related factor 2 (Nrf2) and the heme oxygenase-1 (HO-1) [23]. In addition, EGCG suppressed Aβ-induced cytotoxicity by reducing ROS-induced NF-κB activation and mitogen-activated protein kinase (MAPK) signaling, including c-Jun N-terminal kinase (JNK) and p38 signaling. Taken together these data suggest that EGCG is able to inhibit the neuroinflammatory response of microglia induced by Aβ and to protect against indirect neurotoxicity through several mechanisms.

Previously, *Rezai-Zadeh* et al. demonstrated that GTE reduced the generation of Aβ in murine neuron-like cells (N2a) transfected with the human "Swedish" mutant APP (SweAPP N2a cells) and activated the nonamyloidogenic processing of APP, also promoting its α-secretase cleavage [24]. One of the processes involved in the amyloid formation cascade, is the β-sheet formation. This event is frequently associated with cellular toxicity in many of human protein misfolding diseases, including AD. It has been reported that EGCG was able to interfere with this cascade, by redirection of prone polypeptides' aggregation into off-pathway protein assemblies [25]. In another study, *Bieschke* et al. showed that EGCG converted the large mature Aβ fibrils into smaller forms with no toxicity for mammalian cell [26]. A recent study conducted by *Chesser* et al., proved that EGCG in DIV8 primary rat cortical neurons, was able to enhance the clearance of AD-relevant phosphorylated tau species, indicating that EGCG could be used as an adjuvant agent for AD's treatment [27]. Similar findings were obtained by *Chang* et al. The authors demonstrated that EGCG reduced β-amyloid (Aβ) accumulation in M146 L and CHO cells [28]. Finally, very recently it has been reported that EGCG inhibited β-Amyloid generation and oxidative stress involvement of nuclear receptor peroxisome proliferator-activated receptor gamma (PPARγ) in N2a/APP695 cells [29]. All these data suggest that EGCG may be considered an important agent with neuroprotective properties against AD.

b) **In vivo *preclinical studies: an-update***
The neuroprotective effects of EGCG have been also demonstrated by in vivo experiments on several animal models (Table 2). The first study was reported by *Rezai-Zadeh* et al. [24]. The authors described that EGCG was able to decrease Aβ levels and plaques formation in a transgenic mouse model of "Swedish" mutant APP when was injected intraperitoneally (20 mg/kg). Similar results were obtained by the same group of researchers, when EGCG administered orally in drinking water (50 mg/kg), reduced Aβ deposition in the same mutant mice [30]. In another study based

**Table 2** Pre-clinical in vivo studies on the anti-neurodegenerative properties of EGCG in AD

| Animal models | EGCG dose and route | Effects | Ref |
|---|---|---|---|
| Tg2576 APP mice | 20 mg/kg daily for 4 months (oral gavage) | EGCG impaired Aβ formation by inhibiting APP proteolysis and by inhibiting cAbl/FE65 complex nuclear translocation and GSK3 activation. | [20] |
| Swedish mutant APP-overexpressing mice (Tg APPsw line 2576) | 20 mg/kg (intraperitoneally) | EGCG induced APP processing with reduction of cerebral amyloidosis. | [24] |
| APP transgenic mice | 20 mg/kg/day, for 3 months (oral gavage) | Aβ deposits were reduced by 60% in the frontal cortex and 52% in the hippocampus. | [31] |
| AD mouse model | Nanolipidic particles loaded with EGCG | Improved the bioavailability and α-secretase activity induced by EGCG. | [32] |
| Tg2576 mice | Fish oil (8 mg/kg/day) and EGCG (oral gavage, 62.5 mg/kg/day or 12.5 mg/kg/day) | Fish oil enhanced bioavailability of EGCG versus EGCG treatment alone. Synergetic effect of Fish oil and EGCG on the inhibition of cerebral A β deposits. | [33] |
| Wistar rat model of dementia | 10 mg/kg/day for 4 weeks, oral gavage. ICV infusion of STZ (3 mg/kg) | EGCG completely abrogated the cognitive deficit, S100B content in the hippocampus, AChE activity, glutathione peroxidase activity, NO metabolites, and ROS content | [34] |
| ICR mice model of systemic inflammation | 1.5 and 3 mg/kg for 3 weeks (Oral gavage). LPS (250 µg/kg) intraperitoneal | EGCG prevented LPS-induced memory impairment, apoptotic neuronal cell death, and microglia activation | [19] |
| AD mouse model induced by D-gal | 2 mg/(kg/ day) or 6 mg/(kg/day) for 4 weeks, oral gavage | EGCG decreased the expression of APP and beta-Amyloid in the hippocampus of mice. | [35] |
| APP/PS1 mice | 2 mg/(kg/day) or 6 mg/(kg/day) for 4 weeks, oral gave | EGCG treatment inhibited TNF-α/JNK signaling, increased the phosphorylation of Akt and glycogen synthase kinase-3β. | [37] |
| SAMP8 mice | 5 and 15 mg/kg, for 60 days, intragastric | EGCG induced reduction in Aβ accumulation and increased NEP expression | [28] |

on the generation of transgenic mouse models of AD, *Li* et al., [31] investigated on EGCG (orally 20 mg/kg/day, for 3 months) capacity to interfere with Aβ deposits in different brain areas. Data emerged by immunohistochemistry, showed that Aβ deposits were reduced by 60% in the frontal cortex and 52% in the hippocampus. A reduction of Thioflavine-S histochemistry labelling compact plaques was also detected in both regions. In addition, the percentage of CD45, a marker of microglial activation, was lower than 18% in the cortex and then 28% in the hippocampus respect to those observed in the control cohort. New insights on the role of EGCG in AD's treatment have been reported by *Smith* et al. [32]. The authors engineered nanolipidic EGCG particles to improve oral's bioavailability of EGCG. By using this system in mouse model of AD's disease, the ability of EGCG for the treatment of AD was enhanced more than two-fold respect to treatment with free EGCG.

The role of EGCG in AD's treatment, was also described by *Giunta* et al., in an interesting study in which was used Fish oil (8 mg/kg/day) combined to EGCG (62.5 mg/kg/day or 12.5 mg/kg/day) in a mouse model of AD. Results obtained from these experiments, showed that co-treatment of N2a cells with fish oil and EGCG increased the production of sAPP-alpha respect to either compound alone, indicating that these compounds were able to make

a synergetic action on the inhibition of cerebral Aβ deposits [33].

More recently, *Lee* et al. [19] tested the effects of EGCG on neuroinflammation and amyloidogenesis, in mice with systemic inflammation. The authors demonstrated that EGCG was able to prevent memory impairment induced by lipopolysaccharide (LPS) and apoptotic neuronal cell death. Moreover, EGCG prevented LPS-induced activation of astrocytes and increased cytokines expression (TNF-α, IL-1β, IL-6), suggesting that EGCG could be considered a therapeutic agent for neuroinflammation-associated AD. In animal another model of dementia, generated by infusion of streptozotocin (STZ) into intracerebroventricular (ICV) of rats, *Biasibetti* et al., showed that EGCG (10 mg/kg/day for 4 weeks) completely abrogated the cognitive deficit by influencing the glial-specific calcium binding protein S100B content in the hippocampus, the acetylcholinesterase (AChE) activity, the glutathione peroxidase activity, the nitric oxide (NO) metabolites, and ROS content [34].

*He* et al., by using an AD's mouse model generated by D-gal, showed that EGCG had a protective effect on AD by decreasing the expression of APP and Aβ in the hippocampus of mice [35]. Similarly, *Lin* et al. proved that EGCG impaired the formation of Aβ, through the inhibition of APP proteolysis, cAbl/FE65 complex nuclear translocation and GSK3 activation [20].

Since insulin signaling plays a significant role in the regulation of synaptic activities involved in learning and memory processes, insulin resistance – expressed as increased phosphorylation levels of insulin receptor substrate-1 (IRS-1) - and subsequent alteration in signaling pathways, may contribute to the cognition impairment in AD's patients [36]. Interestingly, *Jia* et al. demonstrated that EGCG reduced the spatial memory impairment (AD-related cognitive deficit) in APP/PS1 mice (bearing brain insulin resistance) by inducing IRS-1 signaling defects in the hippocampus, in a dose dependent manner [37].

In another study, was reported that EGCG reduced Aβ accumulation in vitro and rescued cognitive deterioration in senescence-accelerated mice P8 (SAMP8). The authors showed that EGCG attenuated the cognitive deterioration in AD's mouse model by upregulation of neprilysin (NEP) expression [28]. Taken together, these data strongly suggest that EGCG could be used as a therapeutic agent for the treatment and the prevention of AD.

**Translational perspectives of EGCG's use into clinical practice**

Promising results obtained *by* in vitro and in vivo studies on the use of EGCG as valuable therapeutic options for neurodegenerative disorders and cancer treatments, encourage its commitment to translation into clinical practice [39, 40].

a) *The bioavailability of EGCG in the brain: a discrepancy between animals and humans-based studies*

Despite these encouraging results, there is still a translational gap between in vitro, in vivo and clinical studies with EGCG in neurodegenetative disease treatment. This can be associated to poor data reported on the bioavailability of EGCG in the brain, a feature extremely necessary for its neuroprotrective role. In vivo studies performed on animal models showed that repeated administration of EGCG, increased its accumulation in the brain [41, 42]. Opposite results were obtained in a study performed on six human subjects which assumed green tea by drinking. The products of green tea's metabolism, (i.e. flavan-3-ol methyl-glucuronide and sulfate metabolites) were not able to reach the brain, thus remaining in the bloodstream [43]. These discrepancy can be associated to different causes, as reported by *Mähler* et al.in a review on this topic (i.e. dose, time point of EGCG treatment and different catechin metabolism between animals and humans) [39]. When EGCG is able to reach the brain, it regulates many biological processes and molecular signaling pathways involved in neurodegenerative disorders, included AD, as previously reported based on convincing results of in vitro and in vivo pre-clinical studies [44]. Unfortunately, these mechanisms are not completely elucidated in clinical studies probably due to the absence of standardization of disease severity in humans and in green tea preparations and its derivatives.

This strongly suggest the needing of more detailed and specific studies on EGCG's brain and plasma bioavailability, on its efficacy and safety in patients, and on possible interactions with other drugs.

b) *Clinical trials*

Despite the encouraging data obtained from pre-clinical studies, several pivotal issues, regarding EGCG dose levels and administration frequency as well as genetic and epigenetic modulations involved in the metabolism and distribution of the active compounds in humans, remain to be explored [45].Previous findings from a cross-sectional study showed a negative association between green tea consumption and the prevalence of cognitive impairment in elderly individuals over 70 years old [46]. Thus, there is a discrepancy about the effects of GTE compounds on cognitive functions [47].

Several clinical studies have been performed to evaluate the acute effects of EGCG and other constituents of tea, such as L-theanine, on cognitive function (e.g., attention) and mood. The results obtained, showed that tea consumption had significant acute benefits on mood and work performance and creativity [48, 49]. Another clinical study performed on 27 healthy human adults treated with EGCG (orally administered in a single dose of 135 mg), reported that EGCG was able to modulate cerebral blood flow parameters, without affecting cognitive performance or mood [50]. Similarly, *Scholey* et al. showed that EGCG administration (300 mg) was associated with reduced stress, increased calmness and increased electroencephalographic activity (increased alpha, beta and theta activities) in the midline frontal and central brain regions [51]. *Ide* et al. showed that green tea consumption in subjects with cognitive dysfunction (2 g/day for 3 months, approximately equal to 2 to 4 cups of tea/day) significantly improved cognitive performance [52].

It is of note that the clinical symptoms of AD do not occur immediately. For this reasons, acute results of EGCG or other natural compounds on neurocognitive capacities, cannot be predictive of efficacy in more complex neurodegenerative diseases, such as AD's syndrome. To date, one ongoing clinical trial is investigating on the effects of EGEG in early state of AD patients co-medicated with acetylcholine esterase inhibitors (ClinicalTrials.gov identifier: NCT00951834) [53].

In order to evaluate the clinical effects of EGCG on AD, are necessary: (i) more detailed in vitro and in vitro studies with the purpose of dissect the underlying molecular mechanisms by which EGCG interferes with AD pathogenesis; (ii) clinical studies exploring the long-term effects of EGCG on cognitive functions; (iii) large size epidemiological studies concerning the consumption of EGCG and the progression of AD.

## Conclusions

Several in vitro and pre-clinical studies have demonstrated that EGCG, the principal bioactive component found in green tea, has anti-inflammatory properties by modulating different molecular pathways. Regarding AD's syndrome, in vitro and in vivo studies reviewed here, showed that EGCG mainly induces reduction in Aβ accumulation, by modulating several biological mechanisms. Promising results in the pre-clinical and in recent clinical studies largely encourage EGCG's commitment to translation into a clinical therapeutic approach. However, EGCG dose levels and administration frequency remain to be explored, so more pre-clinical investigations and well-drawn clinical trials are extremely needed.

With the use of different integrated approaches, next studies will shed light on the use of EGCG as a targeted prevention and individualized treatment to patients with AD's disease.

## Abbreviations

AChE: Acetylcholinesterase; AD: Alzheimer's disease; APP: Amyloid precursor protein; Aβ: Amyloid β peptide; BBB: Blood brain barrier; BChE: Butyrylcholinesterase; CNS: Central nervous system; EGCG: (−)-Epigallocatechin-3-O-gallate; GSK-3: glycogen synthase kinase-3; GTE: Green tea extract; HO-1: Heme oxygenase-1; ICV: Intracerebroventricular; IL: Interleukin; iNOS: Inducible nitric oxide synthase; IRS-1: Insulin receptor substrate-1; JNK: c-Jun N-terminal kinase; LPS: Lipopolysaccharide; MAPK: mitogen-activated protein kinase; NEP: Neprilysin; NO: Nitric oxide; NOS: Reactive nitrogen species; Nrf2: Nuclear erythroid-2 related factor 2; PPARγ: peroxisome proliferator-activated receptor gamma; ROS: Reactive oxygen species; S100B: Calcium-binding protein B; SAMP8: Senescence-accelerated mice P8; STZ: Streptozotocin; TNFα: Tumor necrosis factor-α

## Acknowledgments

We are grateful to Dr. Alessandra Trocino and Mrs. Cristina Romano from the National Cancer Institute of Naples for providing excellent bibliographic service and assistance.

## Funding

No funds were used for the preparation of the paper.

## Authors' contributions

The present review was mainly written by MC and SB. MM, VS and AC contributed to revise the manuscript. All authors approved the final version of the manuscript.

## Competing interests

The authors declare that they have no competing interests.

## Author details

[1]Division of Anesthesia and Pain Medicine, Istituto Nazionale Tumori – IRCCS - "Fondazione G. Pascale", Via Mariano Semmola, 80131 Naples, Italy. [2]Division of Infantile Neuropsychiatry, UOMI - Maternal and Infant Health, ASL NA 3 SUD, Torre del Greco, Via Marconi, 80059 Naples, Italy. [3]Division of Anesthesia and Intensive Care, Presidio Ospedaliero "Pineta Grande", Castel Voltuno, 81100 Caserta, Italy.

## References

1. Block ML, Zecca L, Hong JS. Microglia-mediated neurotoxicity: uncovering the molecular mechanisms. Nat Rev Neurosci. 2007;8:57–69.
2. Yadav A, Collman RG. CNS inflammation and macrophage/microglial biology associated with HIV-1 infection. Journal of Neuroimmune Pharmacolog. 2009;4:430–47.
3. Iqbal K. Grundke-Iqbal I Alzheimer neurofibrillary degeneration: significance, etiopathogenesis, therapeutics and prevention. J Cell Mol Med. 2008;12:38–55.
4. Agostinho P, Cunha RA, Oliveira C. Neuroinflammation, oxidative stress and the pathogenesis of Alzheimer's disease. Curr Pharm Des. 2010;16:2766–78.
5. Iadecola C. The overlap between neurodegenerative and vascular factors in the pathogenesis of dementia. Acta Neuropathol. 2010;120:287–96.
6. Cascella M, Muzio MR. Potential application of the Kampo medicine goshajinkigan for prevention of chemotherapy-induced peripheral neuropathy. J Integr Med. 2017;15(2):77–87.
7. Essa MM, Mohammed A, Guillemin G. The Benefits of Natural Products for Neurodegenerative Diseases. 2016. ISBN:978-3-319-28381-4. doi:10.1007/978-3-319-28383-8.
8. Zhao HF, Li N, Wang Q, et al. Resveratrol decreases the insoluble Aβ1-42 level in hippocampus and protects the integrity of the blood-brain barrier in AD rats. Neuroscience. 2015;310:641–9.
9. Cox KHM, Pipingas A, Scholey AB. Investigation of the effects of solid lipid curcumin on cognition and mood in a healthy older population. J Psychopharmacol. 2015;29:642–51.
10. Saad MA, Abdel Salam RM, Kenawy SA, et al. Pinocembrin attenuates hippocampal inflammation, oxidative perturbations and apoptosis in a rat model of global cerebral ischemia reperfusion. Pharmacol Rep. 2015;67:115–22.
11. Chen X, Gawryluk JW, Wagener JF, et al. Caffeine blocks disruption of blood brain barrier in a rabbit model of Alzheimer's disease. J Neuroinflammation. 2008;5:12. doi:10.1186/1742-2094-5-12.
12. Steiner GZ, Yeung A, Liu JX, et al. The effect of Sailuotong (SLT) on neurocognitive and cardiovascular function in healthy adults: a randomised, double-blind, placebo controlled crossover pilot trial. BMC Complement Altern Med. 2015;16:15. doi:10.1186/s12906-016-0989-0.
13. Ahmed HH, Salem AM, Sabry GM, et al. Possible therapeutic uses of Salvia Triloba and Piper nigrum in Alzheimer's disease-induced rats. J Med Food. 2013;16:437–46.
14. Ou H-C, Song T-Y, Yeh Y-C, et al. EGCG protects against oxidized LDL-induced endothelial dysfunction by inhibiting LOX-1-mediated signalling. J Appl Physiol. 2010;108:1745–56.
15. Xu H, Lui WT, Chu CY, et al. Anti-angiogenic effects of green tea catechin on an experimental endometriosis mouse model. Hum Reprod. 2009;24:608–18.
16. Ahn HY, Xu Y, Davidge ST. Epigallocatechin-3-O-gallate inhibits TNFα-induced monocyte chemotactic protein-1 production from vascular endothelial cells. Life Sci. 2008;82:964–8.

17. Lee H, Bae JH, Lee S-R. Protective effect of green tea polyphenol EGCG against neuronal damage and brain edema after unilateral cerebral ischemia in gerbils. J Neurosci Res. 2004;77:892–900.

18. Singh M, Arseneault M, Sanderson T, et al. Challenges for research on polyphenols from foods in Alzheimer's disease: bioavailability,metabolism, and cellular and molecular mechanisms. J Agric Food Chem. 2008;56:4855–73.

19. Lee YJ, Choi DY, Yun YP, et al. Epigallocatechin-3-gallate prevents systemic inflammation-induced memory deficiency and amyloidogenesis via its anti-neuroinflammatory properties. J Nutr Biochem. 2013;24:298–310.

20. Lin CL, Chen TF, Chiu MJ, et al. Epigallocatechin gallate (EGCG) suppresses beta-amyloid-induced neurotoxicity through inhibiting c-Abl/FE65 nuclear translocation and GSK3 beta activation. Neurobiol Aging. 2009;30:81–92.

21. Wang JY. Nucleo-cytoplasmic communication in apoptotic response to genotoxic and inflammatory stress. Cell Res. 2005;15:43–8.

22. Sinha S, Lieberburg I. Cellular mechanisms of beta-amyloid production and secretion. Proc Natl Acad Sci U S A. 1999;96:11049–53.

23. Cheng-Chung Wei J, Huang HC, Chen WJ, et al. Epigallocatechin gallate attenuates amyloid β-induced inflammation and neurotoxicity in EOC 13.31 microglia. Eur J Pharmacol. 2016;770:16–24.

24. Rezai-Zadeh K, Shytle D, Sun N, et al. Green tea epigallocatechin-3-gallate (EGCG) modulates amyloid precursor protein cleavage and reduces cerebral amyloidosis in Alzheimer transgenic mice. J Neurosci. 2005;25:8807–14.

25. Ehrnhoefer DE, Bieschke J, Boeddrich A, et al. EGCG redirects amyloidogenic polypeptides into unstructured, off-pathway oligomers. Nat Struct Mol Biol. 2008;15:558–66.

26. Bieschke J, Russ J, Friedrich RP, et al. EGCG remodels mature α-synuclein and amyloid-β fibrils and reduces cellular toxicity. Proc Natl Acad Sci U S A. 2010;107:7710–5.

27. Chesser AS, Ganeshan V, Yang J, Johnson GV. Epigallocatechin-3-gallate enhances clearance of phosphorylated tau in primary neurons. Nutr Neurosci. 2016;19(1):21–31.

28. Chang X, Rong C, Chen Y, et al. (–)-Epigallocatechin-3-gallate attenuates cognitive deterioration in Alzheimer's disease model mice by upregulating neprilysin expression. Exp Cell Res. 2015;334(1):136–45.

29. Zhang ZX, Li YB, Zhao RP. Epigallocatechin Gallate attenuates β-Amyloid generation and oxidative stress involvement of PPARγ in N2a/APP695 cells. Neurochem Res. 2017;42(2):468–80.

30. Rezai-Zadeh K, Arendash GW, Hou H, Fernandez F, Jensen M, Runfeldt M, et al. Green tea epigallocatechin-3-gallate (EGCG) reduces beta-amyloid mediated cognitive impairment and modulates tau pathology in Alzheimer transgenic mice. Brain Res. 2008;1214:177–87.

31. Li Q, Gordon M, Tan J, et al. Oral administration of green tea epigallocatechin-3-gallate (EGCG) reduces amyloid beta deposition in transgenic mouse model of Alzheimer's disease. Exp Neurol. 2006;198:576.

32. Smith A, Giunta B, Bickford PC, Fountain M, Tan J, Shytle RD. Nanolipidic particles improve the bioavailability and alpha-secretase inducing ability of epigallocatechin-3-gallate (EGCG) for the treatment of Alzheimer's disease. Int J Pharm. 2010;389(1–2):207–12.

33. Giunta B, Hou H, Zhu Y, Salemi J, Ruscin A, Shytle RD, et al. Fish oil enhances anti-amyloidogenic properties of green tea EGCG in Tg2576 mice. Neurosci Lett. 2010;471(3):134–8.

34. Biasibetti R, Tramontina AC, Costa AP, Dutra MF, Quincozes-Santos A, Nardin P, et al. Green tea (–)epigallocatechin-3-gallate reverses oxidative stress and reduces acetylcholinesterase activity in a streptozotocin-induced model of dementia. Behav Brain Res. 2013;236:186–93.

35. He M, Liu MY, Wang S, Tang QS, Yao WF, Zhao HS, et al. Research on EGCG improving the degenerative changes of the brain in AD model mice induced with chemical drugs (article in Chinese). Zhong Yao Cai. 2012; 35(10):1641–4.

36. de la Monte SM. Brain insulin resistance and deficiency as therapeutic targets in Alzheimer's disease. Curr Alzheimer Res. 2012;9:35–66.

37. Jia N, Han K, Kong JJ, Zhang XM, Sha S, Ren GR, et al. (–)-Epigallocatechin-3-gallate alleviates spatial memory impairment in APP/PS1 mice by restoring IRS-1 signaling defects in the hippocampus. Mol Cell Biochem. 2013;380(1–2):211–8.

38. Ali B, Jamal QM, Shams S, et al. In silico analysis of green tea polyphenols as inhibitors of AChE and BChE enzymes in Alzheimer's disease treatment. CNS Neurol Disord Drug Targets. 2016;15:624–8.

39. Mähler A, Mandel S, Lorenz M, et al. Epigallocatechin-3-gallate: a useful, effective and safe clinical approach for targeted prevention and

individualised treatment of neurological diseases? EPMA J. 2013;4(1):5. doi:10.1186/1878-5085-4-5.

40. Bimonte S, Leongito M, Barbieri A, Del Vecchio V, Barbieri M, AlbinoV, et al. Inhibitory effect of (–)-epigallocatechin-3-gallate and bleomycin on human pancreatic cancer MiaPaca-2 cell growth. Infect Agent Cancer. 2015;10:22.

41. Nakagawa K, Miyazawa T. Absorption and distribution of tea catechin, (–)-epigallocatechin-3-gallate, in the rat. J Nutr Sci Vitaminol. 1997;43:679–84.

42. Suganuma M, Okabe S, Oniyama M, Tada Y, Ito H, Fujiki H. Wide distribution of [3H](–)-epigallocatechin gallate, a cancer preventive tea polyphenol, in mouse tissue. Carcinogenesis. 1998;19:1771–6.

43. Wu L, Zhang QL, Zhang XY, Lv C, Li J, Yuan Y, et al. Pharmacokinetics and blood–brain barrier penetration of (+)-catechin and (–)-epicatechin in rats by microdialysis sampling coupled to high-performance liquid chromatography with chemiluminescence detection. J Agric Food Chem. 2012;60:9377–83.

44. Mandel SA, Amit T, Weinreb O, Youdim MB. Understanding the broad-spectrum neuroprotective action profile of green tea polyphenols in aging and neurodegenerative diseases. J Alzheimers Dis. 2011;25:187–208.

45. Szarc vel Szic K, Declerck K, Vidaković M, Vanden Berghe W. From inflammaging to healthy aging by dietary lifestyle choices: is epigenetics the key to personalized nutrition? Clin Epigenetics. 2015;7:33. doi:10.1186/s13148-015-0068-2.

46. Kuriyama S, Hozawa A, Ohmori K, Shimazu T, Matsui T, Ebihara S, et al. Green tea consumption and cognitive function: a cross-sectional study from the Tsurugaya project 1. Am J Clin Nutr. 2006;83:355–61.

47. Molino S, Dossena M, Buonocore D, Ferrari F, Venturini L, Ricevuti G, et al. Polyphenols in dementia: from molecular basis to clinical trials. Life Sci. 2016;161:69–77.

48. Einöther SJ, Martens VE. Acute effects of tea consumption on attention and mood. Am J Clin Nutr. 2013;98(6 Suppl):1700S–8S.

49. Camfield DA, Stough C, Farrimond J, Scholey AB. Acute effects of tea constituents L-theanine, caffeine, and epigallocatechin gallate on cognitive function and mood: a systematic review and meta-analysis. Nutr Rev. 2014;72(8):507–22.

50. Wightman EL, Haskell CF, Forster JS, Veasey RC, Kennedy DO. Epigallocatechin gallate, cerebral blood flow parameters, cognitive performance and mood in healthy humans: a double-blind, placebo-controlled, crossover investigation. Hum Psychopharmacol. 2012;27(2):177–86.

51. Scholey A, Downey LA, Ciorciari J, Pipingas A, Nolidin K, Finn M, et al. Acute neurocognitive effects of epigallocatechin gallate (EGCG). Appetite. 2012;58:767–70.

52. Ide K, Yamada H, Takuma N, Park M, Wakamiya N, Nakase J, et al. Green tea consumption affects cognitive dysfunction in the elderly: a pilot study. Nutrients. 2014;6(10):4032–42.

53. Friedemann P. Sunphenon EGCg (Epigallocatechin-Gallate) in the early stage of Alzheimer's disease - NCT00951834 2009. Available at: https://clinicaltrials.gov/ct2/show/NCT00951834.

# 10

# An update on the management of breast cancer in Africa

V. Vanderpuye[1]* (ID), S. Grover[2], N. Hammad[3], PoojaPrabhakar[4], H. Simonds[5], F. Olopade[6] and D. C. Stefan[7]

## Abstract

**Background:** There is limited information about the challenges of cancer management and attempts at improving outcomes in Africa. Even though South and North Africa are better resourceds to tackle the burden of breast cancer, similar poor prognostic factors are common to all countries. The five-year overall Survival rate for breast cancer patients does not exceed 60% for any low and middle-income country (LMIC) in Africa. In spite of the gains achieved over the past decade, certain characteristics remain the same such as limited availability of breast conservation therapies, inadequate access to drugs, few oncology specialists and adherence to harmful socio-cultural practices. This review on managing breast cancer in Africa is authored by African oncologists who practice or collaborate in Africa and with hands-on experience with the realities.

**Methods:** A search was performed via electronic databases from 1999 to 2016. (PubMed/Medline, African Journals Online) for all literature in English or translated into English, covering the terms "breast cancer in Africa and developing countries". One hundred ninety were deemed appropriate.

**Results:** Breast tumors are diagnosed at earlier ages and later stages than in highincome countries. There is a higher prevalence of triple-negative cancers. The limitations of poor nursing care and surgery, inadequate access to radiotherapy, poor availability of basic and modern systemic therapies translate into lower survival rate. Positive strides in breast cancer management in Africa include increased adaptation of treatment guidelines, improved pathology services including immuno-histochemistry, expansion and upgrading of radiotherapy equipment across the continent in addition to more research opportunities.

**Conclusion:** This review is an update of the management of breast cancer in Africa, taking a look at the epidemiology, pathology, management resources, outcomes, research and limitations in Africa from the perspective of oncologists with local experience.

**Keywords:** Breast cancer, Radiotherapy, Chemotherapy, Targeted therapies, Survival, Hormonal therapy

## Background

Publications on breast cancer in Africa start by describing a large number of patients presenting with advanced disease, limited access to cancer education, screening, and care. We have learned from previous studies that registries are still missing in Africa or are only hospital based in most regions of the continent. The estimates of breast cancer incidence are presented as figures but not with the real data as the current situation, remains still to be determined [1].

Survival is seldom described and if so only selectively in a limited number of countries or centers. Cancer mortality rates in African countries are not comparable to those of high-income countries (HIC) [1], reaching unacceptable high proportions.

The Concorde −2 study of 5-year breast cancer survival from 1995 to 2009 based on the analysis of individual data from 279 population-based registries in 67 countries, reported that, in HIC, age-standardized net survival rates were more than 85%. One country in Africa, Mauritius, a HIC island nation off the coast of Madagascar, had similar survival rates of 87.4% (95% CI:78.1–96.7). North African countries had lower outcomes compared to HIC, for example, 59.8% (95% CI:48.6–71.1) in Algeria, 76.6% (95%

* Correspondence: vanaglat@yahoo.com
[1]National center for Radiotherapy and Nuclear Medicine, Korle-Bu Teaching Hospital, Accra, Ghana
Full list of author information is available at the end of the article

CI:55.5–97.7) in Libya (Benghazi registry) and 68.4% (95% CI:64.5–72.2) in Tunisia. By contrast, data available from three Sub-Saharan countries, South Africa 53.4% (95% CI:35.5–71.3), The Gambia 11.9%(95% CI:0–24.7) and Mali 13.6%(95% CI:0, 0–30.1), were significantly inferior to other countries around the world [1]. More than 50% of African women diagnosed with breast cancer die of the disease [2]. The disease is the most frequent cause of cancer death in less developed regions, causing one in five deaths in African women [3], described as a new "shift" from the previous decade [4]. Breast tumors are diagnosed a decade or two lower on age at diagnosis and present at advanced stages compared to developed countries [5, 6]. A higher prevalence of hormone receptor negative and triple-negative cancers(TNBC) is found in Africa [7]. The paucity of oncology specialist including nurses and surgeons, access to radiotherapy, availability of basic and modern systemic and hormonal therapies and steadfast adherence to negative socio-cultural beliefs is reflected in the observed lower survival rates compared to high-income countries. In spite of the various setbacks, improvements in breast cancer management include the development or adaptation of treatment guidelines, improved pathology services including immunohisto-chemistry testing for hormone receptor testing. The expansion and upgrading of radiotherapy resources, new collaborations fostered between international organizations and African cancer treatment facilities will promote research opportunities and improve outcomes.

Previous reviews were specific to surgery, stage at presentation, pathology services or discussed sub-regions whereas this paper provides an update on the current state of breast cancer management in Africa as whole, looking at epidemiology, clinical presentation, and access to radiotherapy, systemic therapies, pathology services, outcomes and new research.

## Methods

A search was performed via electronic databases (Pubmed, Medline, African Journal online) for literature in English or translated into English covering all aspects of breast cancer in Africa from 1999 to 2016. One thousand three hundred and twenty articles on the subject were retrieved under the terms "breast cancer and Africa or developing countries." Publications with high emphasis on prevention and screening were excluded. Two hundred and twenty-five articles were relevant to the subject under review and One hundred and ninety articles including 15 review articles, were selected.

## Results

The majority of publications were from North and West Africa (60%), others were from East (10%), Central and South Africa (12%). Other publications (31%) broadly discussed breast cancer in larger geographical regions i.e., Sub-Saharan Africa, developing countries in which discussions specific to Africa were highlighted. Publications from authors in developed countries and collaborating international organizations were found in high impact journals whereas publications from local health personnel were found in lower impact journals. There were very few prospective studies and many retrospective studies.

New research findings, epidemiology, practice update, challenges involved in disease control, differences in disease characteristics, management practices, and outcomes are highlighted.

## Epidemiology

Non-communicable diseases, including breast cancer, are on the rise in Africa, presumably due to advances in health care, translating into longer life expectancy and increased detection of cancer. Breast cancer incidence increases with age, and people in Africa are living longer due to better control of human immunodeficiency virus (HIV) and other infectious diseases [8]. This section will discuss prevalence, incidence, and risk factors of breast cancer in Africa. Eleven studies were found on the epidemiology of breast cancer in Africa, including studies from Zimbabwe, Tunisia, Egypt, Morocco, South Africa, and Nigeria.

### Prevalence

Breast cancer is leading cancer among the female population worldwide, as well as in the majority of countries in Africa, according to data from 26 African countries for 2012 [9]. In Africa, breast cancer is responsible for one in four diagnosed cancers and one in five cancer deaths in women [10].

### Incidence

Marked variation exists in the reported incidence of breast cancer worldwide – from 95 to 100 cases per 100,000 persons in North America, Northern Europe, and Australia to 13.5–30 per 100,000 women in sub-Saharan Africa(SSA) [3]. The breast cancer incidence in Africa continues to increase and is projected to double by 2050 [11]. In Zimbabwe, a 4.5% annual increase in breast cancer incidence over the period 1991–2010 has been noted [11]. Within SSA, there is considerable regional variation in the estimated incidence of breast cancer, with 38.9 (per 100,000 women) in Southern Africa, 38.6 in western Africa, 30.4 in eastern Africa, and 26.8 in central Africa [3]. The high rates in southern Africa and urban parts of Africa may be due to better reporting and a higher population of Anglo-Europeans in those areas [12]. Of note, studies from Tunisia, Egypt, and Morocco report that North Africa has a greater proportion of inflammatory breast cancer (IBC) among all breast cancers than elsewhere in the world; however, the incidence of IBC in North Africa is in decline [13–15]. As only a few African countries maintain cancer registries, accurate prevalence figures are unavailable, although the global burden of cancer study (GLOBOCAN) data estimate that in 2012, 94,000 women developed breast cancer [3].

## Risk factors

Several studies have investigated breast cancer risk and various reproductive and anthropometric factors. Use of oral or injectable contraceptives within the previous 10 years significantly increased risk of breast cancer in South Africa, with an odds ratio (OR) of 1.66 and 95% confidence interval (CI) of 1.28–2.16 [16]. Another study in Nigeria found an inverse relationship between age at menarche and breast cancer risk (OR: 0.72; 95% CI: 0.54–0.95) [17]. In a Nigerian study of 1233 breast cancer cases, body mass index (BMI) had an inverse relationship to risk (OR: 1.22; 95% CI: 1.14–1.32) [18]. Also in Nigeria, height, waist circumference (OR: 2.39; 95% CI: 1.59–3.60), and waist-to-hip ratio (OR: 2.15; 95% CI: 1.61–2.85) showed positive correlation to breast cancer [18, 19]. A study for North Africa defines a risk profile in Egyptian and Tunisian women that are more protective about high-income countries. These are a higher mean number of children, younger mean age at first pregnancy, longer mean duration of breastfeeding, lower mean age at menopause, lower prevalence of contraceptive use and lower alcohol consumption [13].

In summary, breast cancer is the most prevalent cancer in African women, although incidence is lower than in high-income countries. Even though the risk factors of breast cancer in Africa are similar to those in high-income countries, the variation in risk factor incidences may account for the differences between African countries and high-income countries.

## Clinical presentation

The clinical presentation of breast cancer in African women is significantly different compared to their counterparts in high-income countries, as well as from Africa.

## Age at presentation

Breast cancer patients in Africa present at a relatively younger age compared to patients in high-income countries [7, 20, 21]. The overall mean age of presentation in West African women is between 35 and 45 years, 10 to 15 years earlier than in women from high-income countries [22]. Similarly, a 3-year retrospective review of 374 breast cancer patients in Kenya showed a median age of 44 years [6], while the mean age in a Tanzanian cancer registry was 44.7 years [23].

## Stage at presentation

The majority of patients in Africa present with advanced stage breast cancer, with 89.6% and 72.8% of breast patients in Kenya and Nigeria respectively presenting with advanced stage disease [6, 24]. These rates are relatively higher than rates of advanced stage breast cancer in high-income countries [25]. Studies in South Africa reported an advanced stage breast cancer incidence of 50 and 55% [25, 26]. However, a Moroccan study reported an incidence of 33% for Stage III and IV breast cancers [27]. Of note, south and northern African patients present at earlier stages compared to the rest of Africa. Table 1. summarizes the data for clinical presentation in the studies reviewed [6, 7, 23–28].

## Receptor status

Breast cancers diagnosed among African women reportedly include a disproportionate number of poor prognosis tumors, including hormone receptor negative, and triple negative. Tumors tend to be larger, with most being >2 cm. Many of the tumors are hormone receptor negative, with reported rates of both estrogen receptor (ER) and progesterone receptor (PR) negativity ranging from 36 to 79% and 30–87% [Table 1]. Few studies report on human epidermal growth factor receptor 2 (HER 2) status as its impact is over shadowed by the high rate of triple negative cancers (TNBC). Over expression of HER 2 is reported in 18% of Malian patients, 26% in South Africa, 22% in Uganda, 17.5% in Sudan, and 27% in Egypt showing differences within the continent [29–33]. Luyeye et al. compared to breast cancer molecular subtypes between Congo and Belgium and found higher Her2 over expression rates in older Congolese women compared to Belgians [34].

Many African women are diagnosed with triple negative tumors [6, 7, 23–28]. Triple-negative breast cancer (TNBC) subtypes account for 12–20% of all breast cancer; however, women of African descent tend to have a high incidence of TNBC translating into poorer outcomes [35]. The proportion of triple-negative breast cancers among all breast cancers is 23 and 28% in Tunisia and Egypt respectively [13, 27].

In summary, there is a lower average age of breast cancer diagnosis and higher stage at presentation in Africa compared to high-income countries. There is a higher proportion of triple-negative breast cancers in Africa compared to other high-income countries.

## Surgical management

Surgery is the primary modality in the management of resectable breast cancer, and when integrated with other therapies plays a significant role in controlling locally advanced or metastatic disease. However, in certain parts of the world including Africa, surgery may be the only

**Table 1** Clinical presentation of breast cancer by study included in this review

| Study | Country | Patients | Reported incidence of advanced stage breast cancer | Median Age at Diagnosis | Receptor Status in HIV-uninfected patients |
|---|---|---|---|---|---|
| Otheino-Abinya [6] | Kenya | 250 | 89.6% | 44 | |
| Ikpat [28] | Nigeria | 300 | | 42.7 | |
| Adebamowo [24] | Nigeria | 250 | 72.8% | 43 | |
| Anyanwu [7] | Nigeria | 179 | 72% | 46.9 | |
| Cubasch [25] | Soweto, South Africa | 1092 | 50% | | ER: 58% |
| | | | | | PR: 47% |
| | | | | | HER2: 22% |
| | | | | | TNBC: 19% |
| Langenhoven [26] | Cape Town, South Africa | 586 | 55% | 56 | ER: 64% |
| | | | | | PR: 51% |
| | | | | | HER2: 36% |
| | | | | | TNBC: 16% |
| Amir [23] | Tanzania | 937 | | 44.7 | |
| Rais [27] | Morocco | 980 | 33% | 46 | TNBC: 16.5% |

treatment option due to limited resources for complimentary adjuvant therapies. The rates of surgical treatment vary across Africa, ranging from 35.2% in Nigeria to 100% in Cameroon; with the majority of countries reporting surgical rates between 48 and 75% compared to over 90% in European countries [26]. The differences in surgical rates could be a result of the high burden of African women presenting with unresectable breast cancer.

## Factors influencing the choice of surgery

The majority of women in developed countries present with early stage disease amenable to breast conserving techniques because of established screening and awareness programs. On the other hand, many women in Africa require radical mastectomy to control their disease [21]. On average, 50–75% of women present with very advanced disease in Africa [36]. Islami et al. reported 74 and 81% advanced stage at presentation in Cote d'Ivoire and the Democratic Republic of Congo respectively [37], Soliman et al. reported 90% of breast cancer patients present with advanced disease in Niger; invariably mastectomy is the most common surgical procedure performed [38]. Reports from Eritrea and Tanzania indicate that up to 99% of patients undergo mastectomy for various reasons including advanced stage and lack of other modalities of treatment [39, 40]. Mastectomy and breast conservation rates in Europe are reported as 30 and 70% respectively, which is in sharp contrast to 85% mastectomy rates in Africa [41]. North America reports rising breast conservation rate (68%) as at 2007 [42].

The indication for breast conserving surgery is limited early resectable disease and dependent on the availability of radiation therapy to sterilize the remaining breast tissue. Borderline resectable tumors can be down staged to allow for breast conservation with neoadjuvant chemotherapy. The poor access to radiation facilities in Africa is a major factor contributing to the limited access to conserving breast surgery in many countries. Even where radiotherapy facilities are available in Africa, very few women are considered candidates for breast conservation despite achieving good response rates to neoadjuvant chemotherapy for various reasons [5]. Maalej et al. reported that even though half of breast cancer patients present with resectable disease in Tunisia, the breast conservation rate was only 17.6% and was dependent on the surgeon's preferences [43].

Egyptian women with early stage disease may be considered poor candidates for breast conservation because of high illiteracy rate and compounding cultural influences. These factors do not allow for regular surveillance of patients following breast conservation required to detect early recurrence in the remaining breast tissue [44].

In a recent review of breast cancer surgery in Africa, Malawi, Ghana, Rwanda and South Africa reported higher rates of lumpectomy (45, 40, 29 and 12% respectively) compared to single digit figures found in other countries [26]. This report may indicate improvement in down staging of tumors, access to care and breast cancer education. Malawi and Rwanda do not have radiotherapy facilities, meaning patients will have to travel to neighboring countries for radiotherapy and would be of interest to know the follow-up data for these patients.

## Quality of surgery

Several authors [45, 46] have discussed the inadequacy of surgical capacities to tackle cancer surgery in LMIC. Resources including skilled personnel are limited to main cities limiting access to the rural poor even though some of the required procedures are basic and could be performed by general surgeons [25]. In a few African countries like Malawi by surgeries are performed by non-physicians, who may not understand the principles underlying the adequacy of axillary dissections, obtaining clear margins and proper fixation of surgical specimens for histological assessment [47]. Economic and political instability on the continent may be a contributing factor to the limited number of trained surgical oncologist by promoting brain drain resulting from not only poor remuneration but also suboptimal resources in the working environment [46]. The continent needs to invest in the training of oncology specialist to improve outcomes [48].

## Factors contributing to poor compliance to surgery

Breast cancer patients in Africa default mastectomy for many reasons which include the fear of mastectomy. The low surgical utilization rates found in some countries could be explained by the lack of awareness in detecting early stage disease, long surgical waiting list leading to the productive use of alternative therapies, a complexity of navigating health care systems, financial constraints and illiteracy [31, 49–52].

Breast cancer surgery is considered demeaning and culturally and spiritually unacceptable [53]. The rate of mastectomy refusal varies within the continent, an example being fewer refusal rates in Eritrea and Cameroon compared to Nigeria [26].

In summary, the quality of breast cancer surgery in Africa is improving but requires an injection of resources starting with a training of surgeons with oncology skills, improving access to care and patient education on the impact of sociocultural myths.

## Systemic therapies

The number of publications documenting and detailing experiences with systemic therapies for breast cancer management in Africa continues to rise in recent years but still considered scare. For this reason, comprehensive comparisons of systemic therapy logistics and outcomes within Africa and the rest of the world was difficult in the absence of rich data.

### Chemotherapy
#### Cost and access to drugs

The cost of newer and more effective systemic therapies for cancer continues to rise. For most of Africa, meager health expenditure budgets, competing for interest and dwindling donor financial support are hindrances to accessing life-saving cancer medication with many low-middle income countries(LMIC) barely satisfying the WHO essential drug list for cancer [54]. Publications from Africa repeatedly demonstrate the limited availability of some core and newer cancer drugs and the unbearable out of pocket payments leading to treatment non –compliance [5, 36, 40]. Breast cancer activist has had little success improving access to drugs by lobbying to reduce a cost of drugs through tax exemptions and ensuring breast cancer screening, diagnosis and treatment are included in national health insurance schemes.

Breast cancer in Africa is characterized by disease in younger women with aggressive disease and poor hormone receptor staining which require the use of second and third generation drugs including Taxane-based chemotherapy [55–58]. These new drugs are considerably expensive with limited access in very few Sub-Saharan African health institutions [59–61]. Patients who are refractory to initial chemotherapy have limited options for subsequent therapies, which are either unavailable or unaffordable. Southern and northern parts of Africa have better access to newer cancer medications and promote the use of national guidelines in an attempt to standardize management of breast cancer in their countries [62].

### Choice of drugs

Most low- and middle-income countries in Africa experience severe limitations with drug access, which unfortunately could foster the influx of cheap, suboptimal or fake drugs. Generic brands of systemic therapies have improved access to life-saving cancer medications with the promise of very low pricing and availability [63].

For each patient, the financial limitations, inconvenient scheduling of cycles, i.e., weekly versus three weekly, and a high cost of supportive therapies needed to reduce toxicity and patient and family beliefs and interferences influences the choice and sequence of treatments [64]. A pilot survey of breast cancer management in sub-Saharan Africa reports that the use of neoadjuvant chemotherapy was more prevalent and could be a result of the high burden of locally reported and or large theater waiting time. In this study cyclophosphamide, adriamycin and five Fluorouracil combination were the commonest protocol prescribed in the neoadjuvant and adjuvant setting [65]. Achieving complete pathological response rates is associated with improved survival in patients who received neoadjuvant chemotherapy. McFarland, et al. in a recent publication, describes improvements in breast cancer pathological response rates over a five-year period following neoadjuvant chemotherapy; from 14 to 43%, with an overall complete response rate of 26.5% [66]. The introduction of newer drugs into neoadjuvant protocols especially Her 2 targeted drugs, Taxanes, and carboplatin for Her2 positive and TNBC subtypes are associated with the recent improvements in pathological response rates. Sule at al., in 2016 published data on 20 patients in Nigeria who received at least five cycles of Taxane- based neoadjuvant chemotherapy, and reported a 67% complete pathological response rate [67]. Other small studies from Africa report complete pathological response rates of 10–35%, none of the studies included Taxanes, carboplatin or Her 2 targets [68–70]. These rates compare favorably with full pathological rates from developed countries before the introduction of Taxanes, carboplatin and targeted therapies [71].

A phase 2 trial conducted in Nigerian patients reported no complete pathological response rate with single neoadjuvant agent capecitabine, but documented a 44% overall response rate [72].

Breast cancer patients in Africa are known to abscond following complete clinical response to neoadjuvant, and this may influence the high mastectomy rate found in some parts of Africa [73].

## Down staging compliance to chemotherapy

In Cameroon, one-third of breast cancer patients delayed the first two cycles chemotherapy at least by 2 weeks and two third cited financial constraints as a compounding factor [74]. The cost was a major factor contributing to high noncompliance rates in other countries [39, 75]. Other than the high cost of chemotherapy, side effects of chemotherapy such as hair loss, nail changes, nausea, vomiting, and infertility is considered culturally unacceptable, driving patients to abscond treatment for traditional and less invasive unorthodox treatments [44, 76].

### Quality of service delivery

The lack of support services to manage toxicities may be a reason to withhold effective chemotherapy protocols even where accessible. In some parts of Africa, the choice and sequencing of chemotherapy protocols is ad hoc. The prescription and administration of systemic therapies are by general physicians, surgeons, and non-oncology nurses, and this negatively impacts optimization of disease control [45]. Low white cell counts levels in Africans may confound the ability to administer full doses of chemotherapy and the use highly myelo-suppressive protocols especially in non-experienced hands, notwithstanding the prohibitive cost of granulocyte stimulating growth factors [77]. The role of specialized oncology nurses is important for cancer control through education, counseling, proper administration of chemotherapy and palliation. Structured oncology nursing training programs are a necessity for Africa and other LMIC to improve the quality of cancer care [78].

## Targeted therapy
### Cost and access to drug

Epidermal Growth Factor Receptors, Vascular Endothelial Growth Factor receptor, Mammalian Target Of Rapamycin inhibitors, cyclin dependent kinases, programmed cell death protein one inhibitor either with single or double blockade of receptors targets are some of the new drugs developed to target the breast cancer cell [79]. The discovery of HER 2 targeted therapy has revolutionized the management of breast cancer. However, the cost of these life-saving drugs remains, unfortunately, astronomical even for high-income countries [80]. In 2015, Trastuzumab was included in the World Health Organisation (WHO) essential drug list for the management of Her2 positive breast cancer. However, the cost-effectiveness of this treatment in most LMIC is under debate [81]. In South and North of Africa where Trastuzumab, a HER 2 targeted drug is easily available, there are serious concerns about access [82].

Biosimilars at markedly reduced cost available to countries like India should be made available to Africa to save precious lives. The astronomical cost of biomarker testing and molecularly targeted drugs brings into question the cost-effectiveness of promoting extensive molecular profiling of breast cancer in Africa other than for research purposes.

## Hormonal therapy

This class of drugs targets the hormone receptor within the breast cancer cell. They are indicated only in hormone receptor positive disease, achieving high response rates, which translate into improved control and survival in the curative or palliative setting. The accuracy of receptor testing is dependent on efficient and reliable pathology services. Countries without these facilities resort to a blind prescription of hormonal therapies.

### Cost and access to drug

Hormonal therapy for breast cancer is one of the most available treatment options even in poorer countries. Many companies supply generic Tamoxifen at a very low cost making it readily available and in some countries available free of charge [83, 84].

Unlike Tamoxifen, the access and availability of aromatase inhibitors is restricted in most of Africa [22, 85].

### Choice of drug

In Africa, patients are more likely to be ER negative, rendering Tamoxifen ineffective in disease control if prescribed for all breast cancer patients [86, 87]. A recent meta-analysis of hormone receptor status of breast cancer patients in Africa indicates that more than half of African women have hormone positive breast cancer, disputing the poor receptor status in the majority of breast cancer cases [85]. However, this finding from the study is debatable and is not evident in clinical practice and will, therefore, require further expanded research. There are detrimental effects of prescribing Tamoxifen for negative receptor disease, and it remains apparent that improving the quality of pathology services is a key to improving survival [10]. Numerous studies have demonstrated improved outcomes with the use of aromatase inhibitors in both premenopausal (following ovarian suppression) and post-menopausal women with receptor positive breast cancer [88, 89]. The acceptance of ovarian suppression in premenopausal young African women is low and a hindrance to prescribing aromatase inhibitors as primary or second line therapy for hormone receptor positive disease. Many African countries currently recognize the importance of receptor testing and are working towards improving pathology services [90]. As an example, Madagascar did not have access to hormone receptor testing until 2011 and are currently reporting a higher ER negative- rates compared to ER-positive disease, defining a better application of targeted therapy [91].

### Compliance to hormone therapy

Non-adherence to hormone treatment is a common worldwide problem and ranges 30–72% for adherence and discontinuation [92].

Small studies from Nigeria and South Africa report 25 and 36% non-adherence rates for Tamoxifen which is comparable to data from developed countries [93, 94].

In summary, the use of systemic therapies to control breast cancer in Africa continues to improve as countries develop and adopt guidelines from developed countries. Sadly, these improvements are evident mainly in the middle and higher income countries in the continent. The impact on outcomes are be dampened by the lack of access to quality medications, unskilled personnel and socio-cultural influences in many countries.

## Radiotherapy
### Access to radiation therapy

The most challenging aspect of providing breast cancer radiotherapy in Africa is access to radiation therapy resources. More than 90% of all radiotherapy equipment is found in South and northern Africa [95]. Twenty-nine countries in Africa have no access to radiation services, and even those with these services face prohibitive maintenance costs and demands for limited skills. There is often extreme pressure on these limited resources, leading to delay in commencement of treatment. With the majority of patients being diagnosed with a locally advanced disease, the inclusion of radiation treatments in the overall management is paramount.

Expanding radiation facilities is a major step to improving outcomes in breast cancer patients with both primary and metastatic disease. Advanced techniques such as conformal and planning techniques used in HIC has been successfully replicated with less sophisticated but modernized Cobalt-60 teletherapy equipment and low energy linear accelerators as a pilot in some countries and has the potential to reduce toxicities associated with breast irradiation [96, 97]. Through partnerships with the International Atomic Energy Agency (IAEA) and other collaborators, many countries are establishing new centers or upgrading existing ones with modern radiotherapy equipment and training of technical staff, which will invariably improve access to radiotherapy services.

### Dose prescription

Treatment protocols for curative breast cancer vary across the continent with some institutions following international standardized protocols of 5 weeks of daily radiation; and in others, shortened hypo-fractionated regimes are adopted in increased throughput of patients on the limited numbers of linear accelerators [98, 99]. Also, hypofractionated regimens are unnecessarily avoided in some instances where access is only to cobalt-60 or low energy linear accelerators due to concerns regarding skin toxicities.

Radiotherapy is a cornerstone of effective palliative care, essential for managing bone pain and unresectable locally advanced disease complicated by ulceration and bleeding. A survey of patterns of palliative radiation has shown that oncologists in Africa conform to cost-effective single fractions in bone metastases but are more likely to use longer fractionation schedules for local disease [100].

### Factors affecting compliance to treatment

Interruption of radiotherapy treatments are a frequent occurrence as the daily costs of traveling for therapy can be significant [101]. Many centers in Africa charge user fees, which for the impoverished lead to a high rate of non-compliance. Data on outcomes the following radiotherapy for breast cancer patients in Africa is lacking, with no particular research being published in the last decade detailing efficacy data, abandonment or cost of treatment.

In summary, the limited radiotherapy access in Africa is a major setback to improving breast cancer outcomes considering the high burden of advanced disease on the continent.

## Managing HIV positive breast cancer in Africa
### Chemotherapy toxicities

Although the cluster of differentiation 4 (CD4) count in HIV-infected patients is not associated with age and stage of breast cancer, CD4 count at diagnosis may affect chemotherapy tolerance [102]. Langenhoven et al., in a South African cohort, reported that more than 84% of breast cancer patients, including 19 who were HIV-infected, who initiated systemic chemotherapy completed it without severe toxicity, regardless of their HIV status [26]. This report was found despite a mean decline in CD4 count during chemotherapy from 477 cells/µL to 333 cells/µL. There was no statistically significant difference in hematologic toxicity requiring dose modification. However, grade 3 or 4 lymphocytopenia developed only in the HIV-infected patients (26.4%; $p = 0.001$). Additionally, there was no data on the HIV-infected patients receiving antiretroviral therapy (ART) concurrently with chemotherapy, with scant details of the ART regimen [26].

These findings suggest that while HIV/AIDS may cause some chemotoxicity in patients with a low CD4 count, a normal CD4 count does not reduce chemotherapy tolerance. Low CD4 count, may have reduced treatment efficacy and treatment adequacy due to poor adherence, dose adjustments, treatment delays and early discontinuation of therapy [103–105].

There are no studies examining treatment outcomes with surgery and radiation therapy in patients with HIV/AIDS and breast cancer in Africa.

In summary, HIV positive breast cancer patients in Africa should be managed like HIV negative patients under proper supervision by skilled clinicians, paying attention to supportive care needs.

## Outcomes

Compared with data on the incidence and overall burden of the disease, there is a significant paucity of data on breast cancer outcomes including overall survival, quality of life and survivorship issues. Large population–based outcome reports are lacking due to various factors such as delay in diagnosis, lack or interruptions of treatment, heterogeneity and difficulty of access to screening, diagnosis and treatment and lack of high-quality population-based cancer registries [106]. Currently available data point to a very high mortality/incidence ratio of 0.55 in Central Africa as compared to 0.16 in the United States [107]. Most publications on Breast cancer treatments and outcomes are from the facility- or hospital-based case series [61]. Nonetheless, these case series provide valuable data. For example, adjuvant, chemotherapy and radiotherapy were given to 44.8 and 11.7% of patients with an overall 5-year survival of 21.8% at the Bugando Medical Center in Tanzania [40]. A retrospective study of 152 patients with triple negative breast cancer in Morocco reported with a 5-year overall survival of 76.5%. The outcome was by literature data from North America and Spain, especially in young age at high-grade diagnosis tumors, advanced stage at

diagnosis, and a short time to relapse [20, 27]. Despite high response rate to chemotherapy, the overall prognosis of this subset of tumors remains poor. A recent publication from Accra, Ghana reports a 5-year overall survival of 91.94% for stage one, 15.09% for stage four and cumulative 5-year overall survival of 47.9% [108].

Increasingly reports and analysis such as treatment rates, rates of treatment adherence, local recurrence and presentation at late stages thought to be of importance in resource constraint regions are being published [40, 100].

Treatment outcomes generated from prospective clinical trials are scarce. Recent efforts to rectify this situation include the study of neoadjuvant Capecitabine chemotherapy in newly diagnosed women with advanced breast cancer in Nigeria [72]. This phase II study indicated that conducting high-quality prospective trials are feasible in resource-constrained settings and highlighted the challenges associated with generating high-quality patient outcome data such as slow accrual leading to early closure.

Poorly kept medical records and losses to follow-up of patients hamper data collection on outcomes. The African Breast Cancer-Disparities in Outcomes (ABC-DO) study is a prospective hospital-based study of overall survival, quality of life (QoL), delays in diagnosis and treatment in five African countries [109]. This study, which is underway utilizes mobile devices to capture the data of 2000 women over 3 years and will overcome traditional barriers to collecting patient-outcome data by harnessing the recent explosion of telecommunication in the continent.

In summary, reported outcomes for breast cancer interventions are scarce but show a positive trend. The poor patient follow-up culture is a major contributing factor to reporting. With improvements in local and collaborative research skills development in Africa, there should be improvements in outcomes data over the next decade.

## Future research

Although there have been significant local and global collaborative efforts to address research needs of breast cancer in Africa, critical research gaps remain in basic, translational, clinical and health services research. Integration of genomic medicine research findings in breast cancer prevention, screening, diagnosis, and treatment is significantly lagging behind in Africa [110]. In addition to research into the different and complex tumor biology of breast cancer in Africa [111], other research priorities including response to treatment, developing validated markers for chemosensitivity and radiosensitivity to guide treatment, understanding the optimal duration, sequencing and logical combinations of treatment for improved personal therapy. LMICs are societies in transition, therefore research in lifestyle changes such as diet and weight [112], hormonal influences and inter-action with other non- communicable diseases(NCD) can shed light on the epidemiology of breast cancer in Africa and elucidate any changing trends in the biology of the disease. Other priorities include psychosocial and cultural dimensions, outcomes and survivorship. Trad-itionally personalized therapy is thought to be of more importance in high-income settings. However, given the cost of access to diagnosis and treatment in resource-limited settings, it is prudent to invest in research informing individualized, outcome-based approach to diagnosis and treatment to maximize rational use of limited resources.

Infrastructural investment enablers for research in breast cancer in Africa will require strategic planning to integrate research in cancer control plans of the contin-ent as a whole in partnership with stakeholders includ-ing the international community. Also needed is the investment in capacity building, training of researchers and health professionals in addition to the creation of innovative programs to encourage collaborative cross-disciplinary working practices [113].

## Summary

The situation in Africa continues to show a slow pro-gression of improved outcomes for breast cancer pa-tients compared with the rest of the developing world. Possible reasons may include the inadequacy of health care infrastructure in many countries, poverty, limited expenditure of health budget on cancer, increasing breast cancer burden with late diagnosis, lack of contin-ued education and awareness programs. Pathology in Africa needs to improve faster than at the present speed and the number of those who have the skills and know-ledge to decipher the diagnosis becomes an urgent issue to address.

However, the outlook on some fronts calls for opti-mism. Many African countries are now working together to create national and international alliances to improve cancer care and therefore breast cancer care should also benefit from a more systematic approach. Increased awareness and education associated with efficient models to facilitate down staging of the disease remain essential in Africa.

## Conclusion

As more and more governments and organizations make finalizing cancer control plans a priority, guidelines and policies for breast cancer care on the continent will con-tinue to improve. The outlook for optimism will keep on increasing as well as the survival and the quality of life for those affected by the disease. Forming consortiums should be fostered, whereby better-resourced regions in Africa could serve as mentors, striving to improve breast cancer survival on the continent.

## Abbreviations

ABC-DO: African Breast Cancer-Disparities in Outcomes; ART: Antiretroviral therapy; BMI: Body mass index; CD 4: Cluster of differentiation 4 is a glycoprotein found on lymphocytes; ER: Estrogen receptor; GLOBOCAN: Global burden of cancer study; Her 2: Human epidermal growth factor receptor 2; HIC: High-income countries; HIV: Human immunodeficiency virus; IAEA: International Atomic Energy Agency; IBC: Inflammatory breast cancer; LMIC: Low-middle income countries; NCD: Non-communicable diseases; PR: Progesterone receptor; QoL: Quality of life; SSA: sub-Saharan Africa; TNBC: Triple negative breast cancer; WHO: World Health Organization

## Acknowledgements

Acknowledgements to Belmira Rodrigues of the AORTIC secretariat for support.

## Funding

No funding was necessary for this publication.

## Authors' contributions

VV Concept development, manuscript design, preparation and final edit. SG manuscript design, preparation and editing of final of manuscript. NH manuscript preparation. CS manuscript preparation and editing of final manuscript. HS, FO, CS, PP – manuscript preparation. All authors read and approved the final manuscript.

## Authors' information

V Vanderpuye Aortic Secretary Treasurer Elect 2016/2017
S Grover Aortic Member
N Hammad Aortic Vice President North America
H Simonds Aortic Member O Olopade Aortic Council Member
Dc Stefan Aortic President Elect 2016/2017.

## Competing interests

The authors declare that they have no competing interest.

## Author details

[1]National center for Radiotherapy and Nuclear Medicine, Korle-Bu Teaching Hospital, Accra, Ghana. [2]Hospital of University of Pennsylvania, Department of Radiation Oncology, (Botswana-UPENN program), 3400 Civic Center Blvd., Philadelphia, PA 19104, USA. [3]Cancer Centre of Southeastern Ontario, Burr 2, Kingston General Hospital, 25 King Street W, Kingston, ON K7L 5P9, Canada. [4]University of Texas Southwestern Medical Center, Dallas, TX, USA. [5]Division of Radiation Oncology, Tygerberg Hospital/University of Stellenbosch, Tygerberg, South Africa. [6]The University of Chicago, 5841 S Maryland Avenue, MC 2115, Chicago, IL 60637, USA. [7]Walter Sisulu University Nelson Mandela Dr, Nelson Mandela Drive, Mthatha 5100, Eastern Cape, South Africa.

## References

1.  Allemani C, Weir HK, Carreira H, Harewood R, Spika D, Wang XS, Bannon F, Ahn JV, Johnson CJ, Bonaventure A, et al. Global surveillance of cancer survival 1995–2009: analysis of individual data for 25,676,887 patients from 279 population-based registries in 67 countries (CONCORD-2). Lancet. 2015; 385:977–1010.

2. Ginsburg OM. Breast and cervical cancer control in low and middle-income countries: human rights meet sound health policy. J Cancer Policy. 2013;1:e35–41.

3. Ferlay JSI, Ervik M, Dikshit R, Eser S, Mathers C, Rebelo M, Parkin DM, Forman D, Bray F. GLOBOCAN 2012 v1.0, Cancer Incidence and Mortality Worldwide IARC CancerBase No. 11 edition. Lyon: International Agency for Research on Cancer; 2013.

4. Jemal A, Bray F, Center MM, Ferlay J, Ward E, Forman D. Global cancer statistics. CA Cancer J Clin. 2011;61:69–90.

5. Anyanwu SN, Egwuonwu OA, Ihekwoaba EC. Acceptance and adherence to treatment among breast cancer patients in Eastern Nigeria. Breast. 2011;20 Suppl 2:S51–53.

6. Othieno-Abinya NA, Nyabola LO, Abwao HO, Ndege P. Postsurgical management of patients with breast cancer at Kenyatta National Hospital. East Afr Med J. 2002;79:156–62.

7. Anyanwu SN. Temporal trends in breast cancer presentation in the third world. J Exp Clin Cancer Res. 2008;27:17.

8. Parkin DM, Nambooze S, Wabwire-Mangen F, Wabinga HR. Changing cancer incidence in Kampala, Uganda, 1991–2006. Int J Cancer. 2010;126:1187–95.

9. Kantelhardt EJ, Cubasch H, Hanson C. Taking on breast cancer in East Africa: global challenges in breast cancer. Curr Opin Obstet Gynecol. 2015;27:108–14.

10. Ferlay J, Shin HR, Bray F, Forman D, Mathers C, Parkin DM. Estimates of worldwide burden of cancer in 2008: GLOBOCAN 2008. Int J Cancer. 2010; 127:2893–917.

11. Chokunonga E, Borok MZ, Chirenje ZM, Nyakabau AM, Parkin DM. Trends in the incidence of cancer in the black population of Harare, Zimbabwe 1991–2010. Int J Cancer. 2013;133:721–9.

12. Parkin DM, Sitas F, Chirenje M, Stein L, Abratt R, Wabinga H. Part I: cancer in indigenous Africans—burden, distribution, and trends. Lancet Oncol. 2008;9:683–92.

13. Corbex M, Bouzbid S, Boffetta P. Features of breast cancer in developing countries, examples from North-Africa. Eur J Cancer. 2014;50:1808–18.

14. Soliman AS, Kleer CG, Mrad K, Karkouri M, Omar S, Khaled HM, Benider AL, Ayed FB, Eissa SS, Eissa MS, et al. Inflammatory breast cancer in North Africa: comparison of clinical and molecular epidemiologic characteristics of patients from Egypt, Tunisia, and Morocco. Breast Dis. 2011;33:159–69.

15. Boussen H, Bouzaiene H, Ben Hassouna J, Dhiab T, Khomsi F, Benna F, Gamoudi A, Mourali N, Hechiche M, Rahal K, Levine PH. Inflammatory breast cancer in Tunisia: epidemiological and clinical trends. Cancer. 2010;116:2730–5.

16. Urban M, Banks E, Egger S, Canfell K, O'Connell D, Beral V, Sitas F. Injectable and oral contraceptive use and cancers of the breast, cervix, ovary, and endometrium in black South African women: case–control study. PLoS Med. 2012;9:e1001182.

17. Huo D, Adebamowo CA, Ogundiran TO, Akang EE, Campbell O, Adenipekun A, Cummings S, Fackenthal J, Ademuyiwa F, Ahsan H, Olopade OI. Parity and breastfeeding are protective against breast cancer in Nigerian women. Br J Cancer. 2008;98:992–6.

18. Ogundiran TO, Huo D, Adenipekun A, Campbell O, Oyesegun R, Akang E, Adebamowo C, Olopade OI. Case–control study of body size and breast cancer risk in Nigerian women. Am J Epidemiol. 2010;172:682–90.

19. Ogundiran TO, Huo D, Adenipekun A, Campbell O, Oyesegun R, Akang E, Adebamowo C, Olopade OI. Body fat distribution and breast cancer risk: findings from the Nigerian breast cancer study. Cancer Causes Control. 2012;23:565–74.

20. Amir H, Makwaya C, Mhalu F, Mbonde MP, Schwartz-Albiez R. Breast cancer during the HIV epidemic in an African population. Oncol Rep. 2001;8:659–61.

21. Edge J, Buccimazza I, Cubasch H, Panieri E. The challenges of managing breast cancer in the developing world—a perspective from sub-Saharan Africa. S Afr Med J. 2014;104:377–9.

22. Fregene A, Newman LA. Breast cancer in sub-Saharan Africa: how does it relate to breast cancer in African-American women? Cancer. 2005;103:1540–50.

23. Amir H, Kaaya EE, Kwesigabo G, Kiitinya JN. Breast cancer before and during the AIDS epidemic in women and men: a study of Tanzanian Cancer Registry Data 1968 to 1996. J Natl Med Assoc. 2000;92:301–5.

24. Adebamowo CA, Adekunle OO. Case-controlled study of the epidemiological risk factors for breast cancer in Nigeria. Br J Surg. 1999;86:665–8.

25. Cubasch H, Joffe M, Hanisch R, Schuz J, Neugut AI, Karstaedt A, Broeze N, van den Berg E, McCormack V, Jacobson JS. Breast cancer characteristics and HIV among 1,092 women in Soweto, South Africa. Breast Cancer Res Treat. 2013;140:177–86.

26. Langenhoven L, Barnardt P, Neugut AI, Jacobson JS. Phenotype and treatment of breast cancer in HIV-positive and -negative women in Cape Town, South Africa. J Glob Oncol. 2016;2(5):284–91.

27. Rais G, Raissouni S, Aitelhaj M, Rais F, Naciri S, Khoyaali S, Abahssain H, Bensouda Y, Khannoussi B, Mrabti H, Errihani H. Triple negative breast cancer in Moroccan women: clinicopathological and therapeutic study at the National Institute of Oncology. BMC Womens Health. 2012;12:35.

28. Ikpat OF, Ndoma-Egba R, Collan Y. Influence of age and prognosis of breast cancer in Nigeria. East Afr Med J. 2002;79:651–7.

29. Ly M, Antoine M, Dembele AK, Levy P, Rodenas A, Toure BA, Badiaga Y, Dembele BK, Bagayogo DC, Diallo YL, et al. High incidence of triple-negative tumors in sub-Saharan Africa: a prospective study of breast cancer characteristics and risk factors in Malian women seen in a Bamako university hospital. Oncology. 2012;83:257–63.

30. McCormack VA, Joffe M, van den Berg E, Broeze N, Silva Idos S, Romieu I, Jacobson JS, Neugut AI, Schuz J, Cubasch H. Breast cancer receptor status and stage at diagnosis in over 1,200 consecutive public hospital patients in Soweto, South Africa: a case series. Breast Cancer Res. 2013;15:R84.

31. Galukande M, Wabinga H, Mirembe F, Karamagi C, Asea A. Molecular breast cancer subtypes prevalence in an indigenous Sub Saharan African population. Pan Afr Med J. 2014;17:249.

32. Awadelkarim KD, Arizzi C, Elamin EO, Hamad HM, De Blasio P, Mekki SO, Osman I, Biunno I, Elwali NE, Mariani-Costantini R, Barberis MC. Pathological, clinical and prognostic characteristics of breast cancer in Central Sudan versus Northern Italy: implications for breast cancer in Africa. Histopathology. 2008;52:445–56.

33. Salhia B, Tapia C, Ishak EA, Gaber S, Berghuis B, Hussain KH, DuQuette RA, Resau J, Carpten J. Molecular subtype analysis determines the association of advanced breast cancer in Egypt with favorable biology. BMC Womens Health. 2011;11:44.

34. Luyeye Mvila G, Batalansi D, Praet M, Marchal G, Laenen A, Christiaens MR, Brouckaert O, Ali-Risasi C, Neven P, Van Ongeval C. Prognostic features of breast cancer differ between women in the Democratic Republic of Congo and Belgium. Breast. 2015;24:642–8.

35. Anders CK, Carey LA. Biology, metastatic patterns, and treatment of patients with triple-negative breast cancer. Clin Breast Cancer. 2009;9 Suppl 2:S73–81.

36. Abdulrahman GO, Rahman GA. Epidemiology of breast cancer in Europe and Africa. J Cancer Epidemiol. 2012;2012:5.

37. Islami F, Lortet-Tieulent J, Okello C, Adoubi I, Mbalawa CG, Ward EM, Parkin DM, Jemal A. Tumor size and stage of breast cancer in Cote d'Ivoire and Republic of Congo—Results from population-based cancer registries. Breast. 2015;24:713–7.

38. Soliman AS, et al. Epidemiologic and Clinical Profiles of Breast Diseases in Niger. Int J Cancer Oncol. 2015;2:1–6.

39. Tesfamariam A, Gebremichael A, Mufunda J. Breast cancer clinicopathological presentation, gravity and challenges in Eritrea, East Africa: Management practice in a resource-poor setting. 2013.

40. Mabula JB, McHembe MD, Chalya PL, Giiti G, Chandika AB, Rambau P, Masalu N, Gilyomai JM. Stage at diagnosis, clinicopathological and treatment patterns of breast cancer at Bugando Medical Centre in north-western Tanzania. Tanzan J Health Res. 2012;14:269–79.

41. Bhikoo R, Srinivasa S, Yu TC, Moss D, Hill AG. Systematic review of breast cancer biology in developing countries (part 1): Africa, the middle East, Eastern Europe, Mexico, the Caribbean and South america. Cancers (Basel). 2011;3:2358–81.

42. Youssef OZ, Azim Jr HA. Understanding the factors associated with the surgical management of early breast cancer. Gland Surg. 2013;2:4–6.

43. Maalej M, Frikha H, Ben Salem S, Daoud J, Bouaouina N, Ben Abdallah M, Ben Romdhane K. Breast cancer in Tunisia: clinical and epidemiological study. Bull Cancer. 1999;86:302–6.

44. Salem AA, Salem MA, Abbass H. Breast cancer: surgery at the South Egypt cancer institute. Cancers (Basel). 2010;2:1771–8.

45. Sullivan R, Alatise OI, Anderson BO, Audisio R, Autier P, Aggarwal A, Balch C, Brennan MF, Dare A, D'Cruz A, et al. Global cancer surgery: delivering safe, affordable, and timely cancer surgery. Lancet Oncol. 2015;16:1193–224.

46. Stefan DC. Cancer care in Africa: An overview of resources. J Glob Oncol. 2015;1(1):30–6.

47. Dare AJ AB, Sullivan R, et al. Surgical Services for Cancer Care. In: Gelband HJP, Sankaranarayanan R, editors. Cancer: Disease Control Priorities, vol. 3. 3rd ed. Washington (DC): The International Bank for Reconstruction and Development/The World Bank; 2015.

48. Cazap E, Magrath I, Kingham TP, Elzawawy A. Structural barriers to diagnosis and treatment of cancer in low- and middle-income countries: the urgent need for scaling up. J Clin Oncol. 2016;34:14–9.

49. Dye TD, Bogale S, Hobden C, Tilahun Y, Hechter V, Deressa T, Bize M, Reeler A. Complex care systems in developing countries: breast cancer patient navigation in Ethiopia. Cancer. 2010;116:577–85.

50. Clegg-Lamptey J, Dakubo J, Attobra YN. Why do breast cancer patients report late or abscond during treatment in ghana? A pilot study. Ghana Med J. 2009;43:127–31.

51. Ezeome ER. Delays in presentation and treatment of breast cancer in Enugu, Nigeria. Niger J Clin Pract. 2010;13:311–6.

52. Brinton L, Figueroa J, Adjei E, Ansong D, Biritwum R, Edusei L, Nyarko KM, et al. Factors contributing todelays in diagnosis of breast cancers in Ghana, West Africa. Breast Cancer Res Treat. 2016:1–0.

53. Tetteh DA, Faulkner SL. Sociocultural factors and breast cancer in sub-Saharan Africa: implications for diagnosis and management. Womens Health (Lond). 2016;12:147–56.

54. Cancer—A Neglected Health Problem in Developing Countries. [http://www.inctr.org/about-inctr/cancer-in-developing-countries/]. Accessed 1 Dec 2016.

55. Azim HA, Abdal-Kader YSED, Mousa MM, Malek RA, Abdalmassih MK, Ibrahim NY. Taxane-based regimens as adjuvant treatment for breast cancer: a retrospective study in egyptian cancer patients. Asian Pac J Cancer Prev. 2015;16:65–9.

56. Sparano JA. Taxanes for breast cancer: an evidence-based review of randomized phase II and phase III trials. Clin Breast Cancer. 2000;1:32–40. discussion 41–32.

57. Ermiah E, Buhmeida A, Abdalla F, Khaled BR, Salem N, Pyrhonen S, Collan Y. Prognostic value of proliferation markers: immunohistochemical ki-67 expression and cytometric s-phase fraction of women with breast cancer in Libya. J Cancer. 2012;3:421–31.

58. Brinton LA, Figueroa JD, Awuah B, Yarney J, Wiafe S, Wood SN, Ansong D, Nyarko K, Wiafe-Addai B, Clegg-Lamptey JN. Breast cancer in Sub-Saharan Africa: opportunities for prevention. Breast Cancer Res Treat. 2014;144:467–78.

59. Balogun OD, Formenti SC. Locally advanced breast cancer—strategies for developing nations. Front Oncol. 2015;5:89.

60. Ogundiran TO, Ayandipo OO, Ademola AF, Adebamowo CA. Mastectomy for management of breast cancer in Ibadan, Nigeria. BMC Surg. 2013;13:59.

61. Kantelhardt EJ, Muluken G, Sefonias G, Wondimu A, Gebert HC, Unverzagt S, Addissie A. A review on breast cancer care in Africa. Breast Care (Basel). 2015;10:364–70.

62. Abulkhair O, Saghir N, Sedky L, Saadedin A, Elzahwary H, Siddiqui N, Al Saleh M, Geara F, Birido N, Al-Eissa N, et al. Modification and implementation of NCCN guidelines on breast cancer in the Middle East and North Africa region. J Natl Compr Canc Netw. 2010;8 Suppl 3:S8–s15.

63. Renner L, Nkansah FA, Dodoo AN. The role of generic medicines and biosimilars in oncology in low-income countries. Ann Oncol. 2013;24 Suppl 5:v29–32.

64. Kingham TP, Alatise OI, Vanderpuye V, Casper C, Abantanga FA, Kamara TB, Olopade OI, Habeebu M, Abdulkareem FB, Denny L. Treatment of cancer in sub-Saharan Africa. Lancet Oncol. 2013;14:e158–167.

65. Vanderpuye VD, Olopade OI, Huo D. Pilot Survey of Breast Cancer Management in Sub-Saharan Africa. J Glob Oncol. 2016:JGO–2016.

66. McFarland DC, Naikan J, Rozenblit M, Mandeli J, Bleiweiss I, Tiersten A. Changes in pathological complete response rates after neoadjuvant chemotherapy for breast carcinoma over five years. J Oncol. 2016;2016:4324863.

67. Sule EA, Nzegwu MA. Attaining pathological complete regression for breast conservation—A pilot experience in a developing country. Ann Med Surg (Lond). 2016;9:61–6.

68. Alawad AA. Evaluation of clinical and pathological response after two cycles of neoadjuvant chemotherapy on Sudanese patients with locally advanced breast cancer. Ethiop J Health Sci. 2014;24:15–20.

69. Abdel-Bary N, El-Kased A, Aiad H. Does neoadjuvant chemotherapy increase breast conservation in operable breast cancer: an Egyptian experience. Ecancermedicalscience. 2009;3:104.

70. Hidar S, Ben Ahmed S, Bouaouina N, Khairi H. Treatment of locally advanced breast cancer: a Tunisian experience. Breast. 2011;20:S30.

71. von Minckwitz G, Untch M, Blohmer JU, Costa SD, Eidtmann H, Fasching PA, Gerber B, Eiermann W, Hilfrich J, Huober J, et al. Definition and impact of pathologic complete response on prognosis after neoadjuvant chemotherapy in various intrinsic breast cancer subtypes. J Clin Oncol. 2012;30:1796–804.

72. Arowolo OA, Njiaju UO, Ogundiran TO, Abidoye O, Lawal OO, Obajimi M, Adetiloye AV, Im HK, Akinkuolie AA, Oluwasola A, et al. Neo-adjuvant capecitabine chemotherapy in women with newly diagnosed locally advanced breast cancer in a resource-poor setting (Nigeria): efficacy and safety in a phase II feasibility study. Breast J. 2013;19:470–7.

73. Adisa AO, Lawal OO, Adesunkanmi AR. Paradox of wellness and nonadherence among Nigerian women on breast cancer chemotherapy. J Cancer Res Ther. 2008;4:107–10.

74. Price AJ, Ndom P, Atenguena E, Mambou Nouemssi JP, Ryder RW. Cancer care challenges in developing countries. Cancer. 2012;118:3627–35.

75. Adisa AO, Gukas ID, Lawal OO, Adesunkanmi AR. Breast cancer in Nigeria: is non-adherence to chemotherapy schedules a major factor in the reported poor treatment outcome? Breast J. 2010;16:206–7.

76. Maree JE, Mulonda J. My experience has been a terrible one, something I could not run away from": Zambian women's experiences of advanced breast cancer. Int J Africa Nurs Sci. 2015;3:24–30.

77. Hershman D, Weinberg M, Rosner Z, Alexis K, Tiersten A, Grann VR, Troxel A, Neugut AI. Ethnic neutropenia and treatment delay in African American women undergoing chemotherapy for early-stage breast cancer. J Natl Cancer Inst. 2003;95:1545–8.

78. Challinor JM, Galassi AL, Al-Ruzzieh MA, Bigirimana JB, Buswell L, So WKW, Steinberg AB, Williams M. Nursing's potential to address the growing cancer burden in low- and middle-income countries. J Glob Oncol. 2016;2:154–63.

79. Munagala R, Aqil F, Gupta RC. Promising molecular targeted therapies in breast cancer. Indian J Pharmacol. 2011;43:236–45.

80. Drucker A, Skedgel C, Virik K, Rayson D, Sellon M, Younis T. The cost burden of trastuzumab and bevacizumab therapy for solid tumours in Canada. Curr Oncol. 2008;15:136–42.

81. Mayor S. WHO includes 16 new cancer drugs on list of essential medicines. Lancet Oncol. 2015;16:757.

82. Aitelhaj M, LKhoyaali S, Rais G, Boutayeb S, Errihani H. First line chemotherapy plus trastuzumab in metastatic breast cancer HER2 positive-Observational institutional study. Pan Afr Med J. 2016;24(324).

83. Kerr DJ, Midgley R. Can we treat cancer for a dollar a day? Guidelines for low-income countries. N Engl J Med. 2010;363:801–3.

84. Shulman LN, Willett W, Sievers A, Knaul FM. Breast cancer in developing countries: opportunities for improved survival. J Oncol. 2010;2010:595167.

85. Kemfang Ngowa JD, Yomi J, Kasia JM, Mawamba Y, Ekortarh AC, Vlastos G. Breast cancer profile in a group of patients followed up at the radiation therapy unit of the Yaounde General Hospital, Cameroon. Obstet Gynecol Int. 2011;2011:143506.

86. Kantelhardt EJ, Zerche P, Mathewos A, Trocchi P, Addissie A, Aynalem A, Wondemagegnehu T, Ersumo T, Reeler A, Yonas B, et al. Breast cancer survival in Ethiopia: a cohort study of 1,070 women. Int J Cancer. 2014;135:702–9.

87. Huo D, Ikpatt F, Khramtsov A, Dangou JM, Nanda R, Dignam J, Zhang B, Grushko T, Zhang C, Oluwasola O, et al. Population differences in breast cancer: survey in indigenous African women reveals over-representation of triple-negative breast cancer. J Clin Oncol. 2009;27:4515–21.

88. Mayer EL, Burstein HJ. Postmenopausal breast cancer: a best endocrine strategy? Lancet. 2015;386:1317–9.

89. Kadakia KC, Henry NL. Adjuvant endocrine therapy in premenopausal women with breast cancer. Clin Adv Hematol Oncol. 2015;13:663–72.

90. Kadzatsa WCE. The Status and Challenges of Cancer Care in Zimbabwe, ASCO Daily News. 2016.

91. Hasiniatsy NR, Vololonantenaina CR, Rabarikoto HF, Razafimanjato N, Ranoharison HD, et al. First results of hormone receptors' status in Malagasy women with invasive breast cancer. Pan Afr Med J. 2014;17(153).

92. Murphy CC, Bartholomew LK, Carpentier MY, Bluethmann SM, Vernon SW. Adherence to adjuvant hormonal therapy among breast cancer survivors in clinical practice: a systematic review. Breast Cancer Res Treat. 2012;134:459–78.

93. Oguntola ASMA, OO Akanbi. Non-adherence to the use of tamoxifen in the first year by the breast cancer patients in an African population. East Cent Afr J Surg. 2011;16.

94. du Plessis M, Apffelstaedt JP. Treatment outcomes of breast carcinoma in a resource-limited environment. S Afr J Surg. 2015;53(2):43–7.

95. Abdel-Wahab M, Bourque JM, Pynda Y, Izewska J, Van der Merwe D, Zubizarreta E, Rosenblatt E. Status of radiotherapy resources in Africa: an International Atomic Energy Agency analysis. Lancet Oncol. 2013;14:e168–175.

96. Krishna GS, Akula RR, Kumar AA, Srinivas V, Ayyangar K, Reddy PY. DVH Analysis of Cobalt-60 treatment plans incorporating a recently developed MLC. Int J Cancer Ther Oncol. 2016;4(3).

97. Cilla S, Kigula-Mugambe J, Digesu C, Macchia G, Bogale S, Massaccesi M, Dawotola D, Deodato F, Buwenge M, Caravatta L, et al. Forward-planned intensity modulated radiation therapy using a cobalt source: a dosimetric study in breast cancer. J Med Phys. 2013;38:125–31.

98. Anderson BO, Shyyan R, Eniu A, Smith RA, Yip CH, Bese NS, Chow LW, Masood S, Ramsey SD, Carlson RW. Breast cancer in limited-resource countries: an overview of the Breast Health Global Initiative 2005 guidelines. Breast J. 2006;12 Suppl 1:S3–15.

99. Smith BD, Bentzen SM, Correa CR, Hahn CA, Hardenbergh PH, Ibbott GS, McCormick B, McQueen JR, Pierce LJ, Powell SN, et al. Fractionation for whole breast irradiation: an American Society for Radiation Oncology (ASTRO) evidence-based guideline. Int J Radiat Oncol Biol Phys. 2011;81:59–68.

100. Scherber S, Soliman AS, Awuah B, Osei-Bonsu E, Adjei E, Abantanga F, Merajver SD. Characterizing breast cancer treatment pathways in Kumasi, Ghana from onset of symptoms to final outcome: outlook towards cancer control. Breast Dis. 2014;34:139–49.

101. Jeremic B, Vanderpuye V, Abdel-Wahab S, Gaye P, Kochbati L, Diwani M, Emwula P, Oro B, Lishimpi K, Kigula-Mugambe J, et al. Patterns of practice in palliative radiotherapy in Africa—case revisited. Clin Oncol (R Coll Radiol). 2014;26:333–43.

102. Latif N, Rana F, Guthrie T. Breast cancer and HIV in the era of highly active antiretroviral therapy: two case reports and review of the literature. Breast J. 2011;17:87–92.

103. Parameswaran L, Taur Y, Shah MK, Traina TA, Seo SK. Tolerability of chemotherapy in HIV-infected women with breast cancer: are there prognostic implications? AIDS Patient Care STDs. 2014;28:358–64.

104. El-Rayes BF, Berenji K, Schuman P, Philip PA. Breast cancer in women with human immunodeficiency virus infection: implications for diagnosis and therapy. Breast Cancer Res Treat. 2002;76:111–6.

105. Ashraff Z, Nallamala S. Breast cancer in a woman with HIV/AIDS: case report and review of literature. J HIV Ther. 2007;12:71–2.

106. Pace LE, Shulman LN. Breast Cancer in Sub-Saharan Africa: Challenges and Opportunities to Reduce Mortality. Oncologist. 2016;21(6).

107. DeSantis CE, Bray F, Ferlay J, Lortet-Tieulent J, Anderson BO, Jemal A. International variation in female breast cancer incidence and mortality rates. Cancer Epidemiol Biomarkers Prev. 2015;24:1495–506.

108. Mensah AC, Yarney J, Nokoe SK, Opoku S, Clegg-Lamptey JN. Survival outcomes of breast cancer in Ghana: an analysis of clinicopathological features. Open Access Library J. 2016;3:1–11.

109. McKenzie F, Zietsman A, Galukande M, Anele A, Adisa C, Cubasch H, Parham G, Anderson BO, Abedi-Ardekani B, Schuz J, et al. African Breast Cancer-Disparities in Outcomes (ABC-DO): protocol of a multicountry mobile health prospective study of breast cancer survival in sub-Saharan Africa. BMJ Open. 2016;6:e011390.

110. Silverstein A, Sood R, Costas-Chavarri A. Breast cancer in Africa: limitations and opportunities for application of genomic medicine. Int J Breast Cancer. 2016;2016:4792865.

111. Newman LA. Disparities in breast cancer and african ancestry: a global perspective. Breast J. 2015;21:133–9.

112. Swinburn BA, Sacks G, Hall KD, McPherson K, Finegood DT, Moodie ML, Gortmaker SL. The global obesity pandemic: shaped by global drivers and local environments. Lancet. 2011;378:804–14.

113. Eccles SA, Aboagye EO, Ali S, Anderson AS, Armes J, Berditchevski F, Blaydes JP, Brennan K, Brown NJ, Bryant HE, et al. Critical research gaps and translational priorities for the successful prevention and treatment of breast cancer. Breast Cancer Res. 2013;15:R92.

# 11

# Mouse mammary tumor-like virus (MMTV) is present in human breast tissue before development of virally associated breast cancer

Teiko Nartey[1], Chiara M. Mazzanti[2], Stella Melana[1], Wendy K. Glenn[3], Generoso Bevilacqua[2], James F. Holland[1], Noel J. Whitaker[3], James S. Lawson[3*] and Beatriz G.T. Pogo[1]

## Abstract

**Background:** There is substantial evidence that a virus homologous to mouse mammary tumor virus (MMTV) may have a role in human breast cancer. The present study indicates that those who developed breast cancer associated with an MMTV-like virus had this virus in their non-cancerous breast tissues years before the cancer developed.

**Methods:** Polymerase chain reaction (PCR) techniques and sequencing were used to identify MMTV-like envelope gene sequences (MMTV-like *env* sequences) in Australian benign breast biopsy specimens from women who several years later developed breast cancer. Murine contamination was excluded by stringent laboratory procedures, and the absence of intracisternal A particle sequences and mitochondrial cyclooxygenase sequences.

**Results:** MMTV-like *env* sequences (also called HMTV sequences to denote their source) were found in 9 of 25 breast cancer specimens (36%). Among 25 non-cancerous breast biopsies of these same patients taken 1 to 11 years earlier, six contained MMTV-like sequences (24%). Five of the six were among the nine virally-associated breast cancers. In two pairs of specimens, benign and malignant, *env* sequences were 97% identical.

**Conclusions:** The identification of MMTV (MMTV-like) sequences in breast tissues prior to the development of MMTV positive breast cancer fulfills a key criterion for a possible causal role for the MMTV-like virus in human breast cancer.

**Keywords:** Benign breast tissues, Breast cancer, Mouse mammary tumor virus, MMTV, Mouse mammary tumor-like virus, MMTV-like, Human mammary tumour virus, HMTV, Morphology, Morphological, Histotype, Histological

## Background

Mouse mammary tumor viruses (MMTV) have a well-documented causal role in mouse mammary tumors in feral and experimental mice [1]. This role of MMTV was first observed by John Bittner in 1936 [2]. These observations led to the search for a similar virus in human breast cancer. Close morphologic and immunologic similarity were repeatedly shown. More recently, near identity of molecular structure to MMTV (90-98%) has

been identified in human breast cancers [3]. The MMTV-like virus in humans is also called human mammary tumor virus (HMTV) [4].

The evidence of a role for an MMTV-like virus in human breast cancer is substantial but incomplete. An essential criterion to establish a causal role of an infectious agent in any disease, including cancer, is evidence of prior infection by the suspect agent [5]. This criterion had not been investigated with respect to MMTV-like virus. MMTV-like *env* sequences have rarely been identified in benign breast tissues [3, 6, 7], nor in the benign breast tissue of individuals with breast cancer containing MMTV-like sequences [8]. For this reason we sought to

* Correspondence: james.lawson@unsw.edu.au
[3]School of Biotechnology and Biomolecular Sciences, University of New South Wales, Sydney, Australia
Full list of author information is available at the end of the article

identify MMTV-like *env* sequences in benign breast biopsy tissues from women who some years later developed MMTV-like positive breast cancer.

The evidence suggestive of a role for an MMTV–like virus in human breast cancer is as follows: (i) a meta-analysis of 22 studies concluded that the identification of MMTV–like gene sequences in breast cancer tissues, was associated with a 15 fold increase in breast cancer [9], (ii) MMTV-like *env* gene sequences were identified in 38% of US human breast tumors but were extremely uncommon in healthy breast tissues [3, 6], (iii) the near complete proviral structure of MMTV-like virus that was 95-98% homologous to MMTV has been identified in human breast tumors [4, 10], (iv) MMTV viral proteins have been identified in human breast cancer [11], (v) Wnt-1 oncogene expression is significantly higher in MMTV-like positive compared to MMTV-like negative breast cancer specimens, which parallels high Wnt-1 expression in MMTV positive mouse mammary tumors [12, 13], (vi) MMTV can infect human cells and randomly integrate its genomic information [14, 15], and produce virus particles [16] (vii) there is increased prevalence of MMTV-like viral sequences in healthy breast tissues (nil), healthy tissue adjacent to breast cancer (19%), breast hyperplasia (27%), ductal carcinoma in situ (82%) [17], (viii) the age standardized rates for breast cancers in five countries of Asia are less frequent (29–43 per 100,000) than in seven countries of Europe, the Americas, and Australia (47–92) [18]. These findings correlate with different burdens of MMTV-like infection in human breast cancers, 0-20% in Asia vs. 27-60%, in the seven countries which are associated with different prevalence of MMTV in the indigenous mouse species [18, 19]. (ix) MMTV–like sequences have been identified in milk from healthy lactating women and three fold positivity in milk from women at high risk for breast cancer [20, 21], (x) MMTV-like sequences have been identified in the saliva of 27% of healthy children, 11% of healthy adults and 57% of adults with breast cancer, which is suggestive of a human to human viral transmission [22] and (xi) MMTV-like viral sequences have been identified in breast cancers which developed in a father, mother and daughter of the same family which is suggestive of an infectious condition [23]. Overall this evidence is consistent with MMTV having similar influences in both human breast cancer and mouse mammary tumors.

If an MMTV-like virus infects human breasts, MMTV-like antibodies should be present in the sera of infected individuals since mice infected with MMTV develop high titers of MMTV specific antibodies. Indeed, MMTV antibodies in human breast cancer have been described [24, 25]. Antibodies were not identified in one recent study, however [26].

## Methods
### Ethics

This project was formally considered and approved by the Human Research Ethics Committees of the several participating institutions.

Twenty five patients were identified for whom both benign breast and subsequent breast cancer specimens were available from the archives of an Australian pathology service (Douglass Hanly Moir – Pathology). All the specimens were formalin fixed and paraffin mounted. Seventeen of these sets of specimens were analysed by polymerase chain reaction (PCR) techniques at the Icahn School of Medicine at Mount Sinai (ISMMS) (New York). Eight additional specimen pairs were analysed by the same PCR techniques but with the cancer tissues microdissected from the specimens at the University of Pisa (UP) (Italy). Eight of the sets of specimens were analysed in both Centers.

### Detection of MMTV-like env sequences

The DNA extraction and detection of MMTV-like *env* sequences were performed by PCR techniques as described by Wang et al. [3]. The primer sequences used in these PCR analyses include part of the MMTV *env* gene, which differs from human endogenous retrovirus 10 (HERV-K10). The same PCR techniques were used in both the ISMMS and UP laboratories with the exception of microdissection of the tumor tissues, that were analysed in the UP laboratory by fluorescence nested PCR. Materials from all patients were not available due to the exhaustion of the blocks. The outcomes from each of the two laboratories are shown in Table 1.

Contamination is a well-known problem with PCR analyses. Therefore, all reagents were shown to be free of MMTV-like sequences before use. PCR products were tested for the presence of murine mitochondrial (MoMt) and genomic DNA to exclude contamination. The methods used were as described by Deligdisch et al. [27] and outlined below:

(i) *Detection of mouse mitochondrial DNA sequences.*
A series of PCR analyses was conducted to detect MoMt contamination by the detection of cytochrome oxidase (*cox-2*) gene as part of the MoMt in any sample DNA in which MMTV *env* sequences were detected. The following primers for *cox-2* were used: mt5982F (5-AGACGCACCTACGGTGAAGA-3) and mt16267R (5-AGAGTTTTGGTTCACGGAA CATGA-3). The product yields an amplicon of 286 base pairs. The semi-nested PCR was done using the primers mt16115F (5-TGCCAAACCCCAAAAA CACT-3) and mt16267R, which results in a 153-bp amplicon. After transfer from the gel to a nylon membrane, the amplicon was detected by

**Table 1** MMTV-like *env* gene sequences in benign breast tissues and subsequent breast cancer in the same patients

| Patient | Age | Diagnosis | MMTV-like New York (ISMMS) by PCR | MMTV-like Pisa (UP) by PCR |
|---|---|---|---|---|
| 1 | 36 | Benign | neg | neg |
|  | 41 | IDC- NST | neg | neg |
| 2 | 72 | Benign |  | neg |
|  | 75 | DCIS- mucinous |  | neg |
| 3 | 33 | Benign | neg | neg |
|  | 44 | IDC/DCIS- NST | neg | neg |
| 4 | 45 | Benign | pos | neg |
|  | 46 | DCIS-cribriform | pos | neg |
| 5 | 50 | Benign | pos | neg |
|  | 60 | ILC-pleomorphic | pos | pos |
| 6 | 62 | Benign | neg |  |
|  | 66 | DCIS- micropapillary | neg |  |
| 7 | 47 | Benign | neg |  |
|  | 56 | IDC-NST | neg |  |
| 8 | 49 | Benign |  | neg |
|  | 52 | IDC- NST |  | neg |
| 9 | 46 | Benign | neg |  |
|  | 53 | IDC-NST | pos |  |
| 10 | 48 | Hyperplasia | pos |  |
|  | 52 | IDC-NST | pos |  |
| 11 | 35 | Benign |  | neg |
|  | 46 | IDC |  | neg |
| 12 | 44 | Benign | neg | neg |
|  | 48 | IDC-NST | neg | neg |
| 13 | 67 | Benign |  | neg |
|  | 75 | IDC-NST |  | neg |
| 14 | 48 | Benign | neg | neg |
|  | 54 | IDC-NST | neg | neg |
| 15 | 42 | Benign |  | neg |
|  | 49 | IDC-NST |  | pos |
| 16 | 42 | Benign |  | neg |
|  | 48 | IDC-NST |  | neg |
| 17 | 39 | Benign | neg |  |
|  | 45 | ILC | neg |  |
| 18 | 53 | Benign | neg |  |
|  | 62 | DCIS | pos |  |
| 19 | 65 | Benign |  | pos |
|  | 67 | IDC-NST |  | neg |
| 20 | 39 | Benign | neg |  |
|  | 44 | DCIS-comedo | neg |  |
| 21 | 55 | Benign |  | neg |
|  | 62 | IDC-NST |  | neg |
| 22 | 37 | Benign | neg | neg |
|  | 39 | IDC-cribriform, mucinous | neg | neg |
| 23 | 39 | Benign | pos | neg |
|  | 42 | DCIS-comedo | pos | neg |
| 24 | 48 | Benign | pos |  |
|  | 54 | DCIS-cribriform | pos |  |
| 25 | 63 | Benign | neg |  |
|  | 67 | IDC-NST | pos |  |

*IDC* invasive ductal carcinoma, *ILC* invasive lobular carcinoma, *DCIS* ductal carcinoma in situ, *NST* no special type, *pos* positive, *neg* negative

**Table 1** MMTV-like *env* gene sequences in benign breast tissues and subsequent breast cancer in the same patients *(Continued)*

hybridization with a MoMt 32P-probe (5-GAAC TAGAATTGATCAGGCAT-3).

(ii) *Detection of murine intracisternal A particle long terminal repeats (IAP)*

IAPs are retrotransposon sequences present at the level of approximately 1000 copies of varying length per mouse genome. Amplification of the IAP sequences was carried out in PCR reactions using the following primers: forward primer (5-ATAA TCTGCCGCATGAGCCAAGG-3) and reverse primer (5-AGGAAGAACACCACAGACCAGA-3) one cycle of 95 °C for 5 min, 35 cycles of 95 °C for 30 s, 58 °C for 30 s, 72 °C for 20 s, and one cycle of 72 °C for 7 min. If present, the products of variable size, reflecting diversity of the IAP sequences, can be visualized on a 2% ethidium bromide stained agarose gel.

## Results

The results from each of the two laboratories are shown in Table 1. Gaps in the results are due to lack of materials due to exhaustion of the blocks. The time between the benign breast biopsy specimen and subsequent breast cancer in the same patients varied from 1 to 11 years.

### Outcomes of PCR analyses

MMTV-like *env* gene sequences were identified in 6 (24%) of 25 benign breast specimens and 9 (36%) of 25 breast cancer specimens. Of the 6 MMTV-like positive benign specimens, 5 later developed (MMTV-like positive) cancer.

Eight sets of benign and later breast cancer blocks were analysed in both the ISMMS and UP laboratories. Negative outcomes of PCR analyses were the same for 5 sets of blocks. MMTV sequences were identified by both laboratories in breast cancer of patient 5. MMTV sequences were identified by the ISMMS lab only (not the UP lab) in patients 4 and 23 breast cancer specimens.

Neither MoMt nor IAP DNA sequences were identified in any of the MMTV-like *env* positive DNAs. This indicates there was no murine DNA contamination.

## Comparison of MMTV env gene sequences in benign and breast cancer specimens within the same patient

Over 97% of the MMTV-like *env* were identical in both the benign breast biopsy and subsequent breast cancer

in 2 selected patients. These sequences are shown in Fig. 1. There are variations in approximately 3% of the sequences between the benign and subsequent breast cancers that developed several years later in the same patients. Such variations could be due to alterations in the MMTV-like genome following integration into the human genome as has been described for murine retroviruses [28] or could also occur during the PCR cycling procedures. These sequence variations indicate that contamination during PCR analyses was unlikely.

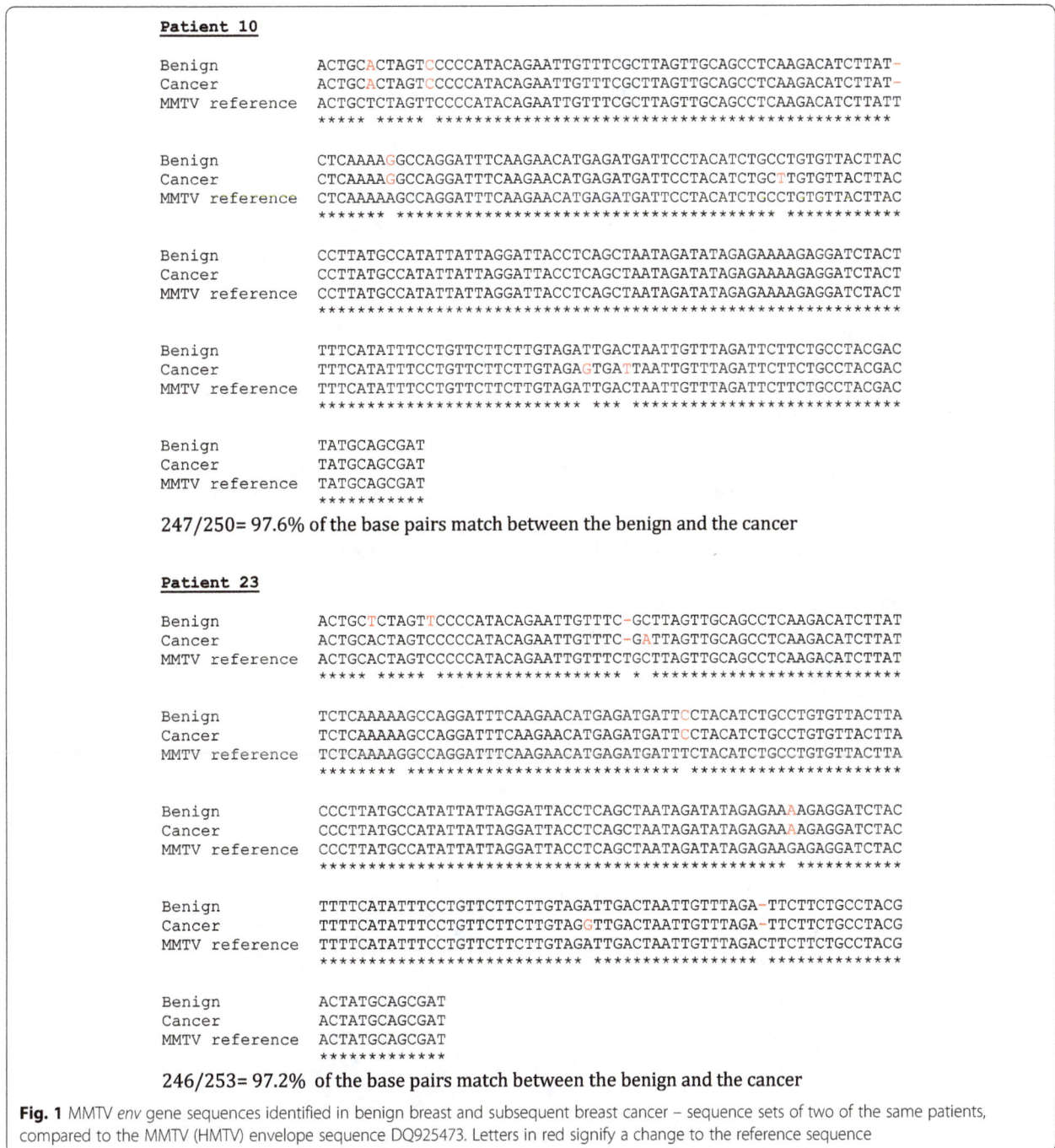

**Fig. 1** MMTV *env* gene sequences identified in benign breast and subsequent breast cancer – sequence sets of two of the same patients, compared to the MMTV (HMTV) envelope sequence DQ925473. Letters in red signify a change to the reference sequence

The morphological (histotype) characteristics in 8 of the 9 MMTV-like sequence positive breast cancers were similar to MMTV positive mouse (C3H strain mice) mammary tumours. These characteristics are shown in Fig. 2.

## Discussion

In this study MMTV-like *env* gene sequences have been identified in benign breast biopsy specimens prior to the subsequent development of MMTV-like *env* positive breast cancer specimens in the same patient. This is consistent with prior infection by MMTV-like virus in breast tissues prior to the development of the same MMTV-like virus positive breast cancer some years later. This finding fulfils one key evidentiary criterion that MMTV-like virus may have a role in some human breast cancers.

## Validity of the data

We consider the data generated in this study to be valid for the following reasons: (i) The study was conducted by PCR with primers based on MMTV-like *envelope* gene sequences as described by Wang et al. [13]. These MMTV *env* gene sequences are unique to the MMTV genome and are not present in human endogenous retrovirus sequences (HERV) and which are commonly identified in studies of the human genome. (ii) Neither MoMt nor IAP DNA sequences were identified in any one of the MMTV-like *env* positive DNAs. This indicates there was no murine DNA contamination. (iii) Variations in approximately 2% of the MMTV *env* sequences of two specimen pairs were identified. This is an indication that contamination during PCR analyses was unlikely. Such variations could be due to alterations in the MMTV genome following integration into the human genome. Variations in sequences can also occur during PCR cycling procedures.

There was one case (case 19 – Table 1) where the earlier biopsy was positive for MMTV-like sequences and the ensuing breast tumor (developing after two years) was negative. In addition the results for cases 4 and 23 are not consistent between the two laboratories. There are several possible reasons: (i) MMTV sequences identified by PCR can be inconsistent and false negatives are possible; (ii) MMTV sequences may be present in some, but not all parts of the tumor; (iii) although unlikely, changes in MMTV *env* sequences may have occurred. The problem of inconsistent outcomes of PCR based analyses has been considered in detail by Vinner et al. [29]. There are particular difficulties in obtaining consistent outcomes from PCR analyses of retroviruses when present in extremely low viral concentrations. While these problems, including the exhaustion of several of the materials, do not invalidate the identification of MMTV in this current study, it would be wise to replicate this study with increased numbers of patients.

It is of interest that MMTV sequences from the long terminal repeat (LTR) section of the MMTV genome have been identified in human breast cancers using Next Generation massive parallel Sequencing (NGS) [30]. These MMTV sequences were highly homologous to the reference MMTV genome based on BLAST technology [31]. These data, based on techniques very different from PCR, confirm the identification of MMTV-like gene sequences in human breast tumors and add validity to PCR based studies that were used in this current investigation. NGS techniques are not as sensitive for the identification of retroviral nucleotide sequences as PCR [29]. This is the reason for the much more frequent identification of MMTV-like nucleotide sequences by PCR compared to NGS.

The identification of MMTV-like *env* gene sequences in 9 (36%) of 25 Australian breast cancer specimens is a similar percentage to previous investigations of Australian breast cancers [7].

It is of considerable interest that the morphology (histotype) of 8 of 9 MMTV-like positive breast cancers was similar to the morphology of MMTV positive

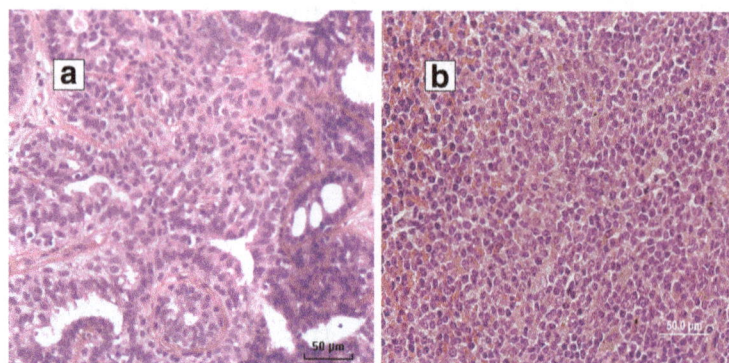

**Fig. 2 a**. MMTV positive human breast cancer. **b**. MMTV positive mouse mammary tumour

mouse mammary tumors. This has been previously observed by Wellings [32] and Lawson et al. [33]. If this observation is confirmed this has important implications as it provides potential evidence that MMTV infections may lead to a specific morphological type of breast cancer.

## Conclusions

The aim of this project has been achieved, namely the identification of MMTV-like sequences in benign breast biopsy tissues from women who several years later developed MMTV-like positive breast cancer. The findings in this study offer an important contribution to the overall body of evidence, which links MMTV-like virus (also called HMTV) to human breast cancer and fulfills a key criterion for a possible causal role for the MMTV-like virus in human breast cancer. Although other viruses and bacteria have been found in human breast cancer, none other is known to have a similar parallel in the animal kingdom. Conclusive proof of HMTV (MMTV-like virus) as a cause of human breast cancer will open a new era for prevention and therapy [34].

## Abbreviations

BLAST technology: Basic Local Alignment Search Tool is an algorithm for comparing primary biological sequence information; cox-2: cytochrome oxidase gene; env sequences: Envelope gene sequences; HERV-K10: Human endogenous retrovirus; HMTV: Human mammary tumor virus; IAP: Intracisternal a particle long terminal repeats; ISMMS: Icahn School of Medicine at Mount Sinai (ISMMS) (New York); LTR: Long terminal repeat section of the MMTV genome; MMTV: Mouse mammary tumor virus; MoMt: Murine mitochondrial DNA; NGS: Next Generation massive parallel Sequencing; PCR: Polymerase chain reaction; UP: University of Pisa, Italy

## Acknowledgements
The archival specimens were provided by Professor Warick Delprado and the Douglass Hanly Moir Pathology Laboratories of Sydney, Australia.

## Funding
The James and Margaret Lawson Research Fund. The T.J. Martell Foundation for Leukemia. Cancer and AIDS Research. The Faith Lynn Price Kash Family Fund. The Derald H. Ruttenberg Foundation.

## Authors' contributions
TN- laboratory analyses; CM – laboratory analyses; SM – laboratory analyses; WG- concepts, histology assessments, data analyses, preparation of the manuscript; GB- concepts, quality control, organisation, preparation of the manuscript; JH- concepts, quality control, preparation of the manuscript; NW- concepts, quality control, data analyses, preparation of the manuscript; JL– initial concept, identification and collection of the specimens, histological assessments, data analyses, preparation of the manuscript; BP– concepts, laboratory analyses, quality control, preparation of the manuscript. All authors read and approved the final manuscript.

## Competing interests
The authors declare that they have no competing interests.

## Author details
[1]Icahn School of Medicine at Mount Sinai, New York, NY, USA. [2]Department of Pathology, University of Pisa, Pisa, Italy. [3]School of Biotechnology and Biomolecular Sciences, University of New South Wales, Sydney, Australia.

## References

1. Ross SR. MMTV infectious cycle and the contribution of virus-encoded proteins to transformation of mammary tissue. J Mammary Gland Biol Neoplasia. 2008;13:299–307.
2. Bittner JJ. Some possible effects of nursing on the mammary gland tumor incidence in mice. Science. 1936;84:162. doi:10.1126/science.84.2172.162.
3. Wang Y, Holland JF, Bleiweiss IJ, Melana S, Liu X, Pelisson I, Cantarella A, Stellrecht K, Mani S, Pogo BG. Detection of mammary tumor virus env gene-like sequences in human breast cancer. Cancer Res. 1995;55:5173–9.
4. Liu B, Wang Y, Melana SM, Pelisson I, Najfeld V, Holland JF, Pogo BG. Identification of a proviral structure in human breast cancer. Cancer Res. 2001;61:1754–9.
5. Hill AB. The environment and disease: Association or causation? Proc R Soc Med. 1965;58:295–330.
6. Etkind P, Du J, Khan A, Pillitteri J, Wiernik PH. Mouse mammary tumor virus-like env gene sequences in human breast tumors and in a lymphoma of a breast cancer patient. Clin Cancer Res. 2000;6:1273–8.
7. Ford CE, Tran DD, Deng YM, Rawlinson WD, Lawson JS. Mouse mammary tumour like virus prevalence in breast tumours of Australian and Vietnamese women. Clin Cancer Res. 2003;9:1118–20.
8. Melana SM, Holland JF, Pogo BG. Search for mouse mammary tumor virus-like env sequences in cancer and normal breast from the same individuals. Clin Cancer Res. 2001;7:283–4.
9. Wang F, Hou J, Shen Q, Yue Y, Xie F, Wang X, Jin H. Mouse mammary tumor virus-like virus infection and the risk of human breast cancer: a meta-analysis. Am J Transl Res. 2014;6:248–66.
10. Melana SM, Nepomnaschy I, Sakalian M, Abbott A, Hasa J, Holland JF, Pogo BG. Characterization of viral particles isolated from primary cultures of human breast cancer cells. Cancer Res. 2007;67:8960–5.
11. Melana SM, Nepomnaschy I, Hasa J, Djougarian A, Djougarian A, Holland JF, Pogo BG. Detection of human mammary tumor virus proteins in human breast cancer cells. J Virol Methods. 2010;163:157–61.
12. Lawson JS, Glenn WK, Salmons B, Ye Y, Heng B, Moody P, Johal H, Rawlinson WD, Delprado W, Lutze-Mann L, Whitaker NJ. Mouse mammary tumor virus-like sequences in human breast cancer. Cancer Res. 2010;70:3576–85.
13. Callahan R, Mudunur U, Bargo S, Raafat A, McCurdy D, Boulanger C, Lowther W, Stephens R, Luke BT, Stewart C, Wu X, Munroe D, Smith GH. Genes affected by mouse mammary tumor virus (MMTV) proviral insertions in mouse mammary tumors are deregulated or mutated in primary human mammary tumors. Oncotarget. 2012;3:1320–34.
14. Indik S, Günzburg WH, Salmons B, Rouault F. Mouse mammary tumor virus infects human cells. Cancer Res. 2005;65:6651–9.
15. Faschinger A, Rouault F, Sollner J, Lukas A, Salmons B, Günzburg WH, Indik S. Mouse mammary tumor virus integration site selection in human and mouse genomes. J Virol. 2008;82:13.
16. Konstantoulas C, Indik S. C₃H strain of mouse mammary tumor viruses like GR strain infects human mammary epithelial cells albeit less efficiently than murine mammary epithelial cells. J Gen Virol. 2015;96:650–62.
17. Mazzanti CM, Al Hamad M, Fanelli G, Scatena C, Zammarchi F, Zavaglia K, Lessi F, Pistello M, Naccarato AG, Bevilacqua G. A mouse mammary tumor virus env-like exogenous sequence is strictly related to progression of human sporadic breast carcinoma. Am J Pathol. 2011;179:2083–90.
18. Stewart BW, Wild CP. World Cancer Report. Lyon, France: IARC, WHO; 2014.
19. Stewart TH, Sage RD, Stewart AF, Cameron DW. Breast cancer incidence highest in the range of one species of house mouse, Mus domesticus. Br J Cancer. 2000;82(2):446–51.
20. Johal H, Ford CE, Glenn WK, Heads J, Lawson JS, Rawlinson WD. Mouse mammary tumor like virus (MMTV) sequences in breast milk from healthy lactating women. Breast Cancer Res Treat. 2011;129:149–55.

21. Nartey T, Moran H, Marin T, Arcaro KF, Anderton DL, Etkind P, Holland JF, Melana SM, Pogo BG. Human Mammary Tumor Virus (HMTV) sequences in human milk. Infect Agent Cancer. 2014;9:20.

22. Mazzanti CM, Lessi F, Armogida I, Zavaglia K, Franceschi S, Al Hamad M, Roncella M, Ghilli M, Boldrini A, Aretini P, Fanelli G, Marchetti I, Scatena C, Hochman J, Naccarato AG, Bevilacqua G. Human saliva as route of inter-human infection for mouse mammary tumor virus. Oncotarget. 2015;6:18355–63.

23. Etkind PR, Stewart AF, Wiernik PH. Mouse mammary tumor virus (MMTV)-like DNA sequences in the breast tumors of father, mother, and daughter. Infect Agent Cancer. 2008;3:2.

24. Witkin SS, Sarkar NH, Good RA, Day NK. An enzyme-linked immunoassay for the detection of antibodies to the mouse mammary tumor virus: application to human breast cancer. J Immunol Methods. 1980;32:85–91.

25. Day NK, Witkin SS, Sarkar NH, Kinne D, Jussawalla DJ, Levin A, Hsia CC, Geller N, Good RA. Antibodies reactive with murine mammary tumor virus in sera of patients with breast cancer: geographic and family studies. Proc Natl Acad Sci U S A. 1981;78:2483–7.

26. Goedert JJ, Rabkin CS, Ross SR. Prevalence of serologic reactivity against four strains of mouse mammary tumour virus among US women with breast cancer. Br J Cancer. 2006;94:548–51.

27. Deligdisch L, Marin T, Lee AT, Etkind P, Holland JF, Melana S, Pogo BG. Human mammary tumor virus (HMTV) in endometrial carcinoma. Int J Gynecol Cancer. 2013;23:1423–8.

28. Monk RJ, Malik FG, Stokesberry D, Evans LH. Direction determination of the point mutation rate of murine retroviruses. J Virol. 1992;66:3683–9.

29. Vinner L, Mourier T, Friis-Nielsen J, Gniadecki R, Dybaker K, Rosenberg J, Langhoff JL, Cruz DF, Fonager J, Izarzugaza JM, Gupta R, Sicheritz-Ponten T, Brunak S, Willerslev E, Nielsen LP, Hansen AJ. Investigation of Human Cancers for Retrovirus by Low-Stringency Target Enrichment and High-Throughput Sequencing. Sci Rep. 2015;5:13201.

30. Larsson lab – http://larssonlab.org/tcga-viruses/report_BRCA.php.

31. Larsson E. Personal communication. Sweden: University of Gottenburg; 2016.

32. Wellings SR. A hypothesis of the origin of human breast cancer from the terminal ductal lobular unit. Pathol Res Pract. 1980;166:515–35.

33. Lawson JS, Tran DD, Carpenter E, Ford CE, Rawlinson WD, Whitaker NJ, Delprado W. Presence of mouse mammary tumour-like virus gene sequences may be associated with specific human breast cancer morphology. J Clin Pathol. 2006;59:1287–92.

34. Braitbard O, Roniger M, Bar-Sinai A, Rajchman D, Gross T, Abramovitch H, La Ferla M, Franceschi S, Lessi F, Naccarato AG, Mazzanti CM, Bevilacqua G, Hochman J. A new immunization and treatment strategy for mouse mammary tumor virus (MMTV) associated cancers. Oncotarget 2016. doi: 10.18632/oncotarget.7762.

# 12

# Interleukin-17F expression is elevated in hepatitis C patients with fibrosis and hepatocellular carcinoma

Ming-Sian Wu[1†], Chun-Hsiang Wang[2†], Fan-Chen Tseng[1], Hsuan-Ju Yang[2], Yin-Chiu Lo[1], Yi-Ping Kuo[1], De-Jiun Tsai[1], Wan-Ting Tsai[1] and Guann-Yi Yu[1,3*]

## Abstract

**Background:** The role of interleukin (IL) 17A in chronic liver diseases had been extensively studied, but the function of IL-17F, which shares a high degree of homology with IL-17A, in the progression of chronic hepatic diseases is poorly understood. The aim of the study was to evaluate the association between IL-17F and liver diseases including, fibrosis and hepatocellular carcinoma (HCC).

**Methods:** Hepatic tumor samples from both hepatitis C virus (HCV) positive and negative patients (without HBV and HCV, NBNC) were examined with quantitative PCR and immunohistochemistry staining for inflammatory cytokine genes expression. In addition, 250 HCV patients naïve for interferon treatment were also subjected to enzyme-linked immunosorbent Assay (ELISA) for their serum cytokine concentrations.

**Results:** Serum IL-17F concentrations were significantly elevated in HCV patients with severe fibrosis stages. In accordance with serum data, IL-17F expression was also found higher in HCV-associated HCC tissues compared with NBNC HCC tissues at both the mRNA and protein levels.

**Conclusions:** Our data suggest that IL-17F might be used as a valuable biological marker than IL-17A during chronic fibrosis progression and HCC development in HCV patients.

**Keywords:** Il-17F, Hepatitis C virus, Fibrosis, Hepatocellular carcinoma

## Background

Approximately 80 million people worldwide have viremic hepatitis C virus (HCV) infection, which causes chronic hepatitis, fibrosis, cirrhosis, and hepatocellular carcinoma (HCC) [1]. The full progression of end-stage liver diseases in HCV-infected patients takes about two to three decades, which provides a window for intervention. Liver fibrosis is a protective response to chronic hepatic injury that leads to accumulation of extracellular matrix proteins [2]. Extensive fibrosis may result in cirrhosis and, in severe cases, lead to liver failure requiring liver transplantation. Severe fibrosis and cirrhosis are the outcome of continuous liver injuries, which can be caused by chronic virus infection or long-term alcohol consumption. Liver fibrosis is one of the known risk factors for HCC [3]. Chronic inflammation caused by innate and adaptive immune responses to HCV infection is involved in the progression of HCV-associated diseases, such as liver cirrhosis and HCC [4, 5]. Identification of factors involved in HCV pathogenesis or biomarkers associated with liver diseases may provide new intervention and treatment approaches for HCV-related diseases.

T helper (Th) 17 cells are a subset of CD4[+] T cells that mediate a protective role against bacterial and fungal infections [6, 7] as well as a pathological role in inflammation-associated diseases, such as autoimmune diseases and cancer [8–10]. Transforming growth factor (TGF)-β, interleukin (IL)-6, IL-21, and IL-23 are the key cytokines for Th17 cell maturation and production of IL-17 family cytokines, the secretion of which is a

* Correspondence: guannyiy@nhri.org.tw
†Equal contributors
[1]National Institute of Infectious Diseases and Vaccinology, National Health Research Institutes, 35 Keyan Road, Zhunan, Miaoli County 35053, Taiwan
[3]Center of Infectious Disease and Signaling Research, National Cheng-Kung University, Tainan 70101, Taiwan
Full list of author information is available at the end of the article

quintessential defining feature for Th17 cells [11–13]. The IL-17 family has six members, including IL-17A–F. IL-17A and IL-17F have high sequence homology and are expressed as homodimers or as an IL-17A + F heterodimer to induce expression proinflammatory cytokines, chemokines, antimicrobial peptides, and matrix metalloproteinases in IL-17 receptor-bearing cells [14].

Th17 cells play an important role in many liver diseases, such as liver fibrosis, alcoholic liver disease, chronic hepatitis B, and autoimmune liver disease [15–18]. The Th17 cell population is increased in chronic hepatitis C patients and Th17 cell abundance correlates positively with liver injury but inversely with HCV RNA load [19]. Although IL-17A had been extensively studied in chronic liver diseases, the function of IL-17F, which shares a high degree of homology with IL-17A, in the progression of chronic hepatic diseases is poorly understood. IL-17F can be secreted by CD8$^+$ T cells, $\gamma\delta$ T cells, NKT cells, LTi-like cells, and epithelial cells in addition to being secreted by Th17 cells (CD4$^+$ T cells) [8, 20]. IL-17F has a weaker receptor binding affinity than IL-17A and therefore induces less expression of proinflammatory cytokines than IL-17A [21]. The aim of this study was to evaluate the association between the expression of IL-17F and HCV-associated diseases by the evaluation of Th17-related cytokine expression in HCC tissue and serum from HCV patients.

## Methods

### HCC cohort

RNA samples derived from cancerous and non-cancerous parts of HCC tissue from patients infected with HCV and controls negative for both HBV and HCV ("non-B, non-C", NBNC) were obtained from the Taiwan Liver Cancer Network (TLCN) [22].

### Treatment naïve HCV cohort

A total of 250 patients who had serologically demonstrated HCV infection and were treated at Tainan Municipal Hospital (TMH), Tainan, Taiwan from 2003 to 2008 were included in our serum cytokine analysis. Baseline sera were collected from the patients within two months before they underwent HCV antiviral therapy. Patients infected with HBV or HIV were excluded from the study. The diagnoses of hepatic steatosis, fibrosis, and HCC of the HCV cohort were independently confirmed by two pathologists at TMH. Based on the METAVIR grading system, liver fibrosis status was classified as: no fibrosis (F0), portal fibrosis without septa (F1), with few septa (F2), with numerous septa but without cirrhosis (F3), and with cirrhosis (F4).

### Serum cytokine detection

IL-6, IL-17A, IL-17F, and IL-21 concentrations in serum samples were measured by enzyme-linked immunosorbent assay (ELISA) according to the manufacturer's instructions. Human IL-6, IL-17A, and IL-17F ELISA kits were purchased from R&D Systems (MN, USA), and the IL-21 immunoassay kit was obtained from eBioscience (CA, USA). The kits' analytic sensitivities were 9.375 pg/mL for IL-6, 15.625 pg/mL for IL-17A, 312.5 pg/mL for IL-17F, and 8 pg/mL for IL-21.

### Cytokine mRNA quantification

Total RNA samples (1 µg) extracted from HCC cancerous and non-cancerous tissues were used for cDNA synthesis with SuperScript-III First-Strand Synthesis System (Invitrogen, Carlsbad, CA). cDNAs were then used as templates in the quantitative-polymerase chain reaction (PCR) with gene specific primers and SYBR green dye to determine quantification cycle (Cq) by Applied Biosystems 7900HT Fast Real-Time PCR System. Primer sequences for human cytokine IL-17A and IL-17F and housekeeping gene ubiquitin C (UBC) [23] were listed in Table 1. Relative cytokine mRNA expression level was normalized to UBC reference gene by the $2^{-\Delta\Delta Cq}$ method [24]. Cytokine mRNA expression with Cq < 35 cycles was counted as positive, and the positive frequency was determined for cancerous and non-cancerous tissue separately for each group.

### IL-17F immunohistochemistry

Paraffin-embedded sections of the HCC cohort were subjected to immunohistochemistry (IHC) by following the protocol described previously with minor modification [25]. In brief, paraffin-embedded sections were deparaffinized and incubated in citrate buffer (pH 6) with 0.05% Tween 20 at 95–98 °C for 20 min. After 3% $H_2O_2$ and 1% bovine serum albumin blocking, slides were incubated with the anti-IL-17F antibody (ab168194, Abcam) overnight at 4 °C, followed by incubation with a secondary antibody (EnVision$^+$ system-HRP-labeled polymer, DakoCytomation) at room temperature for 1 h. The sections were then stained with 3,3′-diaminobenzidine substrate and counterstained with hematoxylin. Samples were considered IL-17F-immunopositive if at least 10% of randomly selected fields contained positive staining signals.

**Table 1** Primer sequences for quantitative RT-PCR

| Gene Name | Oligo sequences |
| --- | --- |
| UBC forward | 5′ CCTGGTGCTCCGTCTTAGAG 3′ |
| UBC reverse | 5′ TTTCCCAGCAAAGATCAACC 3′ |
| IL-17A forward | 5′ AATCTCCACCGCAATGAGGA 3′ |
| IL-17A reverse | 5′ ACGTTCCCATCAGCGTTGA 3′ |
| IL-17F forward | 5′ GAAGCTTGACATTGGCATCA 3′ |
| IL-17F reverse | 5′ GATGCAGCCCAAGTTCCTAC 3′ |

**Table 2** Demographic Summary of TLCN HCC cohort

| Variable | HCV (n = 40) | NBNC (n = 32) |
|---|---|---|
| Age | 66.3 ± 8.4 (59.3–72.0) | 66.0 ± 14.9 (61.0–76.0) |
| Gender | Male:32, Female:8 | Male:22, Female:10 |
| Presence of cirrhosis | 45.0% | 21.9% |
| Tumor size (cm) | 4.5 ± 2.3 (3.0–5.9) | 8.0 ± 5.1 (3.5–11.8) |
| Positive frequency[a] | (Tumor, Non-Tumor) | (Tumor, Non-Tumor) |
| IL-17A | 80.0%, 75.0% | 87.5%, 87.5% |
| IL-17F | 47.5%, 15.0% | 40.6%, 18.8% |

[a]Specific cytokine gene expression was detected by quantitative RT-PCR

## Statistical analyses

Statistical analyses were performed with SPSS software (IBM, NY, USA). Serum cytokine and mRNA expression were across-analyzed with demographic and clinical groups using the Mann-Whitney U test and Kruskal-Wallis tests. The relative distribution of IL-17A and IL-17F mRNA expression in cancerous and noncancerous tissue was analyzed by the Fisher exact test and Mann-Whitney U test. In all cases, $p < 0.05$ was considered statistically significant.

## Results

### IL-17F expression was elevated in HCV-associated HCC

Table 2 listed that the characteristics of the HCV ($N = 40$) and NBNC ($N = 32$) cancer patients from whom paired cancerous and adjacent non-cancerous tissues from TLCN tissue bank were obtained and subjected to quantitative RT-PCR analysis with SYBR dye for IL-17A and IL-17F mRNA detection. IL-17A mRNA was present in more than 75% of RNA samples derived from both cancerous and non-cancerous tissues. In contrast, IL-17F mRNA was expressed only in a portion of HCC samples. As shown in Table 2, the positive frequency was higher in cancerous tissue than in non-cancerous tissue, and notably higher in HCV-infected tissue (47.5% vs. 15%, $p = 0.003$ by Fisher exact test) than in NBNC patients (40.6% vs. 18.8%, $p = 0.1$ by Fisher exact test). Relative IL-17A mRNA expression level demonstrated no differences between cancerous and non-tumor counterpart tissues either derived from HCV-infected patients or NBNC patients. The relative IL-17A and F mRNA expression level in those positive cases did not show a significant difference between HCV and NBNC patients.

IHC revealed IL-17F-immunopositive signals in hepatocytes in HCC tissues (Fig. 1). In total, 85% of the HCC tumor samples from the HCV group and 62% of the HCC tumor samples from NBNC group were positive for IL-17F staining ($p = 0.0002$ by Fisher exact test). In summary, IL-17F expression was higher in HCV-associated HCC tissues compared with NBNC HCC tissues at both the mRNA and protein levels.

### Association of serum IL-17F level with liver fibrosis progression in treatment naïve HCV patient cohort

Due to HCC development is largely confined to patients with liver fibrosis and cirrhosis, a retrospective cohort study was further conducted to determine serum IL-17F expression levels in HCV patients with chronic hepatic diseases. Diagnosis of HCV infection was confirmed in all 250 HCV patients by two sequential tests for HCV antibodies, followed by an HCV RNA assay. The data consisted of 127 men (51%) and 123 women (49%) with

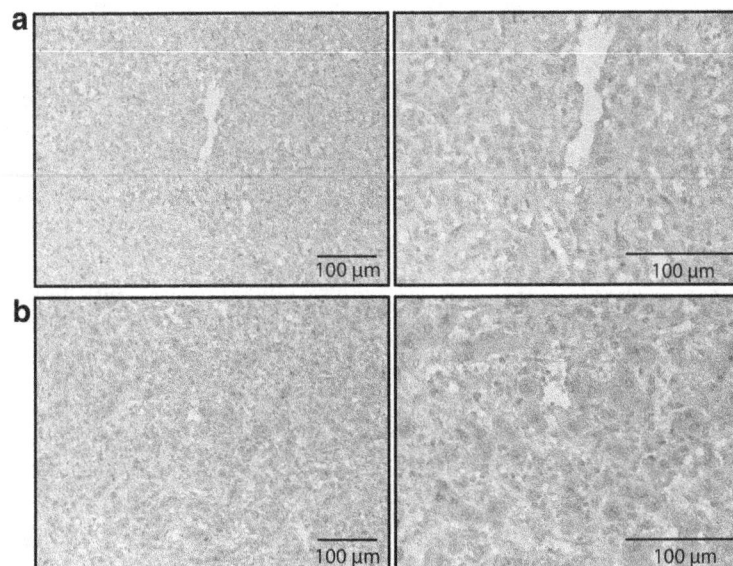

**Fig. 1** Representative images of IL-17F immunohistochemistry staining. Representative images for IL-17F IHC labeling in HCV-infected HCC tumor tissue samples without (**a**) and with (**b**) IL-17F immunopositivity. Magnification in the left column-200X and in the right column-400X

**Table 3** Variables of HCV infected patients from TMH

| Variable | | N | Mean (IQR) | Positive rate |
|---|---|---|---|---|
| Age | | 250 | 56.6 ± 10.5 (51.5–64.8) | |
| Gender | | Male:127, Female:123 | | |
| Steatosis | | 98 (39.2%) | | |
| Fibrosis | F0 | 0 (0%) | | |
| | F1 | 7 (2.8%) | | |
| | F2 | 102 (40.8%) | | |
| | F3 | 94 (37.6%) | | |
| | F4 | 47 (18.8%) | | |
| HCC | | 38 (15.2%) | | |
| IL-17F | | 250 | 1246.7 pg/mL (0–877.7) | 30.4% |
| IL-17A | | 144 | 4.3 pg/mL (0–0) | 6.3% |
| IL-21 | | 137 | 73.2 pg/mL (0–84.7) | 59.9% |
| IL-6 | | 153 | 50.6 pg/mL (0–0) | 20.3% |

a mean age of 56.6 years; 39.2% of the patients had steatosis, 100% had fibrosis, and 15.2% had HCC (Table 3). The distribution of liver fibrosis stage in this cohort was as follows: F1, 7 cases (2.8%); F2, 102 cases (40.8%); F3, 94 cases (37.6%); and F4 (cirrhosis), 47 cases (18.8%). As shown in Table 3, IL-17F ELISAs of 250 serum samples obtained from treatment-naïve HCV patients yielded a mean serum IL-17F concentration of 1246.7 pg/ml. Among the 250 samples, 76 (30.3%) had IL-17F level > 312.5 ng/mL, the lower detection limit of the ELISA. The expression of inflammatory cytokines, IL-17A, IL-21, and IL-6, which are functionally associated with IL-17F were also measured by ELISA. As some serum samples collected from the HCV patients in 2003–2008 were not sufficient for addition ELISAs, the case numbers (N) for these cytokines were less than 250. IL-17A was detected in very few samples (9/144, 6.3%) at a low concentration (mean: 4.3 pg/mL). IL-21 was detected in 82/137 samples (59.9%) at a mean concentration of 73.2 pg/mL, and IL-6 was detected in 31/153 samples (20.3%) at a mean concentration of 50.6 pg/mL.

The correlation efficiency between serum IL-17F levels and chronic hepatic diseases, including hepatitis, steatosis, fibrosis, and HCC was evaluated as shown in Table 4.

Serum alanine aminotransferase (ALT) which is usually elevated during liver inflammation was used as an index for hepatitis in Table 4. When the patients were separated into mild (F1 and F2) and severe (F3 and F4) fibrosis groups for statistical analysis, serum IL-17F level was correlated with fibrotic severity (rho = 0.127, $p$ = 0.045) (Fig.2). Levels of cytokines IL-17A and IL-21 had strong (rho = 0.547, $p$ < 0.0001) and moderate (rho = 0.218, $p$ = 0.011) correlations, respectively, with IL-17F in the HCV patients. However, serum IL-17A and IL-21 level were not significantly associated with fibrosis or other HCV-associated diseases by statistical analyses.

## Discussion

The present study showed that a higher percentage of HCV-associated HCC tissues than of NBNC-HCC tissues were found to have IL-17F mRNA expression. IL-17F mRNA expression was higher in tumor tissue than in non-tumor counterparts. Furthermore, the serum IL-17F levels were elevated in HCV-infected patients with severe liver fibrosis than in patients with mild liver fibrosis.

Chronic HBV, HCV infection and steatohepatitis are common causes of liver fibrosis [26–28]. The relevance of Th17 and IL-17 in liver fibrosis has been studied in human patients and mouse models [29, 30]. Chang et al. showed that circulating and liver-infiltrating Th17 cell levels correlate with severity of liver inflammation [19]. However, serum IL-17A levels are low in HCV patients and appear not to correlate with HCV-related fibrosis [31]. In our HCV cohort study, the mean serum IL-17F level was much higher than that of IL-17A. The severity of liver fibrosis in HCV patients was associated only with IL-17F, but not with IL-17A, suggesting that IL-17F might be a better biomarker than IL-17A for HCV-associated fibrosis progression. The serum IL-17F level did not have a significant correlation with serum alanine aminotransferase activity in the HCV cohort, suggesting that IL-17F elevation was not associated with acute liver inflammation.

IL-17A and IL-17F have highly homologous amino acid sequences, bind the same receptor, and activate similar proinflammatory responses, but these two cytokines differ in tissue distribution and receptor binding affinity [32]. In the present HCV cohort, more serum samples were positive for IL-17F than with IL-17A, and

**Table 4** Correlations of serum IL-17F level with the HCV infection-associated liver diseases and other proinflammatory cytokines

| | | ALT | Steatosis | Fibrosis[c] | HCC | IL-17A | IL-21 | IL-6 |
|---|---|---|---|---|---|---|---|---|
| IL-17F | Correlation Coefficient (r) | −0.094 | 0.012 | 0.127[a] | 0.014 | 0.547[b] | 0.218[a] | 0.009 |
| | Sig. | 0.142 | 0.850 | 0.045 | 0.826 | 0.000 | 0.011 | 0.912 |

[a]Correlation is significant at the 0.05 level (2-tailed)
[b]Correlation is significant at the 0.01 level (2-tailed)
[c] Fibrosis: stage >2
Spearman's rank correlation

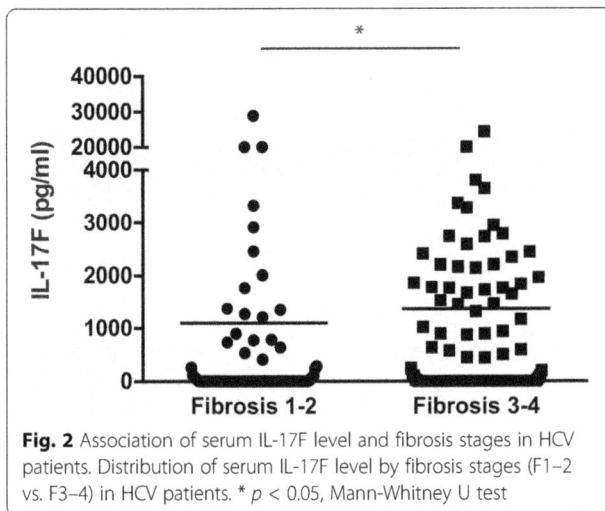

**Fig. 2** Association of serum IL-17F level and fibrosis stages in HCV patients. Distribution of serum IL-17F level by fibrosis stages (F1–2 vs. F3–4) in HCV patients. * $p < 0.05$, Mann-Whitney U test

the mean IL-17F level was much higher than the mean IL-17A level. High levels of IL-17F can be due to a high transcription activity, a long protein half-life, or production by different cell types. Given that the expression of serum IL-17A and IL-21, two key cytokines produced by Th17 cells, was associated with IL-17F expression, it is likely that Th17 cells contribute to IL-17F expression. However, in our IL-17F IHC analysis of HCC tissue sections, IL-17F expression was found mainly in hepatocytes. Serum IL-17F in HCV-infected patients may be produced partially by hepatocytes. The stimuli capable of triggering IL-17F expression in hepatocytes and other cell types and the responses activated by IL-17F-dependent signaling in the liver will need to be addressed further.

A pathological role of IL-17 and Th17 in HCC development has been proposed based on recent studies [29, 33–35]. Proinflammatory, anti-apoptosis, and pro-angiogenesis signals may contribute to the tumor promotion role of Th17 cells and IL-17 in HCC development [29]. The role of IL-17F in HCC remains undetermined. In the present study, we found that IL-17F was elevated in patients with HCV and advanced fibrosis and that IL-17F mRNA was also elevated in HCV-associated tumor tissue. Notably, the IL-17F protein was found mainly in hepatocytes. The exact function of IL-17F in HCC development needs to be clarified with long-term follow-up cohort study.

## Conclusions

The importance of IL-17F in chronic hepatic diseases was poorly investigated; however, we had found Th-17 associated inflammatory cytokine, IL-17F, which took a major part in severe liver fibrosis and HCC symptoms in HCV patients than other inflammatory cytokines, IL-6, and IL-17A. It appears that IL-17F can be a precise biomarker for the diagnosis of liver fibrosis and HCC progression in the future.

### Acknowledgements
We thank Tainan Municipal Hospital and Taiwan Liver Cancer Network for providing patient serum, RNA and tissue sections.

### Funding
This work was supported by National Health Research Institutes (Taiwan), grant number IV-104-pp.-21.

### Authors' contributions
MSW and CHW contributed equally to this work. MSW, CHW, and GYY were in involved in experimental design, data analysis, and manuscript preparation. FCT performed statistical analyses. HJY, YCL, YPK, DJT, and WTT performed related experiments. All authors read and approved the final manuscript.

### Competing interests
The authors declare that they have no competing interests with the contents of this article.

### Author details
[1]National Institute of Infectious Diseases and Vaccinology, National Health Research Institutes, 35 Keyan Road, Zhunan, Miaoli County 35053, Taiwan. [2]Division of Gastroenterology, Tainan Municipal Hospital, Tainan 70173, Taiwan. [3]Center of Infectious Disease and Signaling Research, National Cheng-Kung University, Tainan 70101, Taiwan.

### References
1. Gower E, et al. Global epidemiology and genotype distribution of the hepatitis C virus infection. J Hepatol. 2014;61(1 Suppl):S45–57.
2. Friedman SL. Liver fibrosis – from bench to bedside. J Hepatol. 2003; 38(Suppl 1):S38–53.
3. Fattovich G, et al. Hepatocellular carcinoma in cirrhosis: incidence and risk factors. Gastroenterology. 2004;127(5 Suppl 1):S35–50.
4. Donato F, et al. Alcohol and hepatocellular carcinoma: the effect of lifetime intake and hepatitis virus infections in men and women. Am J Epidemiol. 2002;155(4):323–31.
5. El-Serag HB. Hepatocellular carcinoma and hepatitis C in the United States. Hepatology. 2002;36(5 Suppl 1):S74–83.
6. Tesmer LA, et al. Th17 cells in human disease. Immunol Rev. 2008;223:87–113.
7. Hohl TM, Rivera A, Pamer EG. Immunity to fungi. Curr Opin Immunol. 2006; 18(4):465–72.
8. Komiyama Y, et al. IL-17 plays an important role in the development of experimental autoimmune encephalomyelitis. J Immunol. 2006;177(1):566–73.
9. Miossec P. IL-17 and Th17 cells in human inflammatory diseases. Microbes Infect. 2009;11(5):625–30.
10. Dardalhon V, et al. Role of Th1 and Th17 cells in organ-specific autoimmunity. J Autoimmun. 2008;31(3):252–6.
11. Wei L, et al. IL-21 is produced by Th17 cells and drives IL-17 production in a STAT3-dependent manner. J Biol Chem. 2007;282(48):34605–10.
12. Bettelli E, et al. Reciprocal developmental pathways for the generation of pathogenic effector TH17 and regulatory T cells. Nature. 2006; 441(7090):235–8.
13. Veldhoen M, et al. TGFbeta in the context of an inflammatory cytokine milieu supports de novo differentiation of IL-17-producing T cells. Immunity. 2006;24(2):179–89.
14. Iwakura Y, et al. Functional specialization of interleukin-17 family members. Immunity. 2011;34(2):149–62.
15. Lemmers A, et al. The interleukin-17 pathway is involved in human alcoholic liver disease. Hepatology. 2009;49(2):646–57.
16. Lan RY, et al. Hepatic IL-17 responses in human and murine primary biliary cirrhosis. J Autoimmun. 2009;32(1):43–51.

17. Yasumi Y, et al. Interleukin-17 as a new marker of severity of acute hepatic injury. Hepatol Res. 2007;37(4):248–54.

18. Tan Z, et al. IL-17A plays a critical role in the pathogenesis of liver fibrosis through hepatic stellate cell activation. J Immunol. 2013;191(4):1835–44.

19. Chang Q, et al. Th17 cells are increased with severity of liver inflammation in patients with chronic hepatitis C. J Gastroenterol Hepatol. 2012;27(2):273–8.

20. Takatori H, et al. Lymphoid tissue inducer-like cells are an innate source of IL-17 and IL-22. J Exp Med. 2009;206(1):35–41.

21. Ishigame H, et al. Differential roles of interleukin-17A and -17F in host defense against mucoepithelial bacterial infection and allergic responses. Immunity. 2009;30(1):108–19.

22. Chang IC, et al. The hepatitis viral status in patients with hepatocellular carcinoma: a study of 3843 patients from Taiwan liver cancer network. Medicine (Baltimore). 2016;95(15):e3284.

23. Kim S, Kim T. Selection of optimal internal controls for gene expression profiling of liver disease. BioTechniques. 2003;35(3):456–8. 460

24. Livak KJ, Schmittgen TD. Analysis of relative gene expression data using real-time quantitative PCR and the 2(−Delta Delta C(T)) method. Methods. 2001;25(4):402–8.

25. Grivennikov S, et al. IL-6 and Stat3 are required for survival of intestinal epithelial cells and development of colitis-associated cancer. Cancer Cell. 2009;15(2):103–13.

26. Yilmaz B, et al. Chronic hepatitis B associated with hepatic steatosis, insulin resistance, necroinflammation and fibrosis. Afr Health Sci. 2015;15(3):714–8.

27. Sebastiani G, Gkouvatsos K, Pantopoulos K. Chronic hepatitis C and liver fibrosis. World J Gastroenterol. 2014;20(32):11033–53.

28. Bataller R, Brenner DA. Liver fibrosis. J Clin Invest. 2005;115(2):209–18.

29. Hammerich L, Heymann F, Tacke F. Role of IL-17 and Th17 cells in liver diseases. Clin Dev Immunol. 2011;2011:345803.

30. Meng F, et al. Interleukin-17 signaling in inflammatory, Kupffer cells, and hepatic stellate cells exacerbates liver fibrosis in mice. Gastroenterology. 2012;143(3):765–76. e1–3

31. Foster RG, et al. Interleukin (IL)-17/IL-22-producing T cells enriched within the liver of patients with chronic hepatitis C viral (HCV) infection. Dig Dis Sci. 2012;57(2):381–9.

32. Yang XO, et al. Regulation of inflammatory responses by IL-17F. J Exp Med. 2008;205(5):1063–75.

33. Zhang JP, et al. Increased intratumoral IL-17-producing cells correlate with poor survival in hepatocellular carcinoma patients. J Hepatol. 2009;50(5):980–9.

34. Li J, et al. Interleukin 17A promotes hepatocellular carcinoma metastasis via NF-kB induced matrix metalloproteinases 2 and 9 expression. PLoS One. 2011;6(7):e21816.

35. Kuang DM, et al. Activated monocytes in peritumoral stroma of hepatocellular carcinoma promote expansion of memory T helper 17 cells. Hepatology. 2010;51(1):154–64.

# 13

# Genetic variability in E6, E7 and L1 genes of Human Papillomavirus 62 and its prevalence in Mexico

Cristina Artaza-Irigaray[1,2], María Guadalupe Flores-Miramontes[1,2], Dominik Olszewski[3], María Teresa Magaña-Torres[1], María Guadalupe López-Cardona[4], Yelda Aurora Leal-Herrera[5], Patricia Piña-Sánchez[6], Luis Felipe Jave-Suárez[1*†] and Adriana Aguilar-Lemarroy[1*†] (iD)

## Abstract

**Background:** Human papillomavirus (HPV) is the main etiological agent of cervical cancer, the third most common cancer among women globally and the second most frequent in Mexico. Persistent infection with high-risk HPV genotypes is associated with premalignant lesions and cervical cancer development. HPVs considered as low risk or not yet classified, are often found in coinfection with different HPV genotypes. Indeed, HPV62 is one of the most prevalent HPV detected in some countries, but there is limited information about its prevalence in other regions and there are no HPV62 variants currently described. The aim of this study was to determine the prevalence of HPV62 in cervical samples from Mexican women and to identify mutations in the L1, E6 and E7 genes, which have never been reported in our population.

**Methods:** HPV screening was performed by Cobas HPV Test in women who attended prevention health programs and dysplasia clinics. All HPV positive samples ($n = 491$) and 87 additional cervical cancer samples were then genotyped with Linear Array HPV Genotyping test. Some samples were selected to corroborate genotyping by Next-Generation sequencing. On the other hand, nucleotide changes in L1, E6 and E7 genes were determined using PCR, Sanger sequencing and analysis with the CLC-MainWorkbench 7.6.1 software. L1 protein structure was predicted with the I-TASSER server.

**Results:** Using Linear Array, HPV62 prevalence was 7.6% in general population, 8% in Cervical Intraepithelial Neoplasia grade 1 (CIN1) samples and 4.6% in cervical samples. The presence of HPV62 was confirmed with Next-Generation sequencing. Regarding L1 gene, novel sequence variations were detected, but they did not alter the tertiary structure of the protein. Moreover, several nucleotide substitutions were found in E6 and E7 genes compared to reference HPV62 genomic sequence. Specifically, three non-synonymous sequence variations were detected, two in E6 and one in E7.

**Conclusions:** HPV62 is a frequent HPV genotype found mainly in general population and in women with CIN1, and in 90.5% of the cases it was found in coinfection with other HPVs. Novel nucleotide changes in its *L1*, *E6* and *E7* genes were detected, some of them lead to changes in the protein sequence.

**Keywords:** Cervical cancer, HPV62, E6, E7, L1

* Correspondence: lfjave@yahoo.com; adry.aguilar.lemarroy@gmail.com
†Equal contributors
[1]División de Inmunología, Centro de Investigación Biomédica de Occidente (CIBO), Instituto Mexicano del Seguro Social (IMSS), Guadalajara, Jalisco, Mexico
Full list of author information is available at the end of the article

## Background

Cervical Cancer (CC) is the fourth leading cause of cancer deaths in women worldwide with an estimate of more than 528,000 new diagnosed cases and 266,000 deaths in 2012. More than 85% of deaths occur in developing countries and in particular, in Mexico, CC is the second most frequent cancer leading to 4,769 deaths in 2012 [1]. This pathology is directly associated with HPV (Human Papillomavirus) infection and to date, around 200 HPVs have been described [2, 3]. Mucosal HPVs are grouped into low risk (LR-HPVs) and high risk HPVs (HR-HPVs), the latter being considered the etiologic agents of CC [3]. The *Alphapapillomavirus* genus harbors more than 60 types of HPVs, including the oncogenic HPVs associated to anogenital cancers according to the International Agency for Research on Cancer (IARC): types 16, 18, 31, 33, 35, 39, 45, 51, 52, 56, 58, 59, 66 and 68 [4, 5]. Specifically, HPV16 and HPV18 are found in around 70% of the CC cases worldwide [6, 7].

HPVs have a circular double-stranded 8 kb DNA genome that typically contains eight genes [8]. The L1 gene, which encodes the principal virus capsid protein, is used for the classification and construction of phylogenetic trees as it is well conserved among different HPVs. In 2004, the HPV classification criteria were defined based on differences in the complete L1 Open Reading Frame (ORF): different genera share less than 60% nucleotide sequence identity, HPV species within a genus share between 60 and 70% identity, HPV types share between 71 and 89% nucleotide identity, HPV subtypes differ in 2-10% and HPV variants differ in 1-2% within the L1 ORF [9]. In 2013, the term variant was proposed to also include HPV subtypes. The use of full genome sequence information, instead of the L1 ORF, was recommended to classify a new variant genome. The alignment of complete viral genomes began to define variant lineages and sublineages using differences of 1-10% and 0.5-1%, respectively [10].

HR-HPV genomes encode three oncoproteins —E5, E6 and E7— that contribute to enhanced cell proliferation, initiation and progression of CC [11]. An interesting review contrasts the activities of the human alpha-PV oncoproteins with their non-oncogenic counterparts based on cell culture studies [12]. The comparison of activities of LR- and HR-HPVs would lead to the identification of common activities probably needed for the viral life cycle, while additional functions of HR-HPVs could be crucial for the transformation/immortalization process.

HPV62 was characterized in 2004 by Fu et al. (accession number AY395706) from a cervical sample obtained from a 45-year-old woman with normal cytology [13] and it is considered as a LR-HPV. The E6 (447 bp), E7 (291 bp) and L1 (1512 bp) genes from this HPV62 reference genome (8092 bp) encode for 148, 96 and 503 amino acid proteins, respectively. In a first report including cervical samples from mexican population, HPV62 was mainly detected in coinfection with other HPV genotypes and it was found in 5.1% of HPV positive patients with Cervical Intraepithelial Neoplasia Grade 1 (CIN1) and in 0.8% of HPV positive patients with CC using Linear Array HPV Genotyping test [14]. The aim of this study, was to determine the prevalence of this genotype in a greater number of samples among Mexican women and to detect possible mutations in L1, E6 and E7 genes of the HPV62 circulating in the Mexican population. Until now, only two complete genome sequences have been reported worldwide from 2 patients: the first one in 2004 (AY395706) [13] and the second one very recently uploaded (KU298924.1) [15].

## Methods

### Sample collection

All samples were collected by gynecologists with a cytobrush inserted into the endocervical canal and placed into the transport medium PreservCyt (Hologic, Bedford, MA). Three large groups of samples were included: 1) cervical samples from women (general population), who attended cervical cancer prevention programs; 2) cervical samples with CIN1 from women who attended a Dysplasia Clinic, and 3) cervical samples with CC from women who attended the Oncology Hospital. The first group of samples include women from six different States of the Mexican Republic (Aguascalientes, Colima, Guanajuato, Jalisco, Michoacán, Nayarit and Yucatán), and they were obtained from the Regional Hospital Dr. Valentín Gómez Farías – ISSSTE (Guadalajara, Jalisco). The samples from the second group were recruited at the Dysplasia Clinic of the Regional General Hospital No. 12 Lic. Benito Juárez – IMSS (Mérida, Yucatán), and at the Dysplasia Clinic of the Western National Medical Center – IMSS (Guadalajara, Jalisco). Finally, the last group's samples were obtained exclusively from the Oncology Hospital of the Western National Medical Center – IMSS (Guadalajara, Jalisco). In all cases, the samples were taken as part of the routine diagnosis confirmation and an aliquot of the PreservCyt solution was given for our study, after informed consent was signed. Samples with excess of blood and mucus in the PreservCyt solution, low DNA quantity or quality samples, were eliminated. A total of 2835 samples were screened for HPV; 2399 from general population, 349 from Dysplasia Clinics and 87 from Oncology Hospital. Concerning only the first group of samples, the diagnosis was kept anonymous for this study, as authorized in the ethically approved protocol. However, the diagnosis of the second (CIN1) and third (CC) group of samples was obtained by colposcopic observation and confirmed by histo-pathological analysis.

Samples were collected from July 2014 to July 2016. As detailed in the section of ethical considerations, collection of the samples from the different groups was authorized by the ISSSTE and the National Committee on Health Research and Ethics of the IMSS, for various research protocols.

**HPV screening and genotyping**

The samples from the first and the second group were first screened for HPV positivity with the Cobas HPV Test (Roche Molecular Systems, Inc). Afterwards, all HPV positive samples were genotyped with the Linear Array HPV Genotyping test (LA), Roche Molecular Diagnostics. Additionally, 48 CIN1 samples taken randomly, were genotyped with the 454 Next-Generation Sequencing (NGS) platform to confirm HPV genotyping. Regarding the third group, all CC samples were genotyped with LA and 48 of them were also selected randomly to confirm genotyping with NGS. The set of PGMY11/09 primers (452 bp amplicon from nucleotide 949 to 1400 of L1 ORF) was used for NGS, as previously described [16]. In addition, NGS was also performed using the degenerated FAP primers set [17, 18]. A first conventional Polymerase Chain Reaction (PCR) was done with the primers FAP59 (forward 5′- TAACWG-TIGGICAYCCWTATT - 3′) and FAP64 (reverse 5′-CCWATATCWVHCATITCICCATC - 3′) to amplify a 478 bp fragment from the L1 region. PCR conditions were: 94 °C for 3 min, 35 cycles at 94 °C for 45 s, 50 °C for 30 s and 72 °C for 1 min, finally 72 °C for 10 min. A second PCR was done with the 478 bp amplicon using the following primers: Forward 5′-[Universal Multiplicom tail A: AAGACTCGGCAG-CATCTCCA] − [FAP6085: CCWGATCCHAATMRRT TTGC]-3′. and Reverse 5′ [Universal Multiplicom tail B: GCGATCGTCACTGTTCTCCA] − [FAP64 primer]. The resulting amplicon is of 377 bp (from nucleotide 232 to 607 of L1 ORF). Universal Multiplicom tails A and B were the same used in Cat. no. MR-0020.024 (Multiplicom NV CFTR; Molecular Diagnostics, Niel, Belgium). This second PCR was run under the same conditions as the first PCR, except for the annealing temperature that was changed to 47 °C. Amplicons were visualized by gel electrophoresis in a 1.5% agarose gel. HPV positive samples were selected to undergo further screening by NGS using Multiplex identifiers (MID) barcodes for each sample as described in Flores-Miramontes et al. [16]. Quality control of the obtained sequences was carried out with the online platform Galaxy (version 16.04) and they were analyzed with Roche's GS Reference Mapper Software (version 2.9), using as references all

human papillomavirus sequences from the Papillomavirus Episteme (PaVE) database [3, 19].

**Sanger sequencing for L1, E6 and E7 genes**

E6, E7 and L1 genes were amplified from cervical samples positive to HPV62 by Linear Array using PCR with the following primer pairs specific for each gene of interest (all of them were designed with Oligo v6 software). E6: forward 5′- GGTCAGCACAGTAGCAATGACT-3′ and reverse 5′- CGGGACGCTCTTGTAGGAC- 3′; E7: forward 5′-CAGGAGTGTGGACAGGACGGTA- 3′ and reverse 5′- GCATCGGCCATGTCACTTATG -3′; L1: forward 5′- ACGCCTTCCTTCCCTGCAACTA - 3′ and reverse 5′-CACTGACAAACGCGCACAACAC-3′. The reactions were performed in a final volume of 25 uL containing at least 200 ng of genomic DNA, 200 uM of each dNTP, 1X reaction buffer with 1.8 mM of $MgCl_2$, 12.5 pmol of each primer, and 1.25 units of Fast Start High Fidelity enzyme (Roche Applied Science, Cat. No. 04 738 284 001). PCR conditions were: initial denaturation at 95 °C for 2 min, 35 cycles of 95 °C for 30 s, annealing at 58 °C (*HPV62-E6* and *-E7*) or 62 °C (*HPV62-L1*) for 30 s, elongation at 72 °C for 45 s, and a final extension at 72 °C for 7 min. Afterwards, 5 uL of the PCR products were visualized on 1% agarose gel to corroborate the presence and size of the amplicon, and the other 20 uL were utilized for isopropanol purification. Purified amplicons were sequenced with BigDye Terminator v3.1 Cycle Sequencing Kit (Applied Biosystems, Cat. No. 4337455) using the above mentioned forward primers for E6, E7, and L1 and additional primers designed for L1, which is too long to be sequenced with a single primer (5′-ACACGGAACGCATGGTATGGGC, 5′-GCAGAACCTTATGGCGATTGTA-3′ and 5′-TTG TGCAAAATACAGTTAACCC-3′). Reactions were performed in a final volume of 20 uL with around 50 ng of DNA, 10 pmol of forward primer, 2 uL of 5X Sequencing Buffer, and 4 uL of Ready Reaction Premix. Cycling conditions were set as follows: initial denaturation at 96 °C for 1 min, and 25 cycles at 96 ° C for 10 s, annealing at 50 °C for 5 s, elongation at 60 °C for 4 min. Finally, products were purified with Centri-Sep Spin Columns (ABI, Cat. No. 401762), and sequenced with the ABI PRISM 310 Genetic Analyzer (Applied Biosystems).

**Sequence alignments and L1 protein structure prediction analysis**

To detect genetic mutations or variants in E6, E7 and L1, the obtained gene sequences were aligned to the HPV62 reference sequence (reported as AY395706 in the NCBI database) using the *CLC-MainWorkbench 7.6.1* program (Qiagen). To look for amino acid changes, the DNA sequences were translated into protein with the same software, and aligned to the reference protein. The phylogenetic tree showing alpha-3 group HPVs and all HPV62 sequences obtained in this work, was performed with MEGA v.7.014 software using Maximum Likelihood statistical method.

Finally, the L1 protein structures were predicted with the I-TASSER server (Iterative Threading ASSEmbly Refinement), which identifies structural templates from the Protein Data Bank by multiple threading approach and constructs full-length atomic models by iterative template fragment assembly simulations [20–23]. Protein structure alignment was performed with *CLC MainWorkbench 7.6.1* program.

## Results

### HPV62 prevalence genotyped by Linear Array HPV Genotyping Test

Regarding the first group of cervical samples described in "Methods section" (general population of women who attended cervical cancer prevention health programs), from the 2399 samples screened for HPV positivity by Cobas HPV Test, 291 were HPV positive (12.1%) and 22/291 (7.6%) were HPV62 positive. Concerning the second group (CIN1 samples), from the 349 screened with Cobas, 200 (57.3%) were HPV positive and 16/200 (8%) were HPV62 positive. Finally, the third group of samples (CC samples) showed 100% of HPV positivity with LA, and from those, only 4 samples (4.6%) were HPV62 positive. It is important to highlight that in only 4 samples from the total of 42 HPV62 positive samples, this genotype was found as single infection (exclusively in CIN1 samples), and in the other 38 (90.5%) in coinfection with 1 to 5 additional HPV genotypes (detailed in Table 1).

Interestingly, as depicted in Fig. 1, HPV62 was more frequently found in coinfection with 16, 39, 59, 51 and 83 HPV genotypes.

### HPV genotyping by NGS

To confirm HPV genotyping, 48 CIN1 samples were sequenced with NGS, 8 of them HPV62 positive with Linear Array. In those 8 samples, HPV62 presence was corroborated using NGS; however, 3 additional samples were positive to HPV62 only with the last methodology.

Concerning the presence of HPV62 exclusively in cervical cancer, 48 samples diagnosed with squamous cervical carcinoma were selected for HPV genotyping by NGS (choosing preferentially those that showed more than two HPV genotypes detected by Linear Array). To detect a broader HPV genotype spectrum in those samples, NGS was performed utilizing PGMY11/09 and FAP primer sets. As depicted in Table 2, four of the samples mapped with high identity to HPV62, and they were found in coinfection with additional HPV genotypes,

**Table 1** HPV genotypes detected in coinfection with HPV62 by Linear Array in each of the 38 HPV62 positive samples

GROUP 1 SAMPLES (general population)

| Sample Code | HPV genotypes detected by Linear Array | Sample Code | HPV genotypes detected by Linear Array |
|---|---|---|---|
| GP-1 | **16**, 42, **58**, 81, 83 | GP-12 | **39**, **59**, 61 |
| GP-2 | **31**, **52**, 61, 72, 84 | GP-13 | 42, **45**, 84 |
| GP-3 | **39**, **51**, **56**, **58**, 84 | GP-14 | **16**, **18** |
| GP-4 | 11, **52**, **59**, 83 | GP-15 | **16**, **51** |
| GP-5 | **31**, **39**, *66*, *67* | GP-16 | **16**, **52** |
| GP-6 | **39**, 61, 84, 89 | GP-17 | **31**, **59** |
| GP-7 | **52**, **56**, *70*, 72 | GP-18 | **35**, *67* |
| GP-8 | 11, **16**, **39** | GP-19 | **45**, 72 |
| GP-9 | **16**, **51**, **59** | GP-20 | **51**, **59** |
| GP-10 | *26*, **45**, *66* | GP-21 | **58**, *66* |
| GP-11 | **31**, 72, 83 | GP-22 | **51** |

GROUP 2 SAMPLES (CIN1)

| Sample Code | HPV genotypes detected by Linear Array | Sample Code | HPV genotypes detected by Linear Array |
|---|---|---|---|
| CIN1-1 | **33**, **45**, **59**, 71, 83 | CIN1-7 | **39**, 81 |
| CIN1-2 | **16**, **51**, **59**, 81 | CIN1-8 | **51**, *53* |
| CIN1-3 | 11, *70*, 83 | CIN1-9 | *70*, 83 |
| CIN1-4 | **16**, **39**, *66* | CIN1-10 | **16** |
| CIN1-5 | 61, 72, 84 | CIN1-11 | **59** |
| CIN1-6 | **16**, *53* | CIN1-12 | 89 |

GROUP 3 SAMPLES (CC)

| Sample Code | HPV genotypes detected by Linear Array | Sample Code | HPV genotypes detected by Linear Array |
|---|---|---|---|
| CC-1 | **16**, 54, *70* | CC-3 | **39**, 71 |
| CC-2 | **16**, **18** | CC-4 | **16** |

In bold: HPV genotypes classified as carcinogenic to humans by the IARC (group 1); in italics: possibly carcinogenic to humans (group 2B)

including beta-1 papillomavirus (12, 21 and 118), which were only detected with FAP primers.

### Nucleotide variations in HPV62-L1

To study whether the HPV62 circulating in the Mexican population exhibits nucleotide changes in L1, all HPV62-L1 sequences obtained by NGS with PGMY or FAP primers (independently of the diagnosis of the samples) were aligned to the HPV62 complete genome (AY395706). The contigs were obtained from 11 samples amplified with PGMY primers and 9 samples amplified with FAP primers. Alignment of the eleven HPV62-L1 contigs revealed the presence of 9 mutations distributed among all the samples in the region amplified with

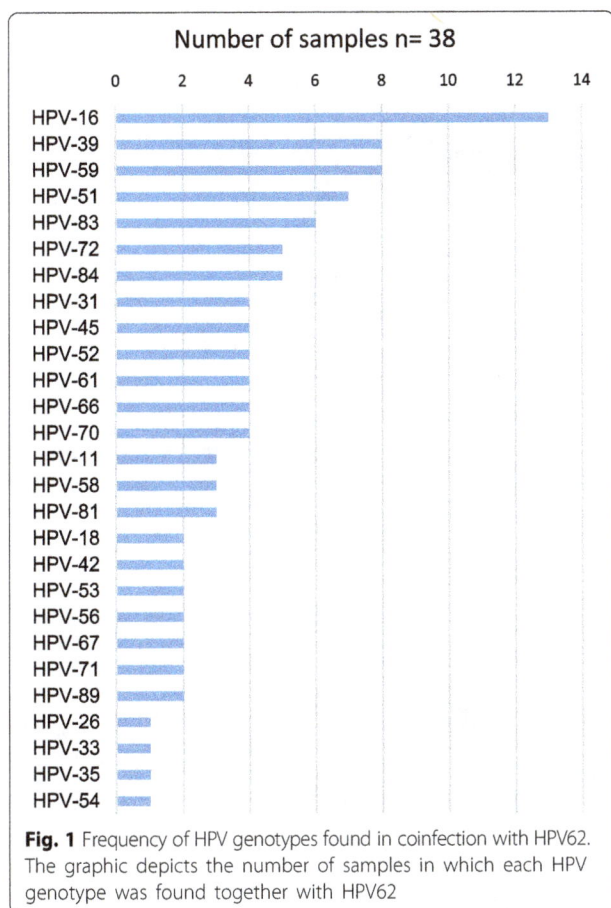

**Fig. 1** Frequency of HPV genotypes found in coinfection with HPV62. The graphic depicts the number of samples in which each HPV genotype was found together with HPV62

PGMY primers. As depicted in Table 3, three out of the nine mutations were non-synonymous. Moreover, nine HPV62-L1 contigs from the region amplified with FAP primers revealed 10 mutations, five of them non-synonymous (Table 3).

To study whether the HPV62 that infects the Mexican population is a variant of the virus, the whole conserved HPV62-L1 ORF (1690 bp amplicon) from genomic DNA of a cervical sample was amplified and sequenced (HPV62-L1 P9). A total of 17 nucleotide changes were detected in HPV62-L1: four non-synonymous c.250A > G (pT84A), c.263C > G (p.A88G), c.1139A > G (p.K380R) and c.1489G > A (p.A497T); and 13 synonymous c.111G > A, c.117C > T, c.126 T > C, c.324C > T, c.627C > T, c.663G > A, c.1014 T > C, c.1017G > A, c.1161C > T, c.1416A > G, c.1425 T > A, c.1443 T > C, c.1497A > C (Fig. 2a). The first 3 amino acid substitutions are in the same spatial region in L1, while the last substitution is in the C-terminal domain, as shown by protein structure prediction (Fig. 2b, c, d). None of the four amino acid changes affect the tertiary structure of the L1 protein according to the predicted models.

### Nucleotide variations in HPV62-E6 and HPV62-E7

The E6 and E7 genes amplified from genomic DNA of 13 cervical samples infected with HPV62 were purified and sequenced to detect nucleotide variations in the HPV62 that circulates in Mexico. Altogether, seven nucleotide changes were identified in HPV62-E6, two of which were non-synonymous and led to an alteration in

**Table 2** HPV genotypes detected in samples from cervical cancer that were positive to HPV62 by NGS

| Sample code | HPV types found by Linear Array | HPV types found by NGS | Reads using FAP primers | Reads using PGMY primers | Total Reads |
|---|---|---|---|---|---|
| CC-1 | 16, 54, 62, 70 | 16 | - | 174 | 174 |
| | | 33 | - | 1 | 1 |
| | | 54 | 776 | 3 | 779 |
| | | 62 | 105 | - | 105 |
| | | 70 | 163 | 348 | 511 |
| | | 118 | 2 | - | 2 |
| CC-2 | 16, 18, 62 | 16 | 9 | 481 | 490 |
| | | 62 | 895 | 3 | 898 |
| CC-3 | 39, 62, 71 | 16 | - | 50 | 50 |
| | | 39 | - | 2 | 2 |
| | | 62 | 1086 | 218 | 1304 |
| | | 71 | - | 98 | 98 |
| | | 81 | 2 | - | 2 |
| CC-5 | 33 | 12 | 21 | - | 21 |
| | | 21 | 1069 | - | 1069 |
| | | 33 | 1 | 507 | 508 |
| | | 62 | 3 | - | 3 |

Reads obtained from each HPV type by using FAP or PGMY11/09 primers are detailed for each sample. Linear Array results are also included

**Table 3** Genetic mutations found in the 5′ and 3′-ends of HPV62-L1

| Nucleotide changes (PGMY primers) | Amino acid change | Number of samples with the mutation n = 11 | Nucleotide changes (FAP primers) | Amino acid change | Number of samples with the mutation n = 9 |
|---|---|---|---|---|---|
| c.969 T > C | | 2 | c.250A > G | p.T84A | 9 |
| c.987A > C * | p.E329D | 3 | c.263C > G | p.A88G | 7 |
| c.1017G > A | | 1 | c.265A > T | p.T89S | 1 |
| c.1071 T > C * | | 3 | c.413C > T | p.A138V | 1 |
| c.1104G > A | | 1 | c.436A > G | p.I146V | 1 |
| c.1236 T > C | | 3 | c.438C > I | | 1 |
| c.1256A > G | p.H419R | 4 | c.468A > G | | 1 |
| c.1279A > G * | p.T427A | 1 | c.495A > T | | 5 |
| c.1287A > G | | 3 | c.495A > G | | 1 |
| | | | c.516C > A | | 1 |

Nucleotide changes are shown in samples amplified with PGMY or FAP primers. The amino acid changes are described for those with non-synonymous mutations. The number of samples that carry each nucleotide change are included. (*) Already reported mutations

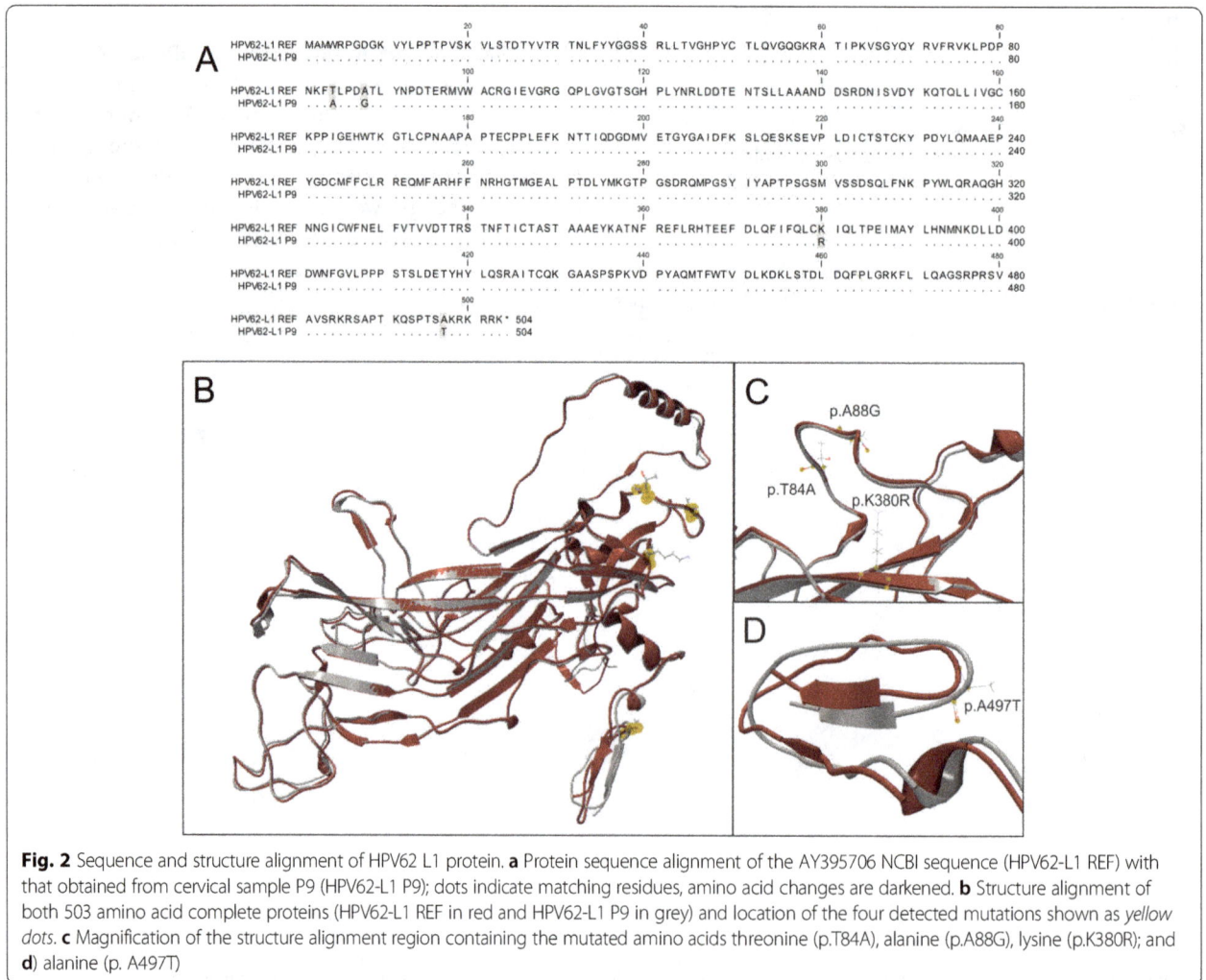

**Fig. 2** Sequence and structure alignment of HPV62 L1 protein. **a** Protein sequence alignment of the AY395706 NCBI sequence (HPV62-L1 REF) with that obtained from cervical sample P9 (HPV62-L1 P9); dots indicate matching residues, amino acid changes are darkened. **b** Structure alignment of both 503 amino acid complete proteins (HPV62-L1 REF in red and HPV62-L1 P9 in grey) and location of the four detected mutations shown as *yellow dots*. **c** Magnification of the structure alignment region containing the mutated amino acids threonine (p.T84A), alanine (p.A88G), lysine (p.K380R); and **d**) alanine (p. A497T)

the protein sequence (c.157C > T, p.R53W and c.404A > G, p.Y135C). Regarding HPV62-E7, three nucleotide changes were detected and one of them affected the protein sequence (c.125C > G, p.A42G) (Table 4). The non-synonymous changes were present in all the samples, while the other nucleotide variations that do not change the amino acid were found only in some of them. The genetic sequences of E6 and E7 from HPV62 amplified from the 13 samples were translated into protein and aligned to the reference sequence for an easier visualization of the nucleotide changes and their location (Fig. 3). Finally, to visualize the relationship between all HPVs from Alpha-3 species and the HPV62 sequences obtained from the 13 cervical samples, a phylogenetic tree was built based on E6/E7 gene sequences (Fig. 4).

## Discussion

A fragment of the L1 ORF —MY09/11 region— of HPV62 was first sequenced in 1994 and the complete genome was isolated and sequenced to characterize the novel HPV type 62 in 2004 [13, 24]. In 2006, the Linear Array HPV Genotyping Test was launched; an assay that identifies up to 37 HPV genotypes in cervical samples, including HPV62. HPV62 belongs to the *Alphapapillomavirus genus*, species 3 group (α-3 group) together with HPV 61, 72, 81, 83, 84, 86, 87, 89, 102 and 114.

In the present study, from 578 HPV positive samples obtained from general population, CIN1 and CC women, the HPV62 frequency found with LA was 7.6, 8, and 4.6%, respectively, showing that this genotype has an important prevalence in Mexico; and it is mainly found in coinfection with HR-HPV genotypes (Table 1 and Fig. 1). Importantly, by using NGS, 11 out of 48 individually sequenced CIN1 samples were also positive for HPV62, despite only 8 of them were positive for this HPV

genotype by Linear Array; moreover, concerning CC samples, only 1 of the 4 HPV62 positive samples detected by NGS, was positive with the last methodology. Therefore, the frequency of HPV62 could be underestimated. It is worth mentioning that, because cervical cancer cells were collected from cervical swabs and not from biopsies, the samples may contain normal cells together with cancer cells, so this could be a limitation of this study, since it is not possible to know which cells each HPV is infecting.

When HPV62 was characterized, it was one of the ten most prevalent HPV types detected in women with normal Pap smears from Costa Rica and New Mexico [13]. Later, more studies supported this finding. In the Italian population, HPV62 was detected in 1.5% of high-grade squamous intraepithelial lesions and also in 1.5% of CC, being the only LR-HPV found in CC samples [25]. There was no HPV62 detection in samples without cervical lesions in both populations. Among LR-HPV types detected in the Northern Indian population, HPV62 was the most common (10.5% of HPV positive samples) and in Egypt HPV62 was also the most prevalent LR-HPV among HPV positive women (17.4 and 9.7% in two different research works) [26–28]. In Thai women, HPV62 is also among the most frequent LR-HPV (11.3% of HPV positive samples) [29]. Another interesting result was found in females from the United States where the most common HPV type was HPV62 (found in 6.5% of all the subjects, where 42.5% are HPV positive) [30]. In Croatian women, HPV62 was among the most prevalent LR-HPVs in women with abnormal cervical cytology (23.3%) [31]. In Northeast Brazil, HPV62 prevalence among the overall population was of 3.6% and in Korea, 2% of atypical squamous cell and low-grade squamous intraepithelial lesions were HPV62 positive [32, 33]. In Mexico, a IMSS Research Network

**Table 4** Nucleotide changes found in *HPV62-E6* and *HPV62-E7* gene sequences from 13 cervical samples infected with HPV62 (P1-P13) compared to the reported HPV62 genome (AY395706, NCBI)

| Mutations | P1 | P2 | P3 | P4 | P5 | P6 | P7 | P8 | P9 | P10 | P11 | P12 | P13 |
|---|---|---|---|---|---|---|---|---|---|---|---|---|---|
| *HPV62-E6* | | | | | | | | | | | | | |
| c.27G > A | ✓ | ✓ | | ✓ | ✓ | ✓ | ✓ | ✓ | ✓ | ✓ | ✓ | ✓ | |
| c.37 T > C | ✓ | ✓ | | ✓ | ✓ | ✓ | | ✓ | ✓ | ✓ | | | |
| c.157C > T* | ✓ | ✓ | ✓ | ✓ | ✓ | ✓ | ✓ | ✓ | ✓ | ✓ | ✓ | ✓ | ✓ |
| c.177 T > C | | | | | | | ✓ | | | | ✓ | | |
| c.199 T > C | ✓ | | | ✓ | | ✓ | | | ✓ | ✓ | | | |
| c.201G > C | ✓ | | | ✓ | | ✓ | | | ✓ | ✓ | | | |
| c.404A > G* | ✓ | ✓ | ✓ | ✓ | ✓ | ✓ | ✓ | ✓ | ✓ | ✓ | ✓ | ✓ | ✓ |
| HPV62-E7 | | | | | | | | | | | | | |
| c.125C > G* | ✓ | | ✓ | ✓ | ✓ | ✓ | ✓ | ✓ | ✓ | ✓ | ✓ | ✓ | ✓ |
| c.183 T > C | | | | | | ✓ | | | | | | | |
| c.199A > C | ✓ | | | ✓ | | ✓ | | | ✓ | ✓ | | | |

(*) Nucleotide substitutions that alter protein sequence

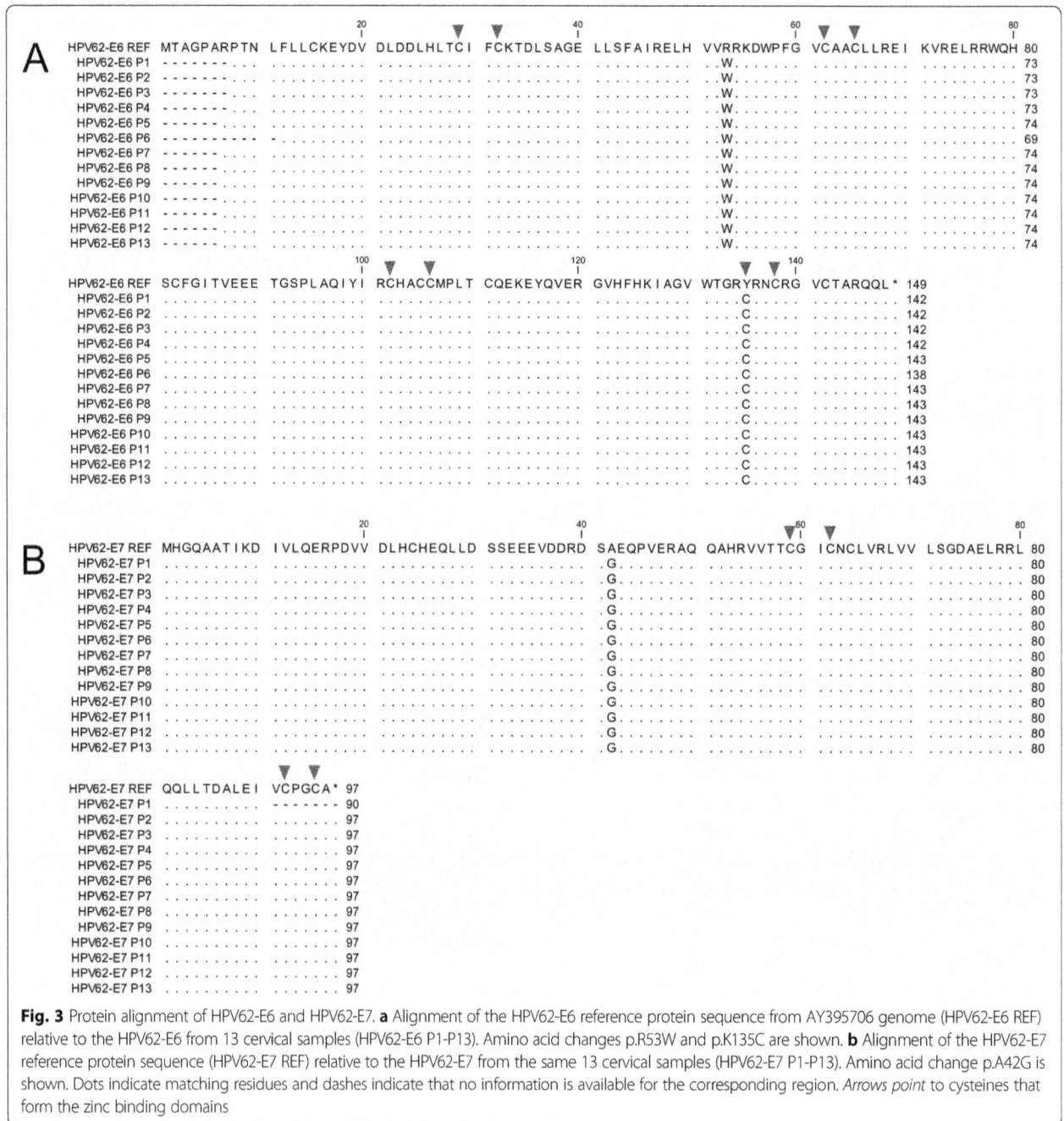

**Fig. 3** Protein alignment of HPV62-E6 and HPV62-E7. **a** Alignment of the HPV62-E6 reference protein sequence from AY395706 genome (HPV62-E6 REF) relative to the HPV62-E6 from 13 cervical samples (HPV62-E6 P1-P13). Amino acid changes p.R53W and p.K135C are shown. **b** Alignment of the HPV62-E7 reference protein sequence (HPV62-E7 REF) relative to the HPV62-E7 from the same 13 cervical samples (HPV62-E7 P1-P13). Amino acid change p.A42G is shown. Dots indicate matching residues and dashes indicate that no information is available for the corresponding region. *Arrows point* to cysteines that form the zinc binding domains

report on HPV, including 822 women, found HPV62 infection in 3.1% of women without cervical lesions, in 5.1% with CIN1, in 6.7% with CIN3 and in 0.8% in CC samples [14].

All these studies agree in the high frequency of HPV62 in cervical samples and its omnipresence in all kind of diagnosed samples; it is therefore of great interest to further study this genotype.

This work describes novel nucleotide changes in the HPV62-L1 complete gene (1512 bp). The 17 variations identified in the L1 ORF amplified from one sample

determine a difference of 1.12% (17/1512 bp) compared to the reference sequence. A nucleotide sequence difference of 1% or more would define a new variant lineage, but according to the recommended new HPV variant classification criteria, the complete genome (and not only the L1 ORF) has to be sequenced [10]. The alignment of 20 HPV62-L1 sequences obtained by NGS using PGMY or FAP primer pairs from 16 cervical samples revealed the presence of a total of 19 mutations, 8 of them being non-synonymous. Interestingly, to our knowledge, only 3 out of the 19 mutations have been

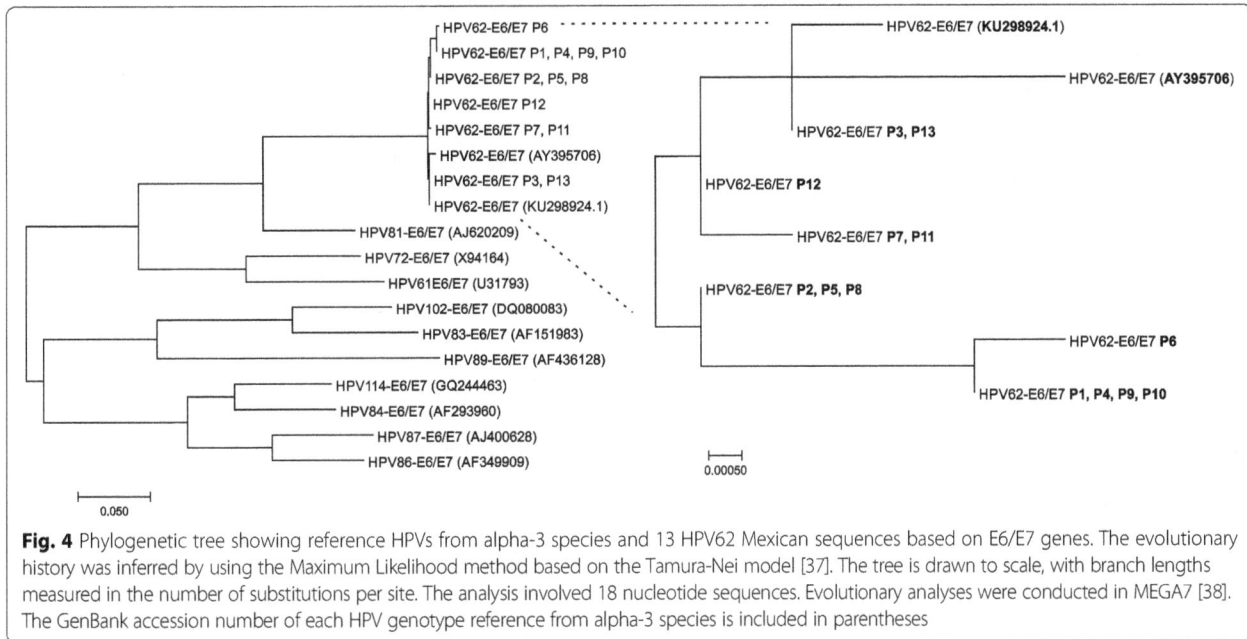

**Fig. 4** Phylogenetic tree showing reference HPVs from alpha-3 species and 13 HPV62 Mexican sequences based on E6/E7 genes. The evolutionary history was inferred by using the Maximum Likelihood method based on the Tamura-Nei model [37]. The tree is drawn to scale, with branch lengths measured in the number of substitutions per site. The analysis involved 18 nucleotide sequences. Evolutionary analyses were conducted in MEGA7 [38]. The GenBank accession number of each HPV genotype reference from alpha-3 species is included in parentheses

previously described [34]. It is worth mentioning that concerning those nucleotide changes, there was not a different distribution between CIN1 and CC samples, the mutations were distributed randomly among them.

Concerning HPV62-E6 and -E7 ORFs, the presence of genetic variations is described for the first time in the present study. Specifically, concerning HPV62-E6, non-synonymous nucleotide changes c.157C > T (p.R53W) and c.404A > G (p.Y135C) were found; additionally, c.125C > G (p.A42G) substitution in HPV62-E7 was found in all the 13 samples under study. However, the c.404A > G (p.Y135C) substitution that leads to a change of a tyrosine by a cysteine in all the 13 analyzed samples is located in a key position essential for the formation of a zinc binding domain which needs two CxxC motifs. Indeed, eight cysteines involved in the formation of two zinc binding sites in E6 protein are conserved among the different HPV types and the seventh cysteine in HPV62 is located in position 135, where a tyrosine was reported instead [12, 35]. HPV62 was originally characterized with the overlapping PCR method and according to the described methodological process, PCR products were visualized with UV illumination in agarose gels before product purification, ligation into pGEM-Teasy vector and sequencing. UV radiation is a strong mutagen that can induce conversion from one base to another [36]. Therefore, the adenine reported in position 404 of the reference genome could probably be due to a spontaneous change caused by UV radiation. The reference AY395706 HPV62 genomic sequence could have been reported with some mistakes and the three non-synonymous changes in E6 and E7 described in

this work might be found of the HPV62 sequence worldwide. Earlier this year, a new complete HPV62 genome sequence has been uploaded in the GenBank database (KU298924.1) [15]; in which some of the nucleotide changes described in the present research are confirmed.

These findings open a new door to the study of LR-HPVs commonly found in HPV positive women. To date, oncogenic HPVs have been studied primarily, thus information on rare or LR-HPVs is limited, although they are often more prevalent than HR-HPVs. When found in coinfection with other HPV types, these non-oncogenic viruses may play an important role in the progression or regression of a cervical lesion, but this remains unstudied. Undoubtedly, more research is needed in this field, particularly with respect to the E5, E6 and E7 proteins and their different domains shared between HR-HPVs and LR-HPVs to understand their way of action. Furthermore, the L1 major capsid protein and its different variants may influence crucial steps of the viral infection cycle due to altered affinity to other proteins.

HPV infection in a single patient often comes along with more than one HPV genotype. Hence, clustering of the different genotypes present in a single sample might be crucial for understanding the roles of each genotype in carcinogenesis. This will lead to a better understanding of possible interactions between HPVs found in coinfections, both low and high risk.

## Conclusions

HPV62 was found in Mexican women who attended their preventive routine check-up and in women with cervical cancer. In the general population and in the CIN1 samples, HPV62 was often present both in single and multiple infection; however, in cervical cancer samples it was only found in coinfections with at least one HR-HPV type. To our knowledge, this is the first study that describes the presence of mutations in HPV62-E6 and -E7 genes. Moreover, newly observed nucleotide changes in the L1 gene were found to alter the L1 protein sequence. Upcoming discoveries in this field will complement the current information on variants of human papillomavirus and on still unclassified genotypes in their carcinogenicity risk to humans.

## Abbreviations
CC: Cervical Cancer; CIN1: Cervical Intraepithelial Neoplasia Grade 1; HR-HPV: High Risk Human Papillomavirus; LR-HPV: Low-Risk Human Papillomavirus; NGS: Next-Generation Sequencing; ORF: Open Reading Frame

## Acknowledgements
CA-I and MGF-M are grateful for a scholarship from Consejo Nacional de Ciencia y Tecnología (CONACyT)- Mexico. PP-S and MTM-T are scholarship holders of the IMSS Foundation and are grateful for their support.

## Funding
This work was supported by Fondo de Investigación en Salud – IMSS, grants numbers FIS/IMSS/PROT/PRIO/14/033 to AA-L and FIS/IMSS/PROT/PRIO/15/046 to LFJ-S.

## Authors' contributions
MGL-C, YAL-H and PP-S were involved in patient interviews and sample recruitment. MGL-C and PP-S performed the Cobas HPV Test, MGF-M and DO conducted the Linear Array HPV test and NGS. CA-I carried out PCR amplifications, Sanger sequencing, the bioinformatics analyses and draft the manuscript; MTM-T gave support with the Sanger sequencing, AA-L and LFJ-S conceived of and designed the study, supervised all experiments and analyses, and wrote the manuscript. All authors read and approved the final manuscript.

## Competing interests
The authors declare that they have no competing interests.

## Author details
[1]División de Inmunología, Centro de Investigación Biomédica de Occidente (CIBO), Instituto Mexicano del Seguro Social (IMSS), Guadalajara, Jalisco, Mexico. [2]Programa de Doctorado en Ciencias Biomédicas, Centro Universitario de Ciencias de la Salud (CUCS), Universidad de Guadalajara, Jalisco, Mexico. [3]Institute of Pharmacy and Molecular Biotechnology, University of Heidelberg, Heidelberg, Germany. [4]Unidad de Medicina Genómica y Genética, Hospital Regional Dr. Valentín Gómez Farías - ISSSTE, Guadalajara, Jalisco, Mexico. [5]Unidad de Investigación Médica Yucatán (UIMY) - IMSS, Mérida, Yucatán, Mexico. [6]Laboratorio de Oncología Molecular, Unidad de Investigación Médica en Enfermedades Oncológicas (UIMEO) - IMSS, Ciudad de Mexico, Mexico.

## References

1. GLOBOCAN. Estimated Cancer Incidence, Mortality and Prevalence Worldwide in 2012. http://globocan.iarc.fr/Pages/fact_sheets_cancer.aspx. Accessed 6 June 2016.
2. Zur Hausen H. Papillomaviruses and cancer: from basic studies to clinical application. Nat Rev Cancer. 2002;2(5):342–50.
3. Pedraza-Brindis EJ, Sanchez-Reyes K, Hernandez-Flores G, Bravo-Cuellar A, Jave-Suarez LF, Aguilar-Lemarroy A, Gomez-Lomeli P, Lopez-Lopez BA, Ortiz-Lazareno PC. Culture supernatants of cervical cancer cells induce an M2 phenotypic profile in THP-1 macrophages. Cell Immunol. 2016;310:42–52.
4. Ma Y, Madupu R, Karaoz U, Nossa CW, Yang L, Yooseph S, Yachimski PS, Brodie EL, Nelson KE, Pei Z. Human papillomavirus community in healthy persons, defined by metagenomics analysis of human microbiome project shotgun sequencing data sets. J Virol. 2014;88(9):4786–97.
5. Bravo IG, Félez-Sánchez M. Papillomaviruses viral evolution, cancer and evolutionary medicine. Evol med public health. 2015;2015(1):32–51.
6. Comprehensive Cervical Cancer Prevention and Control. WHO. 2013.
7. de Sanjose S, Quint WG, Alemany L, Geraets DT, Klaustermeier JE, Lloveras B, Tous S, Felix A, Bravo LE, Shin H-R. Human papillomavirus genotype attribution in invasive cervical cancer: a retrospective cross-sectional worldwide study. Lancet Oncol. 2010;11(11):1048–56.
8. Munoz N, Castellsagué X, de González AB, Gissmann L. HPV in the etiology of human cancer. Vaccine. 2006;24:S1–S10.
9. De Villiers E-M, Fauquet C, Broker TR, Bernard H-U, zur Hausen H. Classification of papillomaviruses. Virology. 2004;324(1):17–27.
10. Burk RD, Harari A, Chen Z. Human papillomavirus genome variants. Virology. 2013;445(1):232–43.
11. Moody CA, Laimins LA. Human papillomavirus oncoproteins: pathways to transformation. Nat Rev Cancer. 2010;10(8):550–60.
12. Klingelhutz AJ, Roman A. Cellular transformation by human papillomaviruses: lessons learned by comparing high-and low-risk viruses. Virology. 2012;424(2):77–98.
13. Fu L, Terai M, Matsukura T, Herrero R, Burk RD. Codetection of a mixed population of candHPV62 containing wild-type and disrupted E1 open-reading frame in a 45-year-old woman with normal cytology. J Infect Dis. 2004;190(7):1303–9.
14. Aguilar-Lemarroy A, Vallejo-Ruiz V, Cortes-Gutierrez EI, Salgado-Bernabe ME, Ramos-Gonzalez NP, Ortega-Cervantes L, Arias-Flores R, Medina-Diaz IM, Hernandez-Garza F, Santos-Lopez G, et al. Human papillomavirus infections in Mexican women with normal cytology, precancerous lesions, and cervical cancer: type-specific prevalence and HPV coinfections. J Med Virol. 2015;87(5):871–84.
15. Siqueira JD, Alves BM, Prellwitz IM, Furtado C, Meyrelles AR, Machado ES, Seuanez HN, Soares MA, Soares EA. Identification of novel human papillomavirus lineages and sublineages in HIV/HPV-coinfected pregnant women by next-generation sequencing. Virology. 2016;493:202–8.
16. Flores-Miramontes MG, Torres-Reyes LA, Alvarado-Ruíz L, Romero-Martínez SA, Ramírez-Rodríguez V, Balderas-Peña LM, Vallejo-Ruíz V, Piña-Sánchez P, Cortés-Gutiérrez EI, Jave-Suárez LF. Human papillomavirus genotyping by linear array and next-generation sequencing in cervical samples from Western Mexico. Virol J. 2015;12(1):161.
17. Forslund O, Antonsson A, Nordin P, Stenquist B, Hansson BG. A broad range of human papillomavirus types detected with a general PCR method suitable for analysis of cutaneous tumours and normal skin. J Gen Virol. 1999;80(Pt 9):2437–43.
18. Li J, Pan Y, Xu Z, Wang Q, Hang D, Shen N, Liu M, Zhang C, Abliz A, Deng Q, et al. Improved detection of human papillomavirus harbored in healthy skin with FAP6085/64 primers. J Virol Methods. 2013;193(2):633–8.
19. Papillomavirus Episteme (PaVE). https://pave.niaid.nih.gov. Accessed 12 July 2016.
20. Roy A, Kucukural A, Zhang Y. I-TASSER: a unified platform for automated protein structure and function prediction. Nat Protoc. 2010;5(4):725–38.
21. Yang J, Yan R, Roy A, Xu D, Poisson J, Zhang Y. The I-TASSER suite: protein structure and function prediction. Nat Methods. 2015;12(1):7–8.
22. I-Tasser Protein Structure and Function Predictions. zhanglab.ccmb.med.umich.edu/I-TASSER/. Accessed 20 July 2016.
23. Zhang Y. I-TASSER server for protein 3D structure prediction. BMC Bioinformatics. 2008;9(1):40.
24. Bernard H-U, Chan S-Y, Manos MM, Ong C-K, Villa LL, Delius H, Peyton CL, Bauer HM, Wheeler CM. Identification and assessment of known and novel human papillomaviruses by polymerase chain reaction amplification,

restriction fragment length polymorphisms, nucleotide sequence, and phylogenetic algorithms. J Infect Dis. 1994;170(5):1077–85.

25. Tornesello ML, Duraturo ML, Botti G, Greggi S, Piccoli R, De Palo G, Montella M, Buonaguro L, Buonaguro FM. Prevalence of alpha-papillomavirus genotypes in cervical squamous intraepithelial lesions and invasive cervical carcinoma in the Italian population. J Med Virol. 2006;78(12):1663–72.

26. Datta P, Bhatla N, Dar L, Patro AR, Gulati A, Kriplani A, Singh N. Prevalence of human papillomavirus infection among young women in North India. Cancer Epidemiol. 2010;34(2):157–61.

27. Shaltout MF, Sallam HN, AbouSeeda M, Moiety F, Hemeda H, Ibrahim A, Sherbini ME, Rady H, Gopala K, DeAntonio R. Prevalence and type distribution of human papillomavirus among women older than 18 years in Egypt: a multicenter, observational study. Int J Infect Dis. 2014;29:226–31.

28. Youssef MA, Abdelsalam L, Harfoush RA, Talaat IM, Elkattan E, Mohey A, Abdella RM, Farhan MS, Foad HA, Elsayed AM. Prevalence of human papilloma virus (HPV) and its genotypes in cervical specimens of Egyptian women by linear array HPV genotyping test. Infect agents cancer. 2016;11(1):1.

29. Kantathavorn N, Mahidol C, Sritana N, Sricharunrat T, Phoolcharoen N, Auewarakul C, Teerayathanakul N, Taepisitpong C, Saeloo S, Sornsamdang G. Genotypic distribution of human papillomavirus (HPV) and cervical cytology findings in 5906 Thai women undergoing cervical cancer screening programs. Infect agents cancer. 2015;10(1):7.

30. Hariri S, Unger ER, Sternberg M, Dunne EF, Swan D, Patel S, Markowitz LE. Prevalence of genital human papillomavirus among females in the United States, the national health and nutrition examination survey, 2003–2006. J Infect Dis. 2011;204(4):566–73.

31. Roksandić-Križan I, Bošnjak Z, Perić M, Đurkin I, Zujić Atalić V, Vuković D. Distribution of Genital Human Papillomavirus (HPV) Genotypes in Croatian Women with Cervical Intraepithelial Neoplasia (CIN)–A Pilot Study. Coll Antropol. 2013;37(4):1179–83.

32. Santos FM, Gurgel A, Lobo C, Freitas A, Silva-Neto J, Silva L. Prevalence of human papillomavirus (HPV), distribution of HPV types, and risk factors for infection in HPV-positive women. Genetics and molecular research. GMR. 2016;15(2):1–9.

33. So KA, Kim MJ, Lee K-H, Lee I-H, Kim MK, Lee YK, Hwang C-S, Jeong MS, Kee M-K, Kang C. The impact of high-risk HPV genotypes other than HPV 16/18 on the natural course of abnormal cervical cytology: a Korean HPV cohort study. Cancer Res Treat. 2016;48(4):1313.

34. Gurgel APAD, Chagas BS, Amaral CMM, Albuquerque EMB, Serra IGSS, Silva Neto JC, Muniz MTC, Freitas AC. Prevalence and genetic variability in capsid L1 gene of rare human papillomaviruses (HPV) found in cervical lesions of women from North-East Brazil. Biomed Res Int. 2013;2013:546354.

35. Thomas M, Narayan N, Pim D, Tomaić V, Massimi P, Nagasaka K, Kranjec C, Gammoh N, Banks L. Human papillomaviruses, cervical cancer and cell polarity. Oncogene. 2008;27(55):7018–30.

36. Rastogi RP, Kumar A, Tyagi MB, Sinha RP. Molecular mechanisms of ultraviolet radiation-induced DNA damage and repair. J Nucleic Acids. 2010;2010:592980.

37. Tamura K, Nei M. Estimation of the number of nucleotide substitutions in the control region of mitochondrial DNA in humans and chimpanzees. Mol Biol Evol. 1993;10(3):512–26.

38. Kumar S, Stecher G, Tamura K. MEGA7: Molecular Evolutionary Genetics Analysis Version 7.0 for Bigger Datasets. Mol Biol Evol. 2016;33(7):1870–4.

# 14

# Safety of new DAAs for chronic HCV infection in a real life experience: role of a surveillance network based on clinician and hospital pharmacist

A. Nappi[1*], A. Perrella[2], P. Bellopede[2], A. Lanza[3], A. Izzi[4], M. Spatarella[1] and C. Sbreglia[2]

## Abstract

**Background:** Direct Antiviral Agents (DAAs) for HCV therapy represents a step ahead in the cure of chronic hepatitis C. Notwithstanding the promising results in several clinical trials, few data are available on adverse effects in real life settings.

**Methods:** We have evaluated 170 patients with persistent infection and on those eligible to treatment we have followed up them through a network managed by clinician and hospital pharmacist.

**Results:** According to our data we have found that 41% (32 out of 78) of enrolled patients experienced adverse reactions, of these 40% were in those under 65 years while 60% was in patients older than 65 years, SVR was achieved in 88% of the patients (including drop-out). We had 4 drop-out treatment due to major adverse reaction (heart and lung related).

**Conclusion:** Even if new antiviral drugs seem to be promising, according to SVR, they require careful follow-up, possibly managed by clinician and hospital pharmacist, to avoid unrecognized side effects which may affect adherence and the real impact of these drugs on chronically infected subjects.

**Keywords:** HCV, DAAs, Antiviral, Adverse drug reactions, Pharmacology, Hepatitis C, SVR

## Background

Hepatitis C virus (HCV) chronically infects approximately 185 million people worldwide and it still represents and important issue in public health. The rate of persistent infection after acute hepatitis ranges from 20 to 40% [1–3]. Once chronically infected patients may undergo antiviral treatment, however in the last decades, according to old antiviral regimen, chronic infection was characterized by low sustained virological response (SVR) [4]. Persistent infection can lead to cirrhosis, liver cancer, and death, and is one of the leading cause of liver transplantation in the European Country [5]. Italy has one of the highest HCV prevalence and according to data managed until 2002 with substantial geographic differences in the prevalence, with a range from 2.6% in the north [5, 6] to 16.2% in the south of Italy, However

other reports suggest a decreasing trend in our country [6, 7].

Despite the lack of recent data, HCV chronic infection still remains an issue in our country. Currently thanks to the direct-acting antivirals (DAA) HCV is treatable and the goal of treatment is to achieve a sustained virological response (SVR), considered to be a functional cure (absence of plasma HCV RNA 12 weeks after completing therapy). [4]. In addition, these new antivirals have been demonstrated to be effective regardless of race, gender, or HIV status, leaving few barriers to treatment having so the potential to reduce long-term costs of complications and interrupt the current global HCV epidemic even if more expansive than previous regimen. [8, 9]. However several drug to drug interactions have been reported for some of these, requiring careful in the management. According to previous studies on first line antiviral as protease inhibitors SVR rates increased with the use of these drugs but so did the adverse events,

* Correspondence: antonellanappi@yahoo.it
[1]Pharmacy Unit, Hospital D. Cotugno – AORN Azienda dei Colli, Naples, Italy
Full list of author information is available at the end of the article

resulting in discontinuation rates of 9–19% in patients on these triple therapy regimens [10]. Therefore the new DAAs seem to have all quality to be considered as a miracle drug [11]. However despite these new drugs has been presented as the new miracle in the infectious disease and been characterized by a very low adverse events rate in the published clinical trials, few data are available on adverse events based real life studies [12]. At the beginning of 2015 when DAAs were available in Campania Region in south Italy, where HCV is epidemic, we decided to assess impact of these new drugs on healthiness of the patients according to their adverse reactions. This kind of approach has been managed trough the creation of a network involving clinician and pharmacist to improve the follow-up of the patients under treatment not only from the efficacy point of view but mainly according to safety of these antivirals. Here we present our analysis and results on a surveillance network based on clinician and pharmacist to evaluate the safety of DAAs for HCV chronic infection in a real life in out-patients clinic of a tertiary care infectious disease division of a regional Hospital Center for Infectious disease in Campania Region.

## Methods

All patients were enrolled in this study according to national guidelines for the evaluation of HCV treatment eligibility assessed following the priority criteria established by the national registry of the Italian Medicines Agency committee (AIFA) (www.agenziafarmaco.gov.it). Data related to the efficacy of the DAAs is not the primary objective of the study therefore they are treated marginally. Data related to adverse drug reactions were collected through standard-of-care operating procedures utilized in a specialty pharmacy setting. These procedures utilized prescription claims software and a clinical assessment management program according to national network for pharmacovigilance (RNF - Rete Nazionale Farmacovigilanza). All patients were counseled prior to receiving their initial prescription according to clinician evaluation in out-patients clinic. Further, during all follow-up a survey based on two simple questions was also proposed and collected by clinician to assess the psychological health status in the course of therapy and to assess possible unrecognized side effects every month during therapy (Fig. 1). All patients were invited to communicate any changes in their health status or wellbeing during the entire treatment period. All concomitant therapies were evaluated and possible drug to drug interactions were assessed according to producer package insert and University of Liverpool web site (http://www.hep-druginteractions.org/). Patients were encouraged to contact their clinicians to report any adverse reaction during treatment. Before the enrollment in any treatment regimen, every patients signed an informed consent under the prescribing physician surveillance. Any enrolled patients performed the following laboratory tests at the following time points: T0 (before starting treatment genotype, initial viral load, HBsAg, Anti-HIV, Haematological, Liver, Renal, Pancreatic Function Test, Cardiological assessment (including Pro-BNP serum levels), at T1 and T3 according to antiviral schedule (on month and three months after starting therapy) Viral load, ETR (the end of treatment) and one month and three months after the end of therapy to evaluate sustained virological response (SVR). Red blood cells count and haemoglobin levels were assessed every week for the first month thereafter every two weeks or according to haematological alterations. Every patient underwent a clinical examination in out-patients clinic and any

---

**Survey for patients undergoing DAAS treatment**

1) Have you experienced any changes in your mood or health body

   during this month?

     i. Yes

     ii. Not

2) If yes please explain which kind of changes you experienced

_____

_____

**Fig. 1** Figure shows the survey proposed by Clinician every month during treatment period. According to possible changes in health status perceived by the patient as well as any relevant clinical and laboratory condition, adverse events notification were reported and discussed with Hospital Pharmacist and entered in the online based Italian system for adverse drug reaction notifications

significant clinical condition was registered and used in case of treatment suspension or antiviral dose adjustment. Adverse events were defined according to FDA regulation (http://www.fda.gov/Safety/MedWatch/HowToReport/ucm053087.htm). All required information for possible adverse drug reaction (ADR) were entered into the RNF home page according to italian surveillance submission form (http://www.agenziafarmaco.gov.it/sites/default/files/tipo_filecb84.pdf). DAAs Regimen according to genotype and Italian National Health system guidelines were as follows: Sofosbuvir + Ribavirin, Sofosbuvir + Simeprevir +/− Ribavirin, Sofosbuvir + Daclatasvir +/− Ribavirin, Ledipasvir + Sofosbuvir +/− Ribavirin and Ombitasvir/Paritaprevir/Ritonavir/Dasabuvir plus ribavirin. Data were extracted and analyzed using Microsoft Excel and GraphPad for Mac Os X.

## Results

A total of 170 subjects were evaluated from March 2015 to March 2016. 104 out 170 were found to be eligible to HCV therapy. 78 out of 104 patients (pts) were enrolled and reached the end of treatment at the moment of our analysis based on the above mentioned antiviral regimens. Sustained virological response (SVR) was reached in 88% of the enrolled patients (percentage is actually including drop-out due to severe adverse reactions with relapse). According to our enrolment protocol to follow-up ADRs, as part of the surveillance network including clinician and hospital pharmacist, we found the following results about demographic, efficacy and safety (also reported in Table 1 and Table 2): 35% of enrolled were < 65 years old while the remaining patients (65%) were ≥ 65 years old. The cohort of subjects ≥ 65 years old had a mean age of 72 years (range, 65–80 years). In the < 65 years old cohort, the mean age was 48 (range, 18–58 years), 59% (n = 17) of the subjects were male. Almost all patients (93%) with age ≥ 65, had Genotype 1b while other genotypes were as follows Genotype 2 (4%), Genotype 3 (3%). In the subjects with age < 65, 86% of the subjects had genotype 1b while the other genotypes were Genotype 2 (6%) and Genotype 3 (15%). Elderly had a higher rate of compensated diagnosed cirrhosis according to Fibroscan as F4 (82% vs. 57%). Adverse events, categorized according to the above reported schedules from FDA and AIFA (Italian Agency for Drugs Administration) were classified as severe, when requiring hospitalization or life-threatening approach or as common when averse events could be managed in out-patients clinic without hospitalization. The most important adverse events are reported in Table 1 and Fig. 2. Basically we had a total of 37 out of 78 enrolled patients (46%) reporting common adverse drug reactions related to all used drugs. Severe adverse events were 11 out 78 pts of these reported ADRs we have that severe were mostly related to Sofosbuvir/Ledipasvir treatment and were related to cardio-pulmunary system. According to our survey we found that majority of the patients experienced asthenia or fatigue were 53% of the enrolled patients, however that adverse events did not require any dose adjustment or have any impact in social life and was considered as minor adverse

**Table 1** Adverse events experienced by patients treated with antiviral schedule regimens

| | SOF/LDV | SOF/DAK | SOF/SIM+/− RBV | SOF/RBV | OMB/PTR/r/DAS +/− RBV |
|---|---|---|---|---|---|
| ENROLLED PTS per regimen | 20 | 15 | 28 | 4 | 11 |
| PTS WITH SERIOUS ADRs | 4 (20%) | 3 (20%) | 1 (4%) | 1 (25%) | 1 (9%) |
| DISCONTINUATION | 3 | 0 | 0 | 0 | 1 |
| DEATHS | 0 | 0 | 0 | 0 | 0 |
| COMMON ADRs | 10 (50%) | 6 (40%) | 12 (43%) | 4 (100%) | 5 (45%) |
| FATIGUE | 6 | 5 | 11 | 4 | 4 |
| HEADACHE | 0 | 0 | 0 | 0 | 0 |
| NAUSEA | 0 | 0 | 0 | 0 | 0 |
| PRURITUS | 0 | 0 | 4 | 0 | 0 |
| INSOMNIA | 1 | 3 | 0 | 0 | 0 |
| DIARRHOEA | 0 | 0 | 0 | 0 | 0 |
| ASTHENIA | 7 | 2 | 11 | 4 | 3 |
| RASH | 0 | 0 | 4 | 0 | 0 |
| IRRITABILITY | 0 | 4 | 0 | 0 | 0 |
| ANAEMIA | 6 | 3 | 12 | 3 | 3 |
| DYSPNOEA | 2 | 0 | 0 | 0 | 1 |

*Common adverse drug reactions are not to single patients, one patient may experience more than one common adverse drug reaction. Data are expressed as absolute number plus percentage

**Table 2** Table shows daemographic data, SVR (in months) and ADRs according to overall enrolled population, genotype (Gt) and disease stage (chirrosis and chronic hepatitis C F3 stage according to metavir)

|  | CHIRROSIS | CHC | TOT |
|---|---|---|---|
| ADRs | 20/51 | 15/27 | 35/78 |
| Sex | M 44 – F 22 | M 14 – F 4 | M 58 - F 26 |
| Age | <65: 10 | <65: 17 | <65: 27 |
|  | >65:41 | >65:11 | >65:51 |
| Genotype in overall population |  |  |  |
| Gt 1 | 38 | 20 | 58 |
| Gt 2 | 9 | 5 | 14 |
| Gt 3 | 4 | 2 | 6 |
| SVR in over all population |  |  |  |
| SVR 3 mts | 44/51 | 25/27 | 69/78 |
| SVR 6 mts | 44/51 | 24/27 | 68/78 |
| RELAPSE | 6/51 | 4/27 | 10/78 |

drug reaction. 12 out 37 adverse events were in patients <65 years old and 25 in those > 65 years old. Major adverse events, according to FDA classification, were about 80% of all reported adverse reactions and were more frequent in those older than 65 years. The majority of ADR for treated patients were found in Sofosbuvir plus Simeprevir (Fig. 3) and in all remaining having Ribavrin as concomitant antiviral, requiring in about 60% of the patients dose reduction.

We had 4 discontinuations during treatment representing 5% of all enrolled cases, two of those were related to heart failure during Sofosbuvir/Ledipasvir plus Ribavirin therapy, one due to allergic reaction to Harvoni and the last one related to pulmonary hypertension with heart failure during Ombitasvir/Paritaprevir/Ritonavir/Dasabuvir plus ribavirin therapy. Of note we had 4 patients during Daklatasvir/Sofosbuvir therapy experiencing change in mood of mild grade, two of them requiring Psychiatric assessment, however none of those patients required therapy suspension. All psychiatric symptoms diminished and disappeared after two weeks from the end of therapy with Daklatasvir/Sofosbuvir.

## Discussion

Despite major progresses have been made in the treatment of chronic hepatitis C, patients should always be managed with caution to avoid the side effects of therapy. Currently the choice of DAAs should be made according to viral genotypes and treatment history to avoid cross-resistance issues [8, 13]. As more safety and efficacy data are becoming available in compensated cirrhosis, antiviral therapy should be considered a priority in these patients and treatment should also be started based on possible adverse reactions and therefore related clinical implications according to age and possible pre-existing factors. In this context, all relevant clinical conditions prior of antiviral treatment should also be careful evaluated being possibly correlated to the onset of adverse events during treatment. For instance, the management of decompensated cirrhotic, could result to be more difficult to manage and to be predictable in its complications as only a few studies of DAA combinations are available [9, 12]. Despite these patients should be treated in an urgent manner, on the other hand they should be managed with caution as at now only few safety data are available for DAAs in real life on the above mentioned clinical condition. Same consideration should also be done for possible cardiovascular system

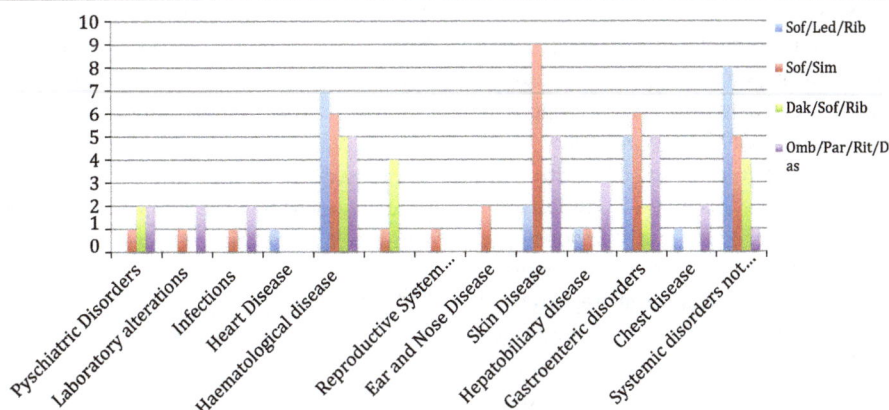

**Fig. 2** Figure represents the frequency (expressed as absolute number) of all adverse drug reactions reported in all patients during treatment follow-up. They are classified according to organ for each single antiviral schedule. According to our findings we had that patients undergoing schedule Simeprevir/Sofosbuvir had a higher frequency of skin disorders, while anaemia and asthenia were most frequently observed in those undergoing Sofosbuvir/Ledipasvir/Ribavirin treatment. Of note the Central Nervous System adverse events related to mood alteration and sleep disorders in those patients under Daklinza/Sofosbuvir antiviral schedule

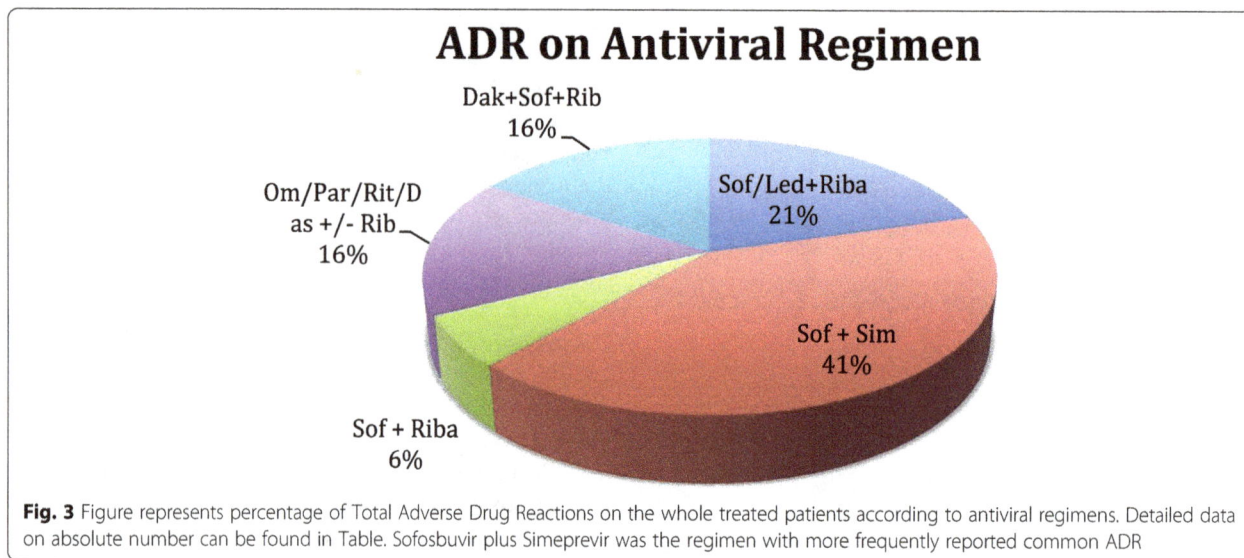

**Fig. 3** Figure represents percentage of Total Adverse Drug Reactions on the whole treated patients according to antiviral regimens. Detailed data on absolute number can be found in Table. Sofosbuvir plus Simeprevir was the regimen with more frequently reported common ADR

adverse events in those patients having cardiac diseases, since the new antivirals seem to be related to the onset of cardiotoxicity, particularly in elder population [13, 14]. In fact, according to our results on adverse events and some literature evidences [13, 14], all patients, particularly those over 65 years, should be referred to a reference centre in case of rapid clinical deterioration. The same caution applies in the pre- and post-transplant setting where drug-to-drug interactions, kidney function and many other factors should be taken into consideration [13]. In our study, we have found a high rate of a total ADR in enrolled patients compared to previous report, particularly we had higher serious adverse events in patients undergoing Sofosbuvir/Ledipasvir, Daclatasvir/Sofosbuvir compared to those reported in published clinical trials [15] particularly in those aged over 65 years. It is of note that in those latter subjects we had the most critical ADR requiring in four cases treatment suspension due to major severe adverse events, life threatening, related to heart function (submitted papers as clinical report). Regarding common adverse events, they have been previously reported to range from 10 to 50% in several clinical trials [15]. In our study of real life we have found a percentage of about 50% with some relevant clinical condition related to mood alterations during Daclatasvir/Sofosbuvir schedule not previously reported in common adverse events at our knowledge. It also should be said that our findings on all reported adverse drug reactions could also be strictly correlated to the presence of a surveillance network based on clinician and pharmacist cooperation. Indeed, one of the most interesting results of our study is mainly the usefulness of that kind of approach to the follow-up based on a network between clinician and pharmacist. Indeed this approach may also justify the evidence of a wider and more detailed assessment of adverse reaction that patients may experience compared to other previous reported paper [12]. Further, it seems also to be really interesting and effectiveness the use of a simple survey as alerting system for clinician and therefore pharmacist for a wide understanding of possible unrecognized adverse events. Certainly, it is our opinion that without this network and that kind of approach, in a real life setting, it would be really hard to identify minor adverse events related to these antivirals that could have important impact on patients. According to previous evidences and our results on possible cardiovascular system adverse events [14–16], a well defined approach and management to this new treatment focusing on ADR according to our network may really be useful for future strategies in treatment schedule in particular setting of patients as our findings on over 65 years old seem to suggest.

## Conclusion

Therefore, in conclusion, even if DAAs seem to be promising for their ability to achieve SVR, a careful and clinician and pharmacist based network should be managed to have a better understanding and follow-up of any significant adverse reaction that may occur particularly on cardiovascular system and in elderly patients. This approach should be used in all real life study to have a wider and better approach to the use of new drugs.

### Abbreviation

ADR: Adverse drug reaction; DAAs: Direct antiviral agents; FDA: Food and drug administration; HCV: Hepatitis C virus; SVR: Sustained virological response

### Acknowledgments

We would like to thanks to all nurses both in out-patient's ward and pharmacy department for their precious help in data collection. In Memory of Oreste Perrella MD PhD who gave a very important contribution to Hospital D Cotugno in terms of Research and Clinical Activity.

### Funding

No to declare.

Safety of new DAAs for chronic HCV infection in a real life experience: role of a surveillance network...

125

## Authors' contributions

The name of the author who is acting as the submission's guarantor is AP and he takes (responsibility for the integrity of the work as a whole, from inception to published article). All authors contributed equally to the papers, particularly AN was involved in adverse drug reactions data collection, writing and results analysis, AP was involved in clinical follow-up, ADR recognizing, writing and results analysis, PB, CS, AI, AGL were involved in clinical follow-up and discussion writing, MS, was involved in adverse drug reaction data analysis and discussion writing. All authors approved the final version of the manuscript.

## Competing interest

The authors declare that they have no competing intersts.

## Author details

[1]Pharmacy Unit, Hospital D. Cotugno – AORN Azienda dei Colli, Naples, Italy. [2]VII Division Infectious Disease and Immunology, Hospital D. Cotugno – AORN Azienda dei Colli, Naples, Italy. [3]I Division Infectious Disease, Hospital D. Cotugno – AORN Azienda dei Colli, Naples, Italy. [4]Hepatology Unit, Hospital A. Cardarelli, Naples, Italy.

## References

1.  Mohd Hanafiah K, Groeger J, Flaxman AD, Wiersma ST. Epidemiology of hepatitis C virus infection: new estimates of age-specific antibody to HCV seroprevalence. Hepatology. 2013;57(4):1333–42.
2.  Armstrong GL, et al. The prevalence of hepatitis C virus infection in the United States, 1999 through 2002. Ann Intern Med. 2006;144(10):705–14.
3.  WHO. Hepatitis C. <http://www.who.int/mediacentre/factsheets/fs164/en/>. Accessed 2 July 2015.
4.  Ghany MG, et al. American association for the study of liver diseases. Diagnosis, management, and treatment of hepatitis C: an update. Hepatology. 2011;49(4):1335–74.
5.  Esteban JI, Sauleda S, Quer J. Changing epidemiology of hepatitis C virus infection in Europe. J Hepatol. 2008;48:148–62.
6.  Mele A, et al. Prevention of hepatitis C in Italy: lessons from surveillance of type-speci c acute viral hepatitis. SEIEVA collaborating group. J Viral Hepat. 2000;7:30–5.
7.  Lavanchy D, Hepatitis C. Virus infection trends in Italy. Hepat Mon. 2012 ;46:7–12.
8.  Gutierrez JA, Lawitz EJ, Poordad F. Interferon-free, direct-acting antiviral therapy for chronic hepatitis C. J Viral Hepat. 2015;22(11):861–70.
9.  Fusco DN, Chung RT. Novel thera- pies for hepatitis C: insights from the structure of the virus. Annu Rev Med. 2012;63:373–87.
10. Fritz SH, Koerner PH, Miller RT, Craft Z. Therapeutic response of triple drug therapy in hepatitis C infection. Gastroenterol Pan- creatol Liver Disord. 2014; 1(1): p.1-6.
11. Momenghalibaf A. Beyond the Hype: What sofosbuvir means—and doesn't—for global hepatitis C treatment. New York: Open Society Foundations; 2013.
12. Saab S, et al. Safety and efficacy of ledipasvir/sofosbuvir for the treatment of genotype 1 hepatitis C in subjects aged 65 years or older. Hepatology. 2016;63(4):1112–9.
13. Omata M, et al. APASL consensus statements and recommendation on treatment of hepatitis C. Hepatol Int. 2016;29:123–31.
14. Padegimas A, et al. Myo-pericarditis Secondary to Ledipasvir-Sofosbuvir Therapy. J Hepatol. 2016;32:p1234–42.
15. Ahmad T, et al. Evaluation of the Incremental Prognostic Cardiac dysfunction associated with a nucleotide polymerase inhibitor for treatment of hepatitis C. Hepatology. 2016;62(2):409–16.
16. Banerjee D, Reddy KR. Review article: safety and tolerability of direct-acting anti-viral agents in the new era of hepatitis C therapy. Aliment Pharmacol Ther. 2016;43:674–96.

# 15

# Association of hepatitis status with surgical outcomes in patients with dual hepatitis B and C related hepatocellular carcinoma

Xiu-Tao Fu[1†], Ying-Hong Shi[1†], Jian Zhou[1,2†], Yuan-Fei Peng[1], Wei-Ren Liu[1], Guo-Ming Shi[1], Qiang Gao[1], Xiao-Ying Wang[1], Kang Song[1], Jia Fan[1,2,3*] and Zhen-Bin Ding[1,3*]

## Abstract

**Background:** The conception that serological hepatitis markers determined surgical prognosis of hepatocellular carcinoma (HCC) associated with hepatitis B (HBV) or hepatitis C (HCV) has been well defined. However, little is known about the relationship between surgical outcomes and serological hepatitis markers in patients with dual HBV and HCV related HCC.

**Methods:** A retrospective analysis of the clinical data of 39 HCC patients with HBV-HCV coinfection who underwent curative hepatectomy between 2001 and 2011 was performed. HBV DNA quantification, expression of HBV antigens, anti-HCV signal-to-cutoff ratio (S/CO) and some clinicopathological characteristics were investigated to show the potential relationship among them and the surgical prognosis.

**Results:** The Cox proportional hazards model identified that HBV DNA quantification of 1,000 IU/mL or higher, HBeAg seropositivity, tumor size of greater than 5 cm, multiple tumors, and vascular invasion were risk factors for HCC prognosis. Thus, HBV DNA quantification, HBsAg level, HBeAg status and HCV-Ab level which may reveal the hepatitis status were further analyzed. The overall survival time in the group with high (≥1,000 IU/mL) HBV DNA quantification was significantly lower than the group with low (<1,000 IU/mL) HBV DNA quantification. Similarly, the high HBsAg level (≥1,000 IU/mL) was associated with poor survival compared with the low HBsAg level. Moreover, HBeAg seropositivity determined a higher cumulative risk for death. However, no significant difference was observed in overall survival time between the groups with low (<10.9 S/CO) and high (≥10.9 S/CO) HCV-Ab level. Compared to HCV-Ab high-level group, the serological HBsAg level was observed significantly higher in HCV-Ab low-level group. Furthermore, the data we analyzed showed these 4 serological hepatitis markers were not correlated with cumulative recurrence rate. On multivariate analysis, none of serological hepatitis markers was an independent prognostic factor for HCC patients with dual hepatitis B and C.

**Conclusion:** Among HCC patients with HBV-HCV coinfection, those who with preoperatively high HBV DNA quantification or HBeAg seropositivity had a short survival time and served as poor survival indicators. Serological expression of HBV status rather than HCV status might potentially dominate the surgical outcomes of the Chinese HCC patients with HBV-HCV coinfection.

**Keywords:** Hepatocellular carcinoma, Hepatitis B, Hepatitis C, Surgical outcomes

* Correspondence: fan.jia@zs-hospital.sh.cn; ding.zhenbin@zs-hospital.sh.cn
†Equal contributors
[1]Liver Cancer Institute, Zhongshan Hospital, and Key Laboratory of Carcinogenesis and Cancer Invasion (Ministry of Education), Fudan University, Shanghai 200032, China
Full list of author information is available at the end of the article

## Background

Hepatocellular carcinoma (HCC) accounts for the second place of the cancer related death [1] and 70–85% of the total liver cancer burden [2] in the world. Curative hepatic resection predominates in the treatment for HCC although several novel treatment options have been applied in the clinical practice in the past few decades [3, 4]. With the recent advances in medicine and technique, overall post-hepatectomy survival rate of HCC patients increased in recent years [5]. Thus, it is extremely important to discover the risk factors for HCC surgical outcomes.

The major risk factors of HCC include alcoholism, cirrhosis, viral hepatitis and fatty liver diseases [2, 6–8]. Hepatitis B virus (HBV) and hepatitis C virus (HCV) are considered to be the main etiological factors for HCC. These two infectious agents are estimated to be responsible for 78% of the HCC cases in the world [9]. HBV-HCV coinfection is thought to be frequent in occurrence, especially in endemic areas, since the virus shares modes of transmission [10].

A retrospective case–control study showed that, compared with non-HBV and non-HCV HCC patients, HBV-HCC patients had significantly worse pre- and postoperative liver function and significantly worse overall survival (OS) and recurrence-free survival (RFS) rates after hepatectomy [11]. Compared with HBV-HCC, HCV-HCC tends to be less differentiated, and to have a higher incidence of vascular invasion and synchronous multicentric recurrence than other HCC types. In addition, HCV-positive livers are more likely to be cirrhotic, have worse liver function, and to be classified as Child B or C which may impact the prognosis of the patients [12, 13].

However, less is known about the clinical characteristics and outcomes of HCC patients with HBV-HCV coinfection. In this retrospective study, we would like to present a detailed clinical data analysis along with their clinic-pathological features. The primary aim of our report was to explore the association between hepatitis status and HCC surgical outcomes in patients with HBV-HCV dual infection which may help to improving the postoperative prognosis.

## Methods

### Study Patients

From 2001 to 2011, a total of 39 patients with chronic HBV and HCV dual infection who underwent curative partial hepatectomy at Liver Cancer Institute, Zhongshan Hospital, Fudan University, China and postoperative pathologically diagnosed as hepatocellular carcinoma were collected in our study. Ethical approval was obtained from the Zhongshan Hospital Research Ethics Committee, and written informed consent was obtained from each patient.

### Data Collection

All patients underwent serological testing 1 week before surgery to determine the hepatitis B surface antigen (HbsAg), hepatitis B e antigen (HbeAg), the α-fetoprotein (AFP) level and liver biochemical tests. Due to technical limitations, 20 patients did not receive quantitative determination of serum HBV-DNA load, and 19 patients only received qualitative detection of HCV-Ab. From 2007, the quantitative determination of HBV-DNA load and HCV-Ab were adopted.

### Clinic-pathological Charicteristics

Clinicopathological characteristics in this study were selected for their potential relation to the prognosis on the basis of the previous studies, including age (≤52 vs >52 years), gender (male vs female), serum AFP concentration (≤20 vs >20 ng/mL), HBsAg level (<1000 vs ≥1000 IU/mL), HBeAg status (positive vs negative), HBV-DNA level (<1000 vs ≥1000 IU/mL), HCV-Ab level (<10.9 S/CO vs ≥10.9 S/CO), severity of cirrhosis (yes vs no), tumor size (≤5 vs >5 cm), number of tumor nodules (single vs multiple), tumor capsule (yes vs no), vascular invasion (yes vs no), differentiation of tumor cells (Edmondson's Classification I/II vs III/IV [14]). The clinicopathological characteristics of the patients were summarized in Table 1.

### Follow-Up

Follow-up was completed in June 15, 2016. Data were obtained at last follow-up for patients without relapse or death. As described in our previous study [15], all patients were monitored prospectively by serum AFP, abdomen ultrasonography, and chest x-ray every 1 to 6 months according to the postoperative time. For patients with test results suggestive of recurrence, computed tomography and/or magnetic resonance imaging were used to verify whether recurrence had occurred. A diagnosis of recurrence was based on typical imaging appearance in computed tomography and/or magnetic resonance imaging scan and an elevated AFP level. OS time was defined as the time period from the date of surgery to the confirmed death date for dead patients or from the date of surgery to the date of last follow-up for surviving patients. RFS was defined as the time period from the date of surgery to confirmed tumor relapse date for relapsed patients or from the date of surgery to the date of last follow-up for nonrecurrent patients.

### Statistical Analyses

Patient OS and RFS rates after surgical resection were calculated using the Kaplan–Meier method. A Chisquare test or Fisher's exact test was performed to compare qualitative variables. The risk factors of OS and RFS after surgery were evaluated by the univariate and

**Table 1** Clinic-pathological characteristics and univariate analysis of factors associated with OS and RFS

| Variable | n | OS HR | OS 95% CI | OS P value | RFS HR | RFS 95% CI | RFS P value |
|---|---|---|---|---|---|---|---|
| Sex (female vs male) | 5 vs 34 | 1.179 | 0.345–4.031 | 0.792 | 1.016 | 0.229–4.509 | 0.984 |
| Age years (≤52 vs >52) | 21 vs 18 | 0.754 | 0.312–1.824 | 0.531 | 1.680 | 0.596–4.732 | 0.326 |
| AFP (ng/ml; ≤20 vs >20) | 13 vs 25 | 1.734 | 0.629–4.778 | 0.287 | 1.214 | 0.414–3.555 | 0.724 |
| HBsAg (IU/mL; <1000 vs ≥1,000) | 6 vs 28 | 5.915 | 0.784–44.637 | 0.085 | 1.561 | 0.340–7.179 | 0.567 |
| HBeAg (negative vs positive) | 33 vs 6 | 8.931 | 2.661–29.982 | 0.000 | 3.361 | 0.848–13.321 | 0.085 |
| HBV-DNA (IU/mL; <1000 vs ≥1,000) | 10 vs 9 | 7.798 | 1.580–38.496 | 0.012 | 2.808 | 0.647–12.186 | 0.168 |
| HCV-Ab (S/CO; <10.9 vs ≥10.9) | 8 vs 12 | 0.579 | 0.152–2.207 | 0.424 | 0.808 | 0.189–3.455 | 0.774 |
| Liver cirrhosis (no vs yes) | 13 vs 26 | 1.245 | 0.478–3.243 | 0.654 | 2.118 | 0.596–7.519 | 0.246 |
| Tumor size (cm; ≤5 vs >5) | 25 vs 14 | 4.336 | 1.753–10.722 | 0.001 | 2.302 | 0.793–6.686 | 0.125 |
| Tumor number (single vs multiple) | 31 vs 8 | 3.155 | 1.145–8.695 | 0.026 | 1.679 | 0.455–6.190 | 0.437 |
| Vascular invasion (no vs yes) | 26 vs 13 | 3.352 | 1.358–8.272 | 0.009 | 3.806 | 13.60–10.646 | 0.011 |
| Capsule (no vs yes) | 12 vs 26 | 1.319 | 0.474–3.670 | 0.596 | 0.775 | 0.259–2.317 | 0.648 |
| Tumor differentiation (I-II vs III-IV) | 21 vs 16 | 0.798 | 0.308–2.068 | 0.642 | 0.664 | 0.221–1.992 | 0.465 |

Note: Univariate analysis, Cox proportional hazards regression model
Abbreviations: *HR*, Hazard ratio; *95% CI*, 95% confidence interval; *AFP*, alpha-fetoprotein; *HCV-Ab*, HCV antibody

the multivariate Cox proportional hazards models. The variables of the multivariate analysis were determined if their *P* values were less than 0.05 during the univariate analysis. The forward LR method was adopted during the multivariate analysis to avoid the multicollinearity. The *P* value for a two-tailed test of less than 0.05 was considered statistically significant. All statistical analyses were performed using SPSS 22.0 for Windows (IBM, Chicago, IL).

## Results

### Overall survival and Recurrence-free survival

From 2001 to 2011, a total of 39 patients with chronic HBV and HCV dual infection who underwent curative hepatectomy at our institute were included in this study. Their postoperative pathological diagnosis was confirmed to be hepatocellular carcinoma. The median overall survival time was 50.1 months and the postoperative 1-, 3-, and 5-year overall survival rates of these patients was 89.6%, 73.3%, and 55.9%, respectively. Afterwards, the median recurrence-free survival time was 45.0 months and the postoperative 1-, 3-, and 5-year recurrence-free survival rates of them was 86.8%, 69.1%, and 53.2%, respectively.

### HBV infection status and patient survival

Kaplan-Meier survival estimates and the log-rank test were used to calculate the factors associated with the OS and RFS for all the patients. Interestingly, OS but not the RFS, was significantly associated with HBV DNA load, HBsAg level and HBeAg status. The overall survival time in the group with high (≥1000 IU/mL) HBV DNA quantification was significantly lower than

the group with low (<1000 IU/mL) HBV DNA quantification (34.33 ± 8.63 vs 110.65 ± 16.50 months; *P* = 0.003, Fig. 1a). Similarly, the high HBsAg level (≥1000 IU/mL) was associated with poor survival compared with the low HBsAg level (79.45 ± 12.88 vs 119.49 ± 16.01 months; *P* = 0.050, Fig. 1c). Moreover, HBeAg seropositivity determined a higher cumulative risk for death (23.59 ± 5.89 vs 107.40 ± 12.07 months; *P* = 0.000, Fig. 1e). Therefore, HBV-DNA, HBsAg and HBeAg which represent the preoperational HBV status impacts OS after curative hepatic resection in these patients.

### HCV infection status and patient survival

HCV-Ab S/CO ratio was found to be highly accurate at predicting HCV viremia. And at an anti-HCV S/CO ratio cutoff value of 10.9, sensitivity and specificity were high [16]. As a result, we selected 10.9 S/CO as the cutoff level for HCV-Ab and categorized these patients into two groups. However, no significant difference was observed in OS and RFS between the groups with low (<10.9 S/CO) and high (≥10.9 S/CO) HCV-Ab level (OS: 43.56 ± 10.32 vs 91.89 ± 15.64 months, *P* = 0.418; RFS: 47.88 ± 12.28 vs 63.797 ± 10.96 months, *P* = 0.773, Fig. 1g, h).

### HCV-Ab level and HBsAg level

Previous cross-sectional and in vitro studies have suggested that HCV coinfection has an inhibitory effect on HBV replication [17, 18], but the in vivo data do not support it [19, 20]. In this study, quantitative analysis indicated that the level of HBsAg was significantly higher in group with low HCV-Ab (<10.9 S/CO) level

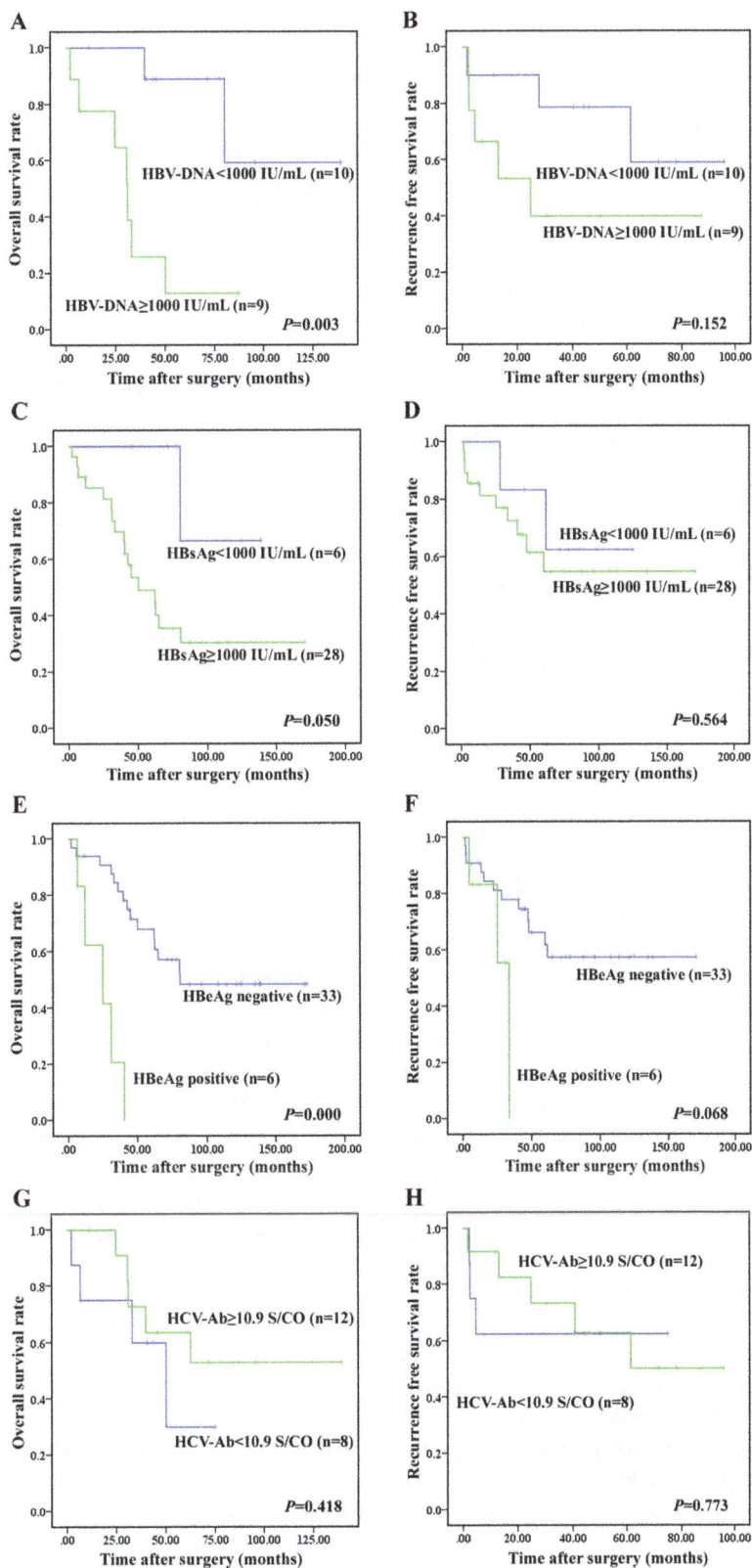

**Fig. 1** (See legend on next page.)

**Fig. 1** Kaplan-Meier survival analysis of hepatitis markers and HCC patients with dual hepatitis B and C. **a**, OS rates between high HBV-DNA level (≥1000 IU/mL, $n = 9$) group and low HBV-DNA level (<1000 IU/mL, $n = 10$); $P = 0.003$; **b**, RFS rates between high HBV-DNA level (≥1000 IU/mL, $n = 9$) group and low HBV-DNA level (<1000 IU/mL, $n = 10$); $P = 0.152$; **c**, OS rates between high HBsAg level (≥1000 IU/mL, $n = 28$) group and low HBsAg level (<1000 IU/mL, $n = 6$); $P = 0.050$; **d**, RFS rates between high HBsAg level (≥1000 IU/mL, $n = 28$) group and low HBsAg level (<1000 IU/mL, $n = 6$); $P = 0.564$; **e**, OS rates between HBeAg positive group ($n = 6$) and HBeAg negative group ($n = 33$); $P = 0.000$; **f**, RFS rates between HBeAg positive group ($n = 6$) and HBeAg negative group ($n = 33$); $P = 0.068$; **g**, OS rates between high HCV-Ab level (≥10.9 S/CO, $n = 12$) group and low HCV-Ab level (<10.9 S/CO, $n = 8$); $P = 0.418$; **h**, RFS rates between high HCV-Ab level (≥10.9 S/CO, $n = 12$) group and low HCV-Ab level (<10.9 S/CO, $n = 8$); $P = 0.773$

than in group with high (≥10.9 S/CO) HCV-Ab level (6696.75 ± 1521.16 vs 3221.99 ± 3104.90; $P = 0.004$).

### Hepatitis status and tumor features

A comparison of hepatitis status (HBsAg, HBeAg, HBV-DNA, and HCV-Ab) between tumor features (tumor size, vascular invasion and TNM stage) revealed that HBeAg-positive patients were more likely to have a larger tumor size (Chi-Square value = 4.712, $P = 0.030$). There was no significant difference between the other groups (Additional file 1: Table S1).

### Other clinicopathological characteristics and patient survival

Worse overall survival was found in association with tumor size of greater than 5 cm (54.13 ± 17.88 vs 118.01 ± 12.79 months; $P = 0.001$, Fig. 2a), multiple tumors (38.00 ± 8.65 vs 107.05 ± 12.62 months; $P = 0.019$, Fig. 2c) and vascular invasion (43.65 ± 7.86 vs 115.89 ± 13.61 months; $P = 0.006$, Fig. 2e). Not tumor size and number, but vascular invasion was significantly correlated with RFS (36.06 ± 8.76 vs 125.01 ± 13.97 months; $P = 0.006$, Fig. 2b, d, f).

### Multivariate logistic regression analysis

All variables with $P < 0.05$ in the univariate analysis were placed into the multivariate Cox regression model. As shown in Table 2, none of serological hepatitis markers was an independent prognostic factor for HCC patients with dual hepatitis B and C.

### Discussion

Hepatocellular carcinoma is one of the most common cancers in China, with a relatively high mortality [6], and curative hepatic resection remains the common treatment in HCC patients. From a global perspective, viral hepatitis is the leading cause for HCC. It is critical to identify risk factors for the outcomes of HCC patients with viral hepatitis. In the present study, we investigated the association between hepatitis status and surgical outcomes in HCC patients with dual HBV-HCV infection.

HCC pathogenesis in HBV monoinfected patients has been studied extensively, and several important viral risk factors which indicate the HBV status have been identified, such as HBsAg level, seropositivity of HBeAg, high viral load. In our previous study [21], high HBsAg level (≥1000 IU/mL) is correlated with more aggressive tumor behavior and serves as a poor survival indicator in patients with surgically resected HBV-related HCC with low HBV load. Here, we continued to use the same standard in order to avoid the influence of HBV-DNA load. Our results demonstrated that the HBsAg level might be a potential risk factor for HCC in patients with dual HBV-HCV infection. HBV-DNA quantification is known to be significantly associated with decreased survival rate in HBV alone infected HCC patients [22]. In present study, similarly, the results demonstrated that high HBV load (≥1000 IU/mL) was correlated with poor surgical outcome of HCC patients with HBV-HCV coinfected. The presence of HBeAg was often used as a criterion for treatment before the introduction of HBV DNA examination [23]. It was reported at our institution that HBeAg seropositivity was an independent factor for overall survival in hepatitis B-related HCC patients after curative resection [24]. The similar conclusion was also identified in this study. Moreover, recent study revealed that HBeAg and its precursors promoted the progress of HCC by interacting with NUMB and decreasing p53 activity [25]. Therefore, in this study, HBeAg positive HCC patients usually had larger tumor compared to HBeAg negative patients. This finding provided some evidence for the association between HBV status and prognosis in HBV-HCV related HCC.

It was reported that the risk of developing HCC in patients with high anti-HCV Ab level is significantly higher than the risk in patients with low level [26]. In HCC patients with HCV monoinfection, recent study strongly suggests that the HCV-Ab level is a predictive factor for HCC recurrence, especially for late recurrence due to presumed multicentric carcinogenesis [27, 28]. And low HCV viral load predicted better long-term surgical outcomes in patients with HCC regardless of the serologic eradication of HCV [29]. Unfortunately, we found the HCV-Ab level was not associated with tumor recurrence or overall survival in HBV-HCV coinfected HCC patients. However, a relation between HBsAg level and anti-HCV Ab level was discovered in these patients. Due to the interaction between HCV and HBV infection, we tentatively put forward that

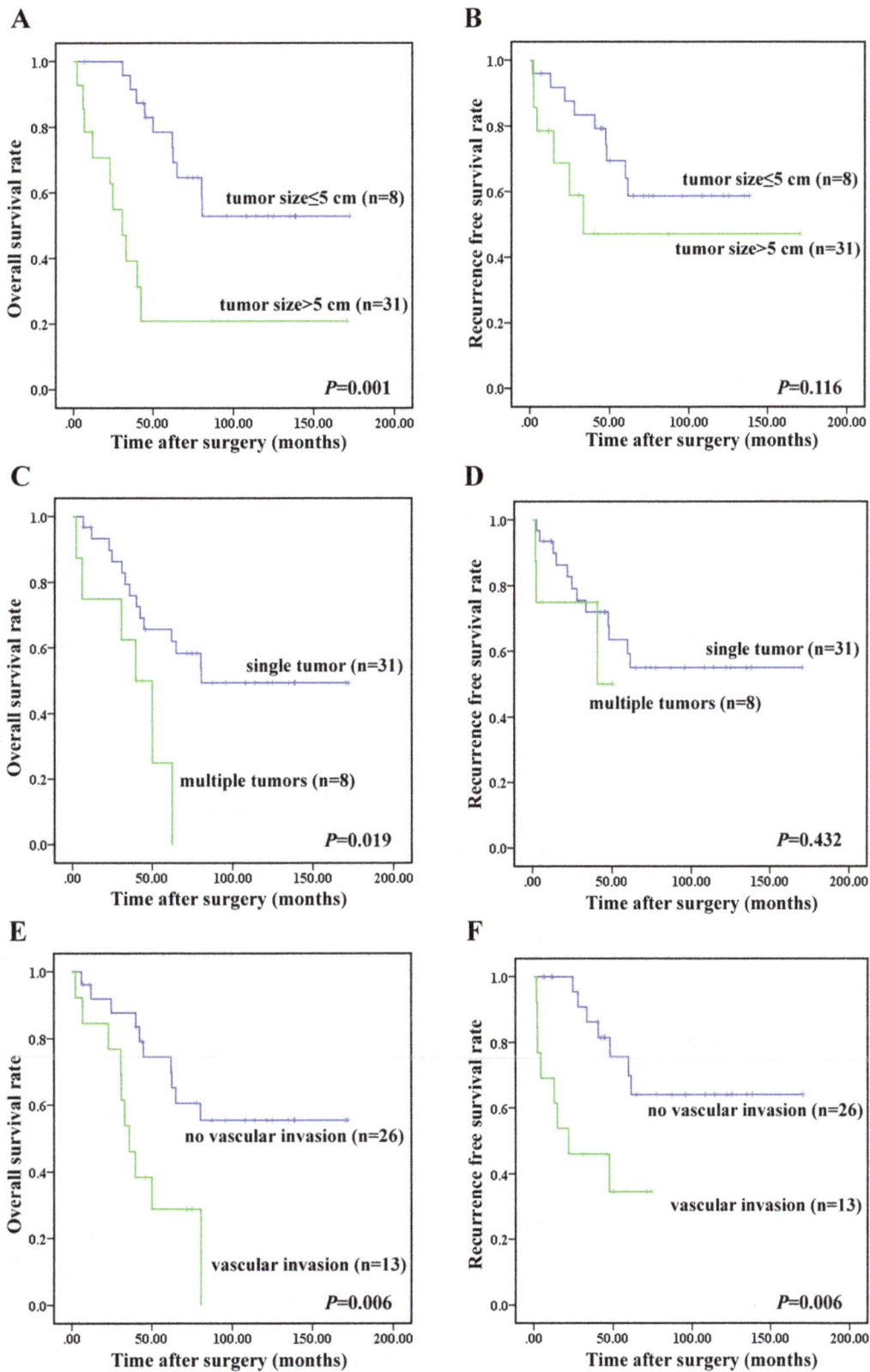

**Fig. 2** (See legend on next page.)

(See figure on previous page.)

**Fig. 2** Kaplan-Meier survival analysis of clinic-pathological characteristics and HCC patients with dual hepatitis B and C. **a**, OS rates between large tumor (>5 cm, n = 8) group and small tumor (≤5 cm, n = 31) group; P = 0.001; **b**, RFS rates between large tumor (>5 cm, n = 8) group and small tumor (≤5 cm, n = 31) group; P = 0.116; **c**, OS rates between single tumor (n = 31) group and multiple tumors (n = 8) group; P = 0.019; **d**, RFS rates between single tumor (n = 31) group and multiple tumors (n = 8) group; P = 0.432; **e**, OS rates between no vascular invasion group (n = 26) and vascular invasion group (n = 13); P = 0.006; **f**, RFS rates between no vascular invasion group (n = 26) and vascular invasion group (n = 13); P = 0.006

HBV status may influence the replication of HCV and play a vital role in coinfected patients, especially in Chinese population. Consequently, further studies are needed to clarify the interaction between the two hepatitis viruses in vivo.

It is well known that specific tumor characteristics were also significantly associated with prognosis of HCC patients [30–33]. Similar to previous studies [34, 35], our research validated that large tumor size, multiple tumors and vascular invasion were significantly associated with poorer prognosis. However, as we can see, the selected serological hepatitis markers including HBsAg, HBeAg and HBV-DNA only correlate with OS, but not RFS. A potential explanation for this discrepancy may be attributed to the high percentage of cirrhosis in dual HBV-HCV infected HCC patients; a number of patients died of impaired liver function or cirrhosis during follow up, which did not allow them to develop multicentric tumor recurrence. However, liver stiffness measurement using elastography-based techniques and indocyanine green kinetics were not applied to quantitatively assess the severity of hepatic cirrhosis and function in our department until 2012, and further study was needed to interpret it.

There are some limitations to our study. First, this retrospective study only enrolled 39 coinfected patients from 2001 to 2011. And the quantitative determination of HBV-DNA and HCV-Ab was adopted to replace previous qualitative detection from 2006. Therefore, we only have HBV-DNA data of 19 cases and HCV-Ab level of 20 cases, which might affect the long-term clinical prognosis analysis. Second, two serological HBV markers (HBeAg and HBV-DNA) that have potential interaction were added into the multivariate analysis. As a result, when multivariate Cox regression model was performed, none of serological hepatitis markers was an independent prognostic factor in these patients.

**Table 2** Multivariate analysis of factors associated with OS

| Variable | OS | | |
|---|---|---|---|
| | HR | 95% CI | P value |
| Tumor size (cm; ≤5 vs >5) | 1.460 | 0.159–13.418 | 0.738 |
| Tumor number (single vs multiple) | 0.882 | 0.154–5.067 | 0.888 |
| Vascular invasion (no vs yes) | 7.612 | 0.771–75.141 | 0.082 |
| HBeAg (negative vs positive) | 7.503 | 0.494–113.848 | 0.146 |
| HBV-DNA (IU/mL; <1000 vs ≥1,000) | 3.235 | 0.378–27.714 | 0.284 |

Finally, determination of serum HCV-RNA load which accurately evaluates the HCV load was not a routine procedure for admitted patient in our department before 2011.

In summary, serological expression of HBV status including HBsAg, HBeAg and HBV-DNA plays a predominant role in prediction of surgical survival in dual HBV and HCV related HCC patients. Our findings suggest that anti-HBV therapy could be a valid strategy for prolonged survival in coinfected HCC patients, especially in Chinese population.

## Conclusions

Our study shows that serological expression of HBV status rather than HCV status might potentially dominate surgical outcomes of the Chinese HCC patients with HBV-HCV coinfection. Anti-HBV therapy could be a valid strategy for prolonged survival in HBV-HCV coinfected HCC patients.

**Abbreviations**

HBeAg: Hepatitis B e Antigen; HBsAg: Hepatitis B Surface Antigen; HBV: Hepatitis B Virus; HCC: Hepatocellular Carcinoma; HCV: Hepatitis C Virus; HCV-Ab: HCV-Antibody; OS: Overall Survival; RFS: Recurrence-Free Survival

**Acknowledgements**

We would like to express our gratitude to Dr. Li Yan for her indefatigable help and support.

**Funding**

This work was supported by the funds from National Natural Science Fund of China (No.81472219 and 81602037).

**Authors' contributions**

FXT, DZB, FJ designed the study and performed the literature review, supervised statistical analysis and interpretation of data and drafted the manuscript; ZJ, SYH contributed to the study design and drafting of the manuscript; LWR, PYF performed the first statistical analyses; SGM, GQ, WXY, KS refined and performed the final statistical analysis, contributed to the study design and drafting of the manuscript. All authors critically revised the manuscript for intellectual and significant contents and approved the final manuscript for submission.

**Competing interests**

The authors declare that they have no competing interests.

**Author details**
[1]Liver Cancer Institute, Zhongshan Hospital, and Key Laboratory of Carcinogenesis and Cancer Invasion (Ministry of Education), Fudan University, Shanghai 200032, China. [2]Institute of Biomedical Sciences, Fudan University, Shanghai 200032, China. [3]Department of Liver Surgery, Zhongshan Hospital, Fudan University, 1609 Xietu Road, Shanghai 200032, China.

**References**

1. Ferlay J, Soerjomataram I, Dikshit R, Eser S, Mathers C, Rebelo M, Parkin DM, Forman D, Bray F. Cancer incidence and mortality worldwide: sources, methods and major patterns in GLOBOCAN 2012. Int J Cancer. 2015;136(5): E359–386.
2. Jemal A, Bray F, Center MM, Ferlay J, Ward E, Forman D. Global cancer statistics. CA Cancer J Clin. 2011;61(2):69–90.
3. Chu KK, Cheung TT. Update in management of hepatocellular carcinoma in Eastern population. World J Hepatol. 2015;7(11):1562–71.
4. Pessaux P. Techniques and innovations in liver surgery. Hepatobiliary surg nutr. 2016;5(4):277–8.
5. Villanueva A, Llovet JM. Liver cancer in 2013: Mutational landscape of HCC-the end of the beginning. Nat Rev Clin Oncol. 2014;11(2):73–4.
6. El-Serag HB. Hepatocellular carcinoma. N Engl J Med. 2011;365(12):1118–27.
7. Yang JD, Roberts LR. Hepatocellular carcinoma: A global view. Nat Rev Gastroenterol Hepatol. 2010;7(8):448–58.
8. Chen CJ, Yu MW, Liaw YF. Epidemiological characteristics and risk factors of hepatocellular carcinoma. J Gastroenterol Hepatol. 1997;12(9–10):S294–308.
9. Perz JF, Armstrong GL, Farrington LA, Hutin YJ, Bell BP. The contributions of hepatitis B virus and hepatitis C virus infections to cirrhosis and primary liver cancer worldwide. J Hepatol. 2006;45(4):529–38.
10. Gaeta GB, Stornaiuolo G, Precone DF, Lobello S, Chiaramonte M, Stroffolini T, Colucci G, Rizzetto M. Epidemiological and clinical burden of chronic hepatitis B virus/hepatitis C virus infection. A multicenter Italian study. J Hepatol. 2003;39(6):1036–41.
11. Li Z, Zhao X, Jiang P, Xiao S, Wu G, Chen K, Zhang X, Liu H, Han X, Wang S, et al. HBV is a risk factor for poor patient prognosis after curative resection of hepatocellular carcinoma: A retrospective case–control study. Medicine. 2016;95(31):e4224.
12. Kanematsu T, Takenaka K, Matsumata T, Furuta T, Sugimachi K, Inokuchi K. Limited hepatic resection effective for selected cirrhotic patients with primary liver cancer. Ann Surg. 1984;199(1):51–6.
13. Li Q, Li H, Qin Y, Wang PP, Hao X. Comparison of surgical outcomes for small hepatocellular carcinoma in patients with hepatitis B versus hepatitis C: a Chinese experience. J Gastroenterol Hepatol. 2007;22(11):1936–41.
14. Edmondson HA, Steiner PE. Primary carcinoma of the liver: a study of 100 cases among 48,900 necropsies. Cancer. 1954;7(3):462–503.
15. Gao Q, Qiu SJ, Fan J, Zhou J, Wang XY, Xiao YS, Xu Y, Li YW, Tang ZY. Intratumoral balance of regulatory and cytotoxic T cells is associated with prognosis of hepatocellular carcinoma after resection. J Clin Oncol Off J Am Soc Clin Oncol. 2007;25(18):2586–93.
16. Seo YS, Jung ES, Kim JH, Jung YK, Kim JH, An H, Yim HJ, Yeon JE, Byun KS, Kim CD, et al. Significance of anti-HCV signal-to-cutoff ratio in predicting hepatitis C viremia. Korean J Intern Med. 2009;24(4):302–8.
17. Liu CJ, Chen PJ, Chen DS. Dual chronic hepatitis B virus and hepatitis C virus infection. Hepatol Int. 2009;3(4):517–25.
18. Chen SY, Kao CF, Chen CM, Shih CM, Hsu MJ, Chao CH, Wang SH, You LR, Lee YH. Mechanisms for inhibition of hepatitis B virus gene expression and replication by hepatitis C virus core protein. J Biol Chem. 2003;278(1):591–607.
19. Bellecave P, Gouttenoire J, Gajer M, Brass V, Koutsoudakis G, Blum HE, Bartenschlager R, Nassal M, Moradpour D. Hepatitis B and C virus coinfection: a novel model system reveals the absence of direct viral interference. Hepatology. 2009;50(1):46–55.
20. Hiraga N, Imamura M, Hatakeyama T, Kitamura S, Mitsui F, Tanaka S, Tsuge M, Takahashi S, Abe H, Maekawa T, et al. Absence of viral interference and different susceptibility to interferon between hepatitis B virus and hepatitis C virus in human hepatocyte chimeric mice. J Hepatol. 2009;51(6):1046–54.
21. Liu WR, Tian MX, Jin L, Yang LX, Ding ZB, Shen YH, Peng YF, Zhou J, Qiu SJ, Dai Z, et al. High levels of hepatitis B surface antigen are associated with poorer survival and early recurrence of hepatocellular carcinoma in patients with low hepatitis B viral loads. Ann Surg Oncol. 2015;22(3):843–50.
22. Yin J, Li N, Han Y, Xue J, Deng Y, Shi J, Guo W, Zhang H, Wang H, Cheng S, et al. Effect of antiviral treatment with nucleotide/nucleoside analogs on postoperative prognosis of hepatitis B virus-related hepatocellular carcinoma: a two-stage longitudinal clinical study. J Clin Oncol Off J Am Soc Clin Oncol. 2013;31(29):3647–55.
23. Milich DR. Do T cells "see" the hepatitis B core and e antigens differently? Gastroenterology. 1999;116(3):765–8.
24. Sun HC, Zhang W, Qin LX, Zhang BH, Ye QH, Wang L, Ren N, Zhuang PY, Zhu XD, Fan J, et al. Positive serum hepatitis B e antigen is associated with higher risk of early recurrence and poorer survival in patients after curative resection of hepatitis B-related hepatocellular carcinoma. J Hepatol. 2007; 47(5):684–90.
25. Liu D, Cui L, Wang Y, Yang G, He J, Hao R, Fan C, Qu M, Liu Z, Wang M, et al. Hepatitis B e antigen and its precursors promote the progress of hepatocellular carcinoma by interacting with NUMB and decreasing p53 activity. Hepatology. 2016;64(2):390–404.
26. Hara M, Mori M, Hara T, Yamamoto K, Honda M, Nishizumi M. Risk of developing hepatocellular carcinoma according to the titer of antibody to hepatitis C virus. Hepato-Gastroenterology. 2001;48(38):498–501.
27. Uemura M, Sasaki Y, Yamada T, Gotoh K, Eguchi H, Yano M, Ohigashi H, Ishikawa O, Imaoka S. Serum antibody titers against hepatitis C virus and postoperative intrahepatic recurrence of hepatocellular carcinoma. Ann Surg Oncol. 2014;21(5):1719–25.
28. Belghiti J, Panis Y, Farges O, Benhamou JP, Fekete F. Intrahepatic recurrence after resection of hepatocellular carcinoma complicating cirrhosis. Ann Surg. 1991;214(2):114–7.
29. Shindoh J, Hasegawa K, Matsuyama Y, Inoue Y, Ishizawa T, Aoki T, Sakamoto Y, Sugawara Y, Makuuchi M, Kokudo N. Low hepatitis C viral load predicts better long-term outcomes in patients undergoing resection of hepatocellular carcinoma irrespective of serologic eradication of hepatitis C virus. J Clin Oncol Off J Am Soc Clin Oncol. 2013;31(6):766–73.
30. Imamura H, Matsuyama Y, Tanaka E, Ohkubo T, Hasegawa K, Miyagawa S, Sugawara Y, Minagawa M, Takayama T, Kawasaki S, et al. Risk factors contributing to early and late phase intrahepatic recurrence of hepatocellular carcinoma after hepatectomy. J Hepatol. 2003;38(2):200–7.
31. Janevska D, Chaloska-Ivanova V, Janevski V. Hepatocellular Carcinoma: Risk Factors, Diagnosis and Treatment. Open access Macedonian j med sci. 2015; 3(4):732–6.
32. Raza A, Sood GK. Hepatocellular carcinoma review: current treatment, and evidence-based medicine. World J Gastroenterol. 2014;20(15):4115–27.
33. Balogh J, Victor 3rd D, Asham EH, Burroughs SG, Boktour M, Saharia A, Li X, Ghobrial RM, Monsour Jr HP. Hepatocellular carcinoma: a review. J hepatocellular carcinoma. 2016;3:41–53.
34. Piardi T, Gheza F, Ellero B, Woehl-Jaegle ML, Ntourakis D, Cantu M, Marzano E, Audet M, Wolf P, Pessaux P. Number and tumor size are not sufficient criteria to select patients for liver transplantation for hepatocellular carcinoma. Ann Surg Oncol. 2012;19(6):2020–6.
35. Gu XQ, Zheng WP, Teng DH, Sun JS, Zheng H. Impact of non-oncological factors on tumor recurrence after liver transplantation in hepatocellular carcinoma patients. World J Gastroenterol. 2016;22(9):2749–59.

# 16

# Clinical and prognostic analysis of 78 patients with human immuno-deficiency virus associated non-Hodgkin's lymphoma in Chinese population

Yang Shen[1†], Renfang Zhang[2†], Li Liu[2], Yinzhong Shen[2], Wei Song[2], Tangkai Qi[2], Yang Tang[2], Zhenyan Wang[2], Liqian Guan[2] and Hongzhou Lu[2*]

## Abstract

**Background:** Human Immuno-deficiency Virus (HIV) associated non-Hodgkin's lymphoma (NHL) was a special group of disease, which manifests distinct clinical features and prognosis as compared with NHLs in patients without HIV. We performed this study to describe the clinical features of the disease and investigated the potential prognostic factors.

**Methods:** HIV-infected patients who were newly diagnosed with NHL were enrolled in this study. The selection of anti-lymphoma treatment regimen was mainly dependent on the pathological subtypes of NHLs. Tumor response was reviewed and classified according to the International Workshop Criteria.

**Results:** A total of 78 patients were enrolled, among whom, 42 (53.8%) were with Diffuse large B cell Lymphoma (DLBCL), and 29 (37.2%) were with Burkitt lymphoma (BL). BL patients presented with higher risk features as compared with DLBCL in terms of numbers of extranodal diseases ($P = 0.004$) and poor Eastern cooperative oncology group (ECOG) score ($P = 0.038$). The estimated 2-year overall survival (OS) and progression free survival (PFS) rate was $74.3 \pm 8.1\%$, $28.9 \pm 11.0\%$, and $54.2 \pm 8.1\%$, $19.2 \pm 7.5\%$ for DLBCL and BL, respectively. In multivariate analysis, international prognostic index (IPI) score was an independent prognostic factor for predicting both OS (OR = 2.172, 95% CI 1.579–2.987, $P < 0.001$) and PFS (OR = 1.838, 95% CI 1.406–2.402, $P < 0.001$).

**Conclusions:** HIV associated NHLs represents a group of heterogeneous aggressive diseases with poor prognosis. IPI parameters were still effective in predicting the prognosis of HIV associated NHLs.

**Keywords:** Human immuno-deficiency virus, Lymphoma, Prognosis, International prognostic index, Prognosis

## Background

Non-Hodgkin's Lymphoma (NHL) is one of the most common types of malignancies with high morbidity and mortality in the patients who were infected by Human Immune-deficiency Virus (HIV) [1]. Generally, HIV associated NHLs present with more aggressive clinical behaviors as compared with general population, exemplified with a huge tumor burden, more extranodal diseases, and a tendency of involving genital system [2, 3]. Fortunately,

although the prognosis of HIV associated NHLs remains very poor, with the introduction of combined antiretroviral therapy (cART) and high dose chemotherapy, a considerable portion of the patients could be cured [4, 5].

The International Prognostic Index (IPI) [6], which includes age, Eastern Cooperative Oncology Group (ECOG) performance status, Lactate Dehydrogenase (LDH) level, Ann Arbor stage, and extranodal involvement, is used extensively for evaluating patients with aggressive lymphomas, especially for those with diffuse large B cell lymphoma (DLBCL) and receive doxorubicin-containing chemotherapy such as R-CHOP [7, 8]. Although its role as prognostic factor in stratification of the NHL patients in daily practice and clinical trial is well established in

* Correspondence: luhongzhou@fudan.edu.cn
†Equal contributors
2Department of Infectious Diseases, Shanghai Public Health Clinical Center, Fudan University, Shanghai 201508, China
Full list of author information is available at the end of the article

general population, its validity remains controversial in HIV associated NHLs.

Another important issue is the complexity of the background of the HIV associated NHLs, such as more aggressive phenotype, immune-deficiency status. What even worse is that treatment factors (cART) also intervene the clinical outcome and prognosis [9–11]. Chronic antigen stimulation (HIV infection) could lead to a polyclonal B-cell expansion and finally promotes the emergence of monoclonal B cells. Both germinal center B cell-like (GCB) active B cell subtype (ABC) could be observed in HIV associated DLBCL. The frequency of double hit mutation could be observed in around 20% in HIV patients with NHLs [12–14]. Thus, a more comprehensive analysis incorporating above mentioned factors is warranted to give more precise stratification of HIV associated NHLs.

In China, with the increasing of incidence of HIV infection in recent years, acquired immunodeficiency syndrome (AIDS) associated NHL became more and more frequently. This subset of the patients might present distinct clinical behavior and treatment outcome as compared with their western counterpart. Hence, we performed this study to describe the clinical features and evaluate the potential prognostic factors of the Chinese AIDS patients with NHLs.

## Methods

### Patients

The HIV-infected patients who were newly diagnosed NHL were consecutively entered in this study from Jan.2002 to May.2015 in Shanghai Public Health Clinical Center. The subtypes of the lymphoma were defined according to the WHO 2008 classification system.

Systemic evaluation of the patients including complete blood cell count (CBC), biochemical parameters, LDH, viral panel (HIV, HBV, and HCV *etc.*), CD4 cell count, bone marrow and radiological examinations, was performed to stage the disease and assess the general and disease status.

### Anti-lymphoma treatment

Sixty-four out of 78 patients received anti-lymphoma treatment, and the regimen for the first line chemotherapy was mainly dependent on the pathological subtypes of lymphomas. For BL and PBL, Hyper-CVAD A (Cyclophosphamide [CTX] 300 mg/m$^2$ Q12h × 6, D1-3, Dexamethasone [DEX] 40 mg/d, D1-4, D11-14, Vincristine [VCR] 1.4 mg/m$^2$, D4, D11, Adriamycin [ADR] 50 mg/m$^2$, D4) and B regimen (Methotrexate 1 g/m$^2$, D1, Ara-C 2 g/m$^2$ Q12h, D2-3) were given alternatively to the patients. For DLBCL, CHOP regimen (CTX 750 mg/m$^2$, D1, ADR 50 mg/m$^2$, D1, VCR 1.4 mg/m$^2$, D1, Prednisone 60 mg/m$^2$, D1) was initially designed for the patients, initiated from Dec.2014, to enhance the efficacy of young high risk patients (age < 60 years, IPI > 1). DA-EPOCH (Etopside 50 mg/m$^2$ D1-4, VCR 0.4 mg/m$^2$ D1-4, ADR 10 mg/m$^2$ D1-4, all above

continuous for 24 h, CTX 750 mg/m$^2$ D5, DEX 40 mg D1-5) was also given to this subgroup of the patients [15]. The patients with FL and IBL received CHOP regimen the same as those with DLBCL. The detailed treatment regimen was depicted in Additional file 1: Table S1. No irradiation therapy was given concurrently during the treatment.

Rituximab 375 mg/m$^2$ was designed to give to the patients with a suitable CD4 cell count (>50 cells/μl) to prevent the deep suppression of both B and T cell immunity. Since rituximab usage is not covered by medical insurance in most provinces in China, the application of treatment with rituximab also depended on patients'

**Table 1** Characteristics of the patients

| Characteristics | DLBCL (n = 42) | BL (n = 29) | PBL and IBL (n = 6) |
|---|---|---|---|
| Age (years) | | | |
| Median | 44 | 54 | 48 |
| Range | 24–73 | 25–73 | 33–74 |
| | P = 0.151 | | |
| Gender (%) | | | |
| Male | 37 (88.1) | 27 (93.1) | 5 (83.3) |
| Female | 5 (11.9) | 2 (6.9) | 1 (6.7) |
| | P = 0.692 | | |
| Ann Arbor stage (%) | | | |
| I, II | 23 (54.8) | 10 (34.5) | 3 (50.0) |
| III, IV | 19 (45.2) | 19 (65.5) | 3 (50.0) |
| | P = 0.146 | | |
| Extranodal diseases (%) | | | |
| 0,1 | 33 (78.6) | 15 (51.7) | 4 (66.7) |
| >1 | 9 (21.4) | 14 (48.3) | 2 (33.3) |
| | P = 0.004 | | |
| LDH | | | |
| Median | 334 | 373 | 283 |
| Range | 139–6016 | 178–5009 | 182–739 |
| | P = 0.257 | | |
| ECOG score (%) | | | |
| 0,1 | 18 (42.9) | 5 (17.2) | 3 (50.0) |
| >1 | 24 (57.1) | 24 (82.8) | 3 (50.0) |
| | P = 0.038 | | |
| IPI (%) | | | |
| 0,1 | 16 (38.1) | 5 (17.2) | 3 (50.0) |
| >1 | 26 (61.9) | 24 (82.8) | 3 (50.0) |
| | P = 0.069 | | |
| CD4 cell count | | | |
| Median | 106 | 108 | 31 |
| Range | 4–483 | 1–549 | 3–69 |
| | P = 0.526 | | |

**Table 2** Baseline characteristics of HIV condition of the patients

| Characteristics | |
|---|---|
| AIDS before lymphoma diagnosis (n, %) | 25 (33) |
| ART at lymphoma diagnosis (n, %) | 17 (22) |
| ART exposure from lymphoma diagnosis (months) | 12 (1–84) |
| Patients with CD4 count <200 cells/uL (n, %) | 59 (75) |
| HIV RNA < 40 copies/ml at lymphoma diagnosis (n, %) | 11 (14) |

willing. Fifty patients had a CD4 count greater than 50 (2 with PBL without CD20 expression), and 20 patients (40%) received rituximab.

The first line treatment regimen was discontinued if patients experienced any severe adverse event or lymphoma progressing. The initiation of the second line or salvage treatment regimen for relapsed and refractory patients was dependent on the decision of the physicians according to the condition of the patients.

### Anti-HIV treatment

ART was given immediately after the diagnosis of HIV with the exception of 5 patients due to rapid progression of lymphoma [16]. They were receiving either a combination of 2 nucleoside reverse transcriptase inhibitors with a protease inhibitor ($n = 1$) or with a non-nucleoside reverse transcriptase inhibitor ($n = 70$), or with an integrase inhibitor ($n = 2$).

### Response assessment

Evaluation of the efficacy was performed one month after completion of all the treatment. Thoracic, abdominal, and pelvic computed tomography scans were performed even if those areas were not initially affected [17, 18]. Interim staging was performed after completion of four cycles of treatment for DLBCL and FL patients. For BL and IBL patients, these evaluations were performed every 2 cycles. Tumor response was based on radiographic review and classified as complete response

(CR), partial response (PR), overall response (OR, CR + PR), stable disease (SD), or progressive disease (PD) according to the International Workshop Criteria [19].

### Statistical analysis

Fisher's Exact P test and one way ANOVA test were used to compare the clinical parameters in different subtypes of lymphoma. All patients entered into the study were followed up. Overall survival (OS) was measured from the date of disease diagnosis to death (failure) or alive at last follow-up (censored). Progression free survival (PFS) was defined as time from disease diagnosis to treatment failure such as relapse, progressive disease, any new anti-lymphoma treatment, and death of any reasons, or alive in CR at last follow-up (censored). Kaplan-Meier analysis was used to calculate the distribution of OS and PFS. Binary logistic regression was used for the multivariate analysis of prognostic parameters for response, while Cox model was used to identify prognostic variables for OS and PFS. A limited backward selection procedure was used to exclude redundant or unnecessary variants. To provide quantitative information on the relevance of results, 95% confidence intervals (95% CIs) of odds ratios (ORs) was calculated. All above statistical procedures were performed with the SPSS statistical software package, version 16.0.

### Results

### Patient characteristics

A total of 78 patients were enrolled, among whom, 42 (53.8%) were with DLBCL, 29 (37.2%) were with Burkitt lymphoma (BL), 5 (6.4%) were with plasmablastic lymphoma (PBL) and 1 (1.3%) was with follicular lymphoma (FL) and angioimmunoblastic lymphoma (IBL), respectively. The median age of the patients was 48 (24–74). A strong tendency of male patients was observed (89.7% vs. 10.3%). The clinical characteristics of the patients were shown in Table 1. The BL patients

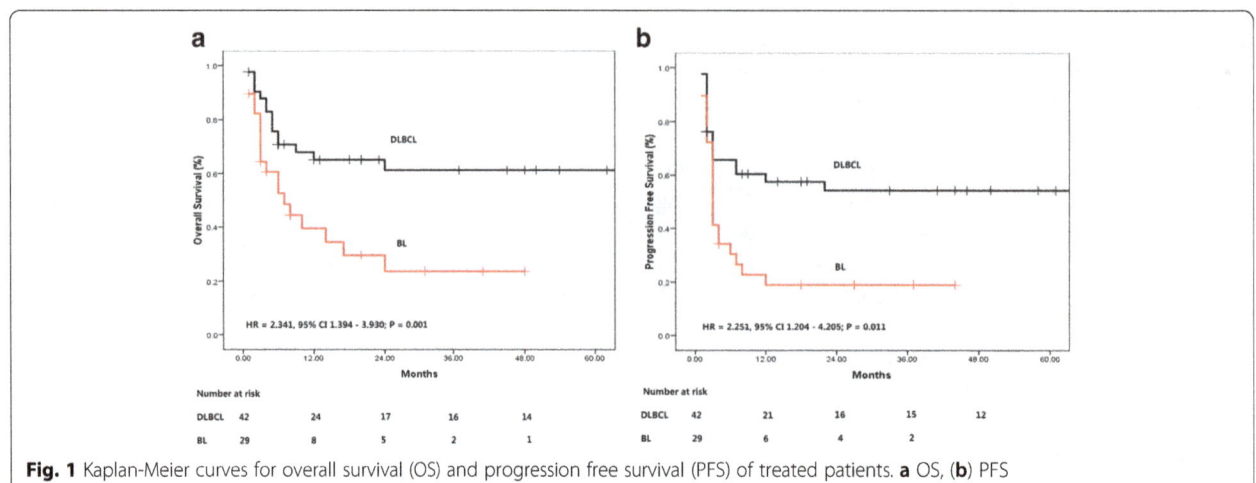

**Fig. 1** Kaplan-Meier curves for overall survival (OS) and progression free survival (PFS) of treated patients. **a** OS, (**b**) PFS

presented with higher risk features as compared with DLBCL patients in terms of numbers of extranodal disease (*P* = 0.004) and poor ECOG score (*P* = 0.038), while age (*P* = 0.151), gender (*P* = 0.692) and CD4 cell count (*P* = 0.526) were distributed equally in the two groups.

33% (25/78) of the patients was confirmed to be infected with HIV before lymphoma diagnosis. 22% (17/78) of them received ART with a median treatment exposure of 12 months before the diagnosis of lymphoma, whereas 78% (61/78) of the patients were ART-naïve. 67% (53/78) of the patients were simultaneously diagnosed of lymphoma and HIV. Notably, 14% (11/78) of the patients had a plasma HIV-1 RNA viral load below 40 copies/ml at the time of lymphoma diagnosis. Table 2 summarized the baseline characteristics of these patients.

### Treatment response

Among 35 DLBCL patients, 22 (62.9%) and 26 patients (74.3%) achieved CR and OR, respectively. For 23 patients with BL, 5 (21.7%) achieved CR while 8 patients (34.8%) achieved OR. One patient with FL achieved PR. None of the patients with PBL and IBL obtained any response.

Further prognostic analysis for CR induction was performed in 58 patients with DLBCL or BL after anti-

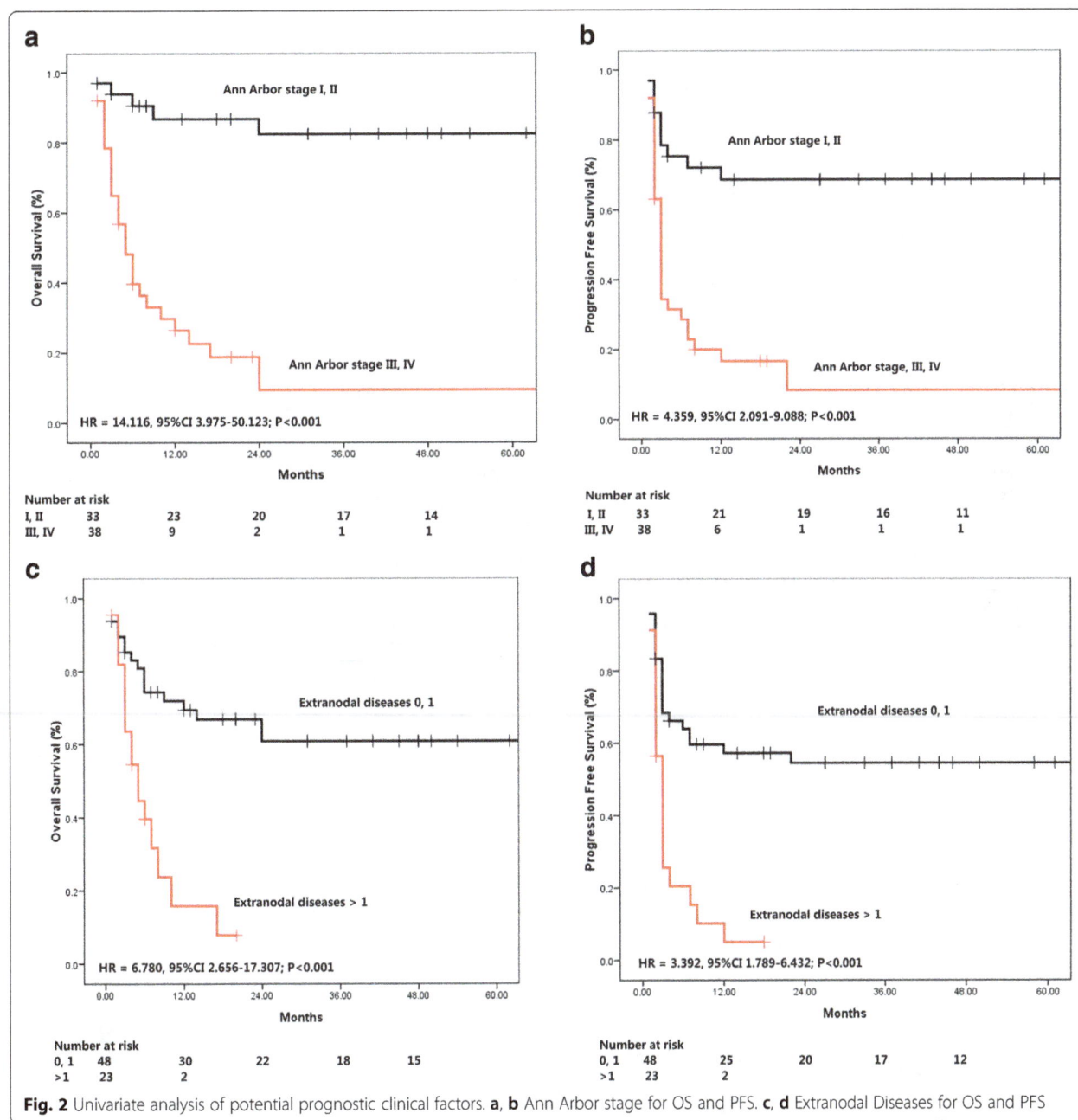

**Fig. 2** Univariate analysis of potential prognostic clinical factors. **a**, **b** Ann Arbor stage for OS and PFS. **c**, **d** Extranodal Diseases for OS and PFS

lymphoma treatment. As shown in Additional file 1: Table S2, in univariate analysis, DLBCL has significant higher CR rate than BL ($P = 0.003$). Ann Arbor stage ($P < 0.001$), number of extranodal disease ($P = 0.001$), ECOG performance status ($P = 0.001$), LDH ($P = 0.008$) and IPI ($P < 0.001$) were proved to be significantly associated the CR induction results.

IPI score and pathological types were entered into multivariate logistic regression analysis. It was proved that pathological types (DLBCL vs. BL, $P = 0.038$, OR = 0.240,

95% CI 0.063–0.925) and IPI score ($P < 0.001$, OR = 0.371, 95% CI 0.229–0.601) were independent prognostic factors of CR (Table 4).

## Survival analysis

Among 64 patients who received anti-lymphoma treatment, the median follow up time was 13.5 months due to the poor prognosis of the patients. The estimated 2 year OS and PFS rate were 74.3 ± 8.1%, 28.9 ± 11.0%, 20.0 ± 17.9%, and 54.2 ± 8.1%, 19.2 ± 7.5%, and 0% for

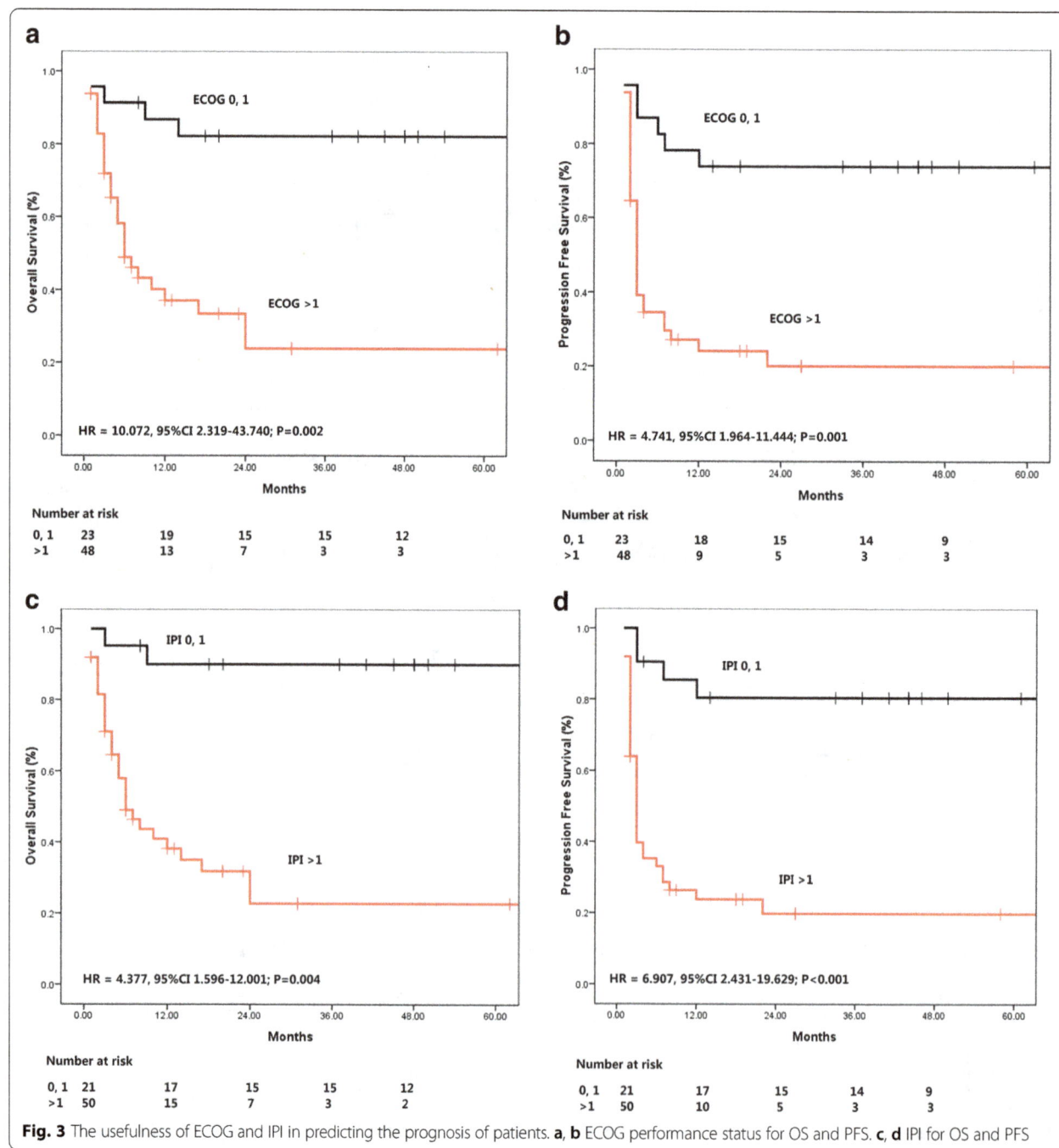

**Fig. 3** The usefulness of ECOG and IPI in predicting the prognosis of patients. **a, b** ECOG performance status for OS and PFS. **c, d** IPI for OS and PFS

**Table 3** The 2 year estimated OS and PFS rate in different subgroups

|  | OS (%) | PFS (%) |
|---|---|---|
| Ann Arbor stage |  |  |
| I, II | 88.6 ± 6.3 | 68.6 ± 8.3 |
| III, IV | 13.0 ± 10.3 | 8.4 ± 6.7 |
| Extranodal diseases |  |  |
| 0, 1 | 71.7 ± 7.8 | 54.5 ± 7.4 |
| > 1 | 10.3 ± 9.5 | 0 |
| ECOG score |  |  |
| 0, 1 | 90.2 ± 6.6 | 73.9 ± 9.2 |
| > 1 | 51.4 ± 9.0 | 20.1 ± 6.7 |
| IPI score |  |  |
| 0, 1 | 95.0 ± 4.9 | 80.4 ± 8.8 |
| > 1 | 49.6 ± 8.8 | 19.9 ± 6.4 |

DLBCL, BL and PBL + IBL, respectively (Fig. 1). One FL patient who achieved PR relapsed after 1 year.

Since a survival plateau could be observed in DLBCL and BL patients (Fig. 1), further prognostic analysis was performed in a group combining the two subsets of the patients. As shown in Figs. 2 and 3, Ann Arbor stage (I, II *vs.* III, IV), number of extranodal diseases (0, 1 *vs.* > 1), ECOG performance status (0,1 *vs.* > 1), and IPI score (0,1 *vs.* > 1) were all significantly associated the survival (OS and PFS) of the patients. LDH as continuous variable, could predict OS (HR = 1.000, 95% CI 1.000–1.001, $P = 0.001$) and PFS (HR = 1.000, 95% CI 1.000–1.001, $P = 0.002$), while CD4 cell count at diagnosis was not associated with the treatment outcome (OS: HR = 1.000, 95% CI 0.996–1.003, $P = 0.824$; PFS: HR = 0.998, 95% CI 0.992–1.005, $P = 0.733$). The estimated 2-year OS and PFS rates were shown in Table 3.

In multivariate analysis, only IPI score was the independent prognostic factor for predicting both OS (OR = 2.172, 95% CI 1.579–2.987, $P < 0.001$) and PFS (OR = 1.838, 95% CI 1.406–2.402, $P < 0.001$) (Table 4).

## Discussion

HIV associated NHL represents a type of aggressive malignancies. Although intensive chemotherapy was given, the prognosis of the disease remained very poor. It was controversial whether some important prognostic factors in HIV negative counterpart such as IPI could still work

in this special group of the patients [20]. In this study, we included a cohort of 78 patients to analyze the characteristics of AIDS associated NHL and to evaluate the prognostic factors of the disease.

Very similar to the normal HIV negative population, the most common subtype of lymphoma observed in HIV-infected patients was also DLBCL (42/78, 53.8%) [21]. As an important trigger of HIV to activate *c-myc*, BL was the second common pathologic subtype of the lymphoma (29/78, 37.2%) among this population. Compared to NHL in general population, AIDS patients with NHL presents with a more aggressive features including advanced Ann Arbor stage, significantly elevated LDH, and poor ECOG performance status, and a high IPI score eventually [2]. Of note, BL patients presented with even higher risk features while compared with those with DLBCL [22]. According to our data, BL patients manifested with the feature of more extranodal diseases ($P = 0.004$) but poorer ECOG scores ($P = 0.038$).

In this study, it was observed that the Chinese NHL patients presented with the characteristics of very low rate of ART exposure prior to the lymphoma diagnosis. Its negative impact on the anti-tumor treatment outcome could not be excluded. The severe immunosuppression status as well as the more aggressive disease phenotypes of these patients all strongly challenged the health care providers. One of the main reasons for the late ART initiation is that most of AIDS patients in China are from low income class, or so called "grass roots", who are often less educated, single or separated from their family to work outside to strive. Although Chinese government have made great efforts to provide the basic education of AIDS, making the free ART publicly available, especially to this population, it seemed that a long way still needs to be run to popularize contemporary knowledge of HIV in such a large country with a huge population. The ignorance of the HIV infection of the patients and the prejudice from their family members should be firstly diminished. In this study, most of the patients came to the hospital not for suspicion of HIV infection, but for the complications, including but not limited to fever, unexplained symptoms and signs, or even hematological events like tumor or pancytopenia.

AIDS patients with DLBCL or BL could still achieve a survival plateau. However, it seemed that this plateau is significantly lower than that of the HIV negative counterpart, especially for BL patients [23]. In this study, the

**Table 4** Multivariate analysis of potential prognostic factors for the patients

| Variables | CR | | OS | | PFS | |
|---|---|---|---|---|---|---|
|  | P | OR (95% CI) | P | OR (95% CI) | P | OR (95% CI) |
| IPI score | <0.001 | 0.371 (0.229–0.601) | <0.001 | 2.172 (1.579–2.987) | <0.001 | 1.838 (1.406–2.402) |
| Pathology subtype (DLBCL vs. BL) | 0.038 | 0.240 (0.063–0.925) | NS | – | NS | – |

2-year OS and PFS rates for DLBCL and BL were 74.3 ± 8.1%, 28.9 ± 11.0%, and 54.2 ± 8.1%, 19.2 ± 7.5%, respectively. High dose chemotherapy other than Hyper-CVAD A and B using the strategy including more anthracyclin (it was observed that most of BL patients progressed while received B regimen), might be designed. As for DLBCL, CHOP is not enough for the HIV-infected patients. An escalated regimen such as DA-EPOCH or CHOP-E should be considered for further clinical trial.

Various prognostic parameters have been used for predicting the treatment outcome of NHL [7, 11, 24]. Among them, the IPI is probably the most commonly used one [25]. Based on IPI, various systems such as FLIPI were designed for some special subtypes of lymphoma [24]. In this study, we have examined the efficacy of IPI parameters in HIV associated NHL (mostly BL and DLBCL). It was encouraging to prove that IPI parameters still worked in such kind of the patients, almost all the IPI parameters were useful in univariate analysis, and IPI was the independent prognostic factor for predicting both OS and PFS. Interestingly, the initial CD4 count before treatment was not associated with the treatment outcome of lymphoma in terms of CR rate, OS or PFS. It was traditionally believed that a low CD4 cell count was associated with death, which was proved in two large studies in pre-cART and early cART eras [26]. We believed that with the wide application of cART treatment, viral load and other related factors were abrogated.

## Conclusion

HIV associated NHLs represents a group of heterogeneous aggressive diseases with poor prognosis. Current anti-lymphoma treatment should be improved in this special group of patients in future clinical practice. IPI still works in the HIV-infected NHL patients in predicting the prognosis during the cART era. However, this study was a retrospective one and the treatment outcome of the patients, especially for BL, need to be further monitored. And the potential usefulness of existing clinical prognostic factors in AIDS patients should be further addressed in future studies.

## Abbreviations

ABC: Activated B-cell subtype; ADR: Adriamycin; BL: Burkitt lymphoma; cART: Combined antiretroviral therapy; CBC: Complete blood cell count; CR: Complete response; CTX: Cyclophosphamide; DEX: Dexamethasone; DLBCL: Diffuse large B cell lymphoma; ECOG: Eastern cooperative oncology group; FL: Follicular lymphoma; HIV: Human immune-deficiency virus; IBL: angioimmunoblastic lymphoma; IPI: International prognostic index; LDH: LactateDehydrogenase; NHL: Non hodgkin's lymphoma; OR: Overall response; ORs: Odds ratios; OS: Overall survival; PBL: Plasmablastic lymphoma; PD: Progressive disease; PR: Partial response; SD: Stable disease; VCR: Vincristine

## Acknowledgements

We are grateful Dr. Yan-Ling Feng for the pathologic reviewing and Dr. Hui Zhang for radiological examinations.

## Funding

This work was supported in part by the National Natural Science Foundation of China (No. 81370653 and 81571977), the 863 project (No.2014AA021403), the Three-Year Action Plan for Public Health (No. 15GWZK0103), and a grant from the Shanghai Municipal Science and Technology Commission (No. 16411960400).

## Authors' contributions

HZL, YS and RFZ conceived and designed the study. YS, RFZ, LL, YZS, WS, TKQ, YT, ZYW and LQG perform the study, collected and entered the data. YS and RFZ analyzed the data. YS and RFZ wrote the manuscript. All authors read and approved the final manuscript.

## Competing interests

The authors declare that they have no competing interests.

## Author details

[1]Department of Hematology, Shanghai Institute of Hematology, Rui Jin Hospital Affiliated to Shanghai Jiao Tong University School of Medicine and Collaborative Innovation Center of Systems Biomedicine, Shanghai Jiao Tong University, Shanghai 200000, China. [2]Department of Infectious Diseases, Shanghai Public Health Clinical Center, Fudan University, Shanghai 201508, China.

## References

1. Gopal S, Patel MR, Yanik EL, Cole SR, Achenbach CJ, Napravnik S, et al. Temporal trends in presentation and survival for HIV-associated lymphoma in the antiretroviral therapy era. J Natl Cancer Inst. 2013;105(16):1221–9.
2. Weiss R, Mitrou P, Arasteh K, Schuermann D, Hentrich M, Duehrsen U, et al. Acquired immunodeficiency syndrome-related lymphoma: simultaneous treatment with combined cyclophosphamide, doxorubicin, vincristine, and prednisone chemotherapy and highly active antiretroviral therapy is safe and improves survival–results of the German Multicenter Trial. Cancer. 2006; 106(7):1560–8.
3. Navarro JT, Vall-Llovera F, Mate JL, Morgades M, Feliu E, Ribera JM. Decrease in the frequency of meningeal involvement in AIDS-related systemic lymphoma in patients receiving HAART. Haematologica. 2008;93(1):149–50.
4. Wolf T, Brodt HR, Fichtlscherer S, Mantzsch K, Hoelzer D, Helm EB, et al. Changing incidence and prognostic factors of survival in AIDS-related non-Hodgkin's lymphoma in the era of highly active antiretroviral therapy (HAART). Leuk Lymphoma. 2005;46(2):207–15.
5. Carroll V, Garzino-Demo A. HIV-associated lymphoma in the era of combination antiretroviral therapy: shifting the immunological landscape. Pathog Dis. 2015;73(7):ftv044.
6. The International Non-Hodgkin's Lymphoma Prognostic Factors Project. A predictive model for aggressive non-Hodgkin's lymphoma. The International Non-Hodgkin's Lymphoma Prognostic Factors Project. N Engl J Med. 1993; 329(14):987–94.
7. Ziepert M, Hasenclever D, Kuhnt E, Glass B, Schmitz N, Pfreundschuh M, et al. Standard International prognostic index remains a valid predictor of outcome for patients with aggressive CD20+ B-cell lymphoma in the rituximab era. J Clin Oncol. 2010;28(14):2373–80.
8. Shen Y, Yao Y, Li JM, Chen QS, You JH, Zhao HJ, et al. Prognostic factors analysis for R-CHOP regimen therapy in diffuse large B cell lymphoma. Zhonghua Xue Ye Xue Za Zhi. 2008;29(4):252–7.
9. Ramaswami R, Chia G, Dalla Pria A, Pinato D, Parker K, Nelson M, et al. Eevolution of HIV associated lymphoma over 3 decades. J Acquir Immune Defic Syndr. 2016;72(2):177–83.
10. Mounier N, Spina M, Gabarre J, Raphael M, Rizzardini G, Golfier JB, et al. AIDS-related non-Hodgkin lymphoma: final analysis of 485 patients treated with risk-adapted intensive chemotherapy. Blood. 2006;107(10):3832–40.

11. Barta SK, Xue X, Wang D, Tamari R, Lee JY, Mounier N, et al. Treatment factors affecting outcomes in HIV-associated non-Hodgkin lymphomas: a pooled analysis of 1546 patients. Blood. 2013;122(19):3251–62.

12. Tohda S. Overview of lymphoid neoplasms in the fourth edition of the WHO classification. Rinsho byori Jpn J Clin Pathol. 2012;60(6):560–4.

13. Alizadeh AA, Eisen MB, Davis RE, Ma C, Lossos IS, Rosenwald A, et al. Distinct types of diffuse large B-cell lymphoma identified by gene expression profiling. Nature. 2000;403(6769):503–11.

14. Li XY, Li JM. Research progress on second-hit in malignant lymphomagenesis–review. Zhongguo Shi Yan Xue Ye Xue Za Zhi. 2010;18(6):1627–31.

15. Dunleavy K, Little RF, Pittaluga S, Grant N, Wayne AS, Carrasquillo JA, et al. The role of tumor histogenesis, FDG-PET, and short-course EPOCH with dose-dense rituximab (SC-EPOCH-RR) in HIV-associated diffuse large B-cell lymphoma. Blood. 2010;115(15):3017–24.

16. Antinori A, Cingolani A, Alba L, Ammassari A, Serraino D, Ciancio BC, et al. Better response to chemotherapy and prolonged survival in AIDS-related lymphomas responding to highly active antiretroviral therapy. AIDS (London, England). 2001;15(12):1483–91.

17. Zhou LL, Wang C, Zhao JH, Yan SK, Gao YR, Cai Q, et al. The role of FDG-PET in staging of lymphoma and evaluation of therapeutic efficiency. Zhonghua Xue Ye Xue Za Zhi. 2009;30(4):233–6.

18. Zhao J, Qiao W, Wang C, Wang T, Xing Y. Therapeutic evaluation and prognostic value of interim hybrid PET/CT with (18)F-FDG after three to four cycles of chemotherapy in non-Hodgkin's lymphoma. Hematology (Amsterdam, Netherlands). 2007;12(5):423–30.

19. Zhou Z, Sehn LH, Rademaker AW, Gordon LI, Lacasce AS, Crosby-Thompson A, et al. An enhanced International Prognostic Index (NCCN-IPI) for patients with diffuse large B-cell lymphoma treated in the rituximab era. Blood. 2014; 123(6):837–42.

20. Luz E, Marques M, Luz I, Stelitano C, Netto E, Araujo I, et al. Survival and prognostic factors for AIDS and Non-AIDS patients with Non-Hodgkin's lymphoma in Bahia, brazil: a retrospective cohort study. ISRN Hematol. 2013;2013:904201.

21. PDQ Adult Treatment Editorial Board. AIDS-Related Lymphoma Treatment (PDQ®): Health Professional Version. PDQ Cancer Information Summaries [Internet]. Bethesda (MD): National Cancer Institute (US); 2002–2015 Apr 2.

22. Lim ST, Karim R, Nathwani BN, Tulpule A, Espina B, Levine AM. AIDS-related Burkitt's lymphoma versus diffuse large-cell lymphoma in the pre-highly active antiretroviral therapy (HAART) and HAART eras: significant differences in survival with standard chemotherapy. J Clin Oncol. 2005;23(19):4430–8.

23. Long JL, Engels EA, Moore RD, Gebo KA. Incidence and outcomes of malignancy in the HAART era in an urban cohort of HIV-infected individuals. AIDS (London, England). 2008;22(4):489–96.

24. Barta SK, Xue X, Wang D, Lee JY, Kaplan LD, Ribera JM, et al. A new prognostic score for AIDS-related lymphomas in the rituximab-era. Haematologica. 2014;99(11):1731–7.

25. Yang S, Yu Y, Jun-Min L, Jian-Qing M, Qiu-Sheng C, Yu C, et al. Reassessment of the prognostic factors of international prognostic index (IPI) in the patients with diffuse large B-cell lymphoma in an era of R-CHOP in Chinese population. Ann Hematol. 2009;88(9):863–9.

26. Bohlius J, Schmidlin K, Costagliola D, Fatkenheuer G, May M, Caro Murillo AM, et al. Prognosis of HIV-associated non-Hodgkin lymphoma in patients starting combination antiretroviral therapy. AIDS (London, England). 2009;23(15):2029–37.

# 17

# Whole-genome analysis of human papillomavirus genotypes 52 and 58 isolated from Japanese women with cervical intraepithelial neoplasia and invasive cervical cancer

Yuri Tenjimbayashi[1,2], Mamiko Onuki[1], Yusuke Hirose[1,2], Seiichiro Mori[2], Yoshiyuki Ishii[2], Takamasa Takeuchi[2], Nobutaka Tasaka[3], Toyomi Satoh[3], Tohru Morisada[4], Takashi Iwata[4], Shingo Miyamoto[1], Koji Matsumoto[1], Akihiko Sekizawa[1] and Iwao Kukimoto[2*] [ID]

## Abstract

**Background:** Human papillomavirus genotypes 52 and 58 (HPV52/58) are frequently detected in patients with cervical intraepithelial neoplasia (CIN) and invasive cervical cancer (ICC) in East Asian countries including Japan. As with other HPV genotypes, HPV52/58 consist of multiple lineages of genetic variants harboring less than 10% differences between complete genome sequences of the same HPV genotype. However, site variations of nucleotide and amino acid sequences across the viral whole-genome have not been fully examined for HPV52/58. The aim of this study was to investigate genetic variations of HPV52/58 prevalent among Japanese women by analyzing the viral whole-genome sequences.

**Methods:** The entire genomic region of HPV52/58 was amplified by long-range PCR with total cellular DNA extracted from cervical exfoliated cells isolated from Japanese patients with CIN or ICC. The amplified DNA was subjected to next generation sequencing to determine the complete viral genome sequences. Phylogenetic analyses were performed with the whole-genome sequences to assign variant lineages/sublineages to the HPV52/58 isolates. The variability in amino acid sequences of viral proteins was assessed by calculating the Shannon entropy scores at individual amino acid positions of HPV proteins.

**Results:** Among 52 isolates of HPV52 (CIN1, $n = 20$; CIN2/3, $n = 21$; ICC, $n = 11$), 50 isolates belonged to lineage B (sublineage B2) and two isolates belonged to lineage A (sublineage A1). Among 48 isolates of HPV58 (CIN1, $n = 21$; CIN2/3, $n = 19$; ICC, $n = 8$), 47 isolates belonged to lineage A (sublineages A1/A2/A3) and one isolate belonged to lineage C. Single nucleotide polymorphisms specific for individual variant lineages were determined throughout the viral genome based on multiple sequence alignments of the Japanese HPV52/58 isolates and reference HPV52/58 genomes. Entropy analyses revealed that the E1 protein was relatively variable among the HPV52 isolates, whereas the E7, E4, and L2 proteins showed some variations among the HPV58 isolates.

**Conclusions:** Among the HPV52/58-positive specimens from Japanese women with CIN/ICC, the variant distributions were strongly biased toward lineage B for HPV52 and lineage A for HPV58 across histological categories. Different patterns of amino acid variations were observed in HPV52 and HPV58 across the viral whole-genome.

**Keywords:** Human papillomavirus, HPV52/58, Cervical cancer, Variant, SNPs

* Correspondence: ikuki@nih.go.jp
[2]Pathogen Genomics Center, National Institute of Infectious Diseases, 4-7-1 Gakuen, Musashi-murayama, Tokyo 208-0011, Japan
Full list of author information is available at the end of the article

## Background

Human papillomaviruses (HPVs) constitute a large family of small DNA viruses, having a circular double-stranded DNA genome of approximately 8000 base pairs [1]. Their genomes share the same genomic organization, and are composed of at least eight coding regions (early genes: E1, E2, E4, E5, E6, and E7; late genes: L1 and L2) and two non-coding regions, including the long control region (LCR). So far, more than 200 different genotypes of HPV have been identified as showing more than 10% differences of the L1 nucleotide sequence in relation to other genotypes [2]. At least 13 genotypes (HPV16, 18, 31, 33, 35, 39, 45, 51, 52, 56, 58, 59, and 68) [3], referred to as "high-risk" HPVs, are recognized as the causative agents of cervical cancer and many other cancers, including vaginal, vulvar, penile, anal, and oropharyngeal cancers [4]. High-risk HPVs preferentially infect basal epithelial cells and induce hyper-proliferative lesions that are clinically manifested as cervical intraepithelial neoplasia grade 1 (CIN1) in the cervix. The majority of such infections are cleared by the host immune system within a few years, and only a small proportion persist and progress further to CIN grade 2 or 3 (CIN2/3). These high-grade lesions eventually develop into invasive cervical cancer (ICC) by accumulating host genetic alternations after years of persistent infection [5].

Among the high-risk HPVs, HPV16 and HPV18 are the most and second most prevalent genotypes in ICC, respectively, in total accounting for about 70% of ICC cases worldwide [6]. Although the high prevalence of HPV16/18 in ICC is common throughout the world, the distribution of other high-risk HPVs in the remaining fraction of ICC shows some region-specific variations [7]. In particular, in East Asian countries including China, Taiwan, South Korea and Japan, HPV52 and HPV58 infections are more prevalent compared to European, North American and African regions [8, 9]. In Japan, HPV52 and HPV58 ranked the second and third, respectively, in CIN2/3 cases, and ranked the third and fourth in ICC cases, accounting for 8–9% and 3–5% of ICC, respectively [10, 11].

HPV genomes with less than 10% differences in their L1 sequences, recognized as intra-type variants, constitutes an additional level of HPV genetic complexity. Based on complete viral genome sequences, intra-type variants are phylogenetically classified into different lineages and sublineages, which are defined as containing 1.0–10.0% and 0.5–1.0% nucleotide variations, respectively [12]. As such, HPV52 is classified into four variant lineages (A, B, C, and D) and seven sublineages (A1, A2, B1, B2, C1, C2, and D), whereas HPV58 consists of four variant lineages (A, B, C, and D) and eight sublineages (A1, A2, A3, B1, B2, C, D1, and D2) [12].

Many lines of evidence attribute a higher risk of progression to ICC to some distinct variant lineages of high-risk HPVs. Intriguingly, recent large-scale studies revealed that different HPV16 variant sublineages were associated with different risks for cervical squamous cell carcinoma or adenocarcinoma [13–15]. A study investigating the worldwide distribution of HPV52 variants also suggested that lineage B (in particular sublineage B2) posed a higher risk for cervical cancer development among the variant lineages [16]. In a study from Taiwan on HPV52 variants, however, lineage C infection posed a higher risk for CIN3/ICC compared to lineage B [17]. Regarding HPV58 variants and their disease association, lineage A was suggested to be more closely associated with persistent infection compared to other lineages [18], and subsequent studies reported that sublineage A1 or A3 might be associated with a risk for CIN3/ICC [17, 19].

While HPV52/58 infections are common in East Asia, comprehensive surveys have not been conducted regarding their variant distributions in Japan. Determining the complete viral genome sequence is the most reliable and accurate procedure to assign HPV variant lineages/sublineages compared with utilizing only limited sequences in the HPV genome, which was generally done in previous studies on HPV52/58 variant classification [17, 20–22]. This study thus aimed to collect the whole-genome sequences of HPV52/58 from Japanese women with CIN/ICC through next generation sequencing techniques and perform in-depth analyses of genetic variations of these particular HPVs.

## Methods

### Study samples

Cervical exfoliated cells were collected in ThinPrep media (Hologic, Bedford, MA) using a cytoblush from Japanese patients diagnosed with CIN1, CIN2, CIN3 or ICC at Keio University Hospital and Tsukuba University Hospital from 2012 to 2016. The total cellular DNA was extracted from the recovered cells on a MagNA Pure LC 2.0 (Roche Diagnostic, Indianapolis, IN), and subjected to PCR with PGMY09/11 primers to amplify HPV L1 DNA, followed by reverse blot hybridization for HPV genotyping, as described previously [23]. Based on the genotyping results, DNA samples positive for HPV52 ($n = 52$) or HPV58 ($n = 47$) were selected for subsequent analyses of the whole-genome sequences of HPV52/58. The study protocol was approved by the Ethics Committees at each hospital and the National Institute of Infectious Diseases, and written informed consent for study participation was obtained from each patient.

**Table 1** HPV52/58 genomes obtained in this study

|  | ID | Histology | HPV type | Age | Length (bp) | Lineage | Accession No. |
|---|---|---|---|---|---|---|---|
| HPV52 | #001 | CIN1 | 52 | 65 | 7960 | B2 | LC270024 |
|  | #002 | CIN1 | 52 | 50 | 7960 | B2 | LC270025 |
|  | #003 | CIN1 | 52 | 30 | 7960 | B2 | LC270026 |
|  | #004 | CIN1 | 51/52 | 31 | 7960 | B2 | LC270027 |
|  | #005 | CIN1 | 52/56 | 24 | 7960 | B2 | LC270028 |
|  | #006 | CIN1 | 52 | 47 | 7960 | B2 | LC270029 |
|  | #007 | CIN1 | 33/52/69 | 31 | 7960 | B2 | LC270030 |
|  | #008 | CIN1 | 45/52/53 | 31 | 7960 | B2 | LC270031 |
|  | #009 | CIN1 | 16/42/52/53 | 41 | 7960 | B2 | LC270032 |
|  | #010 | CIN1 | 52 | 40 | 7960 | B2 | LC270033 |
|  | #011 | CIN1 | 42/52/58 | 23 | 7960 | B2 | LC270034 |
|  | #012 | CIN1 | 52 | 64 | 7960 | B2 | LC270035 |
|  | #013 | CIN1 | 35/52 | 40 | 7960 | B2 | LC270036 |
|  | #014 | CIN1 | 52 | 48 | 7960 | B2 | LC270037 |
|  | #015 | CIN1 | 52 | 45 | 7960 | B2 | LC270038 |
|  | #016 | CIN1 | 52/82 | 24 | 7982** | B2 | LC270039 |
|  | #017 | CIN1 | 45/52 | 31 | 7960 | B2 | LC270040 |
|  | #018 | CIN1 | 31/52 | 30 | 7960 | B2 | LC270041 |
|  | #019 | CIN1 | 52 | 37 | 7960 | B2 | LC270042 |
|  | #020 | CIN1 | 33/52 | 40 | 7960 | B2 | LC270043 |
|  | #021 | CIN2 | 16/52 | 31 | 7960 | B2 | LC270044 |
|  | #022 | CIN2 | 52 | 36 | 7960 | B2 | LC270045 |
|  | #023 | CIN2 | 52 | 28 | 7960 | B2 | LC270046 |
|  | #024 | CIN2 | 52 | 41 | 7960 | B2 | LC270047 |
|  | #025 | CIN2 | 52 | 39 | 7960 | B2 | LC270048 |
|  | #026 | CIN2 | 52 | 53 | 7960 | B2 | LC270049 |
|  | #027 | CIN2 | 52 | 30 | 7960 | B2 | LC270050 |
|  | #028 | CIN2 | 52 | 40 | 7960 | B2 | LC270051 |
|  | #029 | CIN2 | 52/58 | 40 | 7960 | B2 | LC270052 |
|  | #030 | CIN2 | 52 | 37 | 7960 | B2 | LC270053 |
|  | #031 | CIN2 | 52 | 33 | 7960 | B2 | LC270054 |
|  | #032 | CIN3 | 18/52/58 | 36 | 7960 | B2 | LC270055 |
|  | #033 | CIN3 | 52 | 42 | 7960 | B2 | LC270056 |
|  | #034 | CIN3 | 52 | 48 | 7960 | B2 | LC270057 |
|  | #035 | CIN3 | 39/52/82 | 30 | 7960 | B2 | LC270058 |
|  | #036 | CIN3 | 52 | 31 | 7937 | A1 | LC270059 |
|  | #037 | CIN3 | 52 | 37 | 7960 | B2 | LC270060 |
|  | #038 | CIN3 | 52 | 33 | 7903* | B2 | LC270061 |
|  | #039 | CIN3 | 52 | 49 | 7960 | B2 | LC270062 |
|  | #040 | CIN3 | 52 | 36 | 7937 | A1 | LC270063 |
|  | #041 | CIN3 | 52 | 61 | 7960 | B2 | LC270064 |
|  | #042 | ICC (SCC) | 52 | 44 | 7924* | B2 | LC270065 |
|  | #043 | ICC (SCC) | 33/39/52 | 54 | 7921* | B2 | LC270066 |
|  | #044 | ICC (SCC) | 52 | 70 | 7960 | B2 | LC270067 |

**Table 1** HPV52/58 genomes obtained in this study *(Continued)*

| | | | | | | |
|---|---|---|---|---|---|---|
| | #045 | ICC (SCC) | 52 | 68 | 7960 | B2 | LC270068 |
| | #046 | ICC (Ad) | 16/18/52 | 44 | 7960 | B2 | LC270069 |
| | #047 | ICC (SCC) | 52 | 74 | 7960 | B2 | LC270070 |
| | #048 | ICC (SCC) | 16/52 | 47 | 7960 | B2 | LC270071 |
| | #049 | ICC (SCC) | 6/16/52 | 31 | 7960 | B2 | LC270072 |
| | #050 | ICC (SCC) | 52 | 76 | 7960 | B2 | LC270073 |
| | #051 | ICC (SCC) | 52 | 76 | 7960 | B2 | LC270074 |
| | #052 | ICC (SCC) | 52 | 67 | 7960 | B2 | LC270075 |
| HPV58 | #053 | CIN1 | 42/58 | 32 | 7824 | A2 | LC270076 |
| | #054 | CIN1 | 58 | 35 | 7824 | A1 | LC270077 |
| | #055 | CIN1 | 58 | 43 | 7824 | A1 | LC270078 |
| | #056 | CIN1 | 58 | 35 | 7824 | A2 | LC270079 |
| | #057 | CIN1 | 58 | 31 | 7824 | A2 | LC270080 |
| | #058 | CIN1 | 16/58/82 | 27 | 7824 | A1 | LC270081 |
| | #059 | CIN1 | 58 | 36 | 7824 | A2 | LC270082 |
| | #060 | CIN1 | 58 | 48 | 7836 | A3 | LC270083 |
| | #061 | CIN1 | 58 | 34 | 7824 | A1 | LC270084 |
| | #062 | CIN1 | 42/52/58 | 23 | 7824 | A1 | LC270085 |
| | #063 | CIN1 | 58 | 54 | 7814*** | A2 | LC270086 |
| | #064 | CIN1 | 58 | 31 | 7824 | A2 | LC270087 |
| | #065 | CIN1 | 58/68 | 44 | 7824 | A1 | LC270088 |
| | #066 | CIN1 | 58/68 | 44 | 7824 | A2 | LC270089 |
| | #067 | CIN1 | 58 | 30 | 7824 | A2 | LC270090 |
| | #068 | CIN1 | 58 | 39 | 7824 | A1 | LC270091 |
| | #069 | CIN1 | 58 | 36 | 7824 | A2 | LC270092 |
| | #070 | CIN1 | 16/31/52/58/66 | 33 | 7836 | A3 | LC270093 |
| | #071 | CIN1 | 58 | 39 | 7824 | A1 | LC270094 |
| | #072 | CIN1 | 52/58 | 34 | 7824 | A2 | LC270095 |
| | #073 | CIN1 | 58 | 27 | 7824 | A1 | LC270096 |
| | #074 | CIN2 | 16/52/58 | 45 | 7824 | A2 | LC270097 |
| | #075 | CIN2 | 18/52/58 | 36 | 7824 | A1 | LC270098 |
| | #076 | CIN2 | 53/58/84 | 23 | 7824 | A1 | LC270099 |
| | #077 | CIN2 | 58 | 45 | 7824 | A2 | LC270100 |
| | #078 | CIN2 | 58 | 32 | 7824 | A1 | LC270101 |
| | #079 | CIN2 | 58 | 56 | 7823 | A2 | LC270102 |
| | #080 | CIN2 | 58 | 45 | 7823 | A1 | LC270103 |
| | #081 | CIN2 | 58 | 38 | 7824 | A2 | LC270104 |
| | #082 | CIN2 | 58 | 40 | 7820 | C | LC270105 |
| | #083 | CIN2 | 58 | 32 | 7824 | A1 | LC270106 |
| | #084 | CIN2 | 58 | 33 | 7824 | A2 | LC270107 |
| | #085 | CIN2 | 58 | 40 | 7824 | A2 | LC270108 |
| | #086 | CIN3 | 58 | 29 | 7824 | A2 | LC270109 |
| | #087 | CIN3 | 58 | 38 | 7836 | A3 | LC270110 |
| | #088 | CIN3 | 58 | 35 | 7824 | A2 | LC270111 |
| | #089 | CIN3 | 58 | 39 | 7824 | A2 | LC270112 |

**Table 1** HPV52/58 genomes obtained in this study *(Continued)*

| #090 | CIN3 | 58 | 37 | 7824 | A1 | LC270113 |
|------|------|------|------|------|------|------|
| #091 | CIN3 | 58 | 27 | 7824 | A2 | LC270114 |
| #092 | CIN3 | 58 | 34 | 7824 | A1 | LC270115 |
| #093 | ICC (SCC) | 58 | 77 | 7824 | A2 | LC270116 |
| #094 | ICC (Ad) | 16/53/58 | 39 | 7836 | A3 | LC270117 |
| #095 | ICC (SCC) | 58 | 79 | 7824 | A2 | LC270118 |
| #096 | ICC (SCC) | 58 | 48 | 7824 | A1 | LC270119 |
| #097 | ICC (SCC) | 58 | 64 | 7824 | A2 | LC270120 |
| #098 | ICC (SCC) | 58 | 54 | 7824 | A1 | LC270121 |
| #099 | ICC (SCC) | 45/58 | 36 | 7824 | A2 | LC270122 |
| #100 | ICC (SCC) | 58 | 49 | 7836 | A3 | LC270123 |

*CIN* cervical intraepithelial neoplasia, *ICC* invasive cervical cancer, *SCC* squamous cell carcinoma, *Ad* adenocarcinoma. The following sequences were identical: #001, #022 and #033; #004 and #010; #012 and #027; #007 and #018; #020 and #021; #011, #045, #047, and #048; #066, #067, and #084; #058, #068, #075, and #078. *, E2/E4 deletion; **, L2 insertion; ***, E1 deletion

### Viral whole-genome amplification and next generation sequencing

Full-circle PCR or overlapping PCR was performed with PrimeSTAR® GXL DNA polymerase (Takara, Ohtsu, Japan) to amplify the whole-genome sequences of HPV52/58 as described previously [24]. The sequences of PCR primers were as follows: full-circle PCR for HPV52: HPV52-1758F (5′-ACA CAT ATG GTA ATA GAA CCA CCA AAA-3′) and HPV52-1908R (5′-TAT TGT CAA AGC TAT GCT GTA ATA CTG-3′); overlapping PCR for HPV52: HPV52-1758F and HPV52-5968R (5′-TCC AAG CCT GTA CAG GCC CAC ACC AAC-3′); HPV52-5673F (5′-GTG TAC CTG CCT CCT GTA CCT GTC TCT-3′) and HPV52-1908R; full-circle PCR for HPV58: HPV58-1751F (5′-TAC TAT CAA TTC CTG AAA CAT GTA TGA-3′) and HPV58-1889R (5′-AAT CTA TCT ATC CAT TCT GGT GTT G-3′); overlapping PCR for HPV58: HPV58-1751F and HPV58-5846R (5′-GCC TGA TAC CTT GGG AAC TAA TAC TTT-3′); HPV58-5677F (5′-ACC TGC CTC CTG TGC CTG TGT CTA AGG-3′) and HPV58-1889R. The amplified DNA was separated by agarose gel electrophoresis and purified with the Wizard gel purification kit (Promega, Madison, WI). The purified DNA was converted to a short-fragmented DNA library using the Nextera XT DNA sample prep kit (Illumina, San Diego, CA), followed by size selection with SPRIselect (Beckman Coulter, Brea, CA). The multiplexed libraries were analyzed on a MiSeq sequencer (Illumina) with the MiSeq reagent kit v3 (150 cycle). The complete genome sequences of HPV52/58 were de novo assembled from the total read sequences using the Virus-TAP pipeline [25] (https://gph.niid.go.jp/cgi-bin/virustap/index.cgi). The accuracy of the reconstructed whole-genome sequences was verified by read mapping with Burrows-Wheeler Aligner v0.7.12 [26] and subsequent visual inspection by Integrative Genomics Viewer v2.3.90 [27].

### Phylogenetic tree construction

The complete genome sequences of HPV52 ($n = 52$) or HPV58 ($n = 48$) isolates were aligned against each other using MAFFT v7.309 [28] with default parameters, together with the complete genome sequences of HPV52/58 available in GenBank, including HPV52/58 reference genome sequences that represent all variant lineages/sublineages (HPV52: A1, X74481; A2, HQ537739; B1, HQ537740; B2, HQ537743; C1, HQ537744; C2, HQ537746; D, HQ537748; HPV58: A1, D90400; A2, HQ537752; A3, HQ537758; B1, HQ537762; B2, HQ537764; C, HQ537774; D1, HQ537768; D2, HQ537770), and HPV52/58 genome sequences previously determined by us from Japanese CIN1 specimens (HPV52: AB819272, AB819273, AB819274; HPV58: AB819275, AB819276, AB819277, AB819278) [24]. Maximum likelihood trees were constructed using RAxML HPC v8.2.9 [29], employing 1000 bootstrap replicates. Phylogenetic trees were visualized in FigTree v1.4.3.

### Identification of lineage/sublineage-specific SNPs

All the HPV52/58 genome sequences included in the phylogenetic analyses were used to search for viral single nucleotide polymorphisms (SNPs) specific for variant lineages and sublineages. The multiple sequence alignments of the whole-genome sequences of HPV52/58 were sorted according to variant lineage/sublineage and the number of mismatched bases in order to visually differentiate lineage/sublineage-specific SNPs.

### Entropy analysis

Amino acid variations at individual positions of viral proteins were calculated on the basis of Shannon's equation [30]:

$$H(i) = - \sum_{x_i} p(x_i) \log_2 p(x_i)$$

$$(x_i = G, A, I, V, \ldots\ldots),$$

where $H(i)$, $p(x_i)$, and $i$ indicate the amino acid entropy score of a given position, the probability of occurrence of a given amino acid at the position, and the number of positions, respectively. An $H(i)$ score of zero indicates absolute conservation, whereas a score of 4.4 indicates complete randomness. The deduced amino acid sequences of eight HPV proteins (E6/E7/E1/E2/E4/E5/L2/L1) of the HPV52/58 isolates were concatenated and aligned with each other using MAFFT. The entropy calculation was performed on the multiple sequence alignments using R v2.11.1 (https://cran.r-project.org) with bio3d package v1.1–6 [31].

## Statistical analysis

All statistical analyses were performed using R v3.3.2. Fisher's exact test was performed to evaluate a difference in HPV58 A sublineages distribution across histological categories. $P$ value <0.05 was regarded as statistically significant. The relative risk for progression from CIN1 to CIN2/3/ICC among HPV58 A sublineages was estimated by calculating adjusted odds ratio with its 95% confidence interval.

## Results

### Study subjects

The study subjects consisted of 52 HPV52-positive cases (CIN1, $n = 20$; CIN2/3, $n = 21$; ICC, $n = 11$), and 47 HPV58-positive cases (CIN1, $n = 19$; CIN2/3, $n = 20$;

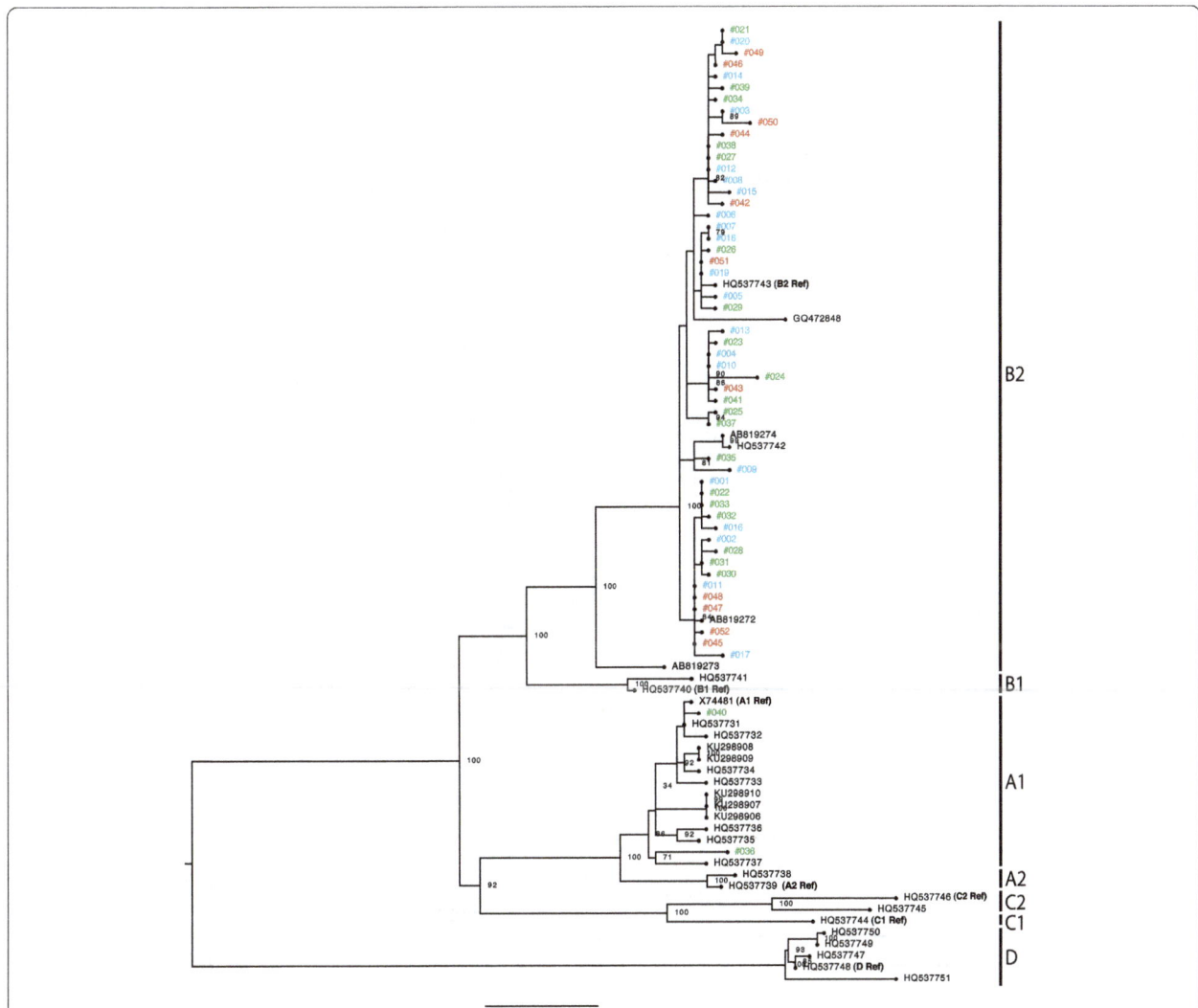

**Fig. 1** Phylogenetic tree based on the analyses of HPV52 whole-genome sequences of 52 isolates and 31 genomes available from GenBank (total 83 sequences). Phylogenetic analyses were conducted using the Maximum likelihood algorithm by RAxML with 1000 bootstrap replicates. The tree is drawn to scale, with branch lengths measured in the number of substitutions per site. The histological grades of cervical specimens from which the isolates were recovered are shown with colored ID: *blue*, CIN1; *green*, CIN2/3; *red*, ICC

ICC, $n = 8$). The mean age ± standard deviation of the cases in each histological grade was as follows: for HPV52: CIN1, 38.6 ± 12.0 years; CIN2/3, 38.6 ± 8.3 years; ICC, 59.2 ± 15.7 years; for HPV58: CIN1, 35.6 ± 7.4 years; CIN2/3, 37.1 ± 7.5 years; ICC, 55.8 ± 16.2 years.

**Phylogenetic analysis of HPV52/58 whole-genomes**

By performing long-range PCR covering viral whole-genomes followed by next generation sequencing analyses, a total of 100 complete genome sequences of 52 isolates of HPV52 and 48 isolates of HPV58 were obtained from the CIN/ICC cases in Japan (Table 1). The lengths of the determined genome sequences ranged from 7903 to 7982-bp for HPV52, and from 7814 to 7836-bp for HPV58.

Nucleotide sequence search for open reading frames (ORFs) identified some deletions and insertions in the viral genes of several HPV52/58 isolates when compared to prototype HPV52/58 genomes (HPV52: X74481; HPV58: D90400) as follows: E2/E4 deletion in three HPV52 isolates (#038, #042, and #043), L2 insertion in one HPV52 isolate (#016), and E1 deletion in one HPV58 isolate (#063). Further, the presence of a premature stop codon was observed in the E4 ORF in one HPV52 isolate (#052) and one HPV58 isolate (#098).

Phylogenetic analyses were conducted with the whole-genome sequences of the HPV52/58 isolates, together with those of reference HPV52/58 genomes that represent individual variant lineages/sublineages. As shown in

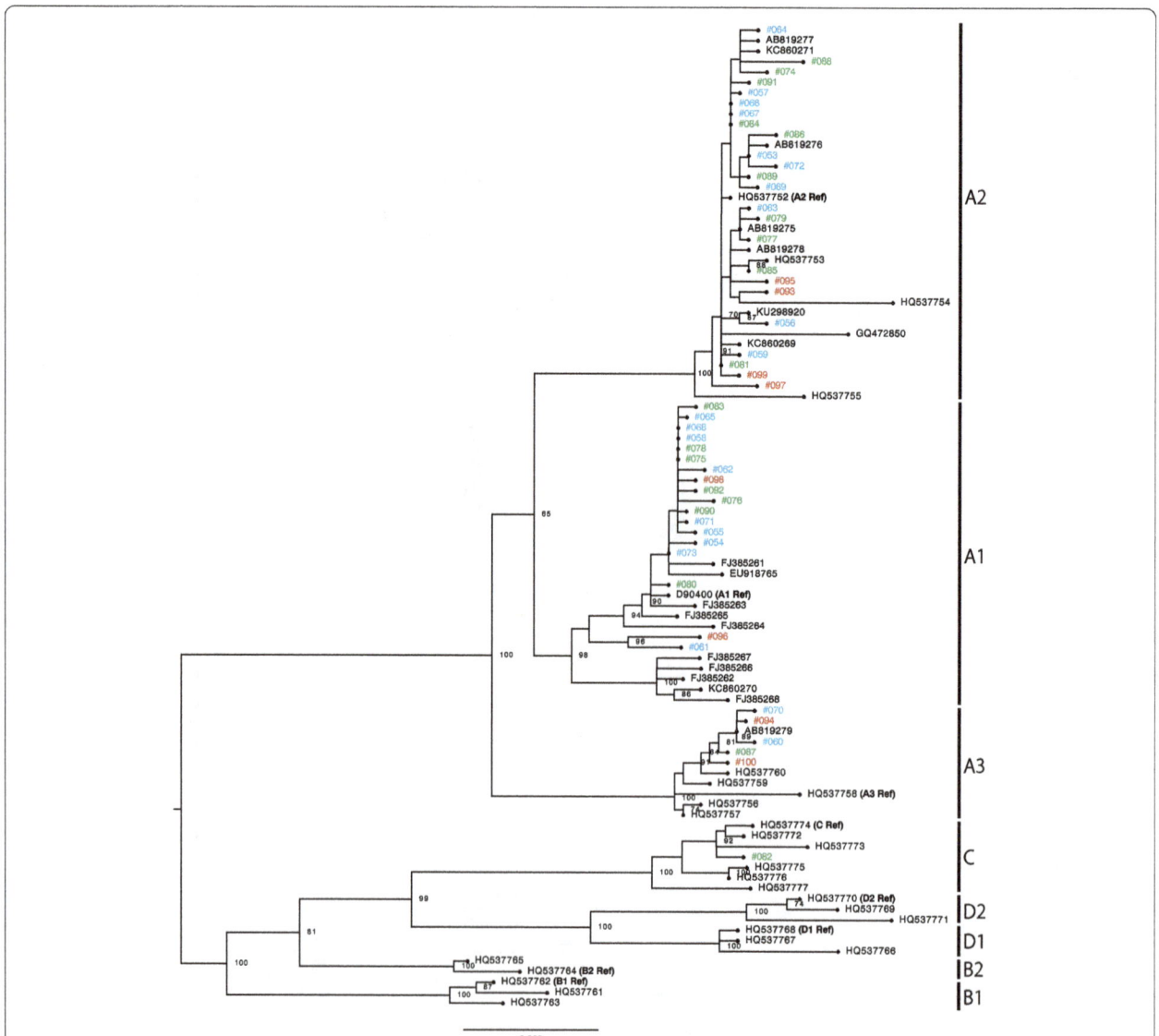

**Fig. 2** Phylogenetic tree based on the analyses of HPV58 whole-genome sequences of 48 isolates and 46 genomes available from GenBank (total 94 sequences). Phylogenetic analyses were conducted using the Maximum likelihood algorithm by RAxML with 1000 bootstrap replicates. The tree is drawn to scale, with branch lengths measured in the number of substitutions per site. The histological grades of cervical specimens from which the isolates were recovered are shown with colored ID numbers: *blue*, CIN1; *green*, CIN2/3; *red*, ICC

Fig. 1, several distinct clusters, including each reference genome, confirmed the presence of four lineages and seven sublineages for HPV52. Among the 52 isolates of HPV52 (CIN1, $n$ = 20; CIN2/3, $n$ = 21; ICC, $n$ = 11), 50 isolates belonged to lineage B (sublineage B2) and two isolates belonged to lineage A (sublineage A1). As shown in Fig. 2, the reference genomes of HPV58 consistently revealed the presence of four lineages and eight sublineages. Among the 48 isolates of HPV58 (CIN1, $n$ = 21; CIN2/3, $n$ = 19; ICC, $n$ = 8), 47 isolates belonged to lineage A (sublineage A1, $n$ = 18; sublineage A2, $n$ = 24; sublineage A3, $n$ = 5) and one isolate belonged to lineage C. Interestingly, one HPV58-positive CIN1 specimen yielded two distinct genome sequences of HPV58 (#065 and #066), and these were classified into two different sublineages (A1 and A2), which indicates co-infections with two closely related sublineages of HPV58 in a single patient. The presence of these two sublineages was further confirmed by cloning and Sanger sequencing of HPV58 PCR products obtained from the original DNA sample (data not shown).

Overall, among the Japanese isolates of HPV52/58, the variant distributions were highly biased toward lineage B (sublineage B2) for HPV52 and lineage A for HPV58. The distributions of HPV52/58 variant lineage/sublineage according to cervical histology status when restricted to single infection (HPV52: $n$ = 33; HPV58, $n$ = 36) are shown in Table 2. Any association of specific lineage/sublineage with a higher risk for CIN2/3 and ICC could not be assessed for the HPV52 isolates, given the dominance of lineage B2 detection across the CIN/ICC cases. The distribution of HPV58 sublineages A1/A2/A3 was almost similar across all histological categories, without a significant difference related to the severity of cervical lesions (Fisher's exact test, $P$ = 0.97). Furthermore, no significant difference in the relative risk for progression from CIN1 to CIN2/3/ICC was observed among HPV58 sublineages A1/A2/A3 (Table 2).

### Lineage/sublineage-specific SNPs in HPV52/58 genomes

Based on multiple sequence alignments of the complete genome sequences of all HPV52/58 genomes included in the phylogenetic analyses above, SNPs discriminating the variant lineages were extracted from the viral whole-genome sequences. Considering the high prevalence of HPV52 lineage B and HPV58 lineage A in Japan, we also searched for SNPs specific for sublineages of these lineages. All viral SNPs specific for HPV52/58 variant lineages/sublineages found in this study are presented in Fig. 3 and listed in Additional file 1.

For HPV52, as shown in Fig. 3a, many lineage D-specific SNPs were densely distributed throughout the whole genome, which reflects the phylogenetic distance of lineage D from other lineages, as shown in Fig. 1. In contrast, SNPs specific for lineages A/B/C were sparsely distributed compared to lineage D, and those specific for lineages B/C were not found in the E6 region, whereas the E7 region and LCR contained at least one SNP for discriminating each HPV52 variant lineage.

For HPV58, as shown in Fig. 3b, while lineage-specific SNPs for lineage A were dispersed across the viral genome, lineages B/C/D showed relatively biased distributions of such SNPs in the whole-genome sequence. In particular, lineage B had only two diagnostic SNPs in the whole genome, which were positioned in the E1 region and LCR.

### Amino acid variation among the HPV52/58 isolates

The variability in amino acid sequences of the viral proteins among the HPV52/58 isolates was examined for each genotype by calculating the Shannon entropy scores. As shown in Fig. 4, the overall levels of amino acid variation were apparently lower in HPV52 than in HPV58, which reflects a close relationship among the HPV52 isolates observed as phylogenetic clusters in Fig. 1. Intriguingly, variable amino acid positions were differently distributed across the viral proteins between the HPV52 and HPV58 isolates. In HPV52, the E1 protein showed relatively high variations among the viral proteins, whereas in HPV58, the E7, E4, and L2 proteins showed higher levels of variation in their amino acid sequences than other proteins. The amino acid positions with the top three entropy scores for each genotype were as follows: HPV52: 423 (Lys or Gln) in E1, 168 (Asn or Thr) in E1, and 429 (Ile or Thr) in E1; HPV58: 63 (Asp, Ser, or Gly) in E7, 39 (Trp, Leu, or Ser) in E4, and 41 (Arg or Gly) in E7.

**Table 2** Distribution of HPV52/58 variant sublineages according to cervical histology status

| | Variant | Total | CIN1 | CIN2 | CIN3 | ICC | Adjusted OR[a] (95% CI) |
|---|---|---|---|---|---|---|---|
| HPV52 | A1 | 2 | 0 | 0 | 2 | 0 | - |
| | A2 | 0 | 0 | 0 | 0 | 0 | - |
| | B1 | 0 | 0 | 0 | 0 | 0 | - |
| | B2 | 31 | 9 | 9 | 6 | 7 | - |
| | C | 0 | 0 | 0 | 0 | 0 | - |
| | D | 0 | 0 | 0 | 0 | 0 | - |
| HPV58 | A1 | 13 | 6 | 3 | 2 | 2 | 1.0 (reference) |
| | A2 | 19 | 7 | 5 | 4 | 3 | 1.47 (0.35–6.17) |
| | A3 | 3 | 1 | 0 | 1 | 1 | 1.71 (0.12–23.9) |
| | B | 0 | 0 | 0 | 0 | 0 | ND |
| | C | 1 | 0 | 1 | 0 | 0 | ND |
| | D | 0 | 0 | 0 | 0 | 0 | ND |

Restricted to cases with HPV52 or HPV58 single infection
OR odds ratio, CI confidence interval, ND not determined
[a]relative risk for progression from CIN1 to CIN2/3/ICC compared to HPV58 sublineage A1

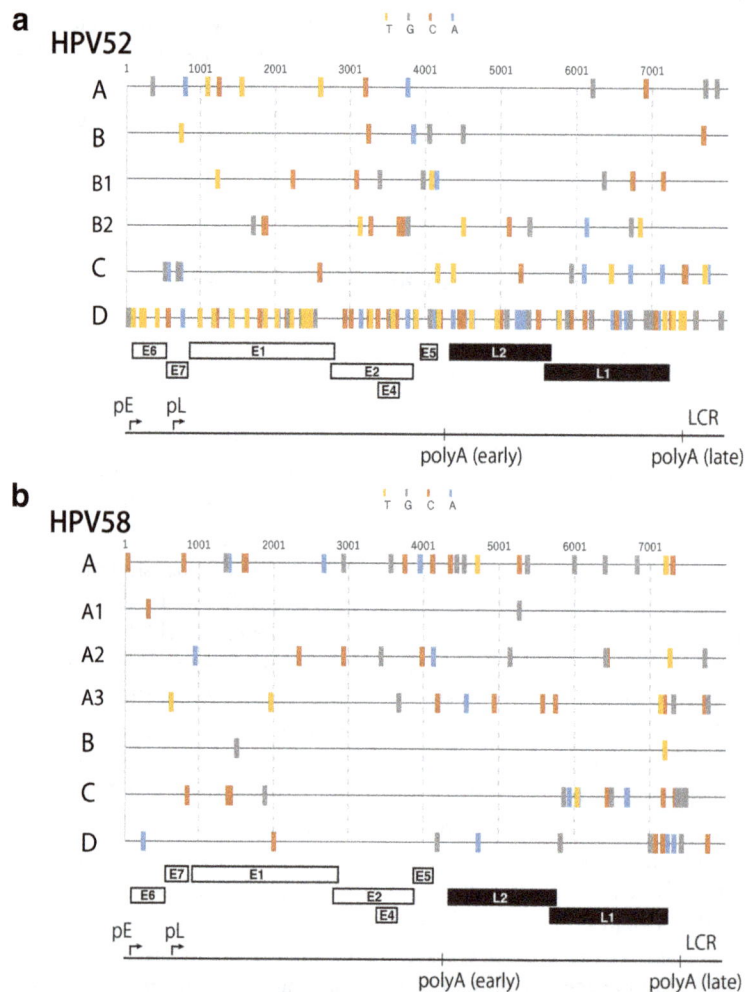

**Fig. 3** Lineage/sublineage-specific SNPs identified from comparisons of whole-genome sequences of the Japanese HPV52/58 isolates and reference HPV52/58 genomes. The positions of specific SNPs for HPV52 lineages A/B/C/D and sublineages B1/B2 (**a**) and for HPV58 lineages A/B/C/D and sublineages A1/A2/A3 (**b**) are indicated with colored bars. The genome organization of HPV52/58 is shown below: pE, the early promoter; pL, the late promoter; LCR, the long control region; polyA (early) and polyA (late), the early and late polyadenylation signals, respectively

## Discussion

By employing next generation sequencing analyses, we are able to report the largest number of complete genome sequences of HPV52/58 in a single study, and have demonstrated variant distributions of HPV52/58 among Japanese women. Intriguingly, lineage B for HPV52 and lineage A for HPV58 were predominantly detected across the CIN/ICC cases in Japan. Moreover, three HPV52 and four HPV58 genome sequences previously determined by us [24] were also included in HPV52 lineage B and HPV58 lineage A, respectively. These findings are in good agreement with a general trend in HPV52/58 variant distributions, suggesting that HPV52 lineage B and HPV58 lineage A are more prevalent in Asia than in Europe, the Americas, and Africa [16, 32]. Further, a high prevalence of lineage B in HPV52-positive cervical specimens was reported in

South Korea [33] and Taiwan [17], and the dominance of lineage A in HPV58-positive specimens was also observed in Taiwan [17], which strongly suggests that such biased distributions of HPV52/58 variant lineages are common among East Asian countries.

In previous studies, a comparison of HPV52/58 variant distributions between different grades of cervical lesions suggested that specific variant lineages, such as HPV52 lineage B [16] and HPV58 lineage A [18], might pose higher risks for cervical cancer development. Meanwhile, because of highly dominant distributions of these HPV52/58 lineages across the CIN/ICC cases in Japan, we were unable to assess a differential risk of these lineages for CIN/ICC progression. Thus, the association of HPV52 lineage B or HPV58 lineage A with cervical cancer development requires further verification with larger sample sizes consisting of mixed distributions of variant lineages.

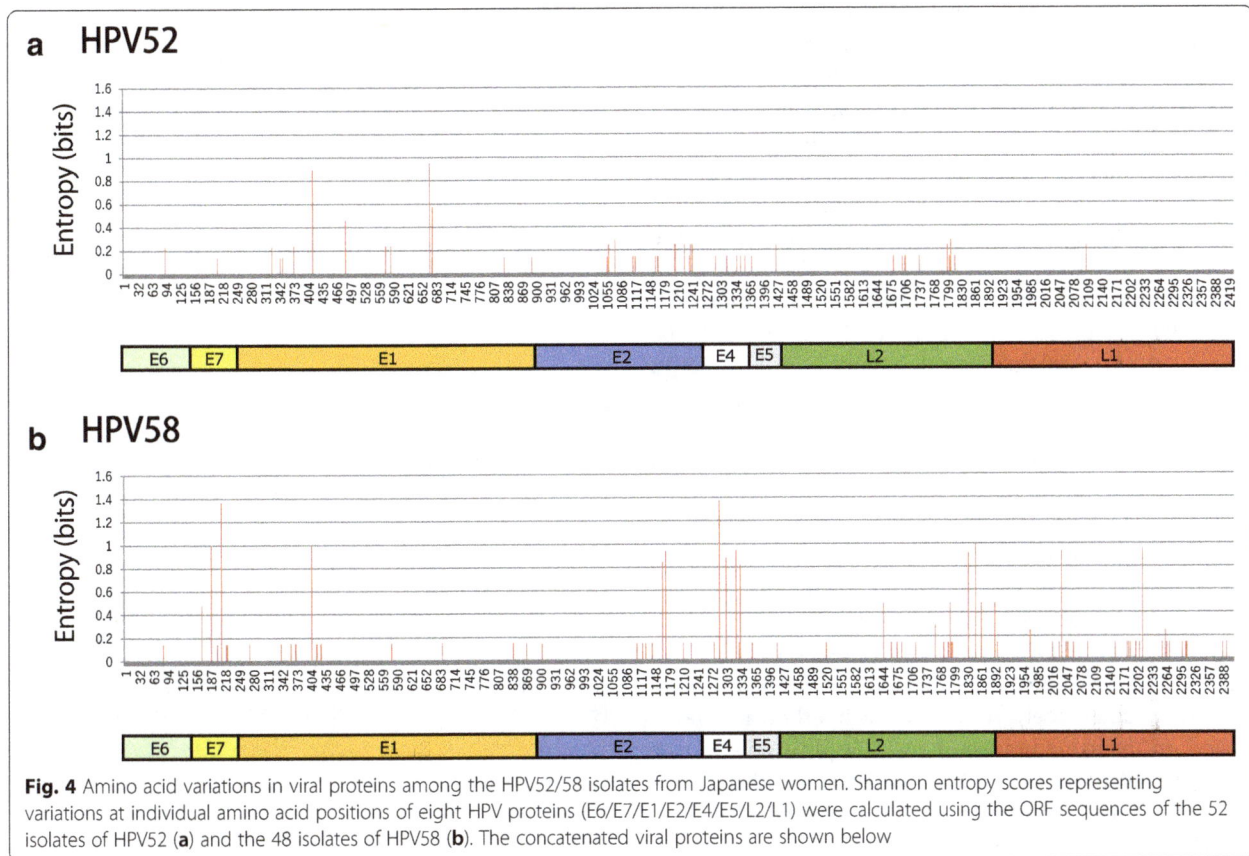

**Fig. 4** Amino acid variations in viral proteins among the HPV52/58 isolates from Japanese women. Shannon entropy scores representing variations at individual amino acid positions of eight HPV proteins (E6/E7/E1/E2/E4/E5/L2/L1) were calculated using the ORF sequences of the 52 isolates of HPV52 (**a**) and the 48 isolates of HPV58 (**b**). The concatenated viral proteins are shown below

Previous studies described E7 T20I/G63S substitutions in HPV58 as a high-risk signature for ICC development [19, 34]. Our phylogenetic analysis demonstrated that all sublineage A3 genomes carried this pair of substitutions; 20I (632 T) was specific to sublineage A3, whereas 63S (760A) was not restricted to sublineage A3 but also found in three lineage B genomes (HQ537761, HQ537762, and HQ537763). The T20I/G63S substitutions were observed in five HPV58 isolates in this study, all of which belonged to sublineage A3, although the small sample size precluded our risk assessment of this variation.

The genomic sequences of several HPV52/58 isolates showed some characteristic features, such as deletions in E2/E4 and E1, and insertion in L2. Intriguingly, all E2/E4 deletions observed in the HPV52 isolates were in-frame deletions (36, 39, and 57 nucleotides deletions), and thus supposed to generate internally deleted E2/E4 proteins, which may have altered biological activities for viral transcription, replication and segregation [35]. Of particular interest, these deleted E2/E4 genes were all recovered from CIN3/ICC samples, supporting a prevailing notion that E2 deletion or inactivation favors cervical cancer progression, because the E2 protein generally represses the viral early promoter responsible for E6/E7 expression, which is required for oncogenic transformation of cervical epithelial cells [1]. The E1 deletion in

HPV58 and the L2 insertion in HPV52, both observed in CIN1 samples, were not in-frame, and were positioned near their N-terminus. These two genetic changes would be expected to abrogate the functions of the corresponding viral proteins, although the consequence of these deletions on the viral life-cycle and cervical carcinogenesis remains unclear.

By comparing the whole-genome sequences of our Japanese HPV52/58 isolates with those of reference HPV52/58 genomes representing all variant lineages/sublineages, we have presented for the first time a comprehensive list of specific SNPs for discriminating their variant lineages/sublineages. In general, these diagnostic SNPs are dispersed throughout the viral genome, as was reported for HPV16 [36] and HPV6 [37]. However, cautions should be exercised because some genomic regions in HPV52/58 lack such diagnostic SNPs for specific lineage/sublineage identification, as visualized in Fig. 3. Although previous variant classification for HPV52/58 mostly depended on partial sequences in E6, E7, E2, L1 or LCR [17, 20–22], the diagnostic SNPs described in this study will be useful for designing new PCR targets and primers to correctly assign variant lineages/sublineages of HPV52/58 in future epidemiological studies.

Previously, a nucleotide substitution in the L1 region of HPV52 (6764 T to C compared to the prototype,

X74481) was reported to generate a mismatched base to the GP6+ primer, one of the consensus primers of GP5 +/6+ PCR to amplify L1 DNA of multiple HPV types [38]. Among the 52 isolates of HPV52 obtained in this study, 49 isolates (all sublineage B2) carried this substitution, whereas three isolates (two sublineage A1 and one sublineage B2) had the prototype nucleotide in this position. Since this substitution precluded the detection of HPV52 by GP5+/6+ PCR, leading to underestimation of HPV52 prevalence [38], other PCR methods, such as PGMY09/11 PCR, should be employed for epidemiological surveys on HPV52 in Japan.

The variability of amino acid residues in viral proteins reflects the degree of non-synonymous substitution in the nucleotide sequences of ORFs, and the higher variation at certain amino acid positions suggests that these positions are either neutral or under diversifying selection pressure during viral evolution. From such an evolutionary point of view, the different patterns of amino acid variations in the viral proteins observed in HPV52 and HPV58 are unexpected because these two viruses are genetically closely related to each other and positioned on the same branch of an HPV phylogenetic tree (*Alphapapillomaviruse-9*) [39]. We speculate that different evolutionary pressures may work on the HPV52/58 genomes, thereby restricting or allowing their genomic diversity in a different manner. Subtle differences in the viral life-cycle or virus/host interactions, such as the host immune response, may exist between these closely related HPVs.

An important unanswered question is why HPV52/58 infections are so common in Asia compared to other parts of the world. During the long history of HPV evolution and spread across the globe, these genotypes might have matched a characteristic property of Asian people through as-yet-unknown mechanisms of viral adaptation. Since HPV52/58 infections pose a significant disease burden of cervical cancer on Asian women, further work based on the viral whole-genome sequences, together with elucidation of the genetic background of Asian people including human leukocyte antigen polymorphism, will be required for a better understanding of cervical carcinogenesis driven by these Asia-prevalent HPVs.

## Conclusions

Among the HPV52/58-positive specimens from Japanese women with CIN/ICC, the variant distributions were strongly biased toward lineage B for HPV52 and lineage A for HPV58 across histological categories. Different patterns of amino acid variations were observed in HPV52 and HPV58 across the viral whole-genome.

## Abbreviations
CIN 1: Cervical Intraepithelial Neoplasia Grade 1; CIN 2: Cervical Intraepithelial Neoplasia Grade 2; CIN 3: Cervical Intraepithelial Neoplasia Grade 3; HPV: Human Papillomavirus; ICC: Invasive Cervical Cancer; LCR: Long Control Region; ORF: Open Reading Frame; SNP: Single Nucleotide Polymorphism

## Acknowledgments
We thank all the patients who participated in this study. We also thank Hironori Sato for his critical comments on the manuscript and Tsuyoshi Sekizuka for his help in sequence alignment analyses.

## Funding
This work was supported by JSPS KAKENHI Grant Numbers 65K10701, 26460564, and 17K11297.

## Authors' contributions
MO, NT, TS, TM, SM, TI, KM, and AS collected clinical specimens. TT, YI, and SM performed HPV genotyping. YT and YH carried out PCR amplification, next generation sequencing, and the bioinformatics analyses. IK conceived of and designed the study, supervised all experiments and analyses, and wrote the manuscript. All authors read and approved the final manuscript.

## Competing interests
The authors declare that they have no competing interests.

## Author details
[1]Department of Obstetrics and Gynecology, Showa University School of Medicine, Tokyo, Japan. [2]Pathogen Genomics Center, National Institute of Infectious Diseases, 4-7-1 Gakuen, Musashi-murayama, Tokyo 208-0011, Japan. [3]Department of Obstetrics and Gynecology, Faculty of Medicine, University of Tsukuba, Tsukuba, Japan. [4]Department of Obstetrics and Gynecology, Keio University School of Medicine, Tokyo, Japan.

## References
1. zur Hausen H. Papillomaviruses and cancer: from basic studies to clinical application. Nat Rev Cancer. 2002;2(5):342–50.
2. Bzhalava D, Eklund C, Dillner J. International standardization and classification of human papillomavirus types. Virology. 2015;476:341–4.
3. Arbyn M, Tommasino M, Depuydt C, Dillner J. Are 20 human papillomavirus types causing cervical cancer? J Pathol. 2014;234(4):431–5.
4. Doorbar J, Egawa N, Griffin H, Kranjec C, Murakami I. Human papillomavirus molecular biology and disease association. Rev Med Virol. 2015;25(Suppl 1):2–23.
5. Moody CA, Laimins LA. Human papillomavirus oncoproteins: pathways to transformation. Nat Rev Cancer. 2010;10(8):550–60.
6. de Sanjose S, Quint WG, Alemany L, Geraets DT, Klaustermeier JE, Lloveras B, Tous S, Felix A, Bravo LE, Shin HR, et al. Human papillomavirus genotype attribution in invasive cervical cancer: a retrospective cross-sectional worldwide study. Lancet Oncol. 2010;11(11):1048–56.
7. Smith JS, Lindsay L, Hoots B, Keys J, Franceschi S, Winer R, Clifford GM. Human papillomavirus type distribution in invasive cervical cancer and high-grade cervical lesions: a meta-analysis update. Int J Cancer. 2007;121(3):621–32.

8.  Li N, Franceschi S, Howell-Jones R, Snijders PJ, Clifford GM. Human papillomavirus type distribution in 30,848 invasive cervical cancers worldwide: variation by geographical region, histological type and year of publication. Int J Cancer. 2011;128(4):927–35.

9.  Chan PK, Ho WC, Chan MC, Wong MC, Yeung AC, Chor JS, Hui M. Meta-analysis on prevalence and attribution of human papillomavirus types 52 and 58 in cervical neoplasia worldwide. PLoS One. 2014;9(9):e107573.

10. Onuki M, Matsumoto K, Satoh T, Oki A, Okada S, Minaguchi T, Ochi H, Nakao S, Someya K, Yamada N, et al. Human papillomavirus infections among Japanese women: age-related prevalence and type-specific risk for cervical cancer. Cancer Sci. 2009;100(7):1312–6.

11. Azuma Y, Kusumoto-Matsuo R, Takeuchi F, Uenoyama A, Kondo K, Tsunoda H, Nagasaka K, Kawana K, Morisada T, Iwata T, et al. Human papillomavirus genotype distribution in cervical intraepithelial neoplasia grade 2/3 and invasive cervical cancer in Japanese women. Jpn J Clin Oncol. 2014;44(10):910–7.

12. Burk RD, Harari A, Chen Z. Human papillomavirus genome variants. Virology. 2013;445(1–2):232–43.

13. Nicolas-Parraga S, Alemany L, de Sanjose S, Bosch FX, Bravo IG, Ris Hpv TT, groups HVs. Differential HPV16 variant distribution in squamous cell carcinoma, adenocarcinoma and adenosquamous cell carcinoma. Int J Cancer. 2017;140(9):2092–100.

14. Hang D, Yin Y, Han J, Jiang J, Ma H, Xie S, Feng X, Zhang K, Hu Z, Shen H, et al. Analysis of human papillomavirus 16 variants and risk for cervical cancer in Chinese population. Virology. 2016;488:156–61.

15. Mirabello L, Yeager M, Cullen M, Boland JF, Chen Z, Wentzensen N, Zhang X, Yu K, Yang Q, Mitchell J, et al. HPV16 Sublineage Associations With Histology-Specific Cancer Risk Using HPV Whole-Genome Sequences in 3200 Women. J Natl Cancer Inst. 2016;108(9):djw100. https://doi.org/10.1093/jnci/djw100.

16. Zhang C, Park JS, Grce M, Hibbitts S, Palefsky JM, Konno R, Smith-McCune KK, Giovannelli L, Chu TY, Picconi MA, et al. Geographical distribution and risk association of human papillomavirus genotype 52-variant lineages. J Infect Dis. 2014;210(10):1600–4.

17. Chang Y-J, Chen H-C, Lee B-H, You S-L, Lin C-Y, Pan M-H, Chou Y-C, Hsieh C-Y, Chen Y-MA, Cheng Y-J, et al. Unique variants of human papillomavirus genotypes 52 and 58 and risk of cervical neoplasia. Int J Cancer. 2011;129(4):965–73.

18. Schiffman M, Rodriguez AC, Chen Z, Wacholder S, Herrero R, Hildesheim A, Desalle R, Befano B, Yu K, Safaeian M, et al. A population-based prospective study of carcinogenic human papillomavirus variant lineages, viral persistence, and cervical neoplasia. Cancer Res. 2010;70(8):3159–69.

19. Chan PK, Zhang C, Park JS, Smith-McCune KK, Palefsky JM, Giovannelli L, Coutlee F, Hibbitts S, Konno R, Settheetham-Ishida W, et al. Geographical distribution and oncogenic risk association of human papillomavirus type 58 E6 and E7 sequence variations. Int J Cancer. 2013;132(11):2528–36.

20. Xin CY, Matsumoto K, Yoshikawa H, Yasugi T, Onda T, Nakagawa S, Yamada M, Nozawa S, Sekiya S, Hirai Y, et al. Analysis of E6 variants of human papillomavirus type 33, 52 and 58 in Japanese women with cervical intraepithelial neoplasia/cervical cancer in relation to their oncogenic potential. Cancer Lett. 2001;170(1):19–24.

21. Bae J-H. Distribution of human papillomavirus type 58 variants in progression of cervical dysplasia in Korean women. J Microbiol Biotechnol. 2009;19(9):1051–4.

22. Chen Q, Luo ZY, Lin M, Yang L, Yang LY, Ju GZ. Evaluation of the genetic variability of human papillomavirus type 52. Int J Mol Med. 2012;30(3):535–44.

23. Kondo K, Uenoyama A, Kitagawa R, Tsunoda H, Kusumoto-Matsuo R, Mori S, Ishii Y, Takeuchi T, Kanda T, Kukimoto I. Genotype distribution of human papillomaviruses in Japanese women with abnormal cervical cytology. Open Virol J. 2012;6:277–83.

24. Kukimoto I, Maehama T, Sekizuka T, Ogasawara Y, Kondo K, Kusumoto-Matsuo R, Mori S, Ishii Y, Takeuchi T, Yamaji T, et al. Genetic variation of human papillomavirus type 16 in individual clinical specimens revealed by deep sequencing. PLoS One. 2013;8(11):e80583.

25. Yamashita A, Sekizuka T, Kuroda M. VirusTAP: viral genome-targeted assembly pipeline. Front Microbiol. 2016;7:32.

26. Li H, Durbin R. Fast and accurate long-read alignment with Burrows-Wheeler transform. Bioinformatics. 2010;26(5):589–95.

27. Thorvaldsdottir H, Robinson JT, Mesirov JP. Integrative Genomics Viewer (IGV): high-performance genomics data visualization and exploration. Brief Bioinform. 2013;14(2):178–92.

28. Katoh K, Asimenos G, Toh H. Multiple alignment of DNA sequences with MAFFT. Methods Mol Biol. 2009;537:39–64.

29. Stamatakis A. RAxML version 8: a tool for phylogenetic analysis and post-analysis of large phylogenies. Bioinformatics. 2014;30(9):1312–3.

30. Shannon CE. The mathematical theory of communication. 1963. MD Comput. 1997;14(4):306–17.

31. Grant BJ, Rodrigues AP, ElSawy KM, McCammon JA, Caves LS. Bio3d: an R package for the comparative analysis of protein structures. Bioinformatics. 2006;22(21):2695–6.

32. Chan PKS, Luk ACS, Park JS, Smith-McCune KK, Palefsky JM, Konno R, Giovannelli L, Coutlee F, Hibbitts S, Chu TY, et al. Identification of human papillomavirus type 58 lineages and the distribution worldwide. J Infect Dis. 2011;203(11):1565–73.

33. Choi YJ, Ki EY, Zhang C, Ho WC, Lee SJ, Jeong MJ, Chan PK, Park JS. Analysis of sequence variation and risk association of human papillomavirus 52 variants circulating in Korea. PLoS One. 2016;11(12):e0168178.

34. Chan PK, Lam CW, Cheung TH, Li WW, Lo KW, Chan MY, Cheung JL, Cheng AF. Association of human papillomavirus type 58 variant with the risk of cervical cancer. J Natl Cancer Inst. 2002;94(16):1249–53.

35. McBride AA. The papillomavirus E2 proteins. Virology. 2013;445(1–2):57–79.

36. Smith B, Chen Z, Reimers L, van Doorslaer K, Schiffman M, Desalle R, Herrero R, Yu K, Wacholder S, Wang T, et al. Sequence imputation of HPV16 genomes for genetic association studies. PLoS One. 2011;6(6):e21375.

37. Jelen MM, Chen Z, Kocjan BJ, Burt FJ, Chan PK, Chouhy D, Combrinck CE, Coutlee F, Estrade C, Ferenczy A, et al. Global genomic diversity of human papillomavirus 6 based on 724 isolates and 190 complete genome sequences. J Virol. 2014;88(13):7307–16.

38. Chan PK, Cheung TH, Tam AO, Lo KW, Yim SF, Yu MM, To KF, Wong YF, Cheung JL, Chan DP, et al. Biases in human papillomavirus genotype prevalence assessment associated with commonly used consensus primers. Int J Cancer. 2006;118(1):243–5.

39. Bernard HU, Burk RD, Chen Z, van Doorslaer K, zur Hausen H, de Villiers EM. Classification of papillomaviruses (PVs) based on 189 PV types and proposal of taxonomic amendments. Virology. 2010;401(1):70–9.

# 18

# Prognostic factors in patients with HBV-related hepatocellular carcinoma following hepatic resection

Narongsak Rungsakulkij[*] (iD), Wikran Suragul, Somkit Mingphruedhi, Pongsatorn Tangtawee, Paramin Muangkaew and Suraida Aeesoa

## Abstract

**Background:** To analyze prognostic factors following hepatic resection in patients with HBV-related hepatocellular carcinoma.

**Methods:** We retrospectively analyzed 217 patients with HBV-related hepatocellular carcinoma who underwent hepatic resection at our hospital between January 2006 and December 2015. Disease-free survival and overall survival rates were analyzed using the Kaplan–Meier method and the log-rank test. The association between recurrence and survival and various clinicopathological factors, including serum alpha-fetoprotein (AFP) level, platelet count, platelet-to-lymphocyte ratio, neutrophil-to-lymphocyte ratio, antiplatelet therapy, antiviral therapy, hepatitis C virus infection, and tumor-related characteristics, were assessed using univariate and multivariate logistic regression analysis.

**Results:** The 1-, 3-, and 5-year overall survival rates were 91, 84, and 79%, respectively, and the recurrence-free survival rates were 72, 51, and 44%, respectively. High post-operative AFP level (hazard ratio [HR] 1.112, 95% confidence interval [CI]: 1.02–1.21, $P = 0.007$), multiple tumors (HR 1.991, 95% CI: 1.11–3.56, $P = 0.021$), and no antiviral treatment (HR 1.823, 95% CI: 1.07–3.09, $P = 0.026$) were independent risk factors for recurrence. High post-operative AFP level (HR 1.222, 95% CI: 1.09–1.36, $P < 0.001$), multiple tumors (HR 2.715, 95% CI: 1.05–7.02, $P = 0.039$), and recurrence (HR 12.824, 95% CI: 1.68–97.86, $P = 0.014$) were independent risk factors for mortality. No other factors analyzed were associated with outcomes in this patient cohort.

**Conclusions:** High post-operative serum alpha-fetoprotein level and multiple tumors, but not inflammatory factors, were risk factors for poor prognosis in HBV-related hepatocellular carcinoma patients after resection.

**Keywords:** Alpha-fetoprotein, Hepatitis B virus, Hepatocellular carcinoma, Risk factors, Survival rate

## Background

Hepatocellular carcinoma (HCC) is the most common type of primary liver cancer worldwide [1]. The Eastern Asia and sub-Saharan Africa are the highest areas in hepatitis B virus (HBV) related HCC [2]. In Thailand, HCC is most frequently caused by chronic HBV infection [3, 4]. Surgical resection is potentially curative for early-stage disease if liver functional reserve is adequate [5], but its outcome in HBV-related HCC patients is generally poor [6]. Cirrhosis, chronic hepatitis [7, 8], and

chronic HBV infection are considered to be poor prognostic factors following hepatic resection in HCC patients [9].

Inflammation is a key contributor to the pathogenesis of HCC in patients with chronic HBV infection [10–12]. Many studies have investigated the utility of inflammatory factors and indices as prognostic markers for HBV-related HCC patients following hepatic resection; however, the results are controversial [13–19]. Recent reports suggest that platelets play a major role in the pathogenesis of HCC in HBV-infected patients [20, 21]. Indeed, antiplatelet therapy reduces the incidence of HCC in an HBV-infected mouse model [22]. In addition, Lee et al. reported that HBV-related HCC patients

* Correspondence: narongsak.run@mahidol.ac.th
Department of Surgery, Faculty of Medicine, Ramathibodi Hospital, Mahidol University, 270 Praram VI Road, Ratchathewi, Bangkok 10400, Thailand

receiving antiplatelet therapy showed better recurrence-free and overall survival after liver resection than untreated patients [23]. Given these observations, we investigated the prognostic value of platelet counts, antiplatelet therapy, inflammatory indices, and various tumor-related characteristics in patients with HBV-related HCC following hepatic resection.

## Methods

A total of 387 consecutive patients underwent liver resection and had pathologically proven HCC at the Department of Surgery, Ramathibodi Hospital, Mahidol University, Bangkok, Thailand between January 2006 and December 2015. All patients were followed-up until December 2017. Of these, we retrospectively analyzed data from the 217 patients with HBV-related HCC. The patients who had HDV co-infection were excluded from the study. All patients underwent preoperative cross-sectional dynamic imaging using either triple-phase CT or magnetic resonance imaging (MRI). Routine blood examinations included complete blood count, coagulogram, liver and kidney function tests, and preoperative serum alpha-fetoprotein (AFP) level. The serum AFP level are measured by electrochemiluminescence immunoassay method, AFP ELISA reagent Roche Elecsys®, Roche Diagnostics USA, Indiana, United State. The neutrophil-to-lymphocyte ratio and platelet-to-lymphocyte ratio were calculated. The prognostic nutritional index was calculated as ([albumin {g/L} + 0.005] × [total lymphocyte count {/μL}]). A preoperative indocyanine green retention test at 15 min (ICG-R15) was performed. The Makuuchi criteria are used for patient selection for curative resection in our center [24]. The extent of liver resection was based on the patient's liver functional reserve as assessed mainly by the Makuuchi criteria, including preoperative ascites volume, Child–Pugh score, ICG-R15 value, and, occasionally, volumetric CT analysis. Liver cirrhosis was defined by the macro or micro nodular surface of the liver intraoperatively.

Pathological specimens were reviewed by a pathologist to confirm the diagnosis of HCC. Patients with combined cholangiocarcinoma and other malignancies were excluded from this study. Microvascular invasion was defined as the presence of tumor cells in the microvasculature. Clinical and pathologic staging was performed according to the American Joint Committee on Cancer staging manual 7th edition [25].

Patients were followed up in outpatient clinics every 3 or 4 months after surgery and routinely underwent imaging studies (ultrasonography, CT, MRI) and blood examinations. Post-operative serum AFP levels were measured within 90 days after hepatic resection. Recurrent disease was defined as the presence of new tumors found by imaging (CT or MRI) during the follow-up period.

### Statistical analyses

Patient characteristics with continuous variables were compared by Student's t-test, and categorical variables were compared with $\chi 2$ or Fisher's exact test. A $P$ value of $< 0.05$ was considered statistically significant. The potential risk factors were analyzed by univariate and multivariate methods using a Cox regression model. Independent risk factors were expressed as hazard ratios (HR) with 95% confidence intervals (CI). Survival analysis was performed using the Kaplan–Meier method and evaluated by the log-rank test. The cut-off value for post-hepatectomy serum AFP level was determined by receiver operating characteristic (ROC) curve analysis with most significance in predicting tumor recurrence after hepatectomy.

## Results

### Patient characteristics and perioperative status

Of the 387 consecutive patients who underwent curative resection for HCC from January 2006 to December 2015, 217 (56.0%) had HBV-related HCC and were evaluated here. The clinicopathological characteristics of this cohort are summarized in Table 1.

### Risk factors associated with disease recurrence

A comparison between patients with and without disease recurrence is shown in Table 2. The recurrence rate following resection was 47.9% (104/217). Compared with the non-recurrence group, the recurrence group had a higher post-operative AFP level (2.8 vs 3.8 ng/mL, $P = 0.045$), was more likely to have multiple tumors (32 vs 16 patients, $P = 0.004$), and was less likely to have received preoperative neoadjuvant treatment (48/92 vs 26/72 patients, $P = 0.04$). Univariate analysis (Table 3) identified the following factors as significantly associated with disease recurrence: post-operative AFP level (HR 1.112, 95% CI: 1.02–1.21, $P = 0.012$), tumor size (HR 1.061, 95% CI: 1.01–1.11, $P = 0.013$), multiple tumors (HR 1.881, 95% CI: 1.23–2.86, $P = 0.003$), microvascular invasion (HR 1.645, 95% CI: 1.02–2.63, $P = 0.037$), stage II or higher (HR 1.553, 95% CI 1.04–2.31, $P = 0.031$), and no antiviral treatment (HR 1.519, 95% CI: 1.01–2.28, $P = 0.045$). In multivariate analysis (Table 3), post-operative AFP (HR 1.112, 95% CI: 1.02–1.21, $P = 0.007$), multiple tumors (HR 1.991, 95% CI: 1.11–3.56, $P = 0.021$), and no antiviral treatment (HR 1.823, 95% CI: 1.07–3.09, $P = 0.026$) remained independent risk factors for recurrence.

### Risk factors associated with mortality

Table 4 shows the comparison of survivors and non-survivors. The survival rate of HBV-related HCC

**Table 1** Clinicopathological features of patients with HBV-related hepatocellular carcinoma

| Characteristic | Value |
|---|---|
| Gender, n (%) (total cohort n = 217) | |
| male | 100 (46.08) |
| female | 117 (53.92) |
| Age (years), mean ± sd | 56.12 (9.78) |
| HBsAg, n (%) | |
| negative | 16 (7.37) |
| positive | 201 (92.62) |
| HBeAg, n (%), n = 119 | |
| negative | 85 (71.43) |
| positive | 34 (28.57) |
| HBV DNA, n (%), n = 103 | |
| negative | 41 (39.81) |
| positive | 62 (60.19) |
| HCV, n (%) | |
| no | 210 (96.77) |
| yes | 7 (3.23) |
| Platelets × 10$^3$ (mm3), median (range) | 190.5 (57, 568) |
| AFP-pre (ng/mL), median (range), n = 185 | 16.8 (0.89, 82,392) |
| AFP-post (ng/mL), median (range), n = 125 | 3.48 (0.83, 19,629) |
| Tumor size (cm), median (range), n = 216 | 4.5 (0.5, 26.5) |
| < 5 | 120 (55.56) |
| ≥ 5 | 96 (44.44) |
| Number of tumors, n (%) | |
| solitary | 166 (77.57) |
| multiple | 48 (22.43) |
| Microvascular invasion, n (%) | |
| no | 170 (79.44) |
| yes | 44 (20.56) |
| Stage, n (%) | |
| I | 138 (63.59) |
| II or higher | 79 (36.41) |
| Resection margin, n (%), n = 185 | |
| free margin | 176 (95.14) |
| positive margin | 9 (4.86) |
| Operation type, n (%) | |
| non-anatomical | 129 (59.45) |
| anatomical | 88 (40.55) |
| Preoperative neoadjuvant, n (%), n = 164 | |
| no | 92 (56.10) |
| yes | 72 (43.90) |
| Platelet-to-lymphocyte ratio, median (range), n = 203 | 101.8 (30.9, 432.8) |
| Prognostic nutritional index, mean ± sd n = 206 | 95.18 (40.21) |
| | 1.77 (0.33, 10.62) |

**Table 1** Clinicopathological features of patients with HBV-related hepatocellular carcinoma (Continued)

| Characteristic | Value |
|---|---|
| Neutrophil-to-lymphocyte ratio, median (range), n = 201 | |
| Antiviral treatment | |
| no | 65 (29.95) |
| yes | 152 (70.05) |
| Antiviral drug, n (%) | |
| Adefovir | 7 (3.23) |
| Lamivudine | 125 (57.60) |
| Tenofovir | 44 (20.28) |
| Entecavir | 20 (9.22) |
| Antiplatelet treatment (ASA + Clopidogrel) | |
| no | 199 (91.71) |
| yes | 18 (8.29) |
| Recurrence, n (%) | |
| no | 113 (52.07) |
| yes | 104 (47.93) |
| Follow-up time (months), median (range) | 36.33 (0.23, 149.07) |

*AFP* alpha-fetoprotein, *ASA* aspirin, *HCV* hepatitis C virus, *sd* standard deviation

patients following hepatectomy was 82.5% (179/217). Compared with the survivor group, non-survivors had significantly higher pre- and post-operative AFP levels (115 vs 14.2 ng/mL, $P = 0.018$ and 13.11 vs 2.8 ng/mL, $P < 0.001$, respectively) and were more likely to have multiple tumors than a solitary tumor (14/48 vs 23/166 patients, $P = 0.013$). Patients undergoing anatomical resection also had a higher mortality rate than those undergoing other operations (22/88 vs 16/129, $P = 0.017$). As shown in Table 5, univariate analysis identified the following factors as significantly associated with survival: post-operative AFP level (HR 1.218, 95% CI: 1.10–1.35, $P < 0.001$), tumor size ≥5 cm (HR 1.679, 95% CI: 1.01–2.77, $P = 0.044$), multiple tumors (HR 2.300 95% CI: 1.18–4.47, $P = 0.014$), anatomical resection (HR 2.443, 95% CI: 1.28–4.65, $P = 0.007$), no antiviral treatment (HR 0.482, 95% CI: 0.25–0.92, $P = 0.027$), and recurrence (HR 2.940, 95% CI: 1.40–6.05, $P = 0.003$). In multivariate analysis, post-operative AFP (HR 1.222, 95% CI: 1.09–1.36, $P < 0.001$), multiple tumors (HR 2.715, 95% CI: 1.05–7.02, $P = 0.039$), and recurrence (HR 12.824, 95% CI: 1.68–97.86, $P = 0.014$) were independent risk factors for death (Table 5).

### Overall survival and recurrence-free survival analysis

The Kaplan–Meier analysis curves for recurrence-free survival (RFS) and overall survival (OS) of all patients are shown in Fig. 1. The overall 1-, 3-, and 5-year overall survival rates were 91, 84, and 79%, respectively, and the RFS rates were 72, 51, and 44%, respectively. As

**Table 2** Clinicopathological features of patients in the non-recurrence and recurrence groups

| Characteristic | Non-Recurrence ($n = 113$) | Recurrence ($n = 104$) | P value |
|---|---|---|---|
| Gender, n (%) (total cohort $n = 217$) | | | |
|    male | 49 (43.36) | 51 (49.04) | 0.402 |
|    female | 64 (56.64) | 53 (50.96) | |
| Age (years), mean ± sd | 56.46 (10.60) | 55.76 (8.86) | 0.604 |
| HCV, n (%) | | | |
|    no | 111 (98.23) | 99 (95.19) | 0.264 |
|    yes | 2 (1.77) | 5 (4.81) | |
| Platelets × 103, median (range), $n = 384$ | 198.5 (57, 465) | 179.5 (76, 568) | 0.068 |
| AFP-pre (ng/mL), median (range), $n = 325$ | 15.2 (0.89, 60,500) | 17.03 (1.1, 82,392) | 0.572 |
| AFP-post (ng/mL), median (range), $n = 226$ | 2.8 (0.83, 5271) | 3.8 (0.9, 19,629) | *0.045* |
| Tumor size (cm), median (range), $n = 386$ | 4.3 (0.6, 26.5) | 5 (0.5, 18) | 0.511 |
|    < 5 | 63 (55.75) | 57 (55.34) | 0.951 |
|    ≥ 5 | 50 (44.25) | 46 (44.66) | |
| Number of tumors, n (%), $n = 382$ | | | |
|    solitary | 94 (85.45) | 72 (69.23) | *0.004* |
|    multiple | 16 (14.55) | 32 (30.77) | |
| Microvascular invasion, n (%), $n = 382$ | | | |
|    no | 89 (80.91) | 81 (77.88) | 0.584 |
|    yes | 21 (19.09) | 23 (22.12) | |
| Stage, n (%) | | | |
|    I | 77 (68.14) | 61 (58.65) | 0.147 |
|    II or higher | 36 (31.86) | 43 (41.35) | |
| Resection margin, n (%), $n = 325$ | | | |
|    free margin | 89 (94.68) | 87 (95.60) | 0.999 |
|    positive margin | 5 (5.32) | 4 (4.40) | |
| Operation type, n (%) | | | |
|    non-anatomical | 69 (61.06) | 60 (57.69) | 0.614 |
|    anatomical | 44 (38.94) | 44 (42.31) | |
| Preoperative neoadjuvant, n (%), $n = 289$ | | | |
|    no | 44 (48.89) | 48 (64.86) | *0.040* |
|    yes | 46 (51.11) | 26 (35.14) | |
| Platelet-to-lymphocyte ratio, median (range), $n = 365$ | 106.6 (46.3, 432.8) | 91.2 (30.9, 290.7) | 0.128 |
| Prognostic nutritional index, median (range), $n = 370$ | 89.12 (0.34, 265.26) | 91.9 (0.41, 245.02) | 0.764 |
| Neutrophil-to-lymphocyte ratio, median (range), $n = 361$ | 1.78 (0.67, 8.11) | 1.76 (0.33, 10.62) | 0.770 |
| Antiviral treatment | | | |
|    no | 30 (26.55) | 35 (33.65) | 0.254 |
|    yes | 83 (73.45) | 69 (66.35) | |
| Antiviral drug | | | |
|    Adefovir | 4 (3.54) | 3 (2.88) | 0.999 |
|    Lamivudine | 66 (58.41) | 59 (56.73) | 0.254 |
|    Tenofovir | 28 (25.66) | 15 (14.42) | 0.021 |
|    Entecavir | 10 (8.85) | 10 (9.62) | 0.846 |

**Table 2** Clinicopathological features of patients in the non-recurrence and recurrence groups *(Continued)*

| Characteristic | Non-Recurrence (*n* = 113) | Recurrence (*n* = 104) | *P* value |
|---|---|---|---|
| Antiplatelet treatment (ASA + Clopidogrel) | | | |
| no | 103 (91.15) | 96 (92.31) | 0.757 |
| yes | 10 (8.85) | 8 (7.69) | |

*AFP* alpha-fetoprotein, *ASA* aspirin, *HCV* hepatitis C virus, *sd* standard deviation
NOTE. Italic font indicates statistical significance

expected, OS was significantly poorer for patients with recurrent compared with non-recurrent disease (Fig. 2). In addition, patients with multiple tumors had poorer OS and RFS than patients with solitary tumors (Fig. 3).

In addition, post-operative AFP was the risk factor of recurrence. Comparison of the patients between high and low post-operative AFP groups. As the first step, the cut-off value for post-AFP was determined by receiver operating characteristic (ROC) curve analysis as shown in Fig. 4. The area under ROC curve was 0.604. The post-operative AFP value 3.5 ng/mL was considered as the optimal cut-off value because of its highest index;

**Table 3** Univariate and multivariate analysis of factors associated with recurrence

| | Univariate | | Multivariate | |
|---|---|---|---|---|
| | HR (95% CI) | *P* value | HR (95% CI) | *P* value |
| Gender (male) | | | | |
| female | 0.894 (0.60–1.32) | 0.574 | | |
| Age (years) | 0.996 (0.97–1.02) | 0.719 | | |
| HCV (no) | | | | |
| yes | 1.473 (0.59–3.62) | 0.399 | | |
| Platelets × 103 (mm3) | 0.987 (0.96–1.01) | 0.367 | | |
| AFP-pre (ng/mL) | 0.996 (0.97–1.01) | 0.665 | | |
| AFP-post (ng/mL) | 1.112 (1.02–1.21) | *0.012* | 1.129 (1.04–1.23) | *0.005* |
| Tumor size (< 5 cm) | 1.061 (1.01–1.11) | *0.013* | | |
| ≥ 5 cm | 1.345 (0.90–1.99) | 0.139 | | |
| Number of tumors (solitary) | | | | |
| multiple | 1.881 (1.23–2.86) | *0.003* | 1.973 (1.15–3.38) | *0.013* |
| Microvascular invasion (no) | | | | |
| yes | 1.645 (1.02–2.63) | *0.037* | | |
| Stage (I) | | | | |
| II or higher | 1.553 (1.04–2.31) | *0.031* | | |
| Resection margin (free margin) | | | | |
| positive margin | 0.977 (0.35–2.66) | 0.964 | | |
| Operation type (anatomical) | | | | |
| non-anatomical | 0.708 (0.47–1.05) | 0.085 | | |
| Preoperative neoadjuvant (no) | | | | |
| yes | 0.828 (0.51–1.34) | 0.450 | | |
| Platelet-to-lymphocyte ratio | 0.913 (0.61–1.34) | 0.648 | | |
| Prognostic nutritional index | 0.959 (0.56–1.61) | 0.875 | | |
| Neutrophil-to-lymphocyte ratio | 1.052 (0.89–1.23) | 0.535 | | |
| Antiviral treatment | | | | |
| no | 1.519 (1.01–2.28) | *0.045* | 1.823 (1.07–3.09) | *0.026* |
| Antiplatelet treatment (ASA + Clopidogrel) | | | | |
| no | 1.018 (0.49–2.09) | 0.961 | | |

*AFP* alpha-fetoprotein, *ASA* aspirin, *CI* confidence interval, *HR* hazard ratio, *HCV* hepatitis C virus
NOTE. Italic font indicates statistical significance

**Table 4** Comparison of clinicopathological features of survivors and non-survivors

| Characteristic | Alive (n = 179) | Dead (n = 38) | P value |
|---|---|---|---|
| Gender, n (%) | | | |
| male | 76 (42.46) | 24 (63.16) | *0.020* |
| female | 103 (57.54) | 14 (36.84) | |
| Age (years), mean ± sd | 56.03 (9.44) | 56.60 (11.39) | 0.742 |
| HCV, n (%) | | | |
| no | 172 (96.09) | 38 (100) | 0.609 |
| yes | 7 (3.91) | 0 | |
| Platelets ×103 (mm3), median (range) | 192 (57, 568) | 185 (91, 332) | 0.485 |
| AFP-pre (ng/mL), median (range), n = 185 | 14.2 (0.89, 82,392) | 115 (1.85, 60,500) | *0.018* |
| AFP-post (ng/mL), median (range), n = 125 | 2.8 (0.83, 5271) | 13.11 (1.19, 19,629) | *0.0003* |
| Tumor size (cm), median (range), n = 216 | 4.3 (0.5, 26.5) | 5.5 (2, 17) | 0.066 |
| < 5 | 103 (57.54) | 17 (45.95) | 0.196 |
| ≥ 5 | 76 (42.46) | 20 (54.05) | |
| Number of tumors, n (%) | | | |
| solitary | 143 (80.79) | 23 (62.16) | *0.013* |
| multiple | 34 (19.21) | 14 (37.84) | |
| Microvascular invasion, n (%) | | | |
| no | 141 (79.66) | 29 (78.38) | 0.861 |
| yes | 36 (20.34) | 8 (21.62) | |
| Stage, n (%) | | | |
| I | 110 (61.45) | 28 (73.68) | 0.155 |
| II or higher | 69 (38.55) | 10 (26.32) | |
| Resection margin, n (%), n = 185 | | | |
| free margin | 144 (96.00) | 32 (91.43) | 0.375 |
| positive margin | 6 (4.00) | 3 (8.57) | |
| Operation type, n (%) | | | |
| non-anatomical | 113 (63.13) | 16 (42.11) | *0.017* |
| anatomical | 66 (36.87) | 22 (57.89) | |
| Preoperative neoadjuvant, n (%) n = 164 | | | |
| no | 71 (53.79) | 21 (65.63) | 0.226 |
| yes | 61 (46.21) | 11 (34.38) | |
| Platelet-to-lymphocyte ratio, median (range), n = 203 | 101.6 (30.9, 432.8) | 107.1 (51.0, 258.9) | 0.339 |
| Prognostic nutritional index, mean ± sd, n = 206 | 97.35 (41.10) | 84.21 (33.78) | 0.082 |
| Neutrophil-to-lymphocyte ratio, median (range), n = 201 | 1.73 (0.33, 10.62) | 2 (0.73, 4.41) | 0.298 |
| Antiviral treatment | | | |
| no | 49 (27.37) | 16 (42.11) | 0.072 |
| yes | 130 (72.63) | 22 (57.89) | |
| Antiplatelet treatment (ASA + Clopidogrel) | | | |
| no | 163 (91.06) | 36 (94.74) | 0.746 |
| yes | 16 (8.94) | 2 (5.26) | |
| Recurrence n (%) | | | |
| no | 103 (57.54) | 10 (26.32) | *0.000* |
| yes | 76 (42.46) | 28 (73.68) | |

*AFP* alpha-fetoprotein, *ASA* aspirin, *HCV* hepatitis C virus, microvascular invasion, *sd* standard deviation

NOTE. Italic font indicates statistical significance

**Table 5** Univariate and multivariate analysis of factors associated with overall survival

| | Univariate | | Multivariate | |
|---|---|---|---|---|
| | HR (95% CI) | P value | HR (95% CI) | P value |
| Gender (male) | | | | |
| female | 0.552 (0.28–1.07) | 0.080 | | |
| Age (years) | 1.002 (0.96–1.04) | 0.890 | | |
| HCV (no) | | | | |
| yes | – | | | |
| Platelets × 103 (mm3) | 0.999 (0.99–1.01) | 0.829 | | |
| AFP-pre (ng/mL) | 1.011 (0.99–1.03) | 0.300 | | |
| AFP-post (ng/mL) | 1.218 (1.10–1.35) | *0.000* | 1.206 (1.08–1.34) | *0.000* |
| Tumor size (< 5 cm) | 1.052 (0.99–1.12) | 0.091 | | |
| ≥ 5 cm. | 1.679 (1.01–2.77) | *0.044* | | |
| Number of tumors (solitary) | | | | |
| multiple | 2.300 (1.18–4.47) | *0.014* | 2.715 (1.05–7.02) | *0.039* |
| Microvascular invasion (no) | | | | |
| yes | 1.598 (0.72–3.54) | 0.249 | | |
| Stage (I) | | | | |
| II or higher | 0.737 (0.35–1.53) | 0.415 | | |
| Resection margin (free margin) | | | | |
| positive margin | 2.140 (0.65–7.05) | 0.211 | | |
| Operation type (anatomical) | | | | |
| non-anatomical | 0.409 (0.21–0.78) | *0.007* | | |
| Preoperative neoadjuvant (no) | | | | |
| yes | 0.958 (0.45–2.01) | 0.910 | | |
| Platelet-to-lymphocyte ratio | 1.003 (0.99–1.01) | 0.195 | | |
| Prognostic nutritional index | 0.991 (0.98–1.00) | 0.065 | | |
| Neutrophil-to-lymphocyte ratio | 1.070 (0.82–1.39) | 0.621 | | |
| Antiviral treatment | | | | |
| no | 0.482 (0.25–0.92) | *0.027* | | |
| Antiplatelet treatment (ASA + Clopidogrel) | | | | |
| no | 1.542 (0.37–6.41) | 0.551 | | |
| Recurrence (no) | | | | |
| yes | 2.940 (1.42–6.05) | *0.003* | 12.824 (1.68–97.86) | *0.014* |

*AFP* alpha-fetoprotein, *ASA* aspirin, *HCV* hepatitis C virus, *sd* standard deviation
NOTE. Italic font indicates statistical significance

the sensitivity and specificity were 56.9 and 58.3%, respectively. The Kaplan-Meier analysis curves for RFS and OS of patients with post-operative AFP level > 3.5 ng/mL had poorer overall and recurrence free survival when compared with post-operative AFP level ≤ 3.5 ng/mL(Fig. 5).

### Outcomes correlation stratified by antiviral treatment in solitary and multiple tumor
The Kaplan-Meier analysis curves for RFS of patients who had soliltary and multiple tumor with or without antiviral treatment (Fig. 6). The RFS in the solitary and multiple tumor groups were not significantly difference with antiviral compared with non-antiviral treatment.

### Discussion
Chronic HBV infection is a major risk factor for the development of HCC, especially in Southeast Asia [26]. The pathogenesis of HBV-induced HCC is complex and involves both direct and indirect mechanisms. The immune response against HBV-infected hepatocytes triggers inflammation and leads to sustained necrosis [12]. Recent work has suggested a role for platelets in

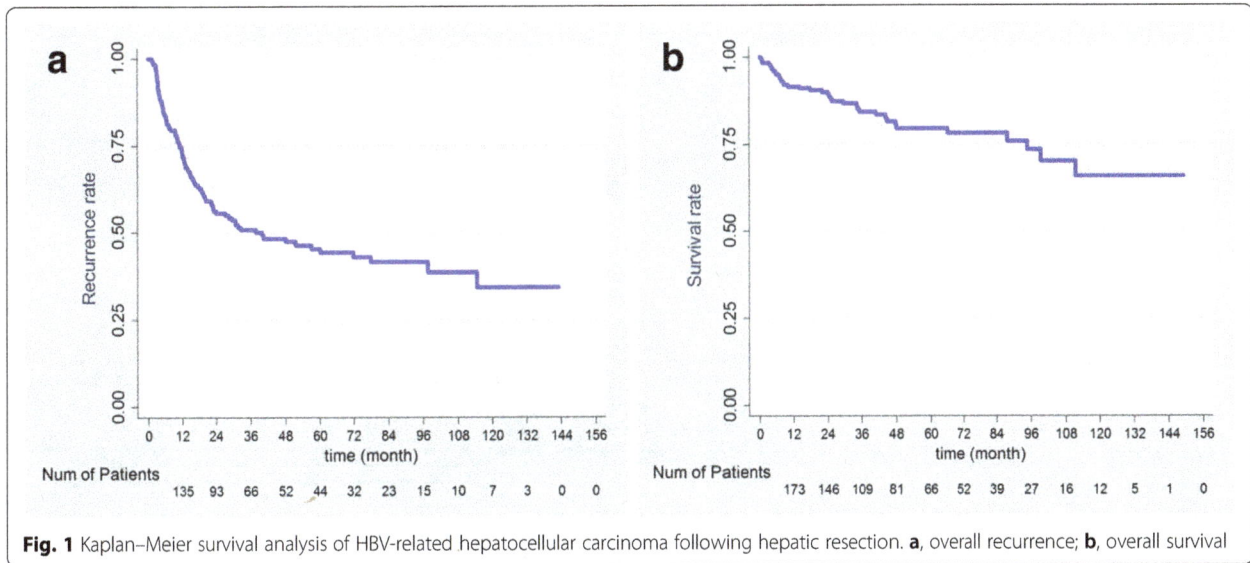

**Fig. 1** Kaplan–Meier survival analysis of HBV-related hepatocellular carcinoma following hepatic resection. **a**, overall recurrence; **b**, overall survival

promoting liver infiltration of cytotoxic T lymphocytes and non-virus-specific inflammatory cells in the pathogenesis of HCC in a HBV transgenic mouse model [20, 27]. In addition, biomarkers such as AFP and inflammatory mediators have been reported to affect the prognosis of HBV-related HCC patients [15, 18, 19, 28–32], although the results are controversial.

In our study, we found that post-operative serum AFP levels and the presence of multiple tumors are predictors of poor prognosis for HBV-related HCC following hepatic resection. AFP is a large glycoprotein produced by the yolk sac and fetal liver. AFP is present in large quantities during gestation and is generally repressed in healthy adults; however, it is re-expressed in a variety of tumors [33, 34]. Several studies have reported correlations between AFP levels and the prognosis of HBV-related HCC patients after curative resection, but most of them measured only preoperative AFP levels and the prognostic impact of AFP levels following hepatic resection was unclear [15, 35–40]. In other studies, post-operative AFP levels were shown to correlate with the prognosis of HCC patients, but the populations in those studies were heterogenous and included both HBV-positive and -negative patients [41–47]. Here, we show for the first time that the post-operative serum AFP level is an independent prognostic factor for survival in HBV-related HCC patients following curative resection. Our results are consistent with a study by Shen et al., who reported that a $\leq 50\%$

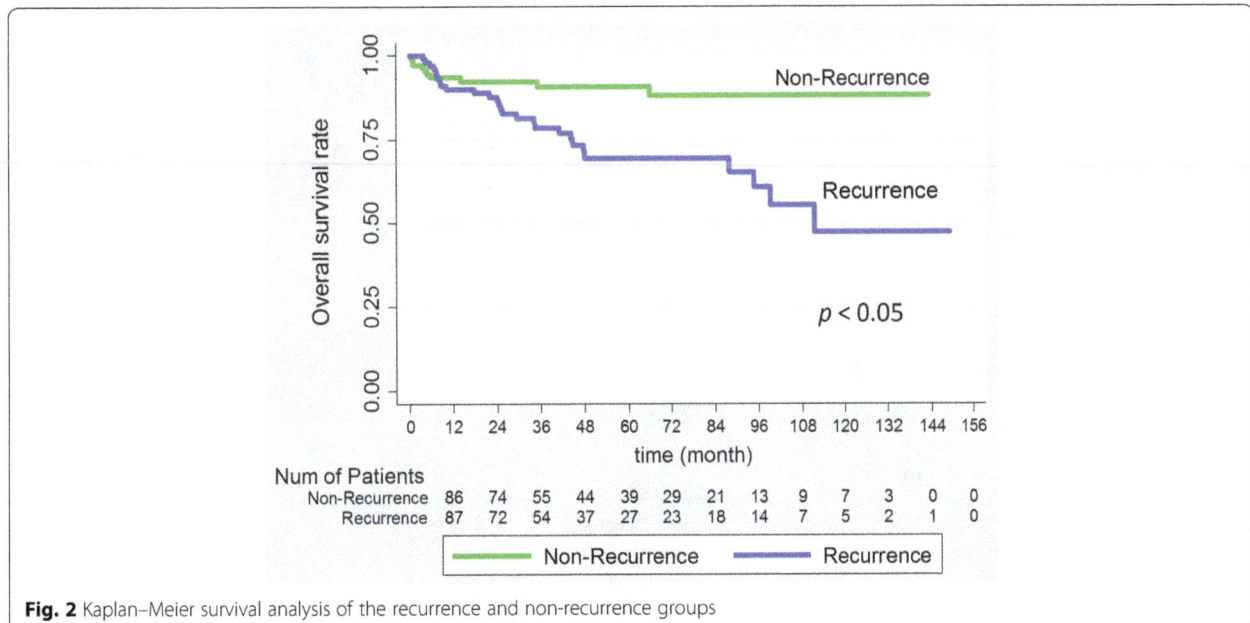

**Fig. 2** Kaplan–Meier survival analysis of the recurrence and non-recurrence groups

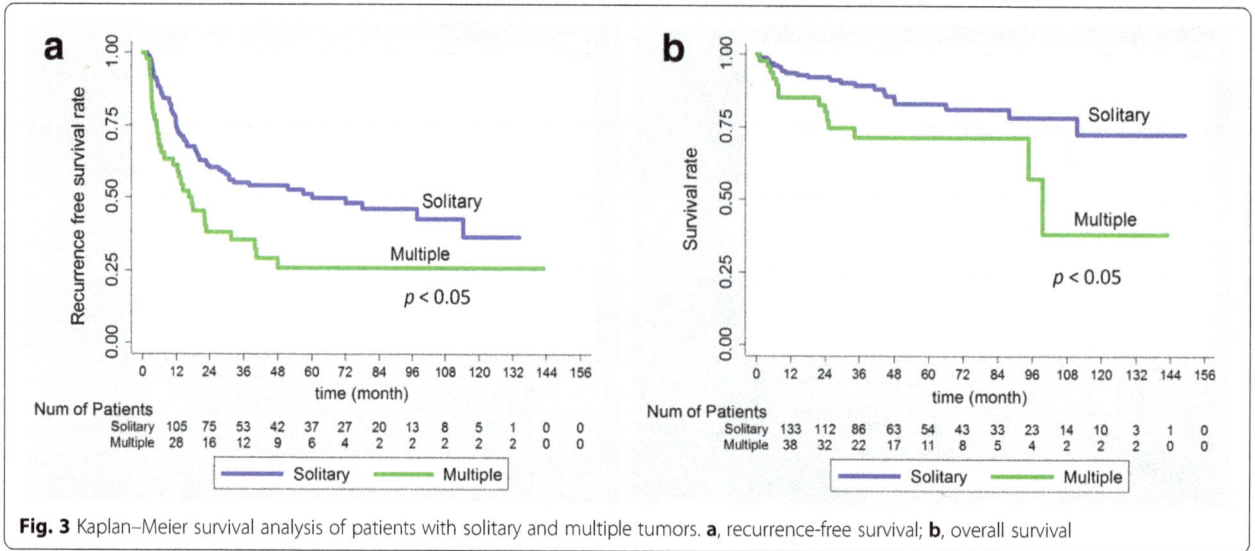

**Fig. 3** Kaplan–Meier survival analysis of patients with solitary and multiple tumors. **a**, recurrence-free survival; **b**, overall survival

difference between pre- and post-operative serum AFP was predictive of poor disease-free and overall survival after hepatectomy in HCC patients, 89.3% of whom had HBV-related HCC [41]. Allard et al. reported that a post-resection AFP level of > 15 ng/mL was a poor predictor of outcome for cirrhotic HCC patients with preoperative AFP levels of > 15 ng/ml [43]. Similarly, Zhang et al. reported that high serum AFP and alpha-fetoprotein-L3 (AFP-L3) levels before and after hepatectomy predicted poor survival [46].

Several potential mechanisms could account for the association between high post-operative serum AFP levels and survival outcome in HBV-related HCC patients. First, although AFP is not present at elevated levels in early-stage HCC and is thus a poor diagnostic biomarker [29, 48, 49], high serum AFP levels may reflect an increasing disease burden due to extrahepatic metastasis, advanced stage, large tumor size, and/or portal vein thrombosis [50]. Ogden et al. and Sung et al. reported that the HBV viral protein HBx dysregulates p53-mediated AFP expression through direct binding to p53, and high HBV integration into the host genome correlated with high serum AFP levels [51, 52]. Moreover, Silva et al. reported that baseline serum AFP levels were higher in HCC patients with more advanced disease and could predict their overall survival, regardless of treatment. Therefore, the patients with high post-operative serum AFP levels in our study may have

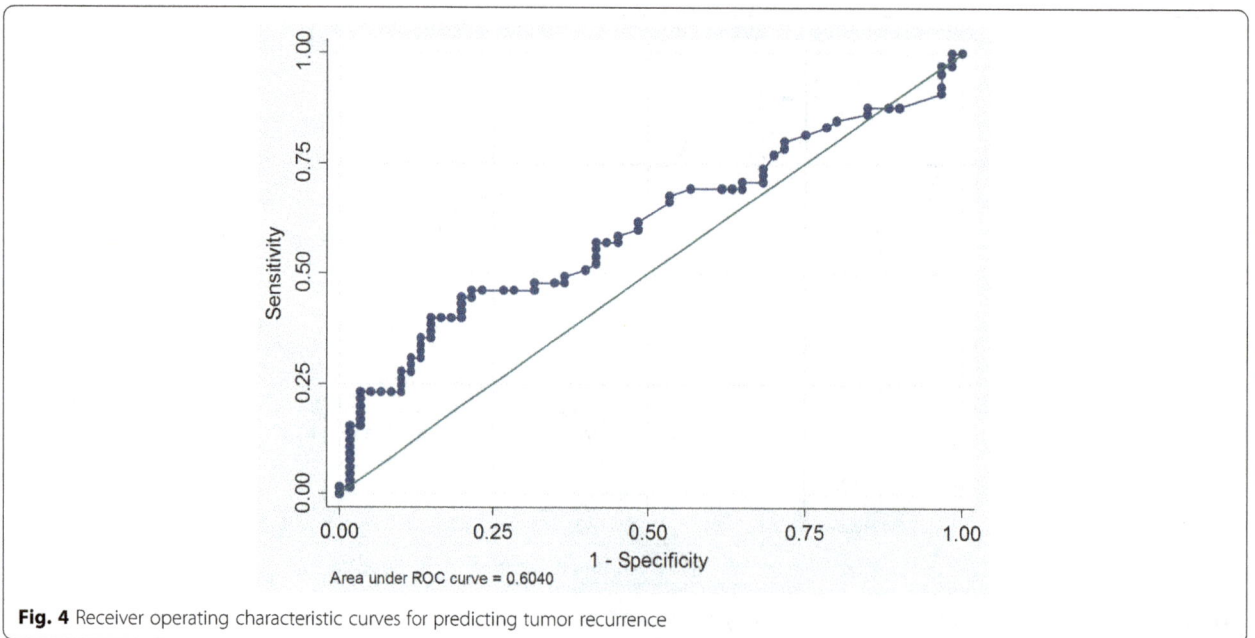

**Fig. 4** Receiver operating characteristic curves for predicting tumor recurrence

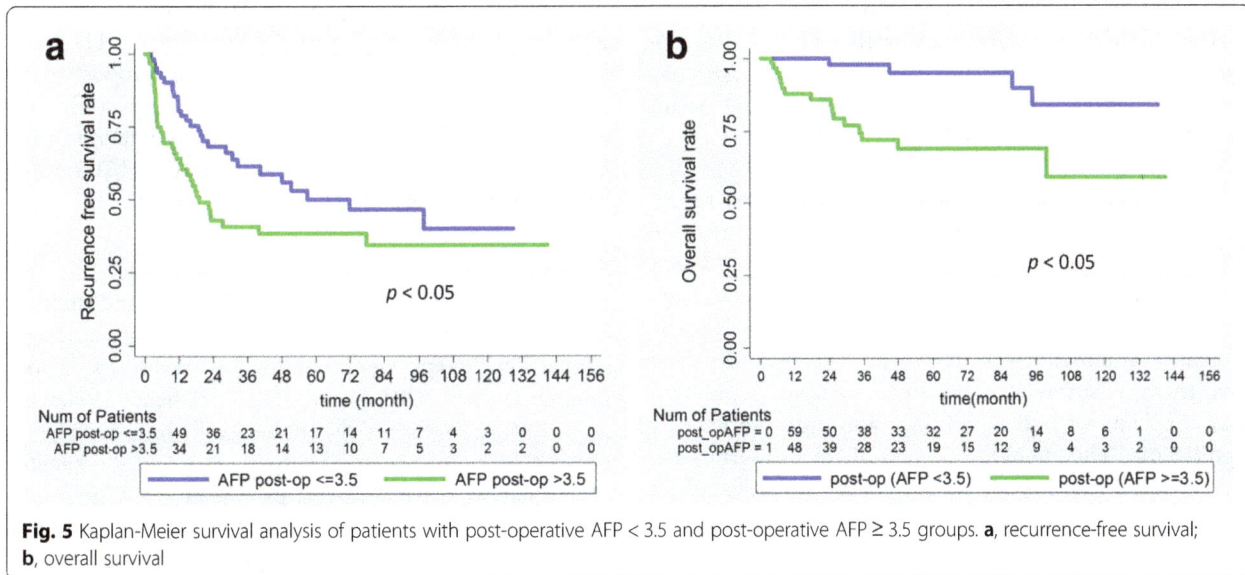

**Fig. 5** Kaplan-Meier survival analysis of patients with post-operative AFP < 3.5 and post-operative AFP ≥ 3.5 groups. **a**, recurrence-free survival; **b**, overall survival

had occult intra- or extrahepatic metastasis [48]. In addition, high serum AFP may be a marker of liver inflammation in patients with chronic liver disorders [10, 12, 50]. Sitia et al. reported that inflammation was a key event in HCC carcinogenesis in HBV transgenic mice and was promoted by lymphocyte infiltration and platelet aggregation [21]. Therefore, ongoing inflammation in patients with high serum AFP could facilitate hepatic carcinogenesis.

In this study, we also found that the presence of multiple HCC tumors is a predictor of recurrence after initial hepatic resection. This is consistent with previous studies showing that multiple tumors is one of the most significant risk factors of early tumor recurrence and poor outcome in HBV-related HCC patients [53–55]. Intrahepatic recurrence is also associated with survival

of HCC patients [56]. In agreement with these observations, our multivariate analysis identified tumor recurrence as an independent predictor of poorer overall survival. Park et al. reported that multiple tumors resulting from intrahepatic metastasis was a strong predictor of early multinodular intrahepatic recurrence in HCC patients following hepatic resection [54]. Hao et al. reported that the presence multiple tumors was significantly associated with intrahepatic metastasis recurrence in HBV-related HCC patients, whereas liver cirrhosis and hepatic inflammation activity were associated with multi-centric recurrence [57]. These authors concluded that intrahepatic and multi-centric metastasis recurrence were mainly caused by tumor-related factors and patient-related factors, respectively [57]. Our results showing that patients with solitary and multiple tumors

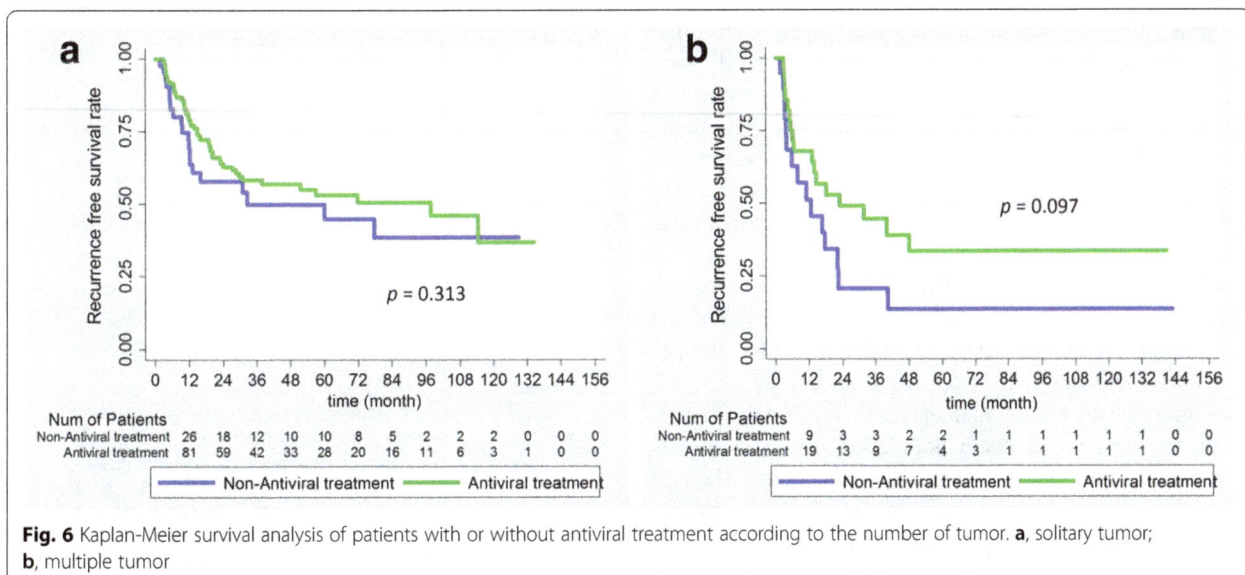

**Fig. 6** Kaplan-Meier survival analysis of patients with or without antiviral treatment according to the number of tumor. **a**, solitary tumor; **b**, multiple tumor

had significantly different recurrence-free and overall survival rates are consistent with this study. We hypothesize that our patients with multiple tumors may have had intrahepatic metastasis and multi-focal occult tumors.

We examined a number of inflammatory markers, including neutrophil-to-lymphocyte ratio, platelet-to-lymphocyte ratio, and prognostic nutritional index, in our patient cohort and found that none of them predicted survival. Antiplatelet therapy also was not a prognostic indicator, although 16 of the 18 patients who received this therapy survived. The small sample population may explain why this finding was not statistically significant. The benefit of antiplatelet therapy in HBV-related HCC patients has been investigated in two large retrospective studies [23, 58]. In a study of Taiwanese patients, Lee et al. found that antiplatelet therapy, including aspirin or clopidogrel, was associated with better recurrence-free survival and overall survival following hepatic resection. However, antiplatelet use significantly increased the risk of upper gastrointestinal bleeding in that study. Lee et al. found that antiplatelet therapy reduced the risk of HCC in South Korean patients whose chronic HBV infection had been effectively suppressed. However, clopidogrel alone with aspirin was found to increase the risk of bleeding [58]. Large-scale prospective studies are clearly needed to unequivocally establish the benefits and risk of complications from antiplatelet therapy.

This study has several limitations. First, it was retrospective in nature. Second, AFP levels in patients with HBV infection could be affected by non-malignancy-related factors such as liver cirrhosis, acute hepatitis, and chronic liver disease [50]. In this study, we included HBV-infected patients with and without cirrhosis and there are seven patients enrolled in the study were co-infected with HBV and HCV. The etiology of HCC among those patients may not due to the chronic HBV infection. Third, there are a number of studies indicating that biomarkers such as protein induced by vitamin K absence-II [32], des-gamma carboxy prothrombin [39], and AFP-L3 [59] may be more accurate prognostic biomarkers than AFP level. However, these tumor markers are not currently measured at our hospital. Fourth, some patients especially in the early period of the study were not treated with anti-viral drugs. Fifth, the patients who neoadjuvant therapy were performed, the AFP level and inflammatory marker levels could be affected. Sixth, the number of death population could be slightly lower than actual due to there are some patients who had recurrence disease have loss to follow-up. Seventh, lamivudine is an anti-HBV drug of modest antiviral effect with low barrier of drug resistance and is no longer suggested

by American Association for the Study of Liver Diseases and European Association of the Study of the Liver as a first-line antiviral option [60, 61]. The proportion of patients with lamivudine treatment in this study was relatively high, which may lead to underestimation of the protective effect of antiviral treatment on HBV related HCC recurrence.

## Conclusions

Post-operative serum alpha-fetoprotein level and multiple tumors, but not inflammatory indices, platelet counts, or antiplatelet therapy, were found to be risk factors of poor prognosis for HBV-related HCC patients following hepatectomy. Prospective studies will be required to clarify the role of platelets in the disease and the benefits of antiplatelet therapy in this patient group. Our results indicate that patients with multiple tumors and high post-operative serum alpha-fetoprotein level should be monitored carefully following hepatic resection.

### Abbreviations
AFP: Alpha-fetoprotein; AFP-L3: Alpha-fetoprotein L3; CI: Confidence intervals; CT: Computed tomography; HBV: Hepatitis B virus; HCC: Hepatocellular carcinoma; HR: Hazard ratio; ICG-R15: Indocyanine green retention at 15 min; MRI: Magnetic resonance imaging

### Acknowledgements
We thank Mr. Napaphat Poprom for reviewing the biostatistical analysis. We thank Edanz Group (https://www.edanzediting.com/ac) for editing a draft of this manuscript.

### Authors' contributions
RN designed the study, collected and interpreted the data, and wrote the paper; SW collected the data and wrote the paper; MS collected and analyzed the data; TP collected and analyzed the data; MP collected the data; and AS analyzed the data. All authors read and approved the final manuscript.

### Competing interests
The authors declare that they have no competing interests.

### References
1.  Torre LA, Bray F, Siegel RL, Ferlay J, Lortet-Tieulent J, Jemal A. Global cancer statistics, 2012. CA Cancer J Clin. 2015;65(2):87–108.
2.  Petruzziello A. Epidemiology of hepatitis B virus (HBV) and hepatitis C virus (HCV) related hepatocellular carcinoma. Open Virol J. 2018;12:26–32.
3.  Chitapanarux T, Phornphutkul K. Risk factors for the development of hepatocellular carcinoma in Thailand. J Clin Transl Hepatol. 2015;3(3):182–8.
4.  Rungsakulkij N, Keeratibharat N, Suragul W, Tangtawee P, Muangkaew P, Mingphruedhi S, Aeesoa S. Early recurrence risk factors for hepatocellular

carcinoma after hepatic resection: experience at a thai tertiary care center. J Med Assoc Thai. 2018;101(1):63–9.

5. Bruix J, Reig M, Sherman M. Evidence-based diagnosis, staging, and treatment of patients with hepatocellular carcinoma. Gastroenterology. 2016;150(4):835–53.

6. Liu W, Zhou JG, Sun Y, Zhang L, Xing BC. Hepatic resection improved the long-term survival of patients with BCLC stage B hepatocellular carcinoma in Asia: a systematic review and meta-analysis. J Gastrointest Surg. 2015;19(7):1271–80.

7. Wang Q, Blank S, Fiel MI, Kadri H, Luan W, Warren L, Zhu A, Deaderick PA, Sarpel U, Labow DM, et al. The severity of liver fibrosis influences the prognostic value of inflammation-based scores in hepatitis B-associated hepatocellular carcinoma. Ann Surg Oncol. 2015;22(Suppl 3):S1125–32.

8. Choi WM, Lee JH, Ahn H, Cho H, Cho YY, Lee M, Yoo JJ, Cho Y, Lee DH, Lee YB, et al. Forns index predicts recurrence and death in patients with hepatitis B-related hepatocellular carcinoma after curative resection. Liver Int. 2015;35(8):1992–2000.

9. Lee JJ, Kim PT, Fischer S, Fung S, Gallinger S, McGilvray I, Moulton CA, Wei AC, Greig PD, Cleary SP. Impact of viral hepatitis on outcomes after liver resection for hepatocellular carcinoma: results from a north american center. Ann Surg Oncol. 2014;21(8):2708–16.

10. Mantovani A, Allavena P, Sica A, Balkwill F. Cancer-related inflammation. Nature. 2008;454(7203):436–44.

11. Seki E, Schwabe RF. Hepatic inflammation and fibrosis: functional links and key pathways. Hepatology. 2015;61(3):1066–79.

12. Levrero M, Zucman-Rossi J. Mechanisms of HBV-induced hepatocellular carcinoma. J Hepatol. 2016;64(1 Suppl):S84–s101.

13. Toyoda H, Kumada T, Kaneoka Y, Osaki Y, Kimura T, Arimoto A, Oka H, Yamazaki O, Manabe T, Urano F, et al. Prognostic value of pretreatment levels of tumor markers for hepatocellular carcinoma on survival after curative treatment of patients with HCC. J Hepatol. 2008;49(2):223–32.

14. Shim JH, Yoon DL, Han S, Lee YJ, Lee SG, Kim KM, Lim YS, Lee HC, Chung YH, Lee YS. Is serum alpha-fetoprotein useful for predicting recurrence and mortality specific to hepatocellular carcinoma after hepatectomy? A test based on propensity scores and competing risks analysis. Ann Surg Oncol. 2012;19(12):3687–96.

15. Yang SL, Liu LP, Yang S, Liu L, Ren JW, Fang X, Chen GG, Lai PB. Preoperative serum alpha-fetoprotein and prognosis after hepatectomy for hepatocellular carcinoma. Br J Surg. 2016;103(6):716–24.

16. Poon RT, Fan ST, Lo CM, Liu CL, Ng IO, Wong J. Long-term prognosis after resection of hepatocellular carcinoma associated with hepatitis B-related cirrhosis. J Clin Oncol. 2000;18(5):1094–101.

17. Tangkijvanich P, Anukulkarnkusol N, Suwangool P, Lertmaharit S, Hanvivatvong O, Kullavanijaya P, Poovorawan Y. Clinical characteristics and prognosis of hepatocellular carcinoma: analysis based on serum alpha-fetoprotein levels. J Clin Gastroenterol. 2000;31(4):302–8.

18. Blank S, Wang Q, Fiel MI, Luan W, Kim KW, Kadri H, Mandeli J, Hiotis SP. Assessing prognostic significance of preoperative alpha-fetoprotein in hepatitis B-associated hepatocellular carcinoma: normal is not the new normal. Ann Surg Oncol. 2014;21(3):986–94.

19. Zhao Z, Liu J, Wang J, Xie T, Zhang Q, Feng S, Deng H, Zhong B. Platelet-to-lymphocyte ratio (PLR) and neutrophil-to-lymphocyte ratio (NLR) are associated with chronic hepatitis B virus (HBV) infection. Int Immunopharmacol. 2017;51:1–8.

20. Iannacone M, Sitia G, Isogawa M, Marchese P, Castro MG, Lowenstein PR, Chisari FV, Ruggeri ZM, Guidotti LG. Platelets mediate cytotoxic T lymphocyte-induced liver damage. Nat Med. 2005;11(11):1167–9.

21. Sitia G. Platelets promote liver immunopathology contributing to hepatitis B virus-mediated hepatocarcinogenesis. Semin Oncol. 2014;41(3):402–5.

22. Sitia G, Aiolfi R, Di Lucia P, Mainetti M, Fiocchi A, Mingozzi F, Esposito A, Ruggeri ZM, Chisari FV, Iannacone M, et al. Antiplatelet therapy prevents hepatocellular carcinoma and improves survival in a mouse model of chronic hepatitis B. Proc Natl Acad Sci U S A. 2012;109(32):E2165–72.

23. Lee PC, Yeh CM, Hu YW, Chen CC, Liu CJ, Su CW, Huo TI, Huang YH, Chao Y, Chen TJ, et al. Antiplatelet therapy is associated with a better prognosis for patients with hepatitis B virus-related hepatocellular carcinoma after liver resection. Ann Surg Oncol. 2016;23(Suppl 5):874–83.

24. Miyagawa S, Makuuchi M, Kawasaki S, Kakazu T. Criteria for safe hepatic resection. Am J Surg. 1995;169(6):589–94.

25. Compton CC, Byrd DR, Garcia-Aguilar J, Kurtzman SH, Olawaiye A, Liver WMK. AJCC Cancer staging atlas: a companion to the seventh editions

of the AJCC Cancer staging manual and handbook. New York: Springer; 2006.

26. Stanaway JD, Flaxman AD, Naghavi M, Fitzmaurice C, Vos T, Abubakar I, Abu-Raddad LJ, Assadi R, Bhala N, Cowie B, et al. The global burden of viral hepatitis from 1990 to 2013: findings from the global burden of disease study 2013. Lancet. 2016;388(10049):1081–8.

27. Sitia G, Iannacone M, Guidotti LG. Anti-platelet therapy in the prevention of hepatitis B virus-associated hepatocellular carcinoma. J Hepatol. 2013;59(5):1135–8.

28. Pang Q, Zhou L, Qu K, Cui RX, Jin H, Liu HC. Validation of inflammation-based prognostic models in patients with hepatitis B-associated hepatocellular carcinoma: a retrospective observational study. Eur J Gastroenterol Hepatol. 2018;30(1):60–70.

29. You DD, Kim DG, Seo CH, Choi HJ, Yoo YK, Park YG. Prognostic factors after curative resection hepatocellular carcinoma and the surgeon's role. Ann Surg Treat Res. 2017;93(5):252–9.

30. Zhu Q, Yuan B, Qiao GL, Yan JJ, Li Y, Duan R, Yan YQ. Prognostic factors for survival after hepatic resection of early hepatocellular carcinoma in HBV-related cirrhotic patients. Clin Res Hepatol Gastroenterol. 2016;40(4):418–27.

31. Giannini EG, Marenco S, Borgonovo G, Savarino V, Farinati F, Del Poggio P, Rapaccini GL, Anna Di Nolfo M, Benvegnu L, Zoli M, et al. Alpha-fetoprotein has no prognostic role in small hepatocellular carcinoma identified during surveillance in compensated cirrhosis. Hepatology. 2012;56(4):1371–9.

32. Kang SH, Kim DY, Jeon SM, Ahn SH, Park JY, Kim SU, Kim JK, Lee KS, Chon CY, Han KH. Clinical characteristics and prognosis of hepatocellular carcinoma with different sets of serum AFP and PIVKA-II levels. Eur J Gastroenterol Hepatol. 2012;24(7):849–56.

33. Gillespie JR, Uversky VN. Structure and function of alpha-fetoprotein: a biophysical overview. Biochim Biophys Acta. 2000;1480(1–2):41–56.

34. Mizejewski GJ. Alpha-fetoprotein structure and function: relevance to isoforms, epitopes, and conformational variants. Exp Biol Med (Maywood). 2001;226(5):377–408.

35. Kim JM, Kwon CH, Joh JW, Park JB, Lee JH, Kim SJ, Paik SW, Park CK, Yoo BC. Differences between hepatocellular carcinoma and hepatitis B virus infection in patients with and without cirrhosis. Ann Surg Oncol. 2014;21(2):458–65.

36. Yang SL, Liu LP, Sun YF, Yang XR, Fan J, Ren JW, Chen GG, Lai PB. Distinguished prognosis after hepatectomy of HBV-related hepatocellular carcinoma with or without cirrhosis: a long-term follow-up analysis. J Gastroenterol. 2016;51(7):722–32.

37. Wu SJ, Lin YX, Ye H, Li FY, Xiong XZ, Cheng NS. Lymphocyte to monocyte ratio and prognostic nutritional index predict survival outcomes of hepatitis B virus-associated hepatocellular carcinoma patients after curative hepatectomy. J Surg Oncol. 2016;114(2):202–10.

38. Li T, Wang SK, Zhou J, Sun HC, Qiu SJ, Ye QH, Wang L, Fan J. Positive HBcAb is associated with higher risk of early recurrence and poorer survival after curative resection of HBV-related HCC. Liver Int. 2016;36(2):284–92.

39. Meguro M, Mizuguchi T, Nishidate T, Okita K, Ishii M, Ota S, Ueki T, Akizuki E, Hirata K. Prognostic roles of preoperative alpha-fetoprotein and des-gamma-carboxy prothrombin in hepatocellular carcinoma patients. World J Gastroenterol. 2015;21(16):4933–45.

40. Franssen B, Alshebeeb K, Tabrizian P, Marti J, Pierobon ES, Lubezky N, Roayaie S, Florman S, Schwartz ME. Differences in surgical outcomes between hepatitis B- and hepatitis C-related hepatocellular carcinoma: a retrospective analysis of a single north American center. Ann Surg. 2014;260(4):650–6. discussion 656-658

41. Shen JY, Li C, Wen TF, Yan LN, Li B, Wang WT, Yang JY, Xu MQ. Alpha fetoprotein changes predict hepatocellular carcinoma survival beyond the Milan criteria after hepatectomy. J Surg Res. 2017;209:102–11.

42. Toyoda H, Kumada T, Tada T, Ito T, Maeda A, Kaneoka Y, Kagebayashi C, Satomura S. Changes in highly sensitive alpha-fetoprotein for the prediction of the outcome in patients with hepatocellular carcinoma after hepatectomy. Cancer Med. 2014;3(3):643–51.

43. Allard MA, Sa Cunha A, Ruiz A, Vibert E, Sebagh M, Castaing D, Adam R. The postresection alpha-fetoprotein in cirrhotic patients with hepatocellular carcinoma. An independent predictor of outcome. J Gastrointest Surg. 2014;18(4):701–8.

44. Toro A, Ardiri A, Mannino M, Arcerito MC, Mannino G, Palermo F, Bertino G, Di Carlo I. Effect of pre- and post-treatment alpha-fetoprotein levels and tumor size on survival of patients with hepatocellular carcinoma treated by resection, transarterial chemoembolization or radiofrequency ablation: a retrospective study. BMC Surg. 2014;14:40.

45. Nobuoka D, Kato Y, Gotohda N, Takahashi S, Nakagohri T, Konishi M, Kinoshita T, Nakatsura T. Postoperative serum alpha-fetoprotein level is a useful predictor of recurrence after hepatectomy for hepatocellular carcinoma. Oncol Rep. 2010;24(2):521–8.

46. Zhang XF, Yin ZF, Wang K, Zhang ZQ, Qian HH, Shi LH. Changes of serum alpha-fetoprotein and alpha-fetoprotein-L3 after hepatectomy for hepatocellular carcinoma: prognostic significance. Hepatobiliary Pancreat Dis Int. 2012;11(6):618–23.

47. Cai ZQ, Si SB, Chen C, Zhao Y, Ma YY, Wang L, Geng ZM. Analysis of prognostic factors for survival after hepatectomy for hepatocellular carcinoma based on a bayesian network. PLoS One. 2015;10(3):e0120805.

48. Silva JP, Gorman RA, Berger NG, Tsai S, Christians KK, Clarke CN, Mogal H, Gamblin TC. The prognostic utility of baseline alpha-fetoprotein for hepatocellular carcinoma patients. J Surg Oncol. 2017;116(7):831–40.

49. Farinati F, Marino D, De Giorgio M, Baldan A, Cantarini M, Cursaro C, Rapaccini G, Del Poggio P, Di Nolfo MA, Benvegnu L, et al. Diagnostic and prognostic role of alpha-fetoprotein in hepatocellular carcinoma: both or neither? Am J Gastroenterol. 2006;101(3):524–32.

50. Wong RJ, Ahmed A, Gish RG. Elevated alpha-fetoprotein: differential diagnosis - hepatocellular carcinoma and other disorders. Clin Liver Dis. 2015;19(2):309–23.

51. Ogden SK, Lee KC, Barton MC. Hepatitis B viral transactivator HBx alleviates p53-mediated repression of alpha-fetoprotein gene expression. J Biol Chem. 2000;275(36):27806–14.

52. Sung WK, Zheng H, Li S, Chen R, Liu X, Li Y, Lee NP, Lee WH, Ariyaratne PN, Tennakoon C, et al. Genome-wide survey of recurrent HBV integration in hepatocellular carcinoma. Nat Genet. 2012;44(7):765–9.

53. Huang G, Lau WY, Zhou WP, Shen F, Pan ZY, Yuan SX, Wu MC. Prediction of hepatocellular carcinoma recurrence in patients with low hepatitis B virus DNA levels and high preoperative hepatitis B surface antigen levels. JAMA Surg. 2014;149(6):519–27.

54. Park JH, Koh KC, Choi MS, Lee JH, Yoo BC, Paik SW, Rhee JC, Joh JW. Analysis of risk factors associated with early multinodular recurrences after hepatic resection for hepatocellular carcinoma. Am J Surg. 2006;192(1):29–33.

55. Zhu WJ, Huang CY, Li C, Peng W, Wen TF, Yan LN, Li B, Wang WT, Xu MQ, Yang JY, et al. Risk factors for early recurrence of HBV-related hepatocellular carcinoma meeting Milan criteria after curative resection. Asian Pac J Cancer Prev. 2013;14(12):7101–6.

56. Hirokawa F, Hayashi M, Miyamoto Y, Asakuma M, Shimizu T, Komedo K, Inoue Y, Uchiyama K. Predictors of poor prognosis by recurrence patterns after curative hepatectomy for hepatocellular carcinoma in child-pugh classification a. Hepato-Gastroenterology. 2015;62(137):164–8.

57. Hao S, Fan P, Chen S, Tu C, Wan C. Distinct recurrence risk factors for intrahepatic metastasis and multicenter occurrence after surgery in patients with hepatocellular carcinoma. J Gastrointest Surg. 2017;21(2):312–20.

58. Lee M, Chung GE, Lee JH, Oh S, Nam JY, Chang Y, Cho H, Ahn H, Cho YY, Yoo JJ, et al. Antiplatelet therapy and the risk of hepatocellular carcinoma in chronic hepatitis B patients on antiviral treatment. Hepatology. 2017;66(5):1556–69.

59. Zhang XF, Lai EC, Kang XY, Qian HH, Zhou YM, Shi LH, Shen F, Yang YF, Zhang Y, Lau WY, et al. Lens culinaris agglutinin-reactive fraction of alpha-fetoprotein as a marker of prognosis and a monitor of recurrence of hepatocellular carcinoma after curative liver resection. Ann Surg Oncol. 2011;18(8):2218–23.

60. Terrault NA, Lok ASF, McMahon BJ, Chang KM, Hwang JP, Jonas MM, Brown RS Jr, Bzowej NH, Wong JB. Update on prevention, diagnosis, and treatment of chronic hepatitis B: AASLD 2018 hepatitis B guidance. Hepatology. 2018;67(4):1560–99.

61. EASL. 2017 clinical practice guidelines on the management of hepatitis B virus infection. J Hepatol. 2017;67(2):370–98.

# 19

# Dissecting the mechanisms and molecules underlying the potential carcinogenicity of red and processed meat in colorectal cancer (CRC)

Marco Cascella[1†], Sabrina Bimonte[1*†] ⓘ, Antonio Barbieri[2†], Vitale Del Vecchio[2†], Domenico Caliendo[1], Vincenzo Schiavone[3], Roberta Fusco[4], Vincenza Granata[4], Claudio Arra[2†] and Arturo Cuomo[1†]

## Abstract

Meat is a crucial nutrient for human health since it represents a giant supply of proteins, minerals, and vitamins. On the opposite hand, the intake of red and processed meat is taken into account dangerous due to its potential of carcinogenesis and cancer risk improvement, particularly for colorectal cancer (CRC), although it has been reported that also the contaminations of beef infected by oncogenic bovine viruses could increase colorectal cancer's risk. Regarding the mechanisms underlying the potential carcinogenicity of red and processed meat, different hypotheses have been proposed. A suggested mechanism describes the potential role of the heterocyclic amines (HACs) and polycyclic aromatic hydrocarbons (PHAs) in carcinogenesis induced by DNA mutation. Another hypothesis states that heme, through the lipid peroxidation process and therefore the formation of N-nitroso compounds (NOCs), produces cytotoxic and genotoxic aldehydes, resulting in carcinogenesis. Furthermore, a recent proposed hypothesis, is based on the combined actions between the N-Glycolylneuraminic acid (Neu5Gc) and genotoxic compounds. The purpose of this narrative review is to shed a light on the mechanisms underlying the potential carcinogenicity of red and processed meat, by summarizing the data reported in literature on this topic.

**Keywords:** Carcinogenesis, Red meat, Processed meat, Heme, Heterocyclic amines, Polycyclic aromatic hydrocarbons, Neu5Gc

## Background

Meat is an important nutrient for human health, since it represents a big source of proteins, minerals and vitamins with poor bioavailability. Red and processed meats, instead, are considered dangerous, due to their potential carcinogenicity. Red meat is a form of unprocessed mammalians muscle, which color is due to the presence of myoglobin [1, 2]. On the other facet, processed meat is identified as a product

* Correspondence: s.bimonte@istitutotumori.na.it
Claudio Arra and Arturo Cuomo are co-last authors.
Marco Cascella, Sabrina Bimonte, Antonio Barbieri, Vitale Del Vecchio contributed equally to this work.
†Equal contributors
[1]Division of Anesthesia and Pain Medicine, Istituto Nazionale Tumori - IRCCS – "Fondazione G. Pascale", Via Mariano Semmola, 80131 Naples, Italy
Full list of author information is available at the end of the article

obtained through several processes such as salting, curing, fermentation or smoking, with the aim of enhancing flavor or improve preservation. Recently, the International Agency for Research on Cancer (IARC) published interesting results on the potential carcinogenicity effects of red and/or processed meat; Bouvard et al. [3] anticipated these data and showed that the processed meat is classified as carcinogenic to human (Group 1), while the red meat is identified as probably carcinogenic to human (Group 2A) (Fig. 1). On the basis of this classification, and from knowledge emerged by epidemiological studies, the intake of meat as a nutrient of a healthy diet for human, has to become a controversial issue [4]. Accumulating studies showed that the consumption of processed meat causes colorectal cancer (CRC), the second most common cause of cancer-related death in affluent

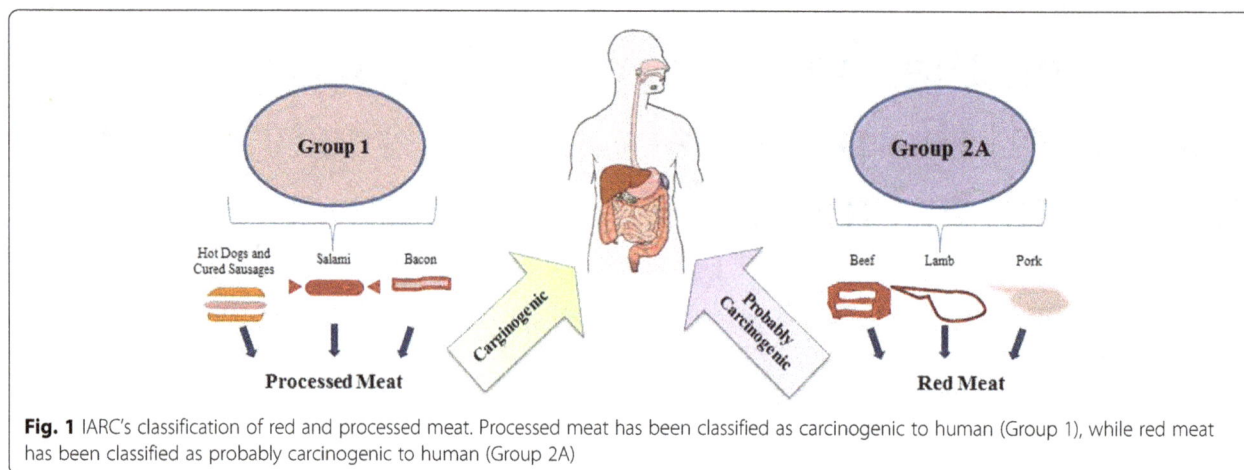

**Fig. 1** IARC's classification of red and processed meat. Processed meat has been classified as carcinogenic to human (Group 1), while red meat has been classified as probably carcinogenic to human (Group 2A)

countries, and stomach cancer, although the evidences for this latter are still not enthusiastic. *Chan* et al. [5] proved evidence that dietary factors, as well as red and processed meat, may be thought of the leading causes of 80% CRC cases. Similar results, obtained by epidemiological studies accumulated over the last decades, confirmed the association of red and processed meat intake and increased risk of CRC [6–9]. Interestingly, *Zu Hausen* et al., suggested that potentially oncogenic thermoresistant bovine viruses, by inducing beef's contaminations provoked infections in the colorectal tract, that combined to chemical carcinogens developed during procedures of cooking, increased the colorectal cancer's risk [10]. The role of red meat consumption as a leading cause of different types of cancer (e.g. pancreatic cancer, prostate cancer, bladder cancer) has been conjointly reported [11–16], although extremely mentioned and contested by the scientific community, since a recent meta-analysis indicated a significantly increased risk (about 22%) of bladder cancer as a result of high processed meat (but not for red meat) consumption [17]. Additionally, in another meta-analysis, *Bylsma and Alexander* concluded that there was no association between red or processed meat intake and prostate cancer, although they found a weak positive summary estimate for processed meats [18]. A detailed summary of recent epidemiological studies on carcinogenicity of consumption of red and processed meat in different types of cancer, including colorectal cancer (CRC), has been recently reported by *Domingo* et al. [19] whereas *Alexander* et al. published a quantitative update on the epidemiological research on the topic [20]. Several molecules have been identified as potential carcinogenic present in red meat or produced by meat processing or by cooking procedure: i) the heterocyclic amines (HACs), as -Amino-3,4- dimethylimidazo quinolone (MeIQ) and 2-Amino-3,8-dimethylimidazo quinoxaline (MeIQx), ii) the N-nitroso-compounds (NOCs), as N-nitrosodimethylamine (NDMA); iii) the polycyclic aromatic hydrocarbons (PAHs), as benzo[a]pyrene (BaP) [17, 21]; iv) the N-glycolylneuraminic acid (Neu5Gc) [22]. In addition,

the carcinogenic role of environmental pollutants (e.g., polychlorinated dibenzo-pdioxins and dibenzofurans, polychlorinated biphenyls, polybrominated diphenyl and polychlorinated diphenyl ethers, polychlorinated naphthalene and perfluoroalkyl substances), which are already present in raw or unprocessed meat, has been also proposed [19]. Furthermore, the carcinogenic role of red and processed meat could be enhanced by other concomitant dietary factors (e.g., high fat and/ or protein intake) and clinical conditions, such as obesity [23, 24]. It is of note that bile acids produced in the gut as a consequence of high fat intake, by damaging the mucosa and the epithelium of colon, leads to cell hyperproliferation and then to colon cancer development [25]. Despite studies on animal models supporting the cancer-promoting effect induced by high fat intake [26], epidemiological studies reported opposite results [27, 28]. Similarly, a high protein intake provokes the formations of metabolites toxic with a great potential of colon carcinogenesis [29], although no data supporting this hypothesis, are available [30]. Others alternative and uncertain hypothesis of mechanisms (e.g., thermoresistant potentially oncogenic bovine viruses [10] and endogenous hormones, [31]) underlying the consumption of red and processed meat and carcinogenesis of CRC, have been reported in the literature and reviewed by *Demeyer* et al. [32]. Our aim is to review the data reported in the literature on the principal mechanisms and molecules involved in carcinogenicity induced by red and processed red meat consumption in CRC, in order to shed a light on the current state of the art on this important issue.

## Mechanisms and molecules involved in the carcinogenicity induced by consumption of red and processed meat

The biological reasons for the association between red and processed meat and cancer- especially CRC- are still unclear, but a large number of molecular mechanisms have been proposed to explain this association. Here, we summarize the most relevant ones, trying to elucidate the current state of scientific knowledge.

### Heterocyclic amines (HCAs)

Heterocyclic amines (HCAs) represent chemical compounds generated in fish and meat by cooked procedures at high temperatures through a specific reaction (i.e. Maillard reaction [33]) between free amino acids and sugars, becoming in this way potentially mutagens to humans [34]. It has been reported that the principals HCAs found in cooked red meat (over a total of 25 identified) are the 2–Amino-3, 8-dimethyl imidazo-[4,5f] quinoxaline (MeIQx) and the 2-Amino-1-methyl6 phenylimidazo [4,5b] pyridine (PhIP) [35]. These compounds, together with amino-3,4- dimethylimidazo[4,5-f] quinoline (MeIQ), have been classified by the IARC as potential carcinogenic to human (Group 2B), while the amino-3-methylimidazo[4,5-f] quinolone (IQ) has been classified as probably carcinogenic to human (Group 2A) [3]. It is of note that HCAs are transformed into mutagens after metabolic activation which regulates their carcinogenicity [8]. Evidences support the hypothesis that the levels of these compounds are high in human organisms after the consumption of cooked red beef [36]. Thanks to in vitro and in vivo pre-clinical studies the metabolism and the molecular pathways of MelQx and PhIP's biotransformation have been largely dissected [37–40]. Specifically, the process of hydroxylation of MelQx and PhIP mediated by the cytochrome P-450, has been identified as the principle pathway [41]. *Schut* et al. [42] showed that HCAs may form DNA adducts. Several epidemiological studies reported a strong association between the HCAs intake and CRC [43–45]. *Le Marchand* et al. confirmed these data as they reported a strong association between MeIQx and rectal cancer [46]. Unfortunately, opposite results have been described probably due to the higher variability of other factors responsible for carcinogenesis (e.g. diet, genetic polymorphisms of the population) used in epidemiological studies [47, 48]. On the basis of these contrasting results, the link between HCAs and cancer risk is not completely clarified [34]. Thus, more studies will be needed.

### The polycyclic aromatic hydrocarbons (PAHs)

Polycyclic aromatic hydrocarbons (PAHs) are considered toxic substances produced by an incomplete combustion of organic compounds such as tobacco, oil, gas. [49]. Regarding the red meat and other foods, PAHs are produced by cooking procedures at high temperatures, such as barbecuing, or by the food's processing by using smoking [50]. The principal PAH (over 100 identified) classified by the IARC as potential carcinogenic to human (Group 1) is the benzo[a]pyrene (BaP) [3]. *Estensen*

et al., in a pre-clinical study conducted on mice with lung tumors, confirmed the carcinogenic role of BaP [51]. This molecule becomes genotoxic after metabolic reaction by which is converted into benzo[a]pyrene diolepoxide (BPDE) [52]. This latter is able to interfere with the bases of DNA, thus resulting in DNA damage which is responsible for cancer promoting [53, 54]. Regarding the carcinogenic mechanism of PAHs, *Phillips* et al., showed that human colon cells are able to metabolize these compounds [50]. *Shimada* et al. demonstrated that the aryl hydrocarbon receptor, a transcription factor activated by ligands like PAH, plays a crucial role within the regulation and therefore the drug metabolizing enzymes (e.g. CYP1A1, CYP1A2, CYP1B1, glutathione S-transferase and UDP-glucoronyltransferase). These enzymes cause toxicity or carcinogenesis through the processing of the toxicants to reactive metabolites that, finally, interact with cellular macromolecules (e.g., DNA adducts) [55]. Similarly, to HCAs, epidemiological studies do not rumor convincing results on the association between dietary BaP intake from meat and cancer appearing (mainly CRC), most likely as a result of the difference in un-supporting factors [56, 57] (e.g. cooking procedures, fat contents) chosen in the populations listed in these studies.

Thus, as for HCAs, additional studies are going to be necessary to ascertain the carcinogenicity of red and processed meat induced by PAHs.

### Heme

Heme represents the prosthetic cluster of myoglobin and hemoglobin [28] and is responsible for the red color of meat, as a results of its elevated concentrations respect to those observed in white meat [58]. Due to many epidemiological [59–61] and pre-clinical studies [62, 63], three mechanisms underlying the association between a consumption of heme and CRC risk, have been elucidated: i) the lipid –peroxidation; ii) the N-nitroso compounds (NOCs) formations; iii) the cytotoxicity. The potential carcinogenicity of heme iron may be associated to its redox properties. By taking part in dangerous free radical-generating reactions with the production of a reactive oxygen species (ROS), heme iron leads to oxidative DNA damage which is considered highly mutagenic [64]. ROS are involved in lipid peroxidation, a complex process which, finally, causes the formation of cytotoxic and genotoxic aldehydes, as malondialdehyde (MDA) and 4-hydroxynonenal (4-HNE) [65]. These aldehydes are able to promote cancer progression, as reported by epidemiological and experimental studies. Thus, lipid peroxidation as thought of one the principal mechanisms underlying the carcinogenicity of red and processed meat induced by heme (Fig. 2).

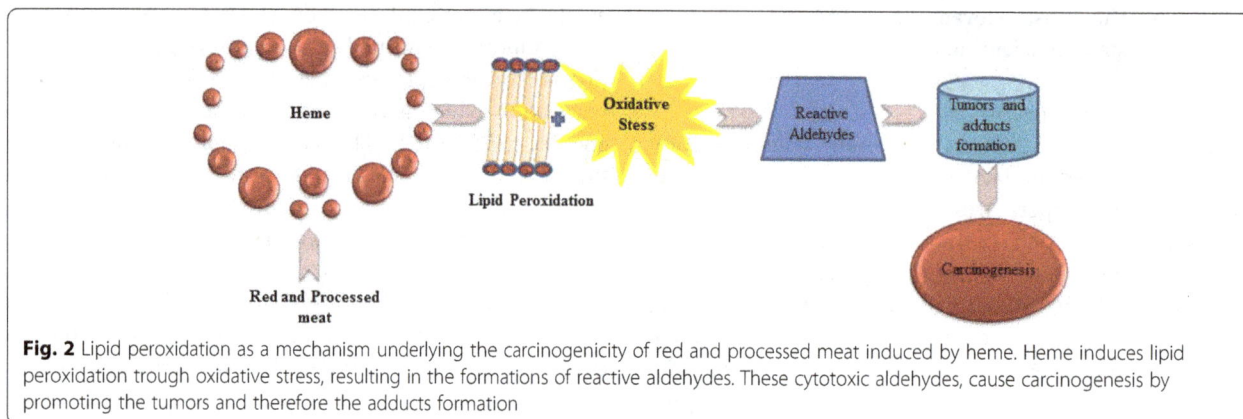

**Fig. 2** Lipid peroxidation as a mechanism underlying the carcinogenicity of red and processed meat induced by heme. Heme induces lipid peroxidation trough oxidative stress, resulting in the formations of reactive aldehydes. These cytotoxic aldehydes, cause carcinogenesis by promoting the tumors and therefore the adducts formation

### The nitrate/nitrite formation and the N-Nitroso compounds (NOCs)

Endogenous NOCs, formed by N-nitrosation process of amines and amides, may be considered important geno-toxins since being to induce DNA mutations [66]. Most NOCs, as well as nitrosamines, nitrosamides, and nitro-soguanidines [67], can yield alkylating agents (N-alkyl-NOCs) throughout metabolism. Plenty of nitrosamines are found in foods, including NDMA, NDEA (Nnitroso-diethylamine), NDBA (N-nitrosodibutylamine), NPIP (N-nitrosopiperidine), NPYR (Nnitrosopyrrolidine), NMOR (N-nitrosomorpholine), NDPhA (Nnitrosodiphenylamine), NPRO (Nnitrosoproline), and NSAR (N- nitrososarco-sine), although not all of these shows carcinogenic effect [3] (See Fig. 3, for IARC's classification of Nitrosamines). Humans may be exposed to two different forms of NOCs: i) exogenous, derived from different sources (e.g., tobacco products, diet, occupational environments and drugs); ii) endogenous nitrosamines and nitrosamides, generated by the reaction of nitrite with the products of amino acid's degradation in the stomach, and accounted for up 75% of the total NOC exposure [68]. Several epidemiological and pre-clinical studies conducted on animal models reported a strong link between endogenous NOCs and CRC.

Regarding CRC, studies demonstrated that N-alkyl-NOCs can induce transitions of DNA's bases (GC → AT) in genes mutated (e.g. *Kras*) in human tumors [69]. Moreover, as shown by *Kuhnle* et al. [70], the presence of nitrosyl heme, which is formed by a nitrosylation or nitrosation in ileum and in faeces, might promote the formation of extremely re-active alkylating agents like diazoacetate. As a consequence, this process ends up in the formation of the NOC DNA ad-duct, named O6-carboxymethyl-2′-deoxy-guanosine (O6CMeG). This compound has been wide studied by *Lewin* et al., as carcinogenetic agent for CRC [71]. DNA damage may be induced by aldehydes with mutagenic ef-fects in microorganism, mammalian, and human cells [72]. For example, *Leuratti* et al. [73], proved evidence that MDA reacts with DNA to form adducts such as 1, N2-

malondialdehyde-deoxyguanosine (M1dG), which has been found at higher levels, in subjects with adenoma compared with adenoma-free subjects. On the other side, the alde-hydes 4-hydroxy-2-nonenal (4-HNE) is weakly mutagenic even though is taken into account the most toxic product of lipid peroxidation. In fact, it may interfere with stress apop-tosis pathway by causing necrosis in human colon carcin-oma cells through the activation of caspase-3 [74]. To overcome the pro-carcinogenic effects of heme, it's been powerfully steered to incorporate in dietary regime a spread of molecules present in fruit and vegetables. As an example, calcium salts and chlorophyll are able to precipitate heme

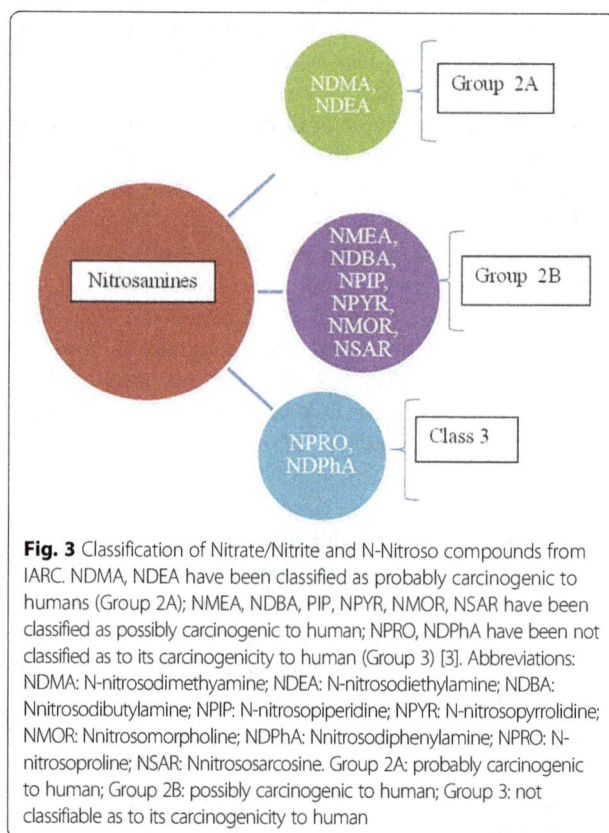

**Fig. 3** Classification of Nitrate/Nitrite and N-Nitroso compounds from IARC. NDMA, NDEA have been classified as probably carcinogenic to humans (Group 2A); NMEA, NDBA, PIP, NPYR, NMOR, NSAR have been classified as possibly carcinogenic to human; NPRO, NDPhA have been not classified as to its carcinogenicity to human (Group 3) [3]. Abbreviations: NDMA: n-nitrosodimethyamine; NDEA: N-nitrosodiethylamine; NDBA: Nnitrosodibutylamine; NPIP: N-nitrosopiperidine; NPYR: N-nitrosopyrrolidine; NMOR: Nnitrosomorpholine; NDPhA: Nnitrosodiphenylamine; NPRO: N-nitrosoproline; NSAR: Nnitrososarcosine. Group 2A: probably carcinogenic to human; Group 2B: possibly carcinogenic to human; Group 3: not classifiable as to its carcinogenicity to human

molecules, whereas vitamins C and E blocked the endogenous formation of NOCs, and several other polyphenols like quercetin, α-tocopherol, or red wine polyphenols, suppressed the lipid peroxidation.

Fewer pre-clinical studies conducted on animal models, showed that heme is able to augment the citoxocity of colon cells, resulting in an increased epithelial proliferation and afterward to cancer occurring [10, 75]. Unfortunately, few epidemiological studies [63, 76] confirmed these knowledges resulting in interpretations that lack of consistency.

### N-glycolylneuraminic acid (Neu5Gc)

Red meat is enriched in glycan's containing a variant of sialic acid, the N-glycolylneuraminic acid (Neu5G). This molecule, not naturally found in human tissues, may be solely assumed by diet regimens containing pork, beef, and lamb [22, 77]. To the current issue, it has been suggested that humans can metabolically incorporate and express Neu5Gc into cell surface glyco-conjugates [78]. Moreover, it has been reported that the incorporation of Neu5Gc into human tissue could be involved in tumor initiation and progression [79]. The mechanism of uptake and incorporation of Neu5Gc into human epithelial was described by *Bardor* et al., 2005) [80]. It is necessary to underline that Neu5Gc-containing glycans act as

"xeno-autoantigens" that may be targeted by naturally circulating anti-Neu5Gc "xeno-autoantibodies". This process ends up in development of xenosialitis, an inflammatory disease that influences cancer formation and progression [81, 82].

Due to the absence of epidemiological data, is suitable to consider the xenosialitis induced by Neu5Gc assumed by red meat consumption, as the only mechanism underlying the association between red meat consumption and increased CRC risk.

### Conclusion

In 2015 the IARC classified the consumption of red meat and processed meat as "probably carcinogenic to humans" (Group 2A), and as "carcinogenic to humans" (Group 1), respectively. A large number of mechanisms have been proposed to elucidate the link between red and processed intake and CRC risk. These mechanisms involve different molecules: i) heme iron, ii) NOCs, iii) HCAs and PAHs; iv) Neu5G, although convincing results have been reported for heme (via lipid peroxidation mechanism) and endogenous NOC. Taking into the account that different compounds could also be present in red and processed red meat, the increased risk for CRC could also be related to multiple carcinogenic compounds (Fig. 4). More studies are going to be necessary

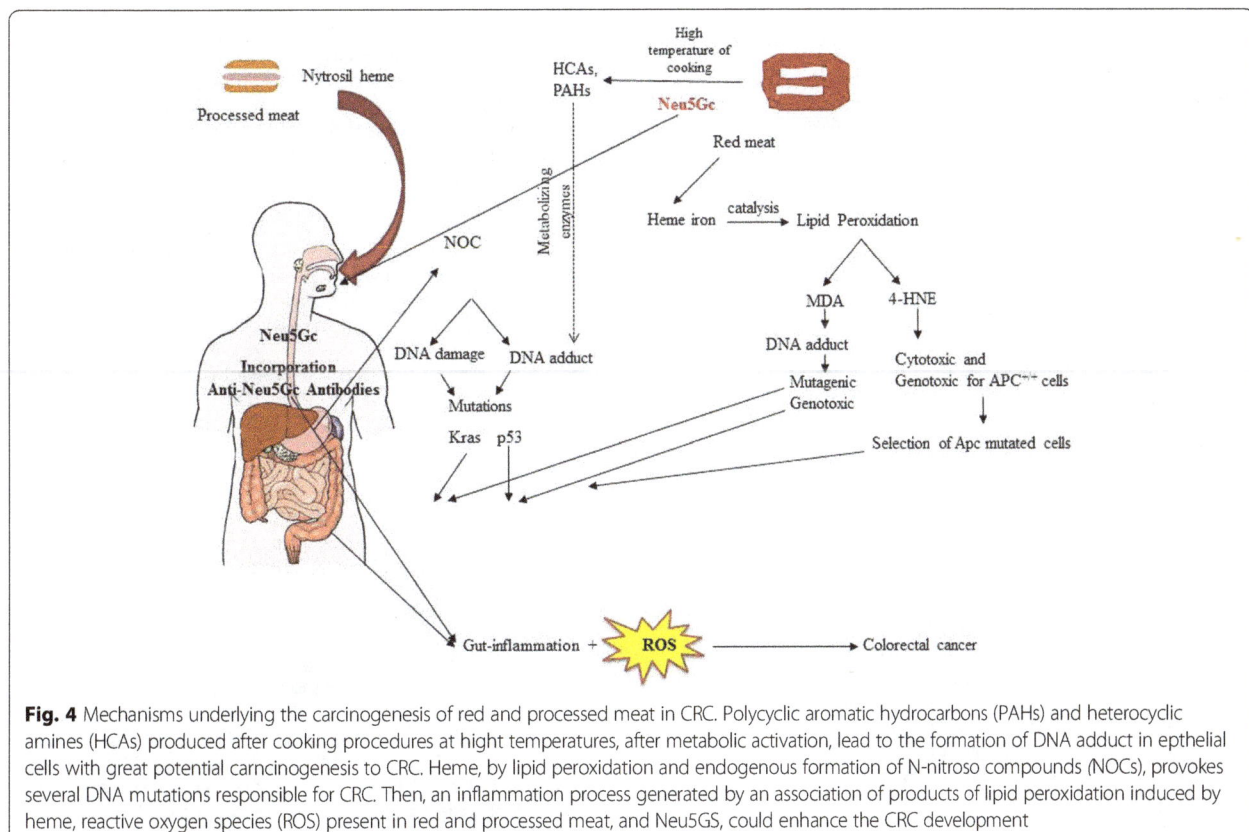

**Fig. 4** Mechanisms underlying the carcinogenesis of red and processed meat in CRC. Polycyclic aromatic hydrocarbons (PAHs) and heterocyclic amines (HCAs) produced after cooking procedures at hight temperatures, after metabolic activation, lead to the formation of DNA adduct in epthelial cells with great potential carncinogenesis to CRC. Heme, by lipid peroxidation and endogenous formation of N-nitroso compounds (NOCs), provokes several DNA mutations responsible for CRC. Then, an inflammation process generated by an association of products of lipid peroxidation induced by heme, reactive oxygen species (ROS) present in red and processed meat, and Neu5GS, could enhance the CRC development

to elucidate the molecular mechanisms underlying the carcinogenicity of red meat and processed meat in CRC and other types of cancer.

## Abbreviations
(Neu5Gc): N-Glycolylneuraminic acid; (NOCs): N-nitroso compounds; 4-HNE: 4-hydroxy-2-nonenal; Bap: Benzo[a]pyrene; CRC: Colorectal cancer; HCAs: Heterocyclic amines; IQ: Amino-3-methylimidazo[4,5 f]quinolone (IQ); M1dg: 1,N2-malondialdehyde-deoxyguanosine; MeIQ: amino-3,4-dimethylimidazo[4,5-f] quinolone; MeIQx: 2–Amino-3,8-dimethylimidazo-[4,5f]quinoxaline; NDBA: N-nitrosodibutylamine; NDEA: Nnitrosodiethylamine; NDMA: N-nitrosodimethyamine; NDPhA: N-nitrosodiphenylamine; NMOR: N-nitrosomorpholine; NPIP: N-nitrosopiperidine; NPRO: N-nitrosoproline; NPYR: N-nitrosopyrrolidine; NSAR: N-nitrososarcosine; O6CMeG: O6-carboxymethyl-2′-deoxy-guanosine; PHAs: Polycyclic aromatic hydrocarbons; PhIP: 2-Amino-1-methyl6 phenylimidazo[4,5b]pyridine; ROS: Reactive oxygen species

## Acknowledgements
We are grateful to Dr. Alessandra Trocino, Mrs. MariaCristina Romano and Mr. Massimiliano Spinelli from the National Cancer Institute of Naples for providing excellent bibliographic service and informatics assistance.

## Funding
No funds were used for the preparation of the paper.

## Authors' contributions
MC, and SB, are the main authors of the manuscript. All authors read and approved the final manuscript.

## Competing interests
The authors declare that they have no competing interests.

## Author details
[1]Division of Anesthesia and Pain Medicine, Istituto Nazionale Tumori - IRCCS – "Fondazione G. Pascale", Via Mariano Semmola, 80131 Naples, Italy. [2]S.S.D. Sperimentazione Animale, Istituto Nazionale Tumori - IRCCS - Fondazione "G. Pascale", Via Mariano Semmola, 80131 Naples, Italy. [3]Division of Anesthesia and Intensive Care, Hospital "Pineta Grande", Castel Volturno, Caserta, Italy. [4]Division of Radiology, "Istituto Nazionale Tumori - IRCCS - Fondazione G. Pascale", Via Mariano Semmola, 80131 Naples, Italy.

## References
1. Lindahl G, Lundstrom K, Tornberg E. Contribution of pigment content, myoglobin forms and internal reflectance to the colour of pork loin and ham from pure breed pigs. Meat Sci. 2001;59:141–51.
2. Sen AR, Muthukumar M, Naveena BM, Ramanna DB. Effects on colour characteristics of buffalo meat during blooming, retail display and using vitamin C during refrigerated storage. J Food Sci Technol. 2014;51:3515–9.
3. Bouvard V, Loomis D, Guyton KZ, Grosse Y, Ghissassi FE, Benbrahim-Tallaa L, Guha N, Mattock H, Straif K. International Agency for Research on Cancer monograph working G: carcinogenicity of consumption of red and processed meat. Lancet Oncol. 2015;16:1599–600.
4. Celada P, Bastida S, Sanchez-Muniz FJ. To eat or not to eat meat. That is the question. Nutr Hosp. 2016;33:177–81.
5. Chan DS, Lau R, Aune D, Vieira R, Greenwood DC, Kampman E, Norat T. Red and processed meat and colorectal cancer incidence: meta-analysis of prospective studies. PLoS One. 2011;6:e20456.
6. Diallo A, Deschasaux M, Latino-Martel P, Hercberg S, Galan P, Fassier P, Allès B, Guéraud F, Pierre FH, Touvier M. Red and processed meat intake and cancer risk: Results from the prospective NutriNet-Santé cohort study. Int J Cancer. 2018;142(2):230-7. https://doi.org/10.1002/ijc.31046. Epub 2017 Oct 16.
7. Boada LD, Henriquez-Hernandez LA, Luzardo OP. The impact of red and processed meat consumption on cancer and other health outcomes: epidemiological evidences. Food Chem Toxicol. 2016;92:236–44.
8. Cross AJ, Sinha R. Meat-related mutagens/carcinogens in the etiology of colorectal cancer. Environ Mol Mutagen. 2004;44:44–55.
9. Kassier SM. Colon Cancer and the consumption of red and processed meat: an association that ismedium, rare or well done? South African Journal of Clinical Nutrition. 2016;29:145–9.
10. zur Hausen H. Red meat consumption and cancer: reasons to suspect involvement of bovine infectious factors in colorectal cancer. Int J Cancer. 2012;130:2475–83.
11. Butler C, Lee Y-CA, Li S, Li Q, Chen C-J, Hsu W-L, Lou P-J, Zhu C, Pan J, Shen H, et al. Diet and the risk of head-and-neck cancer among never-smokers and smokers in a Chinese population. Cancer Epidemiology. 2017;46:20–6.
12. Caini S, Masala G, Gnagnarella P, Ermini I, Russell-Edu W, Palli D, Gandini S. Food of animal origin and risk of non-Hodgkin lymphoma and multiple myeloma: a review of the literature and metaanalysis. Crit Rev Oncol Hematol. 2016;100:16–24.
13. Lippi G, Mattiuzzi C, Cervellin G. Meat consumption and cancer risk: a critical review of published meta-analyses. Crit Rev Oncol Hematol. 2016;97:1–14.
14. Grundy A, Poirier AE, Khandwala F, McFadden A, Friedenreich CM, Brenner DR. Cancer incidence attributable to red and processed meat consumption in Alberta in 2012. CMAJ Open. 2016;4:E768–75.
15. Wu K, Spiegelman D, Hou T, Albanes D, Allen NE, Berndt SI, van den Brandt PA, Giles GG, Giovannucci E, Alexandra Goldbohm R, et al. Associations between unprocessed red and processed meat, poultry, seafood and egg intake and the risk of prostate cancer: a pooled analysis of 15 prospective cohort studies. Int J Cancer. 2016;138:2368–82.
16. Wolk A. Potential health hazards of eating red meat. J Intern Med. 2017;281: 106–22.
17. Li F, An S, Hou L, Chen P, Lei C, Tan W. Red and processed meat intake and risk of bladder cancer:a meta-analysis. Int J Clin Exp Med. 2014;7:2100–10.
18. Bylsma LC, Alexander DD. A review and meta-analysis of prospective studies of red and processed meat, meat cooking methods, heme iron, heterocyclic amines and prostate cancer. Nutr J. 2015;14:125.
19. Domingo JL, Nadal M. Carcinogenicity of consumption of red meat and processed meat: a review of scientific news since the IARC decision. Food Chem Toxicol. 2017;105:256–61.
20. Alexander DD, Weed DL, Miller PE, Mohamed MA. Red meat and colorectal cancer: a quantitative update on the state of the epidemiologic science. J Am Coll Nutr. 2015;34:521–43.
21. Carr PR, Walter V, Brenner H, Hoffmeister M. Meat subtypes and their association with colorectal cancer: systematic review and meta-analysis. Int J Cancer. 2016;138:293–302.
22. Samraj AN, Pearce OM, Laubli H, Crittenden AN, Bergfeld AK, Banda K, Gregg CJ, Bingman AE, Secrest P, Diaz SL, et al. A red meat-derived glycan promotes inflammation and cancer progression. Proc Natl Acad Sci U S A. 2015;112:542–7.
23. Calle EE, Kaaks R. Overweight, obesity and cancer: epidemiological evidence and proposed mechanisms. Nat Rev Cancer. 2004;4:579–91.
24. Jung UJ, Choi MS. Obesity and its metabolic complications: the role of adipokines and the relationship between obesity, inflammation, insulin resistance, dyslipidemia and nonalcoholic fatty liver disease. Int J Mol Sci. 2014;15:6184–223.
25. Bruce WR. Recent hypotheses for the origin of colon cancer. Cancer Res. 1987;47:4237–42.
26. Zhao LP, Kushi LH, Klein RD, Prentice RL. Quantitative review of studies of dietary fat and rat colon carcinoma. Nutr Cancer. 1991;15:169–77.
27. Liu L, Zhuang W, Wang RQ, Mukherjee R, Xiao SM, Chen Z, XT W, Zhou Y, Zhang HY. Is dietary fat associated with the risk of colorectal cancer? A meta-analysis of 13 prospective cohort studies. Eur J Nutr. 2011;50:173–84.
28. Santarelli RL, Pierre F, Corpet DE. Processed meat and colorectal cancer: a review of epidemiologic and experimental evidence. Nutr Cancer. 2008;60:131–44.

29. Corpet DE, Yin Y, Zhang XM, Remesy C, Stamp D, Medline A, Thompson L, Bruce WR, Archer MC. Colonic protein fermentation and promotion of colon carcinogenesis by thermolyzed casein. Nutr Cancer. 1995;23:271–81.

30. Windey K, De Preter V, Verbeke K. Relevance of protein fermentation to gut health. Mol Nutr Food Res. 2012;56:184–96.

31. Toden S, Belobrajdic DP, Bird AR, Topping DL, Conlon MA. Effects of dietary beef and chicken with and without high amylose maize starch on blood malondialdehyde, interleukins, IGF-I, insulin, leptin, MMP-2, and TIMP-2 concentrations in rats. Nutr Cancer. 2010;62:454–65.

32. Demeyer D, Mertens B, De Smet S, Ulens M. Mechanisms linking colorectal cancer to the consumption of (processed) red meat: a review. Crit Rev Food Sci Nutr. 2016;56:2747–66.

33. Zheng W, Lee SA. Well-done meat intake, heterocyclic amine exposure, and cancer risk. Nutr Cancer. 2009;61:437–46.

34. Alaejos MS, Gonzalez V, Afonso AM. Exposure to heterocyclic aromatic amines from the consumption of cooked red meat and its effect on human cancer risk: a review. Food Addit Contam Part A Chem Anal Control Expo Risk Assess. 2008;25:2–24.

35. Puangsombat K, Gadgil P, Houser TA, Hunt MC, Smith JS. Occurrence of heterocyclic amines in cooked meat products. Meat Sci. 2012;90:739–46.

36. Lynch AM, Knize MG, Boobis AR, Gooderham NJ, Davies DS, Murray S. Intra- and interindividual variability in systemic exposure in humans to 2-amino-3,8-dimethylimidazo[4,5-f]quinoxaline and 2-amino-1-methyl-6-phenylimidazo[4,5-b]pyridine, carcinogens present in cooked beef. Cancer Res. 1992;52:6216–23.

37. Yamazoe Y, Abu-Zeid M, Manabe S, Toyama S, Kato R. Metabolic activation of a protein pyrolysate promutagen 2-amino-3,8-dimethylimidazo[4,5-f]quinoxaline by rat liver microsomes and purified cytochrome P-450. Carcinogenesis. 1988;9:105–9.

38. Wallin H, Holme JA, Becher G, Alexander J. Metabolism of the food carcinogen 2-amino-3,8-dimethylimidazo[4,5-f]quinoxaline in isolated rat liver cells. Carcinogenesis. 1989;10:1277–83.

39. Turteltaub KW, Knize MG, Buonarati MH, McManus ME, Veronese ME, Mazrimas JA, Felton JS. Metabolism of 2-amino-1-methyl-6-phenylimidazo[4,5-b] pyridine (PhIP) by liver microsomes and isolated rabbit cytochrome P450 isozymes. Carcinogenesis. 1990;11:941–6.

40. Turesky RJ, Bracco-Hammer I, Markovic J, Richli U, Kappeler AM, Welti DH. The contribution of Noxidation to the metabolism of the food-borne carcinogen 2-amino-3,8-dimethylimidazo[4,5-f]quinoxaline in rat hepatocytes. Chem Res Toxicol. 1990;3:524–35.

41. Hayatsu H, Kasai H, Yokoyama S, Miyazawa T, Yamaizumi Z, Sato S, Nishimura S, Arimoto S, Hayatsu T, Ohara Y. Mutagenic metabolites in urine and feces of rats fed with 2-amino-3,8- dimethylimidazo[4,5-f]quinoxaline, a carcinogenic mutagen present in cooked meat. Cancer Res. 1987;47:791–4.

42. Schut HA, Snyderwine EG. DNA adducts of heterocyclic amine food mutagens: implications for mutagenesis and carcinogenesis. Carcinogenesis. 1999;20:353–68.

43. Helmus DS, Thompson CL, Zelenskiy S, Tucker TC, Li L. Red meat-derived heterocyclic amines increase risk of colon cancer: a population-based case-control study. Nutr Cancer. 2013;65:1141–50.

44. Kampman E, Slattery ML, Bigler J, Leppert M, Samowitz W, Caan BJ, Potter JD. Meat consumption, genetic susceptibility, and colon cancer risk: a United States multicenter case-control study. Cancer Epidemiol Biomark Prev. 1999;8:15–24.

45. Butler LM, Sinha R, Millikan RC, Martin CF, Newman B, Gammon MD, Ammerman AS, Sandler RS. Heterocyclic amines, meat intake, and association with colon cancer in a population-based study. Am J Epidemiol. 2003;157:434–45.

46. Le Marchand L, Hankin JH, Pierce LM, Sinha R, Nerurkar PV, Franke AA, Wilkens LR, Kolonel LN, Donlon T, Seifried A, et al. Well-done red meat, metabolic phenotypes and colorectal cancer in Hawaii. Mutat Res. 2002;506-507:205–14.

47. Nothlings U, Yamamoto JF, Wilkens LR, Murphy SP, Park SY, Henderson BE, Kolonel LN, Le Marchand L. Meat and heterocyclic amine intake, smoking, NAT1 and NAT2 polymorphisms, and colorectal cancer risk in the multiethnic cohort study. Cancer Epidemiol Biomark Prev. 2009;18:2098–106.

48. Tiemersma EW, Voskuil DW, Bunschoten A, Hogendoorn EA, Witteman BJ, Nagengast FM, Glatt H, Kok FJ, Kampman E. Risk of colorectal adenomas in relation to meat consumption, meat preparation, and genetic susceptibility in a Dutch population. Cancer Causes Control. 2004;15:225–36.

49. Mastrangelo G, Fadda E, Marzia V. Polycyclic aromatic hydrocarbons and cancer in man. Environ Health Perspect. 1996;104:1166–70.

50. Phillips DH. Polycyclic aromatic hydrocarbons in the diet. Mutat Res. 1999; 443:139–47.

51. Estensen RD, Jordan MM, Wiedmann TS, Galbraith AR, Steele VE, Wattenberg LW. Effect of chemopreventive agents on separate stages of progression of benzo[alpha]pyrene induced lung tumors in a/J mice. Carcinogenesis. 2004;25:197–201.

52. Yang SK, McCourt DW, Roller PP, Gelboin HV. Enzymatic conversion of benzo(a)pyrene leading predominantly to the diol-epoxide r-7,t-8-dihydroxy-t-9,10-oxy-7,8,9,10- tetrahydrobenzo(a)pyrene through a single enantiomer of r-7, t-8-dihydroxy-7,8-dihydrobenzo(a)pyrene. Proc Natl Acad Sci U S A. 1976;73:2594–8.

53. Phillips DH. Fifty years of benzo(a)pyrene. Nature. 1983;303:468–72.

54. Phillips DH, Grover PL. Polycyclic hydrocarbon activation: bay regions and beyond. Drug Metab Rev. 1994;26:443–67.

55. Shimada T. Xenobiotic-metabolizing enzymes involved in activation and detoxification of carcinogenic polycyclic aromatic hydrocarbons. Drug Metab Pharmacokinet. 2006;21:257–76.

56. Tabatabaei SM, Heyworth JS, Knuiman MW, Fritschi L. Dietary benzo[a]pyrene intake from meat and the risk of colorectal cancer. Cancer Epidemiol Biomark Prev. 2010;19:3182–4.

57. Ferrucci LM, Sinha R, Graubard BI, Mayne ST, Ma X, Schatzkin A, Schoenfeld PS, Cash BD, Flood A, Cross AJ. Dietary meat intake in relation to colorectal adenoma in asymptomatic women. Am J Gastroenterol. 2009;104:1231–40.

58. Schwartz S, Ellefson M. Quantitative fecal recovery of ingested hemoglobin-heme in blood: comparisons by HemoQuant assay with ingested meat and fish. Gastroenterology. 1985;89:19–26.

59. Bastide NM, Pierre FH, Corpet DE. Heme iron from meat and risk of colorectal cancer: a metaanalysis and a review of the mechanisms involved. Cancer Prev Res (Phila). 2011;4:177–84.

60. Qiao L, Feng Y. Intakes of heme iron and zinc and colorectal cancer incidence: a meta-analysis of prospective studies. Cancer Causes Control. 2013;24:1175–83.

61. Gilsing AM, Fransen F, de Kok TM, Goldbohm AR, Schouten LJ, de Bruine AP, van Engeland M, van den Brandt PA, de Goeij AF, Weijenberg MP. Dietary heme iron and the risk of colorectal cancer with specific mutations in KRAS and APC. Carcinogenesis. 2013;34:2757–66.

62. Pierre F, Freeman A, Tache S, Van der Meer R, Corpet DE. Beef meat and blood sausage promote the formation of azoxymethane-induced mucin-depleted foci and aberrant crypt foci in rat colons. J Nutr. 2004;134:2711–6.

63. Sesink AL, Termont DS, Kleibeuker JH, Van der Meer R. Red meat and colon cancer: the cytotoxic and hyperproliferative effects of dietary heme. Cancer Res. 1999;59:5704–9.

64. Fonseca-Nunes A, Jakszyn P, Agudo A. Iron and cancer risk–a systematic review and meta-analysis of the epidemiological evidence. Cancer Epidemiol Biomark Prev. 2014;23:12–31.

65. Betteridge DJ. What is oxidative stress? Metabolism. 2000;49:3–8.

66. Dietrich M, Block G, Pogoda JM, Buffler P, Hecht S, Preston-Martin S. A review: dietary and endogenously formed N-nitroso compounds and risk of childhood brain tumors. Cancer Causes Control. 2005;16:619–35.

67. Lijinsky W. N-Nitroso compounds in the diet. Mutat Res. 1999;443:129–38.

68. Tricker AR. N-nitroso compounds and man: sources of exposure, endogenous formation and occurrence in body fluids. Eur J Cancer Prev. 1997;6:226–68.

69. Bos JL. Ras oncogenes in human cancer: a review. Cancer Res. 1989;49: 4682–9.

70. Kuhnle GG, Story GW, Reda T, Mani AR, Moore KP, Lunn JC, Bingham SA. Diet-induced endogenous formation of nitroso compounds in the GI tract. Free Radic Biol Med. 2007;43:1040–7.

71. Lewin MH, Bailey N, Bandaletova T, Bowman R, Cross AJ, Pollock J, Shuker DE, Bingham SA. Red meat enhances the colonic formation of the DNA adduct O6-carboxymethyl guanine: implications for colorectal cancer risk. Cancer Res. 2006;66:1859–65.

72. Niedernhofer LJ, Daniels JS, Rouzer CA, Greene RE, Marnett LJ. Malondialdehyde, a product of lipid peroxidation, is mutagenic in human cells. J Biol Chem. 2003;278:31426–33.

73. Leuratti C, Watson MA, Deag EJ, Welch A, Singh R, Gottschalg E, Marnett LJ, Atkin W, Day NE, Shuker DE, Bingham SA. Detection of malondialdehyde DNA adducts in human colorectal mucosa: relationship with diet and the presence of adenomas. Cancer Epidemiol Biomark Prev. 2002;11:267–73.

74. Awasthi YC, Sharma R, Cheng JZ, Yang Y, Sharma A, Singhal SS, Awasthi S. Role of 4-hydroxynonenal in stress-mediated apoptosis signaling. Mol Asp Med. 2003;24:219–30.

75. Ijssennagger N, Rijnierse A, de Wit NJ, Boekschoten MV, Dekker J, Schonewille A, Muller M, van der Meer R. Dietary heme induces acute oxidative stress, but delayed cytotoxicity and compensatory hyperproliferation in mouse colon. Carcinogenesis. 2013;34:1628–35.

76. Pierre F, Peiro G, Tache S, Cross AJ, Bingham SA, Gasc N, Gottardi G, Corpet DE, Gueraud F. New marker of colon cancer risk associated with heme intake: 1,4-dihydroxynonane mercapturic acid. Cancer Epidemiol Biomark Prev. 2006;15:2274–9.

77. Chou HH, Takematsu H, Diaz S, Iber J, Nickerson E, Wright KL, Muchmore EA, Nelson DL, Warren ST, Varki A. A mutation in human CMP-sialic acid hydroxylase occurred after the homo-pan divergence. Proc Natl Acad Sci U S A. 1998;95:11751–6.

78. Tangvoranuntakul P, Gagneux P, Diaz S, Bardor M, Varki N, Varki A, Muchmore E. Human uptake and incorporation of an immunogenic nonhuman dietary sialic acid. Proc Natl Acad Sci U S A. 2003;100:12045–50.

79. Samraj AN, Laubli H, Varki N, Varki A. Involvement of a non-human sialic acid in human cancer. Front Oncol. 2014;4:33.

80. Bardor M, Nguyen DH, Diaz S, Varki A. Mechanism of uptake and incorporation of the non-human sialic acid N-glycolylneuraminic acid into human cells. J Biol Chem. 2005;280:4228–37.

81. Padler-Karavani V, Hurtado-Ziola N, Pu M, Yu H, Huang S, Muthana S, Chokhawala HA, Cao H, Secrest P, Friedmann-Morvinski D, et al. Human xeno-autoantibodies against a non-human sialic acid serve as novel serum biomarkers and immunotherapeutics in cancer. Cancer Res. 2011;71:3352–63.

82. Padler-Karavani V, Varki A. Potential impact of the non-human sialic acid N-glycolylneuraminic acid on transplant rejection risk. Xenotransplantation. 2011;18:1–5.

# 20

# Role of BK human polyomavirus in cancer

Jorge Levican[1], Mónica Acevedo[1], Oscar León[1], Aldo Gaggero[1*] and Francisco Aguayo[2,3*]

**Abstract**

Human polyomaviruses (HPyV), which are small DNA viruses classified into the polyomaviridae family, are widely distributed in human populations. Thirteen distinct HPyVs have been described to date. Some of these viruses have been found in human tumors, suggesting an etiological relationship with cancer. In particular, convincing evidence of an oncogenic role has emerged for a specific HPyV, the Merkel cell polyomavirus (MCPyV). This HPyV has been linked to rare skin cancer, Merkel cell carcinoma (MCC). This finding may be just the tip of the iceberg, as HPyV infections are ubiquitous in humans. Many authors have conjectured that additional associations between HPyV infections and neoplastic diseases will likely be discovered. In 2012, the International Agency for Research on Cancer (IARC) evaluated the carcinogenicity of the BK virus (BKPyV), reporting that BKPyV is "possibly carcinogenic to humans." This review explores the BKPyV infection from a historical point of view, including biological aspects related to viral entry, tropism, epidemiology and mechanisms potentially involved in BKPyV-mediated human carcinogenesis. In order to clarify the role of this virus in human cancer, more epidemiological and basic research is strongly warranted.

**Keywords:** Polyomavirus, Cancer, Oncoprotein

## Background

Human polyomaviruses (HPyVs) are small, non-enveloped, double-stranded DNA viruses with approximately 5000-bp genome and icosahedral symmetry. These viruses belong to the polyomaviridae family. The HPyV genome encodes early small-t/large-T antigens as well as late structural proteins called VP1, VP2, VP3, and agnoprotein. The early region, which is transcribed before DNA replication begins, is composed of large T and small t antigen genes and the splice variants $T = 135$, $T = 136$, and $T = 165$ [1]. The late region is transcribed concomitant with DNA replication. The HPyV capsid harbors 72 pentamers of VP1, which interacts with the VP2/VP3 molecules associated with each pentamer [2]. In addition, these viruses encode a pre-miRNA for generation of two mature miRNAs [3, 4]. A non-coding control region (NCCR) is located between the oppositely-oriented transcriptional units that encode for early and late transcripts. The NCCR contains the promoters and enhancers for regulation of gene expression and harbors the replication origin (Ori) [5]. In BKPyV, JCPyV, and SV40, the

agnoprotein is expressed from the 5′region of VP2 open reading frame. It is believed that this protein is involved in various functions related to the HPyV life cycle, such as regulating viral gene expression or inducing viral maturation [6, 7]. A scheme of the BKPyV structure is shown in Fig. 1. The functions of encoded viral products are summarized in Table 1.

In natural hosts, HPyVs establish a productive infection, while in heterologous, non-permissive hosts, the virus establishes latency with potential integration into the host genome (reviewed in [8]). HPyV infection typically occurs early in life, often through fecal-oral transmission, and persists throughout the lifespan [9]. With the development of new high-throughput sequencing techniques, fourteen HPyVs have been described, most of which were discovered in the last few years [10]. As HPyVs are ubiquitous, associations between these viruses and various pathologies are a focus of intensive research, especially the possible contributions of HPyVs to cancer etiology. Four polyomaviruses have been found to show oncogenic potential — SV40, BKPyV, JCPyV, and MCPyV — although there is strong evidence of such a link only in the case of MCPyV. This virus appears to play a role in a rare skin cancer, Merkel cell carcinoma [11]. A carcinogenic role has also been suspected for SV40, but the association remains controversial as no

* Correspondence: agaggero@med.uchile.cl; faguayo@med.uchile.cl
[1]Programa de Virología, Instituto de Ciencias Biomedicas, Facultad de Medicina, Universidad de Chile, Santiago, Chile
[2]Departamento de Oncología Básico clínica, Facultad de Medicina, Universidad de Chile, Santiago, Chile
Full list of author information is available at the end of the article

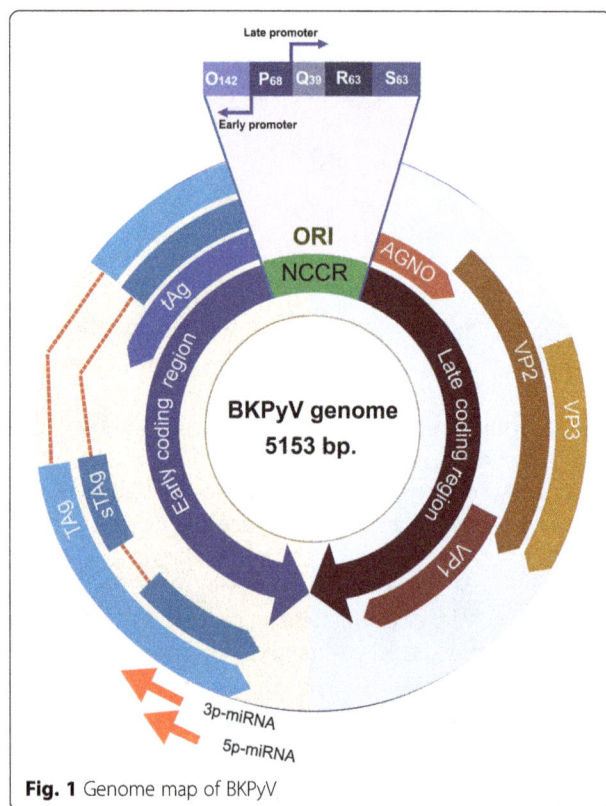

**Fig. 1** Genome map of BKPyV

the ganglioside GD3 is formed, with several points of contact between VP1 and two sialic molecules of a disialic acid ganglioside [14]. This model was tested using site-directed mutagenesis. It was concluded that a specific contact between the terminal sialic acid residue of GD3 and VP1 is essential for virus infection. Previous experiments carried out on African green monkey kidney cells suggest that caveolin is involved in BKPyV entry. However, the entry mechanism of BKPyV was recently re-examined in a primary culture of human renal proximal tubule epithelial cells. Using a siRNA strategy, it was demonstrated that BKPyV entry is caveolin- and clathrin-independent [15]. These findings, along with the fact that virus entry does not require actin polymerization, exclude other known alternative endocytic pathways and suggests that BKPyV utilizes an as-yet-uncharacterized endocytic pathway [15, 16]. After entering the cell, the virus must reach the nucleus for replication. This process depends on acidification and maturation of the endosome and involves retrograde transit of endocytic vesicles to the endoplasmic reticulum (ER) [17, 18]. Once in the ER, partial disassembly occurs. Viral particles escape to the cytoplasm, hijacking ER Derlin family proteins [18]. Finally, the virus enters the nucleus via the importin-α/β pathway, guided by nuclear localization signals present in the minor capsid proteins VP2 and VP3 [19].

### Tropism and epidemiology
BKPyV infection is a widely-distributed strict anthroponosis. The primary infection most often occurs in early childhood, with a seroprevalence of 65–90% in 5–9 year-old children [20]. Following primary infection, BKPyV persists in the kidneys. If the host becomes immunosuppressed, the virus causes significant morbidity. For instance, BKPyV causes hemorrhagic cystitis and nephropathy (BKAN) in bone marrow and renal transplant patients, respectively [21, 22]. BKPyV genomes have also been detected in a wide spectrum of normal

robust evidence has emerged. This virus was initially detected as a contaminant in the poliovirus vaccine, with many infections occurring between 1955 and 1963 [12]. This review evaluates the molecular mechanisms of BKPyV infection and its potential association with cancer.

### BK virus
#### Viral entry
During BKPyV infection, VP1 interacts with the α2, 8-SA-containing b-series gangliosides (GD1b/GT1b) for cell attachment [13]. A crystal-like complex of VP1 and

**Table 1** Function of BKPyV gene products

|  | BKPyV expression products | Function |
| --- | --- | --- |
| Early | Large Tumour Antigen (Tag) | Cell cycle progression, inhibition of apoptosis, viral replication |
|  | truncated Large T antigen (truncTAg) | Cell cycle progression, viral replication |
|  | Minor T Antigen (tAg) | Cell cycle progression |
|  | 3p-miRNA | viral persistence |
|  | 5p-miRNA | viral persistence |
| Late | VP1 | capsid structure (external), viral attachment and entry |
|  | VP2 | capsid structure (internal), involved in viral infectivity |
|  | VP3 | capsid structure (internal), involved in viral infectivity |
|  | Agno protein | Life cycle (assembly, maturation, release) |

tissues including liver, stomach, lungs, parathyroid glands, lymph nodes, brain, peripheral blood mononuclear cells, bladder, uterine cervix, vulva, prostate, lips and tongue [23]. Although the transmission mechanism is not completely elucidated, the high resistance of BKPyV to environmental inactivation and its presence at high concentrations in human sewage and other water sources suggest fecal-oral transmission [24]. In this respect, it was reported that salivary glands and oropharyngeal cells are not involved in BKPyV persistence, suggesting that digestive tract would be important for viral transmission [25]. In addition, Taguchi et al. showed a vertical transmission of this virus only in the case of primary BKV infection of serologically negative pregnant women [26]. Moreover, it was reported the presence of BKPyV in 7 out 10 specimens of aborted fetuses suggesting the possibility of transplacental transmission [27]. Once the virus enters to the body, probably peripheral blood leukocytes (PBLs) transport BKPyV to different sites and organs [28].

Upon BKPyV infection in a permissive host cell, early gene expression leads to DNA replication, followed by late gene expression, production of progeny viral particles and cell death. Permissive cells for viral replication are kidney cells such as Vero (African green monkey kidney) [29], HEK293 (human embryonic kidney cells) [30] or RPTE (primary human renal proximal tubule epithelial cells) [31]. In addition, it has been reported that some salivary glands cells are permissive for BKPyV infection [32].

In a non-permissive cell, BKPyV lytic replication is blocked, and abortive infection may result in oncogenic transformation [33].

Although the oncogenic activity of BKPyV is well-documented in laboratory settings, there is no conclusive evidence of a causal relationship between BKPyV and cancer in human beings. This relationship is difficult to demonstrate in ecological contexts for several reasons: first, the viral agent has a high prevalence in the general population; second, there are a wide range of human tissues in which the virus can be detected; and third, the virus has the ability to remain in a latent state for long periods, with occasional reactivations.

### Role in carcinogenesis

The oncogenic properties of BKPyV are well-demonstrated in in vitro and in vivo experimental models. The transforming activity has been mapped in the early region of the BKPyV genome, which encodes two viral oncoproteins: the large T-antigen (TAg) and the small t-antigen (tAg). These viral products induce alterations in the normal cell cycle, ultimately leading to cell immortalization and neoplastic transformation [34]. In one study, transfection of embryonic fibroblasts or

cells cultured from kidney or brain tissues of diverse mammalian origin with complete or sub-genomic fragments of BKPyV DNA, containing the early coding region, lead to cell transformation [23]. In addition, transformation with a recombinant construct containing the BKPyV TAg gene and the activated c-Ha-ras oncogene-induced neoplastic transformation at early passages in hamster embryo cells with higher efficiency when compared to independently-transfected genes, suggesting a cooperative effect of the two oncogenes in early carcinogenesis [23]. Moreover, continuous expression of functional TAg is required for the maintenance of BKPyV transformation in hamster and mouse cells [23].

BKPyV large TAg is a highly multifunctional protein that can bind various cellular proteins, altering signaling pathways involved in cell cycle control. The most frequently-studied cellular targets of TAg are the p53 family proteins and pRb tumor suppressor proteins. The interaction between BKPyV TAg and p53 results in the inactivation of this protein, interfering with the response to DNA damage and inducing the unscheduled onset of the S-phase [35]. Therefore, BKPyV TAg drives the cell to override a key cell cycle checkpoint, favoring the accumulation of genetic alterations during each cell replication cycle [23, 36, 37]. In addition, the interaction between BKPyV TAg and pRb leads to the release and nuclear translocation of the E2 factor (E2F) family of transcription factors and subsequent expression of genes, inducing quiescent cells to enter the S-phase [37, 38]. The other early gene product of BKPyV, the small tAg, plays an important role in transformation by inhibiting protein phosphatase 2A (PP2A), an essential tumor suppressor in numerous death-signaling pathways. The tAg protein shows two conserved cysteine cluster motifs (CXCXXC) that are thought to be involved in the interaction with PP2A [39]. Indeed, the catalytic (36-kDa) and regulatory (63-kDa) subunits of PP2A have been co-immunoprecipitated with anti-tAg from BKPyV-infected human embryonic kidney (HEK) cells [40]. By inactivating this negative regulator, BKPyV tAg can activate signaling pathways that promote cell proliferation, such as mitogen-activated protein kinase (MAPK) [23, 33, 39].

Early reports demonstrated that BKPyV is highly oncogenic in rodents [41, 42]. Assays conducted in newborn hamsters, mice, and rats inoculated with the virus showed that these animals developed tumors at various locations that contained BKPyV DNA sequences, either integrated into the host genome or in a free episomal form with constitutive TAg expression [23]. In addition, animals injected with BKPyV frequently developed ependymomas, pancreatic islet tumors, osteosarcomas, fibrosarcomas, liposarcomas, osteosarcomas, nephroblastomas and gliomas [23]. Transgenic mice expressing the BKPyV early genome region were found to develop highly tissue-specific tumors. Small et al. showed that these animals developed primary hepatocellular carcinomas and renal tumors [43]. Dalrymple and Beemon also observed two types of alterations: enlarged thymuses and renal adenocarcinomas. Moreover, BKPyV TAg expression in these mice was restricted to the epithelial cells of the kidney tumors and enlarged thymuses [44].

Although the transforming ability of BKPyV is well-documented in experimental rodent models, definitive transforming activity is not always observed in human and primates. The transformation of HEK cells by BKPyV is not efficient and is often abortive, and features of the transformed phenotype are not fully displayed [37, 45]. For instance, BKPyV TAg was able to induce serum-independent growth in BSC-1 African green monkey kidney cells but was unable to induce anchorage-independent growth in soft agar [37]. In addition, BKPyV TAg activity is lower in BKPyV-infected BSC cells than the TAg activity expressed by the SV40 virus under the same conditions. TAg expressed by BKPyV is not sufficient to completely capture the Rb family of proteins. It has been proposed that the difference between SV40 and BKPyV TAg activity may be due to lower expression levels of the BKPyV promoter and enhancer elements, which share only 40% homology with the SV40 promoter region. Alternatively, this finding may be a consequence the greater instability of the BKPyV TAg as compared to SV40 TAg protein [37]. These findings suggest that while BKPyV TAg may modulate cellular growth through direct interactions with critical regulatory proteins, additional events are required for complete transformation. These events could be mutations or alterations of the viral promoter-enhancer elements, leading to increased expression of early genes and a consequent increase in transforming activity [46]. In support of this model, integration of early-region viral sequences into the host genome has been shown to account for the difference between serum-independent growth and full transformation in BKPyV-infected human embryonic kidney cells [47]. This integration event could result in positioning of BKPyV TAg coding sequence under the control of nearby cellular promoter-enhancer elements.

An alternative model for the role of BKPyV TAg in oncogenesis involves the first step in which BKPyV TAg binds to or inactivates tumor suppressor proteins, with a second step leading to cellular oncogene activation. This model is supported by studies showing that human embryonic kidney cells persistently infected with BKPyV exhibited a semi-transformed phenotype and that full

transformation resulted from the additional presence of activated Ha-ras oncogenes [48]. Therefore, p53 inactivation by BK TAg may lead to random mutational events that could activate cellular oncogenes or inactivate other tumor suppressor genes. Moreover, it has been shown that BKPyV TAg induces chromosomal instability in human embryonic fibroblasts, characterized by gaps, breaks, dicentric and ring chromosomes, deletions, duplications and translocations [49]. Consistent with early participation of BKPyV TAg in tumorigenesis, there is evidence that these alterations occur before immortalization [23]. Once chromosomal alterations are fixed into the host cells, viral sequences may be dispensable for the maintenance of transformation and may be lost in the neoplastic tissues.

Various authors have detected BKPyV genetic material in a wide range of human tumors [23, 33]. For instance, the early BKPyV genome region has been detected in brain tumors, osteosarcomas, Ewing's tumors, neuroblastomas and genitourinary tract tissues tumors, including prostatic and bladder cancer [23, 33, 50, 51]. In contrast, other authors reported no association between BKPyV DNA and tumors [33, 52–56]. In any case, the mere presence of BKPyV DNA does not necessarily reflect a neoplastic involvement of the virus. In some cases, BKPyV may not be directly involved in the development of cancer, but instead, play a role as a co-factor in the carcinogenic process. For instance, the virus may co-infect cells that were previously infected by another oncogenic virus, increasing susceptibility to cancer. In fact, HPyVs have been detected in various tissues that are susceptible to transformation by HTLV-I, HCV, HPV, EBV, HHV-8 and HBV [57]. In addition, recent reports have documented the presence of BKPyV DNA in association with HPV16 in high-grade cervical squamous intraepithelial lesions [58]. The association of BKPyV with precancerous cervical lesions suggests that this virus could be involved in HPV16-induced cell transformation. Alternatively, BKPyV might benefit from proliferative enhancement of HPV16-positive cells in precancerous cervical cells. Further experimental studies and clinical observations are needed to verify whether this putative transformation mechanism involving BKPyV and HPV occurs in cervical cancer [58].

Early findings established that BKPyV has a tropism for certain cell types and that this agent can establish a persistent or latent infection in the kidney and urinary tract [59]. Therefore, carcinomas that affect this anatomical zone are likely candidates for associations with BKPyV. Among these diseases, renal cancer, urothelial bladder cancer, and prostatic cancer have been extensively studied [23, 60].

The contribution of BKPyV to the etiology of bladder carcinoma in immunocompetent individuals is not well-established. Some studies demonstrate BKPyV DNA sequences at high frequencies in bladder carcinoma [61, 62]. However, these studies were small case series that either lacked a control group or relied entirely on antibody seroprevalence [63]. In a multi-center study, Polesel et al. found similar a prevalence of the viral DNA in a group of 114 transitional bladder carcinoma cases and a group of 140 hospital controls. This result does not support the role of BKPyV in bladder cancer among immunocompetent individuals [64].

On the other hand, there are reports that link BKPyV with metastatic bladder carcinoma in immunosuppressed transplant recipients [65–67]. In a retrospective study, Roberts et al. reported that while no positive BKPyV TAg urothelial carcinomas were found in a series of non-transplanted patients (0/20), strong nuclear staining for TAg was seen in the urothelial carcinoma of one renal transplant patient [68]. This data indicates that although associations between BKPyV and these tumors are rare, the virus may have a tumorigenic role in some cases. In addition, in a retrospective review of kidney transplant patients, Chen et al. reported that 6/864 patients developed polyomavirus-associated nephropathy (PVAN). Malignancy occurred in 5/6 PVAN patients, suggesting that patients who develop PVAN are at significantly higher risk of developing cancers, including transitional cell bladder carcinoma [66, 69]. Although urothelial carcinomas expressing BK TAg are quite rare [68], these cancers show some distinct features. These tumors are high-grade and invasive. Lesions can arise in the renal allograft or the host urothelial tissue. While TAg is strongly expressed in the tumor cells, the late structural proteins are not expressed, and no viral replication is observed. This finding suggests that the possible oncogenic mechanism involves deregulation of the proliferation inducer TAg [70]. Recent findings using deep sequencing analysis from a high-grade BKPyV-associated tumor expressing TAg have revealed viral DNA integrated into the host genome [71, 72]. While the insertion site seems to be nonspecific, the virus genome linearization break-point was situated in the late gene coding region. This interruption accounts for the blockage of viral replication and suggests a concomitant disruption of regulatory feedback signals that control TAg expression [71, 72]. Moreover, Seo et al., (2008) reported that BKPyV codes a pre-miRNA hairpin at the 3′ end of the late region [73]. The maturation of this element gives rise to two miRNAs, 5p-miRNA and 3p-miRNA, which are perfectly complementary to Tag-coding mRNA. Whether these miRNAs are functional during BKPyV infection and how this regulatory disruption contributes to BKPyV-mediated cell transformation is currently under intense study.

Prostate cancer (PCa) is one of the leading causes of cancer deaths in men worldwide, and its relationship with BKPyV infection has been studied by several groups in recent years [74–80]. Monini et al. detected BKPyV in approximately 60% of cancerous and healthy prostates, and the viral load was found to be significantly higher in neoplastic as compared to non-neoplastic tissue [74]. Das and Russo found similar detection rates in PCa cases, with a significantly lower prevalence in controls [76, 77, 81]. On the other hand, other authors disagree with these results. Lau et al., using in situ, detected BKPyV in only 2/30 prostatic adenocarcinomas, and no TAg expression was detected in neoplastic tissue [79]. Similarly, Sfanos et al. of 338 analyzed total samples from 200 patients for BKPyV DNA and detected only one positive sample [82]. In Chile, our group found only 6/69 (8.7%) BKPyV DNA-positive prostate carcinomas, and the TAg transcripts were detected in 2/6 (33%) of BKPyV positive cases [83]. These apparently contradictory data can be partially explained due to the variable sensitivity and specificity of the detection methods used in each study. However, this finding may also suggest that the virus is dispensable at late stages of the disease, and it may be cleared from the lesion. In this context, it has been postulated that BKPyV constitutes an important factor for early prostate tumorigenesis [77]. Although p53 and pRb proteins are implicated in PCa, there is a low incidence of mutations in these genes during early stages of the disease [84]. This finding has led to the suggestion that a human oncogenic virus such as BKPyV may be implicated in the inactivation of these tumor suppressor proteins at early stages of tumorigenesis [76, 77]. There is growing evidence supporting this model. Using a combination of Laser Capture Microdissection (LCM) and molecular biology techniques, BKPyV DNA has been detected in the epithelial cells of benign and proliferative inflammatory atrophy (PIA) and prostate intraepithelial neoplasia (PIN), entities that have been postulated to be the early transition step toward overt PCa [76, 77, 85, 86]. In addition, using double immunofluorescence labeling with anti-p53 and TAg antibodies in BKPyV positive prostate tumor tissue sections, it has been observed that the two proteins colocalize in the cytoplasm. While the typical localization of both proteins is nuclear, the cytoplasmic localization suggests a functional inactivation mechanism by sequestration [81]. Moreover, p53 genes from atrophic cells expressing TAg are frequently wild-type, whereas tumor cells expressing detectable nuclear p53 contain a mix of wild-type and mutant p53 genes. This finding suggests a possible tumorigenic mechanism in which the TAg inactivates p53 in the atrophic cells, increasing susceptibility to genetic alterations, including tumor suppressor gene mutations that may result in early prostate cancer

**Table 2** Evidences for carcinogenic and non-carcinogenic role of BKPyV

| Evidences of BKPyV carcinogenicity | Evidences for a non-carcinogenic role |
| --- | --- |
| Viral oncogenes are expressed in tumors | Poor and not efficient transforming activity in human cells |
| Tumors developed in in vivo models | Ubiquitous distribution in normal human cells and tissues |
| Transforming properties in in vitro models | Variable BKPyV presence in tumors among different studies |
| BKPyV alterations occur before immortalization | |
| BKPyV genome detected in human tumors | |

progression. This model is consistent with a "hit-and-run" carcinogenesis mechanism [87]. After cell transformation, the loss of BKPyV in the tumor cells could be due to selection against TAg by the immune system, dilution of viral episomes due to lack of replication or pro-apoptotic effects mediated by TAg that are not compatible with the other growth control mutations in the tumor cells, resulting in selection against TAg expression [23, 33, 76, 77, 81]. Nonetheless, the "hit-and-run" mechanism is difficult to defend experimentally. Taken together, a carcinogenic role of this virus has been difficult to demonstrate. Some arguments for a carcinogenic and for a non-carcinogenic role of BKPyV in human cancer are summarized in Table 2.

## Conclusion

The challenge now is to devise investigative strategies that might lead to conclusive evidence that would allow us to confirm or exclude the role of BKPyV in the development of tumors. Thus, more epidemiological and experimental studies are strongly required. In addition, the possibility of interaction with other host-related factors, infectious agents or environmental components for carcinogenesis warrants more investigation.

## Abbreviations
BKPyV: BK polyomavirus; HPyV: Human polyomavirus; PCa: Prostate cancer; SV40: Simian Virus 40; TAg: Major T antigen; tAg: Minor T antigen

## Acknowledgements
Not applicable.

## Funding
This study was supported by FONDECYT Grant 1161219 (FA), FONDECYT Grant 1151250 (OL), FONDECYT Grant 11121411 (MA), U-INICIA Grant 11/08 (MA), Fundación Estudios Biomédicos Avanzados, Facultad de Medicina, Universidad de Chile, and CONICYT-FONDAP Grant 15130011 (FA).

## Authors' contributions
JL, AG, FA: Conceived and designed the manuscript. JL and FA Wrote the manuscript. JL, AG, OL and MA contributed with reading, comments, writing and criticisms. All authors read and approved the final manuscript.

## Competing interests
The authors declare that they have no competing interests.

## Author details
[1]Programa de Virología, Instituto de Ciencias Biomedicas, Facultad de Medicina, Universidad de Chile, Santiago, Chile. [2]Departamento de Oncología Básico clínica, Facultad de Medicina, Universidad de Chile, Santiago, Chile. [3]Advanced Center for Chronic Diseases (ACCDiS), Universidad de Chile, Santiago, Chile.

## References

1. Trowbridge PW, Frisque RJ. Identification of three new JC virus proteins generated by alternative splicing of the early viral mRNA. J Neuro-Oncol. 1995;1(2):195–206.

2. Barouch DH, Harrison SC. Interactions among the major and minor coat proteins of polyomavirus. J Virol. 1994;68(6):3982–9.

3. Lagatie O, Tritsmans L, Stuyver LJ. The miRNA world of polyomaviruses. Virol J. 2013;10:268.

4. Lee S, Paulson KG, Murchison EP, Afanasiev OK, Alkan C, Leonard JH, Byrd DR, Hannon GJ, Nghiem P. Identification and validation of a novel mature microRNA encoded by the Merkel cell polyomavirus in human Merkel cell carcinomas. J Clin Virol. 2011;52(3):272–5.

5. Bethge T, Hachemi HA, Manzetti J, Gosert R, Schaffner W, Hirsch HH. Sp1 sites in the noncoding control region of BK polyomavirus are key regulators of bidirectional viral early and late gene expression. J Virol. 2015;89(6):3396–411.

6. Sariyer IK, Saribas AS, White MK, Safak M. Infection by agnoprotein-negative mutants of polyomavirus JC and SV40 results in the release of virions that are mostly deficient in DNA content. Virol J. 2011;8:255.

7. Khalili K, White MK, Sawa H, Nagashima K, Safak M. The agnoprotein of polyomaviruses: a multifunctional auxiliary protein. J Cell Physiol. 2005; 204(1):1–7.

8. Flippot R, Malouf GG, Su X, Khayat D, Spano JP. Oncogenic viruses: lessons learned using next-generation sequencing technologies. Eur J Cancer. 2016;61:61–8.

9. Martel-Jantin C, Pedergnana V, Nicol JT, Leblond V, Trégouët DA, Tortevoye P, Plancoulaine S, Coursaget P, Touzé A, Abel L, et al. Merkel cell polyomavirus infection occurs during early childhood and is transmitted between siblings. J Clin Virol. 2013;58(1):288–91.

10. Gheit T, Dutta S, Oliver J, Robitaille A, Hampras S, Combes JD, McKay-Chopin S, Le Calvez-Kelm F, Fenske N, Cherpelis B, et al. Isolation and characterization of a novel putative human polyomavirus. Virology. 2017; 506:45–54.

11. Feng H, Shuda M, Chang Y, Moore PS. Clonal integration of a polyomavirus in human Merkel cell carcinoma. Science. 2008;319(5866):1096–100.

12. Dang-Tan T, Mahmud SM, Puntoni R, Franco EL. Polio vaccines, simian virus 40, and human cancer: the epidemiologic evidence for a causal association. Oncogene. 2004;23(38):6535–40.

13. Low JA, Magnuson B, Tsai B, Imperiale MJ. Identification of gangliosides GD1b and GT1b as receptors for BK virus. J Virol. 2006;80(3):1361–6.

14. Neu U, Khan ZM, Schuch B, Palma AS, Liu Y, Pawlita M, Feizi T, Stehle T. Structures of B-lymphotropic polyomavirus VP1 in complex with oligosaccharide ligands. PLoS Pathog. 2013;9(10):e1003714.

15. Zhao L, Marciano AT, Rivet CR, Imperiale MJ. Caveolin- and clathrin-independent entry of BKPyV into primary human proximal tubule epithelial cells. Virology. 2016;492:66–72.

16. Eash S, Atwood WJ. Involvement of cytoskeletal components in BK virus infectious entry. J Virol. 2005;79(18):11734–41.

17. Maru S, Jin G, Desai D, Amin S, Shwetank, Lauver MD, Lukacher AE. Inhibition of retrograde transport limits Polyomavirus infection in vivo. mSphere. 2017;2(6)

18. Jiang M, Abend JR, Tsai B, Imperiale MJ. Early events during BK virus entry and disassembly. J Virol. 2009;83(3):1350–8.

19. Bennett SM, Zhao L, Bosard C, Imperiale MJ. Role of a nuclear localization signal on the minor capsid proteins VP2 and VP3 in BKPyV nuclear entry. Virology. 2015;474:110–6.

20. Siguier M, Sellier P, Bergmann JF. BK-virus infections: a literature review. Med Mal Infect. 2012;42(5):181–7.

21. Hirsch HH, Brennan DC, Drachenberg CB, Ginevri F, Gordon J, Limaye AP, Mihatsch MJ, Nickeleit V, Ramos E, Randhawa P, et al. Polyomavirus-associated nephropathy in renal transplantation: interdisciplinary analyses and recommendations. Transplantation. 2005;79(10):1277–86.

22. Hirsch HH, Randhawa P, Practice AIDCo. BK virus in solid organ transplant recipients. Am J Transplant. 2009;9(Suppl 4):S136–46.

23. Tognon M, Corallini A, Martini F, Negrini M, Barbanti-Brodano G. Oncogenic transformation by BK virus and association with human tumors. Oncogene. 2003;22(33):5192–200.

24. Bofill-Mas S, Pina S, Girones R. Documenting the epidemiologic patterns of polyomaviruses in human populations by studying their presence in urban sewage. Appl Environ Microbiol. 2000;66(1):238–45.

25. Sundsfjord A, Spein AR, Lucht E, Flaegstad T, Seternes OM, Traavik T. Detection of BK virus DNA in nasopharyngeal aspirates from children with respiratory infections but not in saliva from immunodeficient and immunocompetent adult patients. J Clin Microbiol. 1994;32(5):1390–4.

26. Taguchi F, Kajioka J, Shimada N. Presence of interferon and antibodies to BK virus in amniotic fluid of normal pregnant women. Acta Virol. 1985;29(4):299–304.

27. Boldorini R, Allegrini S, Miglio U, Nestasio I, Paganotti A, Veggiani C, Monga G, Pietropaolo V. BK virus sequences in specimens from aborted fetuses. J Med Virol. 2010;82(12):2127–32.

28. Chatterjee M, Weyandt TB, Frisque RJ. Identification of archetype and rearranged forms of BK virus in leukocytes from healthy individuals. J Med Virol. 2000;60(3):353–62.

29. Gardner SD, Field AM, Coleman DV, Hulme B. New human papovavirus (B.K.) isolated from urine after renal transplantation. Lancet. 1971;1(7712):1253–7.

30. Marshall WF, Telenti A, Proper J, Aksamit AJ, Smith TF. Rapid detection of polyomavirus BK by a shell vial cell culture assay. J Clin Microbiol. 1990; 28(7):1613–5.

31. Low J, Humes HD, Szczypka M, Imperiale M. BKV and SV40 infection of human kidney tubular epithelial cells in vitro. Virology. 2004;323(2):182–8.

32. Jeffers LK, Madden V, Webster-Cyriaque J. BK virus has tropism for human salivary gland cells in vitro: implications for transmission. Virology. 2009; 394(2):183–93.

33. Abend JR, Jiang M, Imperiale MJ. BK virus and human cancer: innocent until proven guilty. Semin Cancer Biol. 2009;19(4):252–60.

34. Imperiale MJ. The human polyomaviruses, BKV and JCV: molecular pathogenesis of acute disease and potential role in cancer. Virology. 2000; 267(1):1–7.

35. Papadimitriou JC, Randhawa P, Rinaldo CH, Drachenberg CB, Alexiev B, Hirsch HH. BK Polyomavirus infection and Renourinary tumorigenesis. Am J Transplant. 2016;16(2):398–406.

36. Shivakumar CV, Das GC. Interaction of human polyomavirus BK with the tumor-suppressor protein p53. Oncogene. 1996;13(2):323–32.

37. Harris KF, Christensen JB, Imperiale MJ. BK virus large T antigen: interactions with the retinoblastoma family of tumor suppressor proteins and effects on cellular growth control. J Virol. 1996;70(4): 2378–86.

38. Harris KF, Chang E, Christensen JB, Imperiale MJ. BK virus as a potential co-factor in human cancer. Dev Biol Stand. 1998;94:81–91.

39. White MK, Khalili K. Polyomaviruses and human cancer: molecular mechanisms underlying patterns of tumorigenesis. Virology. 2004;324(1):1–16.

40. Rundell K, Major EO, Lampert M. Association of cellular 56,000- and 32,000-molecular-weight protein with BK virus and polyoma virus t-antigens. J Virol. 1981;37(3):1090–3.

41. Corallini A, Pagnani M, Viadana P, Camellin P, Caputo A, Reschiglian P, Rossi S, Altavilla G, Selvatici R, Barbanti-Brodano G. Induction of malignant subcutaneous sarcomas in hamsters by a recombinant DNA containing BK virus early region and the activated human c-Harvey-ras oncogene. Cancer Res. 1987;47(24 Pt 1):6671–7.

42. Noss G, Stauch G, Mehraein P, Georgii A. Oncogenic activity of the BK type of human papova virus in newborn Wistar rats. Arch Virol. 1981; 69(3–4):239–51.

43. Small JA, Khoury G, Jay G, Howley PM, Scangos GA. Early regions of JC virus and BK virus induce distinct and tissue-specific tumors in transgenic mice. Proc Natl Acad Sci U S A. 1986;83(21):8288–92.

44. Dalrymple SA, Beemon KL. BK virus T antigens induce kidney carcinomas and thymoproliferative disorders in transgenic mice. J Virol. 1990;64(3):1182–91.

45. Portolani M, Borgatti M. Stable transformation of mouse, rabbit and monkey cells and abortive transformation of human cells by BK virus, a human papovavirus. J Gen Virol. 1978;38(2):369–74.

46. Watanabe S, Yoshiike K. Decreasing the number of 68-base-pair tandem repeats in the BK virus transcriptional control region reduces plaque size and enhances transforming capacity. J Virol. 1985;55(3):823–5.

47. Purchio AF, Fareed GC. Transformation of human embryonic kidney cells by human papovarirus BK. J Virol. 1979;29(2):763–9.

48. Pater A, Pater MM. Transformation of primary human embryonic kidney cells to anchorage independence by a combination of BK virus DNA and the Harvey-ras oncogene. J Virol. 1986;58(2):680–3.

49. Trabanelli C, Corallini A, Gruppioni R, Sensi A, Bonfatti A, Campioni D, Merlin M, Calza N, Possati L, Barbanti-Brodano G. Chromosomal aberrations induced by BK virus T antigen in human fibroblasts. Virology. 1998;243(2):492–6.

50. De Mattei M, Martini F, Corallini A, Gerosa M, Scotlandi K, Carinci P, Barbanti-Brodano G, Tognon M. High incidence of BK virus large-T-antigen-coding sequences in normal human tissues and tumors of different histotypes. Int J Cancer. 1995;61(6):756–60.

51. Flaegstad T, Andresen PA, Johnsen JI, Asomani SK, Jørgensen GE, Vignarajan S, Kjuul A, Kogner P, Traavik T. A possible contributory role of BK virus infection in neuroblastoma development. Cancer Res. 1999;59(5):1160–3.

52. Arthur RR, Grossman SA, Ronnett BM, Bigner SH, Vogelstein B, Shah KV. Lack of association of human polyomaviruses with human brain tumors. J Neuro-Oncol. 1994;20(1):55–8.

53. Weggen S, Bayer TA, von Deimling A, Reifenberger G, von Schweinitz D, Wiestler OD, Pietsch T. Low frequency of SV40, JC and BK polyomavirus sequences in human medulloblastomas, meningiomas and ependymomas. Brain Pathol. 2000;10(1):85–92.

54. Greenlee JE, Becker LE, Narayan O, Johnson RT. Failure to demonstrate papovavirus tumor antigen in human cerebral neoplasms. Ann Neurol. 1978;3(6):479–81.

55. Rollison DE, Utaipat U, Ryschkewitsch C, Hou J, Goldthwaite P, Daniel R, Helzlsouer KJ, Burger PC, Shah KV, Major EO. Investigation of human brain tumors for the presence of polyomavirus genome sequences by two independent laboratories. Int J Cancer. 2005;113(5):769–74.

56. Grossi MP, Meneguzzi G, Chenciner N, Corallini A, Poli F, Altavilla G, Alberti S, Milanesi G, Barbanti-Brodano G. Lack of association between BK virus and ependymomas, malignant tumors of pancreatic islets, osteosarcomas and other human tumors. Intervirology. 1981;15(1):10–7.

57. Moens U, Van Ghelue M, Ehlers B. Are human polyomaviruses co-factors for cancers induced by other oncoviruses? Rev Med Virol. 2014;24(5):343–60.

58. Comar M, Bonifacio D, Zanconati F, Di Napoli M, Isidoro E, Martini F, Torelli L, Tognon M. High prevalence of BK polyomavirus sequences in human papillomavirus-16-positive precancerous cervical lesions. J Med Virol. 2011; 83(10):1770–6.

59. Chesters PM, Heritage J, McCance DJ. Persistence of DNA sequences of BK virus and JC virus in normal human tissues and in diseased tissues. J Infect Dis. 1983;147(4):676–84.

60. Abend JR, Joseph AE, Das D, Campbell-Cecen DB, Imperiale MJ. A truncated T antigen expressed from an alternatively spliced BK virus early mRNA. J Gen Virol. 2009;90(Pt 5):1238–45.

61. Monini P, de Lellis L, Rotola A, Di Luca D, Ravaioli T, Bigoni B, Cassai E. Chimeric BK virus DNA episomes in a papillary urothelial bladder carcinoma. Intervirology. 1995;38(5):304–8.

62. Fioriti D, Pietropaolo V, Dal Forno S, Laurenti C, Chiarini F, Degener AM. Urothelial bladder carcinoma and viral infections: different association with

human polyomaviruses and papillomaviruses. Int J Immunopathol Pharmacol. 2003;16(3):283–8.

63. Newton R, Ribeiro T, Casabonne D, Alvarez E, Touzé A, Key T, Coursaget P. Antibody levels against BK virus and prostate, kidney and bladder cancers in the EPIC-Oxford cohort. Br J Cancer. 2005;93(11):1305–6.

64. Polesel J, Gheit T, Talamini R, Shahzad N, Lenardon O, Sylla B, La Vecchia C, Serraino D, Tommasino M, Franceschi S. Urinary human polyomavirus and papillomavirus infection and bladder cancer risk. Br J Cancer. 2012;106(1):222–6.

65. Geetha D, Tong BC, Racusen L, Markowitz JS, Westra WH. Bladder carcinoma in a transplant recipient: evidence to implicate the BK human polyomavirus as a causal transforming agent. Transplantation. 2002;73(12):1933–6.

66. Chen CH, Wen MC, Wang M, Lian JD, Cheng CH, Wu MJ, Yu TM, Chuang YW, Chang D, Shu KH. High incidence of malignancy in polyomavirus-associated nephropathy in renal transplant recipients. Transplant Proc. 2010;42(3):817–8.

67. Pino L, Rijo E, Nohales G, Frances A, Ubre A, Arango O. Bladder transitional cell carcinoma and BK virus in a young kidney transplant recipient. Transpl Infect Dis. 2013;15(1):E25–7.

68. Roberts IS, Besarani D, Mason P, Turner G, Friend PJ, Newton R. Polyoma virus infection and urothelial carcinoma of the bladder following renal transplantation. Br J Cancer. 2008;99(9):1383–6.

69. Gupta G, Kuppachi S, Kalil RS, Buck CB, Lynch CF, Engels EA. Treatment for presumed BK polyomavirus nephropathy and risk of urinary tract cancers among kidney transplant recipients in the United States. Am J Transplant. 2018;18(1):245–52.

70. Müller DC, Rämö M, Naegele K, Ribi S, Wetterauer C, Perrina V, Quagliata L, Vlajnic T, Ruiz C, Balitzki B, et al. Donor-derived, metastatic urothelial cancer after kidney-transplantation associated with a potentially oncogenic BK polyomavirus. J Pathol; 2017;244(3):265–70.

71. Kenan DJ, Mieczkowski PA, Burger-Calderon R, Singh HK, Nickeleit V. The oncogenic potential of BK-polyomavirus is linked to viral integration into the human genome. J Pathol. 2015;237(3):379–89.

72. Kenan DJ, Mieczkowski PA, Latulippe E, Côté I, Singh HK, Nickeleit V. BK Polyomavirus genomic integration and large T antigen expression: evolving paradigms in human Oncogenesis. Am J Transplant. 2017;17(6):1674–80.

73. Seo GJ, Fink LH, O'Hara B, Atwood WJ, Sullivan CS. Evolutionarily conserved function of a viral microRNA. J Virol. 2008;82(20):9823–8.

74. Monini P, Rotola A, Di Luca D, De Lellis L, Chiari E, Corallini A, Cassai E. DNA rearrangements impairing BK virus productive infection in urinary tract tumors. Virology. 1995;214(1):273–9.

75. Balis V, Sourvinos G, Soulitzis N, Giannikaki E, Sofras F, Spandidos DA. Prevalence of BK virus and human papillomavirus in human prostate cancer. Int J Biol Markers. 2007;22(4):245–51.

76. Das D, Shah RB, Imperiale MJ. Detection and expression of human BK virus sequences in neoplastic prostate tissues. Oncogene. 2004;23(42):7031–46.

77. Das D, Wojno K, Imperiale MJ. BK virus as a cofactor in the etiology of prostate cancer in its early stages. J Virol. 2008;82(6):2705–14.

78. Fioriti D, Russo G, Mischitelli M, Anzivino E, Bellizzi A, Di Monaco F, Di Silverio F, Giordano A, Chiarini F, Pietropaolo V. A case of human polyomavirus Bk infection in a patient affected by late stage prostate cancer: could viral infection be correlated with cancer progression? Int J Immunopathol Pharmacol. 2007;20(2):405–11.

79. Lau SK, Lacey SF, Chen YY, Chen WG, Weiss LM. Low frequency of BK virus in prostatic adenocarcinomas. APMIS. 2007;115(6):743–9.

80. Zambrano A, Kalantari M, Simoneau A, Jensen JL, Villarreal LP. Detection of human polyomaviruses and papillomaviruses in prostatic tissue reveals the prostate as a habitat for multiple viral infections. Prostate. 2002;53(4):263–76.

81. Russo G, Anzivino E, Fioriti D, Mischitelli M, Bellizzi A, Giordano A, Autran-Gomez A, Di Monaco F, Di Silverio F, Sale P, et al. p53 gene mutational rate, Gleason score, and BK virus infection in prostate adenocarcinoma: is there a correlation? J Med Virol. 2008;80(12):2100–7.

82. Sfanos KS, Sauvageot J, Fedor HL, Dick JD, De Marzo AM, Isaacs WB. A molecular analysis of prokaryotic and viral DNA sequences in prostate tissue from patients with prostate cancer indicates the presence of multiple and diverse microorganisms. Prostate. 2008;68(3):306–20.

83. Rodriguez H, Levican J, Munoz JP, Carrillo D, Acevedo ML, Gaggero A, Leon O, Gheit T, Espinoza-Navarro O, Castillo J, et al. Viral infections in prostate carcinomas in Chilean patients. Infect Agents Cancer. 2015;10:27. https://infectagentscancer.biomedcentral.com/track/pdf/10.1186/s13027-015-0024-y?site=infectagentscancer.biomedcentral.com.

84. Dong JT. Prevalent mutations in prostate cancer. J Cell Biochem. 2006;97(3):433–47.

85. De Marzo AM, Meeker AK, Zha S, Luo J, Nakayama M, Platz EA, Isaacs WB, Nelson WG. Human prostate cancer precursors and pathobiology. Urology. 2003;62(5 Suppl 1):55–62.

86. Delbue S, Matei DV, Carloni C, Pecchenini V, Carluccio S, Villani S, Tringali V, Brescia A, Ferrante P. Evidence supporting the association of polyomavirus BK genome with prostate cancer. Med Microbiol Immunol. 2013;202(6):425–30.

87. Ambinder RF. Gammaherpesviruses and "hit-and-run" oncogenesis. Am J Pathol. 2000;156(1):1–3.

# 21

# Negative effect of hepatitis in overall and progression-free survival among patients with diffuse large B-cell lymphoma

Mubarak M. Al-Mansour[1,2*], Saif A. Alghamdi[2], Musab A. Alsubaie[2], Abdullah A. Alesa[2] and Muhammad A. Khan[2]

## Abstract

**Background:** Hepatitis B virus (HBV) is one of the most prevalent and serious infections worldwide. HBV reactivation is a serious complication for lymphoma patients who are being treated with rituximab-containing regimen. Since the impact of HBV has not been fully evaluated on the prognosis of diffuse large B cell lymphoma (DLBCL), this study examined the effect of the hepatitis infection on the progression-free survival (PFS) and overall survival (OS) in patients with DLBCL who received rituximab-containing chemotherapy.

**Methods:** This retrospective cohort study was conducted at Princess Noorah Oncology Center, Jeddah by reviewing all medical records of 172 DLBCL diagnosed patients and recieved Rituximab-containing chemotherapy dated from January 2009 to February 2016.

**Results:** Out of 172 patients, 53 were found positive in hepatitis serology. The 12 of those were HBsAg-positive and 41 were HBcAb-positive. Hepatitis reactivation was observed in 1% of the patients (i.e., 2 out of 172) and both of them were HBsAg-positive. Thus, the risk of hepatitis reactivation among the HBsAg-positive patients was 17% (i.e., 2 out of 12). The predicted 3-year PFS for HBsAg-positive and HBcAb-positive were 52% (± 8%), while 76% (± 4) for HBsAg-negative and HBcAb-negative patients. On the other hand, the predicted 3-year OS for HBsAg and HBcAb-negative group is 93% (±3) while for HBsAg-positive and HBcAb-positive is 77% (±7), respectively.

**Conclusion:** The present study demonstrated a low HBV reactivation rate of 1% exclusively in 2 patients with HBsAg-positive status diagnosed with DLBCL and receiving R-CHOP chemotherapy.

**Keywords:** Hepatitis B virus reactivation, Lymphoma, Diffuse large B-cell lymphoma

## Background

Hepatitis B virus (HBV) is one of the most prevalent and serious infections worldwide. It is estimated that more than one third of the world population has been infected with HBV and one million die annually from HBV-related liver disease [1, 2]. Therefore, HBV is considered a major health risk. HBV reactivation is a serious complication for lymphoma patients who are being treated with rituximab containing regimen [3–5]. The risk is higher for patients who are HBsAg-positive at presentation, and ranges from 26 to 53%, while the risk is approximately 2 to 20% for HBcAb-positive patients [6–8]. While the risk of reactivation and the role of prophylactic antiviral were described in the literature, nevertheless, the impact of HBsAg-positive or HBcAb-positive status on the DLBCL prognosis has not been fully evaluated. Hence, this study examined the effect of hepatitis infection on the progression-free survival (PFS) and overall survival (OS) in patients with DLBCL who received R-CHOP chemotherapy.

## Methods

This retrospective cohort study was conducted at Princess Noorah Oncology Center, Jeddah by reviewing all medical records of patients diagnosed with DBCL between January 2009 and February 2016. Patients at the age of over 16 years with histopathologically proven

* Correspondence: drmubarak55@hotmail.com
[1]Princess Noorah Oncology Center, King Abdulaziz Medical City, Ministry of National Guard Health Affairs-Western Region (WR), PO Box 9515, Jeddah 21423, Kingdom of Saudi Arabia
[2]College of Medicine (COM), King Saud Bin Abdulaziz University for Health Sciences (KSAU-HS), Jeddah, Saudi Arabia

$CD20^+$ and received frontline Rituximab-containing chemotherapy were included for this study. Patients with primary central nervous system (CNS) lymphoma, and patients who did not completed the total cycles of chemotherapy or only received palliative chemotherapy were excluded. Three reviewers conducted the case identification and data capturing using a computerized datasheet. A total of 172 patients were then identified and became eligible for this study.

## Data collected

The collected data includes patients' demographic information, performance status, International Prognostic Index (IPI) score. The datasheet also comprised of disease characteristics, including stage, B-symptoms bone marrow involvement, and site of extranodal involvement. A complete history of the chemotherapy course and follow-up were noted as well. Patients were analyzed before and after chemotherapy for HBV serology including hepatitis B surface-antigen (HBsAg), hepatitis B envelope-antigen (HBeAg), and hepatitis B core-antibody (HBcAb IgM and HBcAb IgG). Viral load (HBV-DNA), liver profile (alanine aminotransferase [ALT], aspartate aminotransferase [AST], and total bilirubin [TB] levels) were also obtained before and after the chemotherapy. Prophylaxis to HBV with Entecavir (0.5 mg orally everyday) or Lamivudine (100 mg orally everyday) was started one week before the chemotherapy in patients with positive HBsAg and HBcAb and some patients with only positive HBcAb, and was ended 6 months after completion of the chemotherapy regimen. Date of HBV reactivation and patients post treatment status were recorded.

## Statistical method

Patients were categorized into HBsAg and/or HBcAb-negative and HBsAg-positive and/or HBcAb-positive groups. Patients characteristics and other variables were compared as follows. A student's t-test was used for continuous variables between the two groups. A $X^2$ test was used for a category or ordinal variables. Fisher's exact test was used when a small sample size existed. Progression-free survival (PFS) and overall survival (OS) were estimated by using the Kaplan-Meier method [9]. PFS was defined as from the date of diagnosis to the date of relapse or the date of the last follow-up. OS was defined as from the time of diagnosis to the date of death from any cause or the date of the last follow-up. Survival curves differences were analyzed using the two-tailed log-rank test [10]. Univariate analysis by using Cox's proportional hazards model was utilized to determine risk factors that affect PFS. Variables significantly identified in univariate analysis were tested in multivariate anvalysis by using Cox's proportion

hazard model. All statistical tests were two-sided, and a $P$ value $< 0.05$ was considered statistically significant. Analyses were performed by use of the SPSS statistical package (IBM Corp., Released 2012, IBM SPSS Statistics for Windows, Version 21.0. Armonk, NY: IBM Corp).

## Definition of HBV reactivation

The researchers define HBV reactivation as a 10-folds or more increase in the HBV-DNA when compared to baseline during rituximab-containing chemotherapy or within 1 year after the final course of chemotherapy. Hepatitis attributable to HBV reactivation is defined as a threefold or more increase in ALT above the normal range or an increase in ALT to more than 100 U/L [11, 12].

## Results

### Patients characteristics

A total of 172 patients with biopsy proven DLBCL were identified. The median age was 58 years (18–85). Majority of patients were males (55%). In addition, 70% were diagnosed with advanced stage III-IV, and B symptoms were seen in 52%. Moreover, 77% of patients had ECOG performance status 0–2, and high-intermediate to high risk international prognostic index (IPI) was noted in 27% of patients. Extranodal involvement was reported in 58%. The most common sites of extranodal sites were liver (16%), bone (13%), lung (11%), stomach (9%), and bone marrow (9%). CNS involvement was observed in 8%. Majority of patients were treated with R-CHOP chemotherapy (89%). Patients clinical characteristics are presented in Table 1.

### Hepatitis serology status

Fifty-three of the patients were found positive in hepatitis. The 12 of those are HBsAg-positive and 41 are HBcAb-positive patients.

The proportion of HBsAg-positive patients who were HBcAb-positive was 7% (12/172), and the proportion HBsAg-negative patients who were HBcAb-positive was 26% (41/160).

### Type of prophylaxis

At the time of the diagnosis, all HBsAg-positive patients ($n = 12$) were given antiviral therapy with either Entecavir ($n = 9$) or Lamivudine ($n = 3$). Among the 41 HBcAb-positive, 28 patients received prophylactic antiviral therapy with either Entecavir ($n = 17$) or Lamivudine ($n = 11$), and 13 patients did not receive any prophylaxis therapy.

### Hepatitis reactivation

Hepatitis reactivation was observed in 1% (2 of 172 patients). Patients who developed hepatitis reactivation were HBsAg-positive. Thus, the risk of hepatitis

**Table 1** Clinical characteristics

| Characteristic | All Patients (N = 172) | | HBsAg and HBcAb Negative (n = 119) | | HBsAg or HBcAb Positive (n = 53) | | P |
|---|---|---|---|---|---|---|---|
| | No. | % | No. | % | No. | % | |
| Age, years | | | | | | | |
| Median (range) | 58 (18–85) | | 57 (18–85) | | 62 (32–85) | | 0.02 |
| Age groups, years | | | | | | | |
| < 60 | 96 | 56 | 75 | 63 | 21 | 40 | 0.004 |
| ≥ 60 | 76 | 44 | 44 | 37 | 32 | 60 | |
| Sex | | | | | | | 0.17 |
| Male | 95 | 55 | 62 | 52 | 33 | 62 | |
| Female | 77 | 45 | 57 | 48 | 20 | 38 | |
| Ann Arbor stage | | | | | | | |
| I | 10 | 6 | 8 | 7 | 2 | 4 | 0.60 |
| II | 42 | 24 | 31 | 26 | 11 | 21 | |
| III | 20 | 12 | 12 | 10 | 8 | 15 | |
| IV | 100 | 58 | 68 | 57 | 32 | 60 | |
| B symptoms | | | | | | | |
| No | 82 | 48 | 58 | 51 | 24 | 45 | 0.67 |
| Yes | 90 | 52 | 61 | 49 | 29 | 55 | |
| Performance status 2–4 | 84 | 49 | 53 | 45 | 31 | 58 | 021 |
| Extranodal | | | | | | | |
| No | 73 | 42 | 52 | 44 | 21 | 40 | 0.61 |
| Yes | 99 | 58 | 67 | 56 | 32 | 60 | |
| Serum LDH > Normal International prognostic index | | | | | | | |
| Low | 62 | 38 | 46 | 39 | 15 | 28 | 0.10 |
| Low-intermediate | 57 | 35 | 35 | 29 | 11 | 21 | |
| High-intermediate | 30 | 18 | 23 | 19 | 14 | 26 | |
| High | 15 | 9 | 15 | 13 | 13 | 24 | |
| Liver cirrhosis | | | | | | | |
| No | 170 | 99 | 118 | 99 | 52 | 98 | 0.55 |
| Yes | 2 | 1 | 1 | 1 | 1 | 2 | |
| Baseline liver function | | | | | | | |
| ALT> UNL | 14 | 8 | 10 | 8 | 4 | 8 | 0.78 |
| AST > UNL | 8 | 5 | 6 | 5 | 2 | 4 | 0.53 |
| Bilirubin >UNL | 6 | 3.5 | 5 | 4 | 1 | 2 | 0.39 |
| Type of prophylaxis | | | | | | | |
| NO | 132 | 77 | 119 | 100 | 13 | 25 | |
| Entecavir | 26 | 15 | 0 | 0 | 26 | 49 | |
| Lamivudine | 14 | 8 | 0 | 0 | 14 | 26 | 0.00 |
| Chemotherapy | | | | | | | |
| R-CHOP | 153 | 89 | 124 | 106 | 89 | 89 | 0.39 |
| R-CVP | 12 | 7 | 14 | 6 | 5 | 11 | |
| R-CEOP | 3 | 2 | 2 | 3 | 3 | 0 | |
| R-EPOCH | 4 | 2 | 0 | 4 | 3 | 8 | |

**Table 1** Clinical characteristics *(Continued)*

| Characteristic | All Patients (N = 172) | | HBsAg and HBcAb Negative (n = 119) | | HBsAg or HBcAb Positive (n = 53) | | P |
|---|---|---|---|---|---|---|---|
| | No. | % | No. | % | No. | % | |
| Consolidation radiotherapy | | | | | | | |
| Yes | 17 | 10 | 12 | 10 | 5 | 9 | 0.89 |
| No | 155 | 90 | 107 | 90 | 48 | 91 | |
| No. of cycles | | | | | | | |
| Median | 6 | | 6 | | 6 | | 0.40 |
| Range | 1–11 | | 3–11 | | 1–8 | | |

reactivation among the HBsAg-positive was 17% (2 of 12 patients). None of the HBcAb-positive patients developed hepatitis reactivation regardless of the prophylaxis therapy. Hepatitis reactivation occurred after R-CHOP chemotherapy in two patients. One patient received a total of 6 cycles R-CHOP chemotherapy and developed hepatitis reactivation after 6 months from the last cycle of chemotherapy, whereas the second patient received a total of 6 cycles R-CHOP chemotherapy and developed hepatitis reactivation one year after completion of R-CHOP chemotherapy. For the two patients, the only marker for HBV reactivation, which is HBV-DNA, was elevated greater than 10-folds from the baseline. None of the two patients developed hepatitis with increased liver enzymes. Both patients were on Entecavir therapy before initiation of chemotherapy. The first patient developed a relapsed disease three years after the completion of R-CHOP chemotherapy. He was treated with salvage chemotherapy ESHAP for 6 cycles, and he is in remission and alive. The second patient is in remission and alive. Both patients didn't experience any more episodes of HBV reactivation.

**Hepatitis reactivation risk factors**

Several clinical and treatment-related factors were tested to identify if theres any clinical significant difference between those who developed hepatitis reactivation (n = 2) and those who did not (n = 51), and all of them were not significant.

**Survival analysis**

The median follow time was 34 months. Out of 172 patients, 50 patients (29%) had relapsed or progressive disease post primary therapy. Twenty seven patients were HBsAg-negative and HBcAb-negative, and 23 patients were either HBsAg-positive or HBcAb-positive. Out of the 23 patients, 4 patients among the HBsAg-positive had relapsed and one patient had progressive disease. Out of the remaining 18 patients with HBcAb-positive, six patients had relapsed disease and 12 patient had progressive disease. Thus, the risk of relapse or progression was 23% among the HBsAg-negative/HBcAb-negative patients (27/119). For HBsAg-positive or HBcAb-positive patients, the risk of relapse was 43% (23/53). Treatment outcomes are presented in Table 2.

The median PFS for all patients was not reached with an estimated 3-year rate of 70% (± 4%). The predicted 3-year PFS for HBsAg-positive and/or HBcAb-positive were 52% (± 8%). However, the predicted 3-year PFS was 76% (± 4) for HBsAg and HBcAb-negative patients. The median OS for the whole group likewise not reached, the predicted 3-year OS was 93% (±3) and 77% (±7) for HBsAg and HBcAb-negative group and HBsAg-positive and/or HBcAb-positive group, respectively. There was significant difference in PFS (P = 0.009; Fig. 1) or OS (P = 0.012; Fig. 2) rates in HBsAg and HBcAb-positive patients as compared to HBsAg and HBcAb-negative patients, respectively. Out of all patients, 16 patients have died, 7 patients in the HBsAg-negative and

**Table 2** Treatment Outcomes

| Outcome | All Patients (N = 172) | | HBsAg/HBcAb Negative (n = 119) | | HBsAg/HBcAb Positive (n = 53) | | P |
|---|---|---|---|---|---|---|---|
| | No. | % | No. | % | No. | % | |
| Response | | | | | | | |
| CR/PR | 122 | 71 | 92 | 77 | 30 | 57 | 0.022 |
| PD/RD | 29 | 17 | 16 | 14 | 13 | 24 | |
| Disease relapse | 21 | 12 | 11 | 9 | 10 | 19 | |
| Predicted 3-year PFS (± SE) | 67% (± 4%) | | 76% (± 4%) | | 52% (± 8%) | | 0.009 |
| Death | 16 | 9 | 7 | 6 | 9 | 17 | 0.21 |
| Predicted 3-year OS (± SE) | 88% (± 3%) | | 93% (± 3%) | | 77% (± 7%) | | 0.012 |

*Abbreviations*: *CR/PR* Complete response/partial response, *PD/RD* Progressive disease/refractory disease

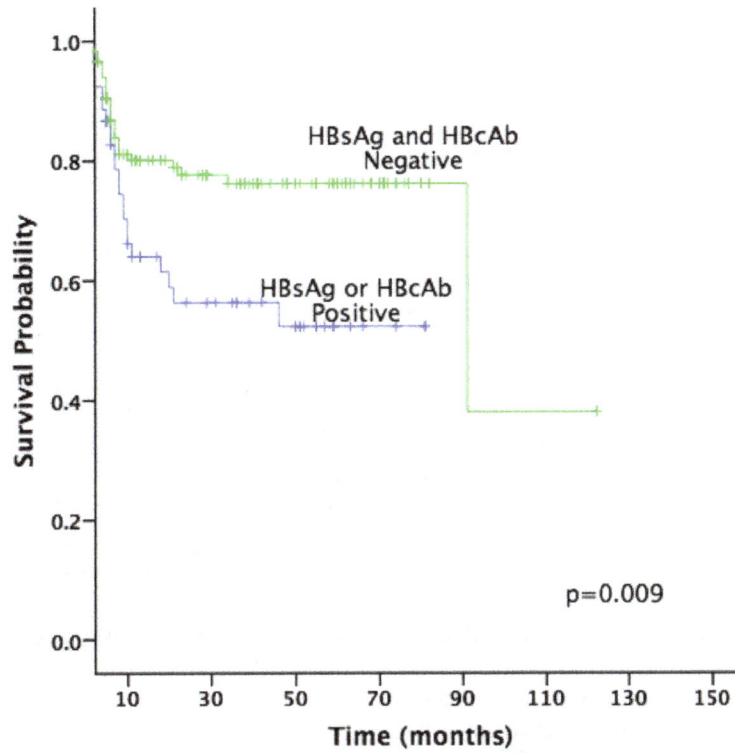

**Fig. 1** Progression-free survival of HBsAg and HBcAb negative and HBsAg or HBcAb positive groups (two-sided $p = 0.009$)

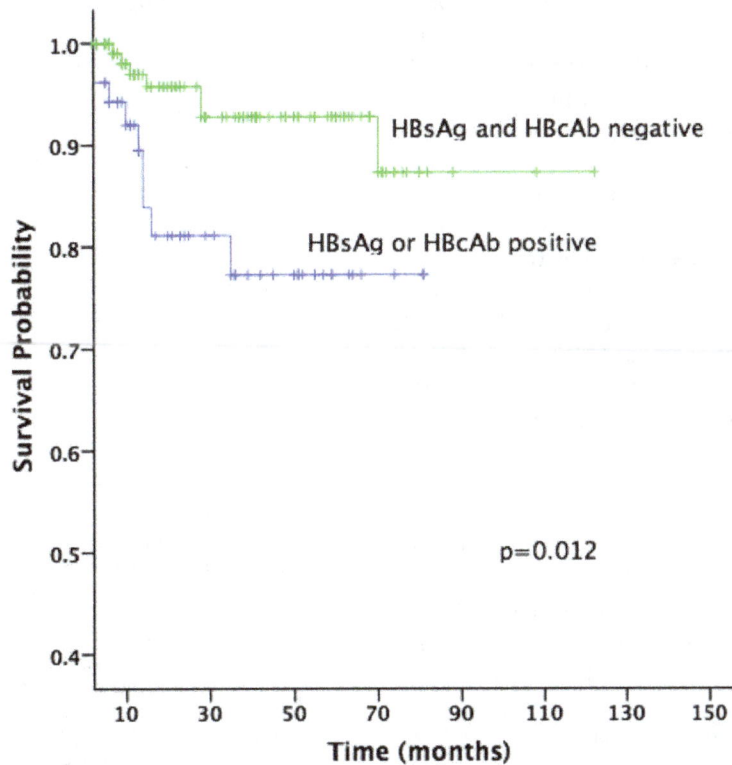

**Fig. 2** Overall survival of HBsAg and HBcAb negative and HBsAg or HBcAb positive groups (two-sided $p = 0.012$)

HBcAb-negative group, and 9 patients in the HBsAg-positive or HBcAb-positive group (Table 2).

In univariate analysis, clinical characteristics such as stage, IPI, extranodal involvement, poor performance status and HBsAg-positive and/or HBcAb-positive status were factors significantly affected the PFS. However, in multivariate analysis, HBsAg-positive and/or HBcAb-positive and poor performance status were the two independently factors that affected the PFS (HR = 0.55; 95%CI: 0.31–0.99; $p$ = 0.046) and (HR = 1.65; 95%CI: 1.09–2.49; $p$ = 0.016), respectively. For OS, clinical factors such as stage, IPI, extranodal involvement, poor performance status and HBsAg-positive and/or HBcAb-positive were also found to be significant on univariate analysis. On multivariate analysis, the HBsAg-positive and/or HBcAb-positive status was the only factor independently affected the OS (HR = 0.32; 95% CI: 0.12–0.88; $p$ = 0.028).

## Discussion

The prevalence of the chronic hepatitis infection (HBsAg-positive) in our patients with DLBCL was 7%. This is lower compared to other reports from China where the prevalence of the chronic hepatitis infection in DLBCL patients ranges from 8.6 to 30.2% [13].

Among our patients with HBsAg-negative, the prevalence of HBcAb-positive was 26%. Data from other countries demonstrated variable prevalence rate compared to our results. Some of those studies reported higher prevalence rate (34 to 44%) of resolved hepatitis infection in DLBCL patients, and other studies showed lower rate ranging from 2 to 20.1% [13, 14].

The risk of the hepatitis reactivation in our study was 1% for the whole group (2 out of 172). The two patients who developed hepatitis reactivation were HBsAg-positive at the time of the diagnosis with their lymphomas, and both received anti-viral treatment before initiation of the Rituximab based chemotherapy. This risk was similar to other studies in the Rituximab based therapy era. In addition, since HBV reactivation in our patients was observed 6 months to 1 year after the cessation of chemotherapy, several studies found out that cessation of rituximab-CHOP chemotherapy and antiviral such as lumivadine resulted in delayed HBV reactivation [15, 16]. Thus, prophylactic antiviral therapy was recommended to extend to at least one year after discontinuation of chemotherapy [17].

There were no patients (0%) who developed HBV reactivation in HBsAg-negative and HBcAb-positive group. This finding is consistent with the multicenter study conducted by Ji et al. [18] but in contrast with the result reported in the study of Yeo et al. (2.2 to 23.8%) [19]. The discrepancy could be explained by giving prophylactic anti-viral therapy for 68% of our patients before initiation of chemotherapy. Other explanation could be the protective immunity for the previously resolved infection, which can be confirmed by the presence of the anti-hepatitis B surface antibody (HBsAb), but unfortunately this data is missing in our study.

In this retrospective study, we demonstrated a negative impact on PFS and OS in DLBCL patients with either HBsAg-positive or HBcAb-positive serology (Figs. 1 and 2). Despite the low risk of HPV reactivation, the risk of relapse was higher in HBsAg-positive and/or HBcAb-positive group (43%) as compared to HBsAg-negative and HBcAb-negative group (23%), with a decrease in the 3-year PFS from 76 to 52%, and a decrease in the 3-year OS from 93 to 77% (Table 2). It is indeed that hepatitis infection is a significant factor that affects the survival of DLBCL patients. Although factors other than hepatitis infection were also described in literature, the exact mechanism and impact of these factors during chemotherapy remains unclear. This study, therefore, suggests to define recommendations and improvements on measures to prevent HBV reactivation among DLBCL patients.

## Limitations

One of the limitations of the study was its retrospective nature in which we reviewed the charts of the patients. Moreover, the sample size was small and some of the data was not found in patients' charts like HBsAb which would have helped us in better result depiction.

## Conclusion

The present study demonstrated a low HBV reactivation rate of 1% exclusively in two DLBCL patients with HBsAg-positive status. We have also demonstrated that HBV has an negative impact on the PFS and the OS of DLBCL patients. HBV reactivation in DLBCL patients receiving rituximab based chemotherapy in our study was less than what is reported in the literature.

## Abbreviations

ALT: Alanine aminotransferase; ALT: Alanine Transaminae; AST: Aspartate aminotransferase; CR: Complete response; DLBCL: Diffuse Large B Cell Lymphoma; ECOG: Eastern Cooperative Oncology Group; ESHAP: Etopside, Solu-Medrol (Methylprednisolone), High-dose Ara-C (Cytarabine), Platinum (Cisplatin); HBcAb: Hepatitis B core-antibody; HBeAg: Hepatitis B envelope-antigen; HBsAg: Hepatitis B surface-antigen; HBV: Hepatitis B virus; HBV-DNA: Hepatitis B Virus DNA; IgG: Immunoglobulin G; IgM: Immunoglobulin M; IPI: International Prognostic Index; OS: Overall survival; PD: Progressive disease; PFS: Progression free survival; PR: Partial response; R-CEOP: Rituximab,Cyclophosphamide, Etoposide, Oncovin (Vincristine) Prednisolone; R-CHOP: Rituximab, Cyclophosphamide, Hydroxydaunomycin (Doxorubicin Hydrochloride), Oncovin (vincristine), Prednisone; R-CVP: Rituximab,Cyclophosphamide, Vincristine,Prednisone; RD: Refractory disease; R-EPOCH: Rituximab, Etoposide, Prednisone, Oncovin (Vincristine), Cyclophosphamide, Hydroxydaunorubicin (Doxorubicin Hydrochloride); TB: Total bilirubin; ULN: Upper Limit of Normal

## Authors' contributions

MMA carried out the conception and design of the study, analysis and interpretation, writing the manuscript, critical revision and assume the general responsibility and guarantees the scientific integrity of the study. SAA helped to draft the study, conducted the data collection, data analysis. MAA participated in data collection, statistics and data analysis. AAA participated in data collection and statistical analysis. MAK helped to draft and finalized manuscript, and performed the statistics and also data analysis. All authors read and approved the final manuscript.

## Competing interests

The authors declare that they have no competing interest.

## References

1. Pungpapong S, Kim WR, Poterucha JJ. Natural history of hepatitis B virus infection: an update for clinicians. Mayo Clin Proc. 2007 Aug;82(8):967–75.
2. Lee W. Hepatitis B virus infection. N Engl J Med. 1997;337:1733–45.
3. Yeo W, Chan PK, Zhong S, et al. Frequency of hepatitis B virus reactivation in cancer patients undergoing cytotoxic chemotherapy: a prospective study of 626 patients with identification of risk factors. J Med Virol. 2000;62(3):299–307.
4. Su WP, Wen CC, Hsiung CA, et al. Long-term hepatic consequences of chemotherapy-related HBV reactivation in lymphoma patients. World J Gastroenterol. 2005;11(34):5283–8.
5. Evens AM, Jovanovic BD, Su YC, et al. Rituximab-associated hepatitis B virus (HBV) reactivation in lymphoproliferative diseases: meta-analysis and examination of FDA safety reports. Ann Oncol. 2011;22(5):1170–80.
6. Yeo W, Zee B, Zhong S, et al. Comprehensive analysis of risk factors associating with hepatitis B virus (HBV) reactivation in cancer patients undergoing cytotoxic chemotherapy. Br J Cancer. 2004;90(7):1306–11.
7. Yeo W, Chan PK, Hui P, et al. Hepatitis B virus reactivation in breast cancer patients receiving cytotoxic chemotherapy: a prospective study. J Med Virol. 2003;70(4):553–61.
8. Lau GK, Yiu HH, Fong DY, et al. Early is superior to deferred preemptive lamivudine therapy for hepatitis B patients undergoing chemotherapy. Gastroenterology. 2003;125(6):1742–9.
9. Kaplan EL, Meier P. Nonparametric estimation from incomplete observations. J Am Stat Assoc. 1958;53:457–81.
10. Mantel N. Evaluation of survival data and two new rank order statistics arising in its consideration. Cancer Chemother Rep. 1966;50(3):163–70.
11. Lok AS, Liang RH, Chiu EK, et al. Reactivation of hepatitis B virus replication in patients receiving cytotoxic therapy. Report of a prospective study Gastroenterology. 1991;100(1):182–8.
12. Yeo W, Chan PK, Ho WM, et al. Lamivudine for the prevention of hepatitis B virus reactivation in hepatitis B s-antigen seropositive cancer patients undergoing cytotoxic chemotherapy. J Clin Oncol. 2004;22:927–34.
13. Marcucci F, Mele A, Spada E, Candido A, Bianco E, Pulsoni A, et al. High prevalence of hepatitis B virus infection in B-cell non-Hodgkin's lymphoma. Haematologica. 2006;91(4):554–7.
14. Wang F, Xu RH, Han B, et al. High incidence of hepatitis B virus infection in B-cell subtype non-Hodgkin lymphoma compared with other cancers. Cancer. 2007;109(7):1360–4.
15. Perceau G, Diris N, Estines O, et al. Late lethal hepatitis B virus reactivation after rituximab treatment of low-grade cutaneous B-cell lymphoma. Br J Dermatol. 2006;155:1053–6. 33
16. Dai MS, Chao TY, Kao WY, et al. Delayed hepatitis B virus reactivation after cessation of preemptive lamivudine in lymphoma patients treated with rituximab plus CHOP. Ann Hematol. 2004;83(12):769 74.
17. Law MF, Lai HK, Chan HN, et al. The impact of hepatitis B virus (HBV) infection on clinical outcomes of patients with diffuse large B-cell lymphoma. Eur J Cancer Care (Engl). 2015;24(1):117–24.
18. Ji D, Cao J, Hong X, et al. Low incidence of hepatitis B virus reactivation during chemotherapy among diffuse large B-cell lymphoma patients who are HBsAg-negative/ HBcAb-positive: a multicenter retrospective study. Eur J Haematol. 2010;85(3):243–50.
19. Yeo W, Chan TC, Leung NW, et al. Hepatitis B virus reactivation in lymphoma patients with prior resolved hepatitis B undergoing anticancer therapy with or without rituximab. J Clin Oncol. 2009;27(4):605–11.

# 22

# Hepatitis C Virus (HCV) genotypes distribution among hepatocellular carcinoma patients in Southern Italy

Arnolfo Petruzziello[1][*] ⓘ, Samantha Marigliano[1], Giovanna Loquercio[1], Nicola Coppola[2], Mauro Piccirillo[3], Maddalena Leongito[3], Rosa Azzaro[4], Francesco Izzo[3] and Gerardo Botti[1]

## Abstract

**Background:** Hepatocellular carcinoma (HCC) is one of the major cause for cancer in the world. Aim of this case-control study was to investigate the distribution pattern of HCV genotypes among HCC patients and suggest whether infection with specific subtypes may be associated with an increased risk of progression to cancer.

**Methods:** 152 HCC anti-HCV positive patients, fulfilling the criteria from the Barcelona 2000 EASL conference, and 568 patients HCV chronically infected but without HCC as control group were included in the study. Serum of each patient was evaluated for viral load estimation and genotyping.

**Results:** Males with HCC significantly showed to have quite 2 times higher risk of exposure to HCV infection (OR = 1.72; 95% CI = 1.15–2.58). Moreover, HCC was significantly associated with older age. In fact, > 50 years older patients showed to have a higher risk of developing HCC (OR = 17.4; 95% CI = 4.24 to 71.36) compared to younger patients.

HCV RNA rate was significantly higher (83.7%) among HCC patients than in the control group (61.4%, $p < 0.001$) and the most prevalent genotype was 1b (68.0% in HCC vs 54.4% in the control group, $p < 0.005$). HCC patients significantly have a risk of exposure to HCV 1b infection almost 2 times greater than the control group (OR = 1.8; 95% CI = 1.11–2.82). The multivariate-adjusted OR (95% CI) of developing HCC for HCV 1b comparing to non-1b was 1.65 (1.16–2.33).

**Conclusions:** Our study detected a significantly higher rate of HCV RNA positivity and a higher rate of HCV 1b infection in HCC patients, suggesting the strict association between subtype 1b infection and HCC. A prospective study with larger number of samples would be needed to confirm our results.

**Keywords:** Hepatocellular carcinoma, HCV, HCV genotypes, Italy, Risk factors, Liver cancer, Viral load

## Background

Hepatocellular carcinoma (HCC) is one of the most common causes of morbidity worldwide [1–3], accounting for about 7% of all cancers [4] and over 80% of primary liver cancer [5, 6]. A recent estimate indicates that it is the fifth and the seventh most common cancer in males and females respectively [2], with approximately one million deaths per year, especially in developing countries [7, 8] and represents one of the major dreaded complication of chronic liver disease, frequently associated with compensated cirrhosis. It has been reported that approximately 3–4% of HCV chronically infected patients with underlying cirrhosis will develop HCC on average 30 years after infection [9–11].

Globally, three main epidemiological zones have been defined according to the age-adjusted HCC incidence per 100,000 inhabitants per year: low (< 5%), intermediate (5% to 15%), and high (>15%) [12], with a geographical distribution that varies throughout the world, ranging from 2.1 per 100,000 in Central America to 35.5 per 100,000 in Eastern Asia [13].

---
* Correspondence: a.petruzziello@istitutotumori.na.it
[1]Virology and Molecular Biology Unit, Department of Diagnostic Pathology, Istituto Nazionale Tumori, Fondazione "G. Pascale" IRCCS Italia, Via Mariano Semmola, 80131 Naples, Italy
Full list of author information is available at the end of the article

It has been suggested that a strict geographical correlation exists between the incidence of HCC and the prevalence of chronic HBV infection (especially in Eastern Asia and South East Asia where the incidence is more than 8%) and HCV infection, suggesting that these two viral infections could be the most important risk factors associated with HCC [8].

In countries where HCV infection is endemic (Japan or some areas of Southern Italy), a high prevalence of HCV infection has been reported among people with HCC [14, 15]. Several studies found a three-fold increase in HCV-related HCC, whereas the rate of HCC associated with HBV or alcohol-induced liver disease and idiopathic cirrhosis remained stable [2, 16].

It has been suggested that incidence of HCC is expected to significantly increase in the next decades, although the incidence of newly acquired HCV infections has been gradually decreasing [17]. The rate of progression from chronic hepatitis to HCC is variable and numerous factors have been identified as important predictors of progression, some related to the host (older age, longer duration of infection, male sex or alcohol consumption >50 g/day), others to environment (viral genotype/subtype or viral load) [2, 18, 19]. While alcohol and other risk factors are proposed to cause HCC because they cause cirrhosis, the carcinogenic role of HCV is still controversial, since HCV infection has been also described in HCC patients without cirrhosis [20–22].

HCV is characterized by a high degree of heterogeneity. At present, it is classified into seven recognized genotypes on the basis of sequence of the viral genome [23–26], each differing at 30–35% of nucleotide sites [27]. The geographic distribution of HCV genotypes is rather complex [28]. The so called "epidemic subtypes" —specifically 1a, 1b, 2a, and 3a— are widely distributed worldwide and account for a great proportion of the totality of HCV cases, especially in high income countries [29–32]. The so called "endemic" strains, instead, are comparatively more rare and have been restricted for long time in specific regions, as West Africa, Southern Asia, Central Africa and South Eastern Asia [33, 34].

If considered in an international context, Italy shows a moderate prevalence of anti-HCV in the population, except for the Southern regions where the infection is endemic and the HCV prevalence ranges from 6% to 12% [35, 36]. As we previously described, genotype 1b, historically the most prevalent not only in Italy but in the whole of Europe, is the most common genotype also in Southern Italy, followed by genotype 2 [37, 38].

Despite several published studies showing that patients infected with HCV genotype 1b may have a higher risk of developing HCC than those infected with other genotypes [39–41], other authors did not confirm this result [42, 43]. As a consequence, no consensus has yet

emerged and the role of HCV genotypes in both accelerating the progression of the disease and as a risk factor for HCC remains to be established.

The aim of this case-control study was to investigate the distribution pattern of HCV genotypes in HCC patients and identify whether infection with specific HCV genotypes may be associated with an increased risk of HCC development.

## Methods
### Study population and sample collection

A total of 152 HCC cases (105 males and 47 females, with a Male/female ratio of 2.23:1), all coming from different regions of Southern Italy and collected during the period between February 2012 and November 2014, were recruited among patients referred to the Hepatobiliar and Pancreatic Unit, Department of Surgical Oncology, Istituto Nazionale Tumori – IRCCS, Fondazione "Pascale", Naples, Italy and Section of Infectious Diseases, Department of Public Health, Università "Luigi Vanvitelli", Naples, Italy. The diagnoses of HCC and chronic hepatitis were based on the criteria from the Barcelona 2000 EASL Conference and from the recommendation of AASLD 2009 updated guidelines [44]. Majority of these patients were ≥50 years (98.7% with a mean age of 73 years) and 95.4% of them had underlying cirrhosis at presentation and 83.5% serum level of alpha-fetoprotein exceeding 6 ng/mL. Cirrhosis was diagnosed based on morphological and clinical criteria, as well as ultrasound or Computed Tomography (CT), according to standard definitions [45]. All 152 patients were tested for HCV-RNA and only anti-HCV/HCV-RNA positive patients (103/152) were selected and used for the genotype characterization (73 males and 30 females, with a Male/female ratio of 2.4:1). Among them, the percentage of untreated and treated patients (with IFN therapy) were similar (48% and 52%, respectively). No sustained virological response (SVR) was described among treated patients.

Five hundred sixty eight age matched patients (320 males and 248 females, with a Male/female ratio of 1.30:1) chronically HCV infected but without HCC diagnosis were collected in the same period from the Virology Ambulatory, IRCCS "Fondazione G. Pascale", Naples, Italy and Section of Infectious Diseases, Università "Luigi Vanvitelli", Naples, Italy and used as control group. Majority of these patients were ≥50 years (81.1%, with a mean age of 65 years). Three hundred fourty nine of them (61.4%) that showed HCV-RNA positivity were selected and subsequently used for the characterization of the genotype. The percentage of untreated and treated (with IFN therapy) patients were similar (46.5% and 53.5%, respectively). Only 9% of the treated patients showed a sustained virological response (SVR).

No DAA treated patients were selected in the HCC and control groups.

The demographic details and risk factors of the two groups are described in Table 1. A large number of HCC patients (48.0%) and of control subjects (45.9%) were in the 50 to 70 years age group, while younger patients (<50 years) were most common among control subjects (18.9 vs 1.3%) and older ones (>70 years) among HCC patients (50.7 vs 35.2%).

Alcohol intake was considered significant in case of consumption of about 1 glass of wine/ day (approximately 8 g/day for men and 6 g/day for women for at least 5 years) while cigarette consumption if over 15 cigarettes/day for almost 5 years. No alcoholic patients were included in the study. Analysis of the main modality of infection (surgery, dental therapy, blood transfusion or sexual intercourses) showed no significant differences between the two groups (data not shown).

Only patients negative for HIV, HBV and HDV infections and with no clinical or serological sign of other chronic liver disease (autoimmune disease, non-alcoholic steatohepatitis, etc.) were enrolled in both groups.

A written informed consent was obtained from all the subjects and the study protocol, conformed to the ethical guidelines of the declaration of Helsinki was approved by the Ethics committee of our Institute.

**Table 1** Baseline characteristics and risk factors of HCC and control group patients

| Characteristics | HCC (n = 152) | | Control Group (n = 568) | |
|---|---|---|---|---|
| | n. | % | n. | % |
| Male | 105 | 69.1[A] | 320 | 56.4[A] |
| Female | 47 | 30.9 | 248 | 43.6 |
| M/F ratio | 2.23 | | 1.30 | |
| Median BMI (range) kg/m$^2$ | 26 (21–32) | | 25.5 (20–38) | |
| Mean Age (range), years | 73 (55–91) | | 65 (45–85) | |
| < 50 years | 2 | 1.3 | 107 | 18.9 |
| 50–70 years | 73 | 48.0 | 261 | 45.9 |
| > 70 years | 77 | 50.7[B] | 200 | 35.2[B] |
| Alcohol consumption* | 74 | 48.7 | 289 | 50.8 |
| Cigarettes smoking^ | 60 | 39.5 | 201 | 35.4 |
| Serum levels of AST (> 45 U/L) | 94 | 61.8 | 352 | 61.9 |
| Serum levels of ALT (> 45 U/L) | 89 | 58.5 | 325 | 57.2 |
| ALP levels (> 250 U/L) | 71 | 46.7 | 261 | 45.9 |
| Albumin levels (< 3.5 g/L) | 81 | 53.3 | 280 | 49.2 |
| Bilirubin levels (> 1.2 mg/dL) | 91 | 59.8 | 301 | 52.9 |

*Alcohol intake was considered only in case of consumption of 8 g/day by men and 6 g/day by women for at least 5 years
^ Cigarette consumption was considered significant if over 15 cigarettes/day for almost 5 years
[A] = $\chi^2$:7.06; $p < 0.01$; OR: 1.72; 95% C.I = 1.15–2.58
[B] = $\chi^2$:12.08; $p < 0.001$; OR: 1.88; 95% C.I = 1.31–2.71

Blood samples for serological and molecular analysis were collected and all the participants were interviewed using a questionnaire including biochemical, clinical and risk factors information.

### Serological analysis

All the plasma samples from the HCC patients and the control group were analyzed for estimation of serum levels of liver function tests (albumin, bilirubin, alkaline phosphatase (ALP), alanine aminotransferase (ALT), aspartate aminotransferase (AST), and a-fetoprotein), using a Cobas c-501 automated immunoassay system (Roche Diagnostic) and the presence of anti-HCV antibodies by means of the Vitros-ECi test (Ortho Clinical Diagnostics), used according to the manufacturers' instructions. The Ortho-Clinical Vitros ECi test employs chemiluminescent technology and results are reported as signal-to-cut off (S/Co). Results greater than or equal to 1.00 were considered reactive for HCV antibodies. Specificity and sensitivity of the test were, respectively, 99.97 and 100%.

Nevertheless what we previously described [46] and the CDC recommendations [47] stating that anti-HCV positive samples with S/Co ratios of ≥8.0 can be reported as positive without further supplemental testing, we decided to include in the study only repeatedly anti-HCV reactive samples with S/Co ratios of ≥8.0 confirmed by a third generation immunoblot assay Innolia HCV Score (Fujirebio Europe N.V.) .

### HCV molecular analysis

Only anti-HCV/RIBA HCV positive samples were subsequently tested for the presence of HCV-RNA and its quantification was performed via COBAS Ampliprep/ Taqman HCV 48 (Roche Diagnostics System Inc.), which exploits a polymerase chain reaction in Real time (RT-PCR). Linear range of quantification of the test was 1.50 E + 01 to 6.90 E + 07 HCV RNA IU/mL, using the accuracy acceptance criterion of +/− 0.3 log$^{10}$. Specificity of the test was 100% and its detection limit was 15 IU/mL.

HCV genotyping was performed using the Versant HCV Genotype Assay 2.0 LiPA test (Siemens Healthcare Diagnostics), which involves the amplification and hybridization of viral genome fragments, the latter by means of genotype-specific probes adsorbed onto nitrocellulose strips. The various steps were performed by Auto-LiPA, a fully automated system for complete genotyping. Specificity and sensitivity of this test are, respectively, 96% and 99.4%, and its detection limit is 15 IU/mL.

The limitations of the test LiPA are well known, especially concerning its inability to correctly discriminate the subtypes 2a and 2c of the genotype 2 and subtype 1c of genotype 1, as demonstrated using a restriction fragment length polymorphism (RFLP) analysis [48].

Anyway, its degree of specificity is similar to that of RFLP analysis and, as previously reported, comparable to that of the direct sequencing test Trugene, with an accuracy of 76 and 74%, respectively, even though the InnoLiPA confirms its less subtype discriminating power in subtyping genotype 2 [49, 50].

## Statistical analysis

For the case control study, the odds ratio (OR) with 95% confidence interval for the risk factors of HCC were calculated by logistic regression using the SAS statistical package. Statistical analysis of the data was performed using SPSS for Windows, version 16. The data are presented as mean and standard deviation and categorical variables in absolute number and percentage. Frequency tables were analysed using the $\chi^2$ tests with the Pearson correlations being used to assess the significance of the correlation between the categorical variables. In all tests, $p$-values <0.05 were regarded as statistically significant. A two-proportion hypothesis test was applied to correct any variability between the studied groups.

To further evaluate the independence of HCV genotype on the risk of HCC, the multivariate OR (95% CI) was examined in relation to HCV genotype (1b and non-1b) and IFN responder and not responder patients.

## Results

As shown in Table 1, the main risk factors (alcohol consumption and cigarette smoking) and liver function parameters (AST/ALT, albumin, bilirubin, and ALP levels) did not show significant variations between HCC and the control group. Even if our population did not include alcoholic patients, we also analysed our data excluding patients with alcohol intake and no significant differences were observed (data not shown).

A significantly higher rate of males (105/152), instead, was shown among patients with HCC (69.1%) respect to the control group (320/568, 56.4%) ($\chi^2$:7.06; $p < 0.01$). Males with HCC showed to have quite 2 times risk of exposure to HCV infection (OR = 1.72; 95% CI = 1.15–2.58).

In addition, a significantly higher rate of older patients was observed in the HCC group both considering the threshold age at 50 years (150/152; 98.6% in HCC group and 461/ 568; 81.1% in the control group, $\chi^2$: 28.65; $p < 0.001$) and at 70 years (77/152; 50.7% in HCC group and 200/568; 35.2% in the control group, $\chi^2$:12.08; $p < 0.001$) (Table 1). This finding suggests that 50 years old patients had 17 times higher risk of developing HCC (OR = 17.4; 95% CI = 4.24 to 71.36) and 70 years old patients about 2 times higher risk (OR 1.88; 95% CI = 1.31–2.71). These data were also confirmed by using the two-proportion hypothesis test, Z test (data not shown).

Specific HCV RNA positive rate was found significantly higher (83.7%) among HCC patients (103/152) if compared to the control group (349/568; 61.4%) ($\chi^2$: 12.49; $p < 0.001$), suggesting that HCC patients have a risk of active infection 1 and half times higher than patients without HCC (OR:1.31; 95% C.$I$ = 0.90–1.92) (Fig. 1).

No significant differences in viral load (>2.0 E + 05 IU/mL) was found between HCC patients and the control group (Table 2).

The most prevalent genotype in HCC patients was 1b found in 70/103 HCC patients (67.9%) vs 190/349 (54.4%) in the control group ($\chi^2$: 7.33 p < 0.001). HCC patients have a risk to be infected by genotype 1b quite 2 times greater than patients of the control group (OR:1.77;95% C.$I$ = 1.11–2.82) (Table 3) and after adjusting for age and sex, patients HCV 1b infected showed a similar fold risk of HCC (OR:1.65; 95% C.$I$ = 1.16–2.33), if compared to those with HCV non-1b infection, showing that HCV 1b subtype may be an independent risk factor for HCC (Table 4).

In order to completely remove the potential confounding effect of SVR, a separate multivariate analysis excluding patients who had achieved SVR was also provided. In this analysis, genotype 1b remained independently associated with HCC development (data not shown).

## Conclusion

Hepatocellular carcinoma (HCC), with its incidence of more than 5% of all the cancers globally, is the sixth most common cancer and the third leading cause of cancer-related deaths worldwide [6, 51], especially in Japan and Eastern Asia where the age-adjusted annual death rate due to primary liver cancer has increased from approximately 10 per 100,000 in 1975 to 27.5 in 2002, probably for the increased diffusion of HCV infection [52].

Despite of the recent therapeutic efforts, HCC still remains one of the higher malignant neoplasia, with an

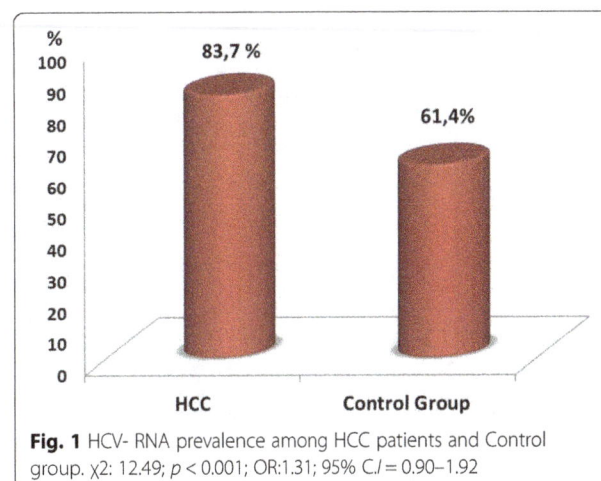

**Fig. 1** HCV- RNA prevalence among HCC patients and Control group. χ2: 12.49; $p < 0.001$; OR:1.31; 95% C.$I$ = 0.90–1.92

**Table 2** HCV RNA viral load among HCC and control group patients

| HCV RNA (IU/mL) | HCC ($n = 103$) | | Control group ($n = 349$) | |
|---|---|---|---|---|
| | n. | % | n. | % |
| $< 2.0 E + 10^5$ | 24 | 23.7 | 88 | 25.2 |
| $2.0 E + 10^5 - 6.0 E + 10^5$ | 17 | 16.5 | 67 | 19.2 |
| $> 6.0 E + 10^5$ | 62 | 59.8 | 194 | 55.6 |

average survival rates of less than 1 year. Such a high mortality seems to be related to the fact that the majority of HCC patients are generally diagnosed at an advanced stage of the disease, especially for the complexity of the prevention and early detection [18]. It is clear, thus, how the identification of prognostic factors associated with tumor development may be extremely important for the timely referral of patients eligible for curative treatment in order to prevent HCC development.

HCV infection is well known globally as one of the main risk factor in HCC development [6, 53] and the recent increase of the incidence of this neoplasia, especially in developed countries, like the United States, is probably related to a substantial increase in HCV circulation [54]. The rate of HCC progression varies greatly among patients with chronic HCV infection and this is probably due to the existence of a complex interplay between host, viral and environmental factors [55], including older age, male gender, alcohol intake and HCV infection [2, 9, 18].

Our study confirms that males with HCC significantly show to have quite 2 times risk of exposure to HCV infection (OR = 1.72; 95% CI = 1.15–2.58) and, furthermore, that older patients have 17 times higher risk of developing HCC if older than 50 years and about 2 times higher risk of developing HCC if older than 70 years, supporting the idea that HCC is age-related and that

**Table 3** Genotype distribution among HCC patients and control group

| Genotype | HCC group | | Control group | |
|---|---|---|---|---|
| | n. | % | n. | % |
| 1 | 77 | 74.7 | 212 | 60.8 |
| 1a | 4 | 3.9 | 9 | 2.6 |
| 1b | 70 | 67.9[A] | 190 | 54.4[A] |
| 1 | 3 | 2.9 | 13 | 3.8 |
| 2 | 21 | 20.4 | 123 | 35.2 |
| 2a/2c | 16 | 15.5 | 100 | 28.7 |
| 2 | 4 | 3.9 | 23 | 6.5 |
| 2a | 1 | 1.0 | 0 | 0 |
| Other genotypes | 5 | 4.9 | 14 | 4.0 |
| Total | 103 | 100 | 349 | 100 |

[A]$\chi^2$:7.33; $p < 0.001$; OR: 1.77; 95% C.I = 1.11–2.82

**Table 4** Odds ratios of genotypes associated with HCC

| Genotype | Crude OR (95% CI) | Age–sex-adjusted OR (95% CI) |
|---|---|---|
| Non 1b | 1.00 | 1.00 |
| 1b | 1.77 (1.11–2.82) | 1.65 (1.16–2.33) |

older age acts as independent factors in HCC development [2, 18, 56, 57], probably because malignant transformation usually occurs after two or more decades from the onset of HCV infection [18]. Instead, no correlation was found between the HCC and the control group regarding liver biochemical parameters, risk factors (alcohol consumption or smoking) or other modality of infection.

Regarding the association between HCV infection and HCC, as recently reported [36], Italy shows a moderate prevalence of anti-HCV in the general population (approximately 2.0%), except for some Southern areas where the prevalence greatly increases ranging from 6% to 12% with an average viraemic rate estimated at over 70% [36]. As we previously reported [58], confirming several other studies [9, 59–61], anti-HCV incidence in our area is significantly greater among HCC patients, suggesting that these patients significantly have an higher risk of exposure to HCV infection if compared to the general population. Nevertheless, although some authors have suggested the central role of HCV in hepatocarcinogenesis [62–64], the mechanism of virus related carcinoma is not yet fully understood, even if it is clear that HCV, alone or in conjunction with other risk factors can contribute to the epidemiological heterogeneity of this neoplasia, as demonstrated by the findings of HCV RNA in liver tissue among HCC patients anti- HCV negative [65].

Although HCV viral load may be considered as an important prognostic variable, whose knowledge might be useful in the treatment decision to eradicate HCV infection and thus reduce or prevent HCC progression [9, 16, 17], its correlation with HCC progression still remains controversial. Even if it has been suggested a possible direct oncogenic effect of HCV, maybe related to genetic mutations [66] or to some cellular deregulation effects, no consensus has emerged yet.

Although our study is simply a retrospective analysis and prevents us to make any hypothesis about mechanisms of HCC progression, our data clearly shows that a significantly higher percentage of HCC patients (83.7%) shows HCV-RNA in their sera compared to the control group (61.4%) ($p < 0.001$), suggesting that HCC patients have a risk of HCV active infection almost 1 and half times higher than patients without HCC, even if we did not find any correlation between high levels of viremia and advanced liver stage, as reported by other authors [38, 67].

The role of genotypes 1b and 3 in increasing the risk of HCC development has been widely questioned recently and even though numerous studies have often suggested their association with the HCC carcinogenetic progression [68–74], especially in patients with underlying cirrhosis, [38–41, 75–77], probably for the strict correlation existing between these subtypes and liver damage, no consensus has emerged yet. Whether HCV 1b genotype contains specific nucleotide sequences that may be associated with direct pathogenesis or may trigger a stronger inflammatory response still needs to be extensively investigated. This has prevented the International health organizations up to now to adopt HCV genotyping as a globally prevention tool in an international program of HCC eradication [78].

Although in our area, as we previously reported [37, 38], genotype 1b is the most common subtype, our data show that its prevalence in HCC patients is significantly higher (67.9%) if compared to the control group (54.4%) ($p < 0.001$), suggesting that HCC patients have a risk to be infected by subtype 1b quite 2 times greater than patients without HCC. Although a minority of treated control group patients achieved SVR, in order to minimize the potential confounding effect of SVR, we adjusted the estimates for SVR achievement, and we also provided a separate multivariate analysis that excluded all patients who had achieved SVR. These data confirmed that genotype 1b was independently associated with the development of HCC.

In conclusion, our study detects a significantly higher rate of HCV RNA positivity in HCC patients than in control group. Furthermore, HCC patients harbours a higher rate of HCV 1b than general population, not influenced by the use of antiviral treatment as the multivariate analysis showed.

Despite of its limitations related to the absence of a prospective study and data regarding the impact of HCV subtype on the fibrosis stages, our data suggest the strict association existing between HCV genotype 1b and HCC. A prospective study with larger number of samples will be needed to confirm our results, especially considering the introduction of the new direct acting antiviral (DAA) therapies.

## Abbreviations

AFP: α- fetoprotein; CDC: Centers for Disease Control; ECi: Enhanced Chemiluminescent immunoassay; HBV: Hepatitis B virus; HCC: Hepatocellular Carcinoma; HCV: Hepatitis C Virus; IU/mL: International Units per Milliliter; LiPA: Line Probe Assay; NIDD: Non-insulin-dependent diabetes; RNA: Ribonucleic Acid; RT-PCR: Reverse transcription polymerase chain reaction; S/Co: Signal-to-cutoff; SPSS: Software package used for statistical analysis; SVR: Sustained virological response

## Acknowledgements

Special thanks to Rita Guarino and to all the patients who consented to enable us to conduct this study.

## Funding

The authors declare no study sponsors involvement in the study design, in the collection, analysis and interpretation of data, in the writing of the manuscript and in the decision to submit the manuscript for publication.

## Authors' contributions

AP, SM and GL acquired the data; AP drafted the article and contributed to conception and design and SM assisted him; MP and ML assisted in clinical database generation and first line interaction; RA, GB and FI contributed to critical revision for important intellectual content; all authors approved the final version to be published.

## Competing interests

The authors declare that they have no competing interests.

## Author details

[1]Virology and Molecular Biology Unit, Department of Diagnostic Pathology, Istituto Nazionale Tumori, Fondazione "G. Pascale" IRCCS Italia, Via Mariano Semmola, 80131 Naples, Italy. [2]Section of Infectious Diseases, Department of Mental Health and Public Medicine, University of Naples "Luigi Vanvitelli", Naples, Italy. [3]Hepatobiliar and Pancreatic Unit, Department of Surgical Oncology, Istituto Nazionale Tumori - Fondazione "G. Pascale" , IRCCS Italia, Naples, Italy. [4]Transfusion Service, Department of Hemathology, Istituto Nazionale Tumori - Fondazione "G. Pascale" , IRCCS Italia, Naples, Italy.

## References

1. Perz JF, Armstrong GL, Farrington LA, et al. The contributions of hepatitis B virus and hepatitis C virus infections to cirrhosis and primary liver cancer worldwide. J Hepatol. 2006;45:529–38.
2. Sherman M. Hepatocellular carcinoma: epidemiology, risk factors and screening. Sem Liv Dis. 2005;25:143–54.
3. Parkin DM, Bray F, Ferlay J, Pisani P. Global cancer statistics. Am Canc J Clin. 2002;55:77–108.
4. Aghemo A, Colombo M. Hepatocellular carcinoma in chronic hepatitis C: from bench to bedsite. Semin Immunopathol. 2013;35:111–20.
5. Sangiovanni A, Del Ninno E, Fasani P, et al. Increased survival of cirrhotic patients with a hepatocellular carcinoma detected during surveillance. Gastroenterol. 2004;126:1005–14.
6. Peng C, You C, Meiu XS, et al. icluster and pathway enrichment analysis of HCV induced cirrhosis and hepatocellular carcinoma. Asian Pac J Canc Prev. 2012;13:3741–5.
7. Mori M, Hara M, Wada I, et al. Prospective study of hepatitis B and C viral infections, cigarette smoking, alcohol consumption, and other factors associated with hepatocellular carcinoma risk in Japan. Am J Epidemiol. 2000;151:131–9.
8. Levrero M. Viral hepatitis and liver cancer: the case of hepatitis C. Oncogene. 2006;25:3834–47.
9. Jin Hu F, Jian-Bing W, Yong J, et al. Attributable causes of liver cancer. Asian Pac J Can Prev. 2013;14:7251–6.
10. Lee CM, Lu SN, Hung CH, Tung WC, Wang JH, Tung HD, et al. Hepatitis C virus genotypes in southern Taiwan : prevalence and clinical implications. Trans R Soc Trop Med Hyg. 2006;100:767–74.
11. Benvegnù L, Gios M, Boccato S, Alberti A. Natural history of compensated viral cirrhosis: a prospective study on the incidence and hierarchy of major complications. Gut. 2004;53:744–9.
12. Kumar M, Kumar R, Hissar SS, et al. Risk factors analysis for hepatocellular carcinoma in patients with and without cirrhosis: a case control study of 213 hepatocellular carcinoma. J Gastroenterol Hepatol. 2007;22:1104–11.
13. Oyunsuren T, Kurbanov F, Tanaka Y, et al. High frequency of hepatocellular carcinoma in Mongolia; association with mono-, or co-infection with hepatitis C, B, and delta viruses. J Med Virol. 2006;78:1688–95.

14. Takeshi T, Kazuhiro N, Akiko S, et al. Incidence of hepatocellular carcinoma in chronic hepatitis B and C: a prospective study of 251 patients. Hepatol. 2012;27:797–804.

15. Tornesello ML, Buonaguro L, Tatangelo F, et al. Mutations in TP53, CTNNB1 and PIK3CA genes in hepatocellular carcinoma associated with hepatitis B and hepatitis C virus infections. Genomics. 2013;102:74–83.

16. El Sarag HB. Mason AC: "Risk factors for the rising rates of primary liver cancer in the United States". Arch Int Med. 2000;160(21):3227–30.

17. Rathi PK, Luucinda LH, Lauren EE, Stanley ML, David RM. Hepatitis C virus infection causes cell cycle arrest at the level of initiation of mitotis. J Virol. 2011;85:7989–8001.

18. Savino B, Daniela S, Piero LA, et al. Critical reappraisal of risk factors for occurence of hepatocellular carcinoma in patients with hepatitis C virus. Hep Med. 2011;3:21–8.

19. Chakravarti A, Dogra G, Verma V, Srivastava AP. Distribution pattern of HCV genotypes and its association with virals load. Indian J Med Res. 2011;133: 326–31.

20. Amarapurkar DN, Patel ND, Kamani PM. Impact of diabetes mellitus on outcome of HCC. Ann Hepatol. 2008;7:148–51.

21. Idilman R, De Maria N, Colantoni A, et al. Pathogenesis of hepatitis B and C-induced hepatocellular carcinoma. J Viral Hep. 1998;5:285–99.

22. De Mitri MS, Poussin K, Baccarini P, et al. HCV-associated liver cancer without cirrhosis. Lancet. 1995;345:413–5.

23. Timm J, Roggendorf M. Sequence diversity of hepatitis C virus: implications for immune control and therapy. World J Gastroenterol. 2007;13:4808–17.

24. Ford N, Kirby C, Singh K, Mills EJ, Cooke G, Kamarulzaman A, duCros P. Chronic hepatitis C treatment outcomes in low- and middle-income countries: a systematic review and meta-analysis. Bull World Health Organ. 2012;90:540–50.

25. Ford N, Singh K, Cooke GS, Mills EJ, von Schoen-Angerer T, Kamarulzaman A, du Cros P. Expanding access to treatment for hepatitis C in resource-limited settings: lessons from HIV/AIDS. Clin Infect Dis. 2012;54:1465–72.

26. Simmonds P, Alberti A, Alter HJ, Bonino F, Bradley DW, Brechot C, Brouwer JT, Chan SW, Chayama K, Chen DS. A proposed system for the nomenclature of hepatitis C viral genotypes. Hepatology. 1994;19:1321–4.

27. Anderson JC, Simonetti J, Fisher DG, Williams J, Yamamura Y, Rodriguez N, Sullivan DG, Gretch DR, McMahon B, Williams KJ. Comparison of different HCV viral load and genotyping assays. J Clin Virol. 2003;28:27–37.

28. Petruzziello A, Marigliano S, Loquercio G, Cozzolino A, Cacciapuoti C. Hepatitis C Virus (HCV) infection: an epidemiology up-date of the circulation of HCV genotypes. World J Gastroenterol. 2016;22(34):7824–40.

29. Smith DB, Bukh J, Kuiken C, Muerhoff AS, Rice CM, Stapleton JT, Simmonds P. Expanded classification of hepatitis C virus into 7 genotypes and 67 subtypes: updated criteria and genotype assignment web resource. Hepatol. 2014;59: 318–27.

30. Smith DB, Pathirana S, Davidson F, Lawlor E, Power J, Yap PL, Simmonds P. The origin of hepatitis C virus genotypes. J Gen Virol. 1997;78(2):321–8.

31. Pybus OG, Cochrane A, Holmes EC, Simmonds P. The hepatitis C virus epidemic among injecting drug users. Inf Gen Evol. 2005;5:131–9.

32. Magiorkinis G, Magiorkinis E, Paraskevis D, Ho SY, Shapiro B, Pybus OG, Allain JP, Hatzakis A. The global spread of hepatitis C virus 1a and 1b: a phylodynamic and phylogeographic analysis. PLoS Med. 2009;6:1000–198.

33. Simmonds P. The origin and evolution of hepatitis viruses in humans. J Gen Virol. 2001;82:693–712.

34. Pybus OG, Barnes E, Taggart R, Lemey P, Markov PV, Rasachak B, Syhavong B, Phetsouvanah R, Sheridan I, Humphreys IS, Lu L, Newton PN, Klenerman P. Genetic history of hepatitis C virus in East Asia. J Virol. 2009;83:1071–82.

35. Marascio N, Liberto M, Barreca G, Zicca E, Quirino A, Lamberti A, et al. Update on epidemiology of HCV in Italy: focus on the Calabria Region. BMC Infect Dis. 2014;14(5):S2.

36. Petruzziello A, Marigliano S, Loquercio G, Cacciapuoti C. Hepatitis C Virus (HCV) genotypes distribution: an epidemiological up-date in Europe. Infect Agent Cancer. 2016;12(11):53.

37. Petruzziello A, Coppola N, Diodato AM, Iervolino V, Azzaro R, et al. Age and gender distribution of hepatitis C virus genotypes in the metropolitan area of Naples. Intervirology. 2013;56(3):206–12.

38. Petruzziello A, Coppola N, Loquercio G, Marigliano S, Giordano M, et al. Distribution pattern of Hepatitis C Virus (HCV) genotypes and correlation

with viral load and risk factors in chronic positive patients. Intervirology. 2014;57:311–31.

39. Savino B, Crosignani A, Maisonneuve P, et al. Hepatitis C virus Genotype 1b as a major risk factor associated with Hepatocellular carcinoma in patients with cirrhosis: a seventeen- year prospective cohort study. Hepatol. 2007; 46(5):1350–6.

40. Lee MH, Yang HI, Lu SN, et al. Hepatitis C virus genotype 1b increases cumulative lifetime risk of hepatocellular carcinoma. Intern J Cancer. 2014; 135:1119–26.

41. Raimondi S, Savino B, Mondelli MU, Maisonneuve P. Hepatitis C virus genotrype 1b as a risk factor for hepatocellular carcinoma development: a meta analysis. J Hepatol. 2009;50:1142–54.

42. Fattovich G, Stroffolini T, Xagni I, Donato F. Hepatocellular carcinoma in cirrhosis incidence and risk factors. Gastroenterol. 2004;127:S35–50.

43. Benvegnù L, Pontisso P, Cavalletto D, Noventa F, Alberti A. Lack of correlation between hepatitis C virus genotypes and clinical course of hepatitis C virus- related cirrhosis. Hepatol. 1997;25:211–5.

44. Bruix J, Sherman M, Llovet JM, et al. Clinical management of hepatocellular carcinoma. Conclusions of the Barcelona-2000 EASL conference. J Hepatol. 2001;35:421–3.

45. Leevy CM, Sherlock S, Tygstrup N, et al. Diseases of the Liver and Biliary Tract. Standardization of Nomenclature, Diagnostic Criteria and Prognosis. New York: Raven Press; 1994. p. 61–2.

46. Petruzziello A, Coppola N, Fraulo M, Loquercio G, Azzaro R, et al. Ortho Vitros enhanced chemiluminescence assay for the detection of hepatitis C virus antibodies. Determination of a borderline range. AJMR. 2013;7:2359–64.

47. Centers for disease Control and Prevention: Guideline for laboratory testing and result reporting of antibody to hepatitis C virus (anti-HCV). Morb Mortal Wkly Rep Recomm Rep. 2003;52:1–13.

48. Buoro S, Pizzighella S, Boschetto R, Pellizzari L, et al. Typing of hepatitis C virus by a new method based on restrivction fragment length polymorphism. Intervirology. 1999;42:1–8.

49. Stuyver I, Wyseur A, Van Arnhem W, Lunel F, et al. Hepatitis C virus genotyping by means of 59-UR/core line probe assay and molecular analysis of untypeable samples. Virus Res. 1995;38:137–57.

50. Halfon P, Trimoulet P, Bourliere M, Khiri H, et al. Hepatitis C virus genotyping based on 5′ non coding sequence analysis (Trugene). J Clin Microbiol. 2001;39:1771–3.

51. Yang JD, Roberts LR. Hepatocellular carcinoma: a global view. Nat Rev Gastroenterol Hepatol. 2010;7:448–58.

52. Tanaka Y, Hanada K, Mizokami M, et al. Inaugural article: a comparison of the molecular clock of hepatitis C virus in the US and Japan. Proc Nat Ac Sci USA. 2002;99:15584–9.

53. Samreen B, Khaliq S, Ashfaq UA, et al. Hepatitis C virus entry: role of host and viral factors. Inf Gen Evol. 2012;12:1699–709.

54. Davila JA, Morgan RO, Shaib Y, KA MG, El-Serag HB. Hepatitis C infection and the increasing incidence of hepatocellular carcinoma: a population-based study. Gastroenterol. 2004;127:1372–80.

55. David RM, Stanley ML. Virus-specific Mechanisms of carcinogenesis in hepatitis C virus associated liver cancer. Oncogene. 2011;28:1969–83.

56. Hirakawa M, Ikeda K, Arase Y, et al. Hepatocarcinogenesis following HCV RNA eradication by interferon in chronic hepatitis patients. Int Med. 2008;47: 1637–43.

57. Jen-Eing J, Meng-Feng T, Hey-Ru T, et al. Impact of hepatitis B and hepatitis C on adverse hepatitis fibrosis in hepatocellular carcinoma related to betel quid chewing. Asian Pac J Canc Prev. 2014;15:637–42.

58. Petruzziello A, Marigliano S, Loquercio G, Guarino R, Izzo F, Cacciapuoti C. Hepatitis C Virus (HCV) genotype 1b as a risk factor for hepatocellular carcinoma development in chronic HCV positive patients in Southern Italy. J Liver. 2016;5:2(Suppl).

59. Ruiz J, Sangro B, Cuende JI, et al. Hepatitis B and C viral infections in patients with hepatocellular carcinoma. Hepatol. 1992;16:637–41.

60. Takano S, Yokosuka O, Imazeld F, et al. Incidence of hepatocellular carcinoma in chronic hepatitis B and C: a prospective study of 251 patients. Hepatol. 1995;21:650–5.

61. Donato F, Tagger A, Gelatti U, et al. Alcohol and hepatocellular carcinoma: the effect of lifetime intake and hepatitis virus infections in men and women. Am J Epidemiol. 2002;155:323–31.

62. Koike K. Hepatitis C virus contributes to hepatocarcinogenesis by modulating metabolic and intracellular signaling pathways. J Gastroenterol Hepatol. 2007;22:108–11.

63. Farinati F, Cardin R, Bortolami M, et al. Hepatitis C virus: From oxygen free radicals to hepatocellular carcinoma. J Viral Hepat. 2007;14:821–9.

64. Abd El-Rahman NZ, Nabawy Z, Auhood AMN, et al. Disease progression from chronic hepatitis C to cirrhosis and hepatocellular carcinoma is associated with increasing DNA promoter methylation. Asian Pac J Canc Prev. 2013;14:6721–6.

65. Esaki T, Suzuki N, Yokoyama K, et al. Hepatocellular carcinoma in a patient with liver cirrhosis associated with negative serum HCV tests but positive liver tissue HCV RNA. Int Med. 2004;43:279–82.

66. Moutaz D, Aliaa A. Hepatocellular carcinoma in hepatitis c genotype 4 after viral clearance and in absence of cirrhosis: two case reports. Case Report Cases. 2009;2:7927.

67. Berry V, Arora R, Paul P. Hepatitis C-clinical outcome and. Diagnosis. J K Sci. 2005;7:129–32.

68. Lee MH, Yang HI, Lu SN, Jen CL, You SL, Wang LY, L'Italien G, Chen CJ, Yuan Y, REVEAL-HCV Study Group. Hepatitis C virus genotype 1b increases cumulative lifetime risk of hepatocellular carcinoma. Int J Cancer. 2014; 135(5):1119–26.

69. Korba B, Shetty K, Medvedev A, Viswanathan P, Varghese R, Zhou B, Roy R, Makambi K, Ressom H, Loffredo CA. Hepatitis C virus Genotype 1a core gene nucleotide patterns associated with hepatocellular carcinoma risk. J Gen Virol. 2015;96(9):2928–37.

70. Bruno S, Crosignani A, Maisonneuve P, Rossi S, Silini E, Mondelli MU. Hepatitis C virus genotype 1b as a major risk factor associated with hepatocellular carcinoma in patients with cirrhosis: a seventeen-year prospective cohort study. Hepatology. 2007;46(5):1350–6.

71. Tanaka K, Ikematsu H, Hirohata T, Kashiwagi S. Hepatitis C virus infection and risk of hepatocellular carcinoma among Japanese: possible role of type 1b (II) infection. J Natl Cancer Inst. 1996;88(11):742–6.

72. Hung CH, Chen CH, Lee CM, Wu CM, Hu TH, Wang JH, Yen YH, Lu SN. Association of amino acid variations in the NS5A and E2-PePHD region of hepatitis C virus 1b with hepatocellular carcinoma. J Viral Hepat. 2008;15(1): 58–65.

73. Toyoda H, Kumada T, Kaneoka Y, Maeda A. Amino acid substitutions in the hepatitis C virus core region are associated with postoperative recurrence and survival of patients with HCV genotype 1b-associated hepatocellular carcinoma. Ann Surg. 2011;254(2):326–32.

74. Le Guillou-Guillemette H, Ducancelle A, Bertrais S, Lemaire C, Pivert A, Veillon P, Bouthry E, Alain S, Thibault V, Abravanel F, Rosenberg AR, Henquell C, André-Garnier E, Petsaris O, Vallet S, Bour JB, Baazia Y, Trimoulet P, André P, Gaudy-Graffin C, Bettinger D, Larrat S, Signori-Schmuck A, Saoudin H, Pozzetto B, Lagathu G, Minjolle-Cha S, Stoll-Keller F, Pawlotsky JM, Izopet J, Payan C, Lunel-Fabiani F. Identification of a duplicated V3 domain in NS5A associated with cirrhosis and hepatocellular carcinoma in HCV-1b patients. J Clin Virol. 2015;69:203–39.

75. Parkin DM, Bray F, Ferlay J, Pisani P. Global cancer statistics, 2002. Am Canc J Clin. 2005;55:74–108.

76. Nkontchou G, Ziol M, Aout M, Lhabadie M, et al. HCV genotype 3 is associated with a higher hepatocellular carcinoma incidence in pactients with ongoing virsal C cirrhosis. J Viral Hep. 2011;18:e516–22.

77. Kanwal F, Kramer JR, Ilyas J, Duan Z, El-Serag H. HCV Genotype 3 is associated with an increased risk of cirrhosis and hepatocellular carcinoma in a National Samples of US Veterans with HCV. Hepatol. 2014;60:98–105.

78. Bruix J, Sherman M. Management of hepatocellular carcinoma. Practice Guidelines Committee, American Association for the Study of Liver Diseases. Hepatol. 2005;42:1208–36.

# 23

# Prevalence of "unclassified" HPV genotypes among women with abnormal cytology

Clorinda Annunziata[1], Giovanni Stellato[2], Stefano Greggi[2], Veronica Sanna[3], Maria Pia Curcio[3], Simona Losito[3], Gerardo Botti[3], Luigi Buonaguro[1], Franco Maria Buonaguro[1] and Maria Lina Tornesello[1*]

## Abstract

**Background:** High risk human papillomaviruses (HPVs) have been unequivocally recognised as the necessary cause of squamous intraepithelial lesions (SIL) and invasive carcinoma of the cervix. The distribution and the role of unclassified risk HPV genotypes in cervical neoplasia has not been fully elucidated.

**Methods:** Liquid-based cytological samples were collected from 337 women referred for colposcopy following an abnormal cytological diagnosis. HPV DNA was detected by broad-spectrum PCR and genotypes identified by nucleotide sequencing analysis and reverse line blot (RLB).

**Results:** The overall frequency of HPV infection was 36.5% (35 out of 96) in samples negative for intraepithelial lesions or malignancy (NILM), 80% (181 out of 226) in low grade SIL and 93.3% (14 out of 15) in high grade SIL ($P <$ 0.001). Thirty-five different genotypes were identified among the 230 HPV-positive cases. The Group 1 oncogenic viruses (HPV16, 18, 31, 33, 35, 39, 45, 51, 52, 56, 58 and 59) were found in 21.9, 46.5, and 86.7% of NILM, low grade SIL and high grade SIL, respectively. The Group 2A, including the probably oncogenic virus HPV68, was found in 1 and 0.8% of NILM and low grade SIL, respectively. The Group 2b possibly oncogenic HPVs (HPV34, 53, 66, 67, 70, 73, 82 and 85) were found in 4.2, 21.7 and 26.7% of NILM, low grade SIL and high grade SIL, respectively. The unclassified viruses (HPV12, 42, 54, 55, 61, 62, 81, 83, 84, 89, 90, 91) were detected in 8.3 and 14.6% of NILM and low grade SIL, respectively, and never in high grade SIL.

**Conclusions:** Group 1 HPVs were mainly prevalent in high grade SIL and low grade SIL while Group 2B were equally distributed among the two groups. The dominant frequency of unclassified HPVs in low grade SIL and NILM and their rarity in high grade SIL suggests their marginal role in cervical neoplasia of the studied population.

**Keywords:** Human papillomavirus, Cervix carcinoma, Squamous intraepithelial neoplasia

## Background

Human papillomaviruses (HPVs) of the genus alpha represent the most common sexually transmitted viruses infecting mucosal epithelial cells of male and female genital tract [1–3]. Alpha HPVs currently comprise 62 genotypes classified in 15 species on the basis of their phylogenetic similarity [4–6]. The oncogenic risk of mucosal HPVs has been established by large epidemiological studies investigating the different prevalence of specific genotypes in normal cytology, in low and high grade cervical intraepithelial lesions (SIL) and in cervical

carcinoma [7–9]. Twelve viruses (HPV16, 18, 31, 33, 35, 39, 45, 51, 52, 56, 58 and 59) have been found significantly associated with cervical carcinoma and classified as Group 1 "carcinogenic to humans", one virus (HPV68) as Group 2A "probably carcinogenic to humans", 12 viruses (HPV26, 53, 66, 67, 70, 73, 82, 30, 34, 69, 85, 97) as Group 2B "possibly carcinogenic to humans" and two viruses (HPV6 and 11) as Group 3 "unclassifiable as to carcinogenicity in humans" [10]. Several other HPV genotypes are unclassified regarding to their epidemiologic oncogenic risk although few of them have been shown to bind and to ubiquitinate p53 oncosuppressor with the same efficiency as the Group 1 oncogenic viruses [11, 12].

* Correspondence: m.tornesello@istitutotumori.na.it
[1]Molecular Biology and Viral Oncology Unit, Istituto Nazionale Tumori IRCCS "Fondazione G. Pascale", via M Semmola, 80131 Naples, Italy
Full list of author information is available at the end of the article

A meta-analysis of HPV genotype distribution among 115,789 women positive for HPV infection, including normal cytology, atypical squamous cells of undetermined significance (ASCUS), low grade SIL, high grade SIL and invasive cervical cancer cases, showed limited difference in the prevalence of Group 1 HPV type distribution among all groups while HPV16, HPV18 and 45 were relatively high frequent in cervical carcinoma [7]. Moreover, a large meta analysis, comprising above one million women with normal cervical cytology, showed that Group 1 HPV genotypes were found to be the most common viruses in the general female population worldwide, accounting for 70% of HPV infections in normal cytological samples [13]. Some HPV genotypes belonging to the Groups 2A and 2B, namely HPV26, 67, 68, 69, 73 and 82, were found also relatively common in invasive cervical cancer compared to normal cytology [2]. Conversely, Group 2A/2B HPV53 and 66 were found more common in normal cytology and low grade SIL than in invasive cervical cancer. Among viruses with unclassified risk the HPV61, 62, 84 and 89 have been found to be relatively uncommon in normal cytology and invasive cancer and more frequent in low grade SIL [2].

In Italy, several studies evaluating the HPV prevalence and genotype distribution have been performed among women enrolled in organized and in opportunistic screening programs [14–17]. All the studies confirmed the high prevalence of Group 1 HPV genotypes, particularly HP16, 31 and 18 in SIL and invasive cervical cancer [17–19]. However, some unclassified HPVs have been also found to be relatively common in women with normal cytology. In particular, Tornesello et al. observed that several unknown risk viruses were present in low-grade SIL (HPV30, 32), in high-grade SIL (HPV62, 90), and in a small percentage of cervical carcinoma (HPV62) [16, 20]. More recently, Del Prete et al. reported that among 2149 women enrolled in Apulia region the HPV42 was the most common genotype followed by HPV16 with frequency rates of 10.7 and 8.9%, respectively [21].

In the present study we aimed to expand previous analyses on the distribution of alpha HPV genotypes among Italian women referred to the colposcopy outpatient clinic of the Istituto Nazionale Tumori of Napoli after an abnormal cytological diagnosis. We used broad spectrum amplification technology followed by nucleotide sequencing analysis in order to identify known and unknown HPV genotypes infecting the analyzed women population. All HPVs not included in the Group 1, 2A, 2B and 3 have been designed as unclassified HPVs in the present study.

## Methods

### Patients and samples

Cervical cytological samples were collected in liquid-based PreservCyt (Hologic Inc., Marlborough, MA) from 337

Italian women which following a primary abnormal cytological test were referred for a colposcopy examination and directed biopsy at the Istituto Nazionale Tumori "Fond Pascale" from January 2015 to December 2017. All women enrolled in the study self-reported to be not HIV positive or pregnant. Cytology results were recorded according to the Bethesda system as negative for intraepithelial lesions and malignancy (NILM), low grade squamous intraepithelial lesion (SIL) and high grade SIL. Histological diagnoses were available for 224 women and cervical lesions were classified as cervical intraepithelial neoplasia of grade 1, 2 and 3 (CIN1, 2 and 3).

This study was approved by the Institutional Scientific Board of the Istituto Nazionale Tumori "Fond Pascale", and it is in accordance with the principles of the Declaration of Helsinki. All patients provided written informed consent.

### DNA isolation

PreservCyt specimens were vortexed briefly, divided into two 2-ml aliquots and centrifuged 5 min at 12′000 g. The cell pellet was washed twice with phosphate buffered saline (PBS Buffer, 137 mM NaCl, 2.7 mM KCl, 8 mM Na2HPO4, and 2 mM KH2PO4, pH 7.4) and resuspended in 100 μl of lysis buffer (50 mM Tris-HCl pH 8.5, 1 mM EDTA, 0.5% Tween20) containing proteinase K (200 μg per ml). Cell lysates were digested at 60 °C for 30 min. DNA was purified by phenol and phenol-chloroform-isoamyl alcohol (25:24:1) extraction and concentrated by ethanol precipitation in 0.3 M sodium acetate (pH 4.6). The quantity of isolated DNA was assessed using the spectrophotometer Nanodrop 2000C (Thermo Fisher Scientific, Waltham, MA).

### Broad spectrum HPV amplification and genotyping

Nucleic acid integrity was assessed by PCR amplification of TP53 gene exon 7 which rendered all 337 samples suitable for further analysis [22]. HPV detection was carried out by nested PCR using the MY09/11 consensus primer pairs [23] for the outer reaction (~ 450 bp) and the MGP primer system [24] for the inner reaction (~ 150 bp) [25]. The method has been evaluated 95% proficient for detection of HPV16, 18, 31, 33, 35, 39, 45, 52, 56, 58, 59, 66 and 68b with a specificity above 97% using a proficiency panel of HPV plasmids in the context of the 4th WHO HPV LabNet Proficiency Study for Evaluating HPV DNA Typing Methods (2010), [26]. A negative control sample, made of a reaction mixture without template DNA, was included in every set of five clinical specimens for each PCR run.

The amplified DNA was subjected to electrophoresis on a 7% polyacrylamide gel followed by staining with ethidium bromide and image analysis by the Gel Doc gel imaging system (Bio-Rad Laboratories Inc., Hercules,

CA). HPV genotypes were identified by direct automated DNA sequencing analysis of MGP amplified products using both the forward GP5+ and the reverse GP6+ oligoprimers [27] at Eurofins Genomics GmbH (Ebersberg, DE). HPV genotypes were identified by alignment of HPV sequences with those present in the GenBank database using the BLASTn software (http://www.ncbi.nlm.nih.gov/blast/html). The DNA samples showing multiple peaks on the pherograms, compatible with multiple infections, were re-amplified using for the inner reaction biotinylated GP5+/GP6+ primers and resulting amplimers subjected to the reverse line blot assay (Qiagen Manchester Ltd., UK) for the detection of 18 HPV genotypes as described previously [28].

### Statistical analyses

The statistical analysis was performed using the Epi Info 6 Statistical Analysis System Software (Version 6.04b, 1997, Centers for Disease Control and Prevention, USA). Unpaired $t$ test was used for comparisons of continuous variables (i.e. age); Yates-corrected $\chi^2$ test and, where appropriate, two-sided Fisher's exact test were used for comparison of categorical data. Differences were considered to be statistically significant when $P$ values were less than 0.05.

### Results

The study included 337 women with a mean age of 37.6 ($\pm$ 10.9) years diagnosed with normal cytology ($n = 96$), low grade SIL ($n = 226$) and high grade SIL ($n = 15$). The histological analysis was available for 224 women and rendered 82 NILM, 129 CIN1 and 13 CIN2/3 diagnoses, respectively (Table 1). Overall HPV DNA sequences were detected in 230 out of 337 (68.3%) samples (Table 1). The mean age of HPV-negative and HPV-positive women was 38.5 ($\pm$11.8) and 37.2 ($\pm$10.6) years, respectively.

**Table 1** Cytological and histological diagnosis of cervical scrapes and biopsies stratified by HPV status

|  | Cases n (%) | HPV positive n (%) | HPV negative n (%) |
|---|---|---|---|
| Cytology | 337 | 230 (68.3) | 107 (31.8) |
| NILM* | 96 (28.5) | 35 (15.2) | 61 (57.0) |
| LSIL* | 226 (67.1) | 181 (78.7) | 45 (42.1) |
| HSIL* | 15 (4.5) | 14 (6.1) | 1 (0.9) |
| Histology[a] | 224 | 161 (71.9) | 63 (28.1) |
| NILM* | 82 (36.6) | 54 (65.8) | 28 (34.2) |
| CIN1* | 129 (57.6) | 95 (73.6) | 34 (26.4) |
| CIN2/CIN3* | 13 (5.8) | 12 (92.3) | 1 (7.7) |

*NILM negative for intraepithelial lesions or malignancy, LSIL low grade SIL; HSIL high grade SIL; CIN1, 2 and 3 cervical intraepithelial neoplasia grade 1, 2 or 3
[a]The HPV status of each histological biopsy has been determined on the corresponding cytological sample

Among analyzed samples, 41.3% were positive for Group 1 HPV genotypes, 0.9 and 16.9% for Group 2A and Group 2B, respectively, and 2.7% for Group 3 HPV genotypes. Unclassified viruses were found in 12.2% of samples and represented 17.8% of all infections (Table 2).

The most common genotypes were HPV16 (11.9%), HPV31 (5.3%), HPV18 (3.9%), HPV33 (3.3%), HPV52 (3%), HPV56 (3%) HPV58 (2.4%) and HPV59 (2.1%) belonging to Group1; HPV53 (6.5%) and HPV66 (6.2%) of the Group 2; HPV6 (2.4%) of the Group 3 and unclassified HPV type 81 (2.1%). The frequency of all other genotypes was below 2% of all HPV infections (Table 2).

The higher prevalence of HPVs (71.3%) was observed among women in the age group 18–30, $P = 0.659$. Single HPV infections were found in 59.8 and 63.4% of the women aged 18–30 and $\geq$ 31 years, respectively. Multiple infections were observed in 11.5 and 4.5% of women aged 18–30 and $\geq$ 31 years, respectively. HPV16 was the most common type found in the two age groups (11.5 and 11.9%, respectively) followed by HPV66 (8.1 and 5.5%), HPV31 (6.9 and 4.5%), HPV 53 (5.8 and 8.4%), HPV58 (5.8% in 18–30 age group), HPV18 (4.6 and 4%) and HPV56 (4.6 and 2.5%).

According to cervical cytology, the prevalence of HPV infection was 36.5, 80 and 93.3% in patients with NILM, low grade SIL and high grade SIL respectively (Table 2). Group 1 HPV genotypes were detected in 21.9, 46.5, and 86.7% of NILM, low grade SIL and high grade SIL, respectively. Group 2B HPV genotypes were identified in 4.2, 21.7 and 26.7% of NILM, low grade SIL and high grade SIL. Group 3 HPV types were detected in 2.1 and 3.1% of NILM and low grade SIL but in none high grade SIL. Moreover, unclassified HPV types were found in 8.3 and 14.6% of NILM and low grade SIL, respectively, but not in high grade SIL (Table 2). Figure 1 shows the relative frequency of Group 1, 2A and 2B as well as of unclassified HPV genotypes among all HPV-positive NILM, low grade SIL and high grade SIL.

Multiple infections containing at least one HPV genotype of Group 1 were found in 4.5% of cases, while those containing no high risk HPV genotypes represented 1.5% of all analyzed samples. Multiple infections were observed in 2.1% of NILM, 6.6% of low grade SIL and 20% of high grade SIL.

HPV types targeted by the nonavalent HPV vaccine (HPV6, 11, 16, 18, 31, 33, 45, 52 and 58) were detected, alone or in association with other genotypes in 17.7% (17/96), 40.3% (91/226) and 53.3% (8/15) of NILM, low grade SIL and high grade SIL, respectively.

### Discussion

This study provides a comprehensive information on the HPV prevalence and genotype distribution among a cohort of Italian women which were referred to a single

**Table 2** Frequency of group 1, 2A, 2B, 3 and unclassified HPV genotypes among NILM, low grade SIL and high grade SIL

| Species | HPV genotype[a] | All samples $n = 337$ (%) | NILM $n = 96$ (%) | LSIL $n = 226$ (%) | HSIL $n = 15$ (%) |
|---|---|---|---|---|---|
| | HPV Negative | 107 (31.8) | 61 (63.5) | 45 (20.0) | 1 (6.7) |
| | HPV Positive | 230 (68.3) | 35 (36.5) | 181 (80.0) | 14 (93.3) |
| | Group 1 | | | | |
| A9 | HPV16 | 40 (11.9) | 5 (5.2) | 30 (13.3) | 5 (33.3) |
| A7 | HPV18 | 13 (3.9) | 2 (2.1) | 10 (4.4) | 1 (6.7) |
| A9 | HPV31 | 18 (5.3) | 0 | 17 (7.5) | 1 (6.7) |
| A9 | HPV33 | 11 (3.3) | 1 (1.0) | 9 (3.9) | 1 (6.7) |
| A9 | HPV35 | 2 (0.6) | 0 | 1 (0.4) | 1 (6.7) |
| A7 | HPV39 | 7 (2.1) | 1 (1.0) | 5 (2.2) | 1 (6.7) |
| A7 | HPV45 | 7 (2.1) | 0 | 7 (3.1) | 0 |
| A5 | HPV51 | 6 (1.8) | 0 | 5 (2.2) | 1 (6.7) |
| A9 | HPV52 | 10 (3.0) | 4 (4.2) | 6 (2.7) | 0 |
| A6 | HPV56 | 10 (3.0) | 3 (3.1) | 5 (2.2) | 2 (13.3) |
| A9 | HPV58 | 8 (2.4) | 3 (3.1) | 5 (2.2) | 0 |
| A7 | HPV59 | 7 (2.1) | 2 (2.1) | 5 (2.2) | 0 |
| | Total Group 1 | 139 (41.3) | 21 (21.9) | 105 (46.5) | 13 (86.7) |
| | Group 2A | | | | |
| A7 | HPV68 | 3 (0.9) | 1 (1.0) | 2 (0.8) | 0 |
| | Group 2B | | | | |
| A6 | HPV53 | 22 (6.5) | 2 (2.1) | 19 (8.4) | 1 (7.1) |
| A6 | HPV66 | 21 (6.2) | 1 (1.0) | 17 (7.5) | 3 (21.4) |
| A9 | HPV67 | 3 (0.9) | 0 | 3 (1.3) | 0 |
| A7 | HPV70 | 5 (1.5) | 0 | 5 (2.2) | 0 |
| A11 | HPV73 | 2 0.6) | 0 | 2 (0.9) | 0 |
| A5 | HPV82 | 2 (0.6) | 1 (1.0) | 1 (0.4) | 0 |
| A11 | HPV34 | 1 (0.3) | 0 | 1 (0.4) | 0 |
| A7 | HPV85 | 1 (0.3) | 0 | 1 (0.4) | 0 |
| | Total Group 2B | 57 (16.9) | 4 (4.2) | 49 (21.7) | 4 (26.7) |
| | Group 3 | | | | |
| A10 | HPV6 | 8 (2.4) | 2 (2.1) | 6 (2.7) | 0 |
| A10 | HPV11 | 1 (0.3) | 0 | 1 (0.4) | 0 |
| | Total Group 3 | 9 (2.7) | 2 (2.1) | 7 (3.1) | 0 |
| | Unclassified | | | | |
| A3 | HPV81 | 7 (2.1) | 1 (1.0) | 6 (2.7) | 0 |
| A1 | HPV42 | 5 (1.5) | 0 | 5 (2.2) | 0 |
| A3 | HPV62 | 6 (1.8) | 1 (1.0) | 5 (2.2) | 0 |
| A10 | HPV55 | 4 (1.2) | 1 (1.0) | 3 (1.3) | 0 |
| A3 | HPV89 | 4 (1.2) | 3 (3.1) | 1 (0.4) | 0 |
| A8 | HPV91 | 4 (1.2) | 0 | 4 (1.8) | 0 |
| A13 | HPV54 | 3 (0.9) | 0 | 3 (1.3) | 0 |
| A14 | HPV90 | 3 (0.9) | 1 (1.0) | 2 (0.9) | 0 |
| A3 | HPV84 | 2 (0.6) | 1 (1.0) | 1 (0.4) | 0 |
| A3 | HPV61 | 1 (0.3) | 0 | 1 (0.4) | 0 |

**Table 2** Frequency of group 1, 2A, 2B, 3 and unclassified HPV genotypes among NILM, low grade SIL and high grade SIL (Continued)

| Species | HPV genotype[a] | All samples n = 337 (%) | NILM n = 96 (%) | LSIL n = 226 (%) | HSIL n = 15 (%) |
|---|---|---|---|---|---|
| A3 | HPV83 | 1 (0.3) | 0 | 1 (0.4) | 0 |
| B1 | HPV12 | 1 (0.3) | 0 | 1 (0.4) | 0 |
| | Total Unclassified | 41 (12.2) | 8 (8.3) | 33 (14.6) | 0 |

[a]Type-specific prevalence includes HPVs in single or multiple infections

Centre for colposcopy following a diagnosis of abnormal cytology. As expected, the overall prevalence of high risk HPVs (Group 1), particularly HPV16, was significantly higher among high grade SIL (86.7%) compared to low grade SIL (46.5%) and NILM (17.7%), $P < 0.001$. Moreover, the probably and possibly carcinogenic HPVs (Group 2A and 2B) were found in 5.2, 22.6 and 26.7% of NILM, low grade SIL and high grade SIL, respectively.

As expected, the infection rates of both high and low risk viruses observed in our study are comparable to that obtained in other studies including Italian women participating in opportunistic screenings but higher than those observed among Italian women attending organized cervical cancer screening programs [17, 19].

Interestingly, we have identified 12 unclassified genotypes in 8.3% of NILM and in 14.6% of low grade SIL but in none of high grade SIL. The inverse correlation between infection frequency and disease severity suggests a limited role for such viruses in cervical carcinogenesis in the analyzed population. Among the unclassified HPVs the genotypes 81, 42, 62 and 91 were the most frequent being found in 2.7, 2.2, 2.2 and 1.8% of low grade SIL, respectively, while the genotype 89 was the most frequent (3.1%) among NILM cases. Despite the low rate of unclassified HPV genotypes in high grade SIL among the women included in the present study, it is important to report that unclassified HPV 54, 61, 62 and 81 represented 27.8% of all infections among HIV-positive Italian women diagnosed with high grade SIL, suggesting that compromised immune system could be not able to limit the "weak oncogenic" activity of some unclassified viruses [29]. Accordingly, Garbuglia et al. found that HPV62 and HPV81 were associated, as single infections, with 9.1 and 4.5% of high grade SIL, respectively, among HIV-positive women [30]. However, the frequency of unclassified HPV genotypes and their oncogenic risk remains underestimated because they are not included in the HPV assays commonly used to detect and characterize HPV genotypes in the majority of studies performed among HIV-negative and HIV-positive women [31, 32].

Cell transformation by HPVs mainly relies on the ability of the viral E6 protein to bind and degrade the p53 oncosuppressor. Mesplède et al. (2012) by performing a quantitative measurement of p53 degradation by the E6 of 29 different HPV genotypes showed that all Group 1 HPVs and several Groups 2A and 2B genotypes (HPV26, 30, 34, 53, 66, 68, 69, 70, 73, 82, 97) were able to suppress p53 by binding and degradation [12]. Studies evaluating the ability of E6 proteins encoded by unclassified HPVs to bind p53 are warranted in order to understand the oncogenic potential of such viruses.

According to our results, the dynamic of unclassified HPVs seems to be stable over the years. In fact, a previous study performed in 2006 in our Centre showed that HPV62 and 81 were the most common unclassified genotypes among SIL samples [16, 20].

In the present study, multiple infections were more frequent in low grade (6.6%) and high grade SIL (20%) than in NILM (2.1%). The majority of such infections (75%) contained at least one HPV genotype of Group 1, while in the remaining 25% various combinations of low risk and unknown risk HPV genotypes were detected. Previous studies showed that multiple HPV infections are not associated to the severity of cervical lesions since they were as common in ICC or HSIL as in LSIL or NILM [33]. However, the coinfections of HPV16 and HPV68 caused a significant increase in the risk of high grade SIL and invasive cervical cancer (OR = 16.5, $P$ = 0.0002) compared to that found for HPV16 (OR = 1.9, $P$ = 0.003) or HPV68 (OR = 3.5, $P$ = 0.38) as single infections, suggesting a synergistic effect between the two viruses [33].

Vaccination against high risk HPVs represents a primary prevention measure for anogenital cancers and squamous intraepithelial lesions caused by those HPV types. The recently licensed nonavalent HPV vaccine targets the seven high-risk HPV genotypes most frequently detected in invasive cervical cancer worldwide (HPV16, 18, 31, 33, 45, 52 and 58) and the low risk HPV genotypes 6 and 11 causing benign genital papillomas [34–36]. Considering the frequency of these nine HPVs among the analyzed women, the use of nonavalent vaccine would be able to prevent more than 50% of HPV infections. In particular, vaccination would prevent 40.3 and 53.3% of low grade SIL and high grade SIL, respectively.

An important limitation of this study was that the self-referred women to the gynecologic center were likely not representative of the general population. Indeed, the HPV prevalence in this cohort was much

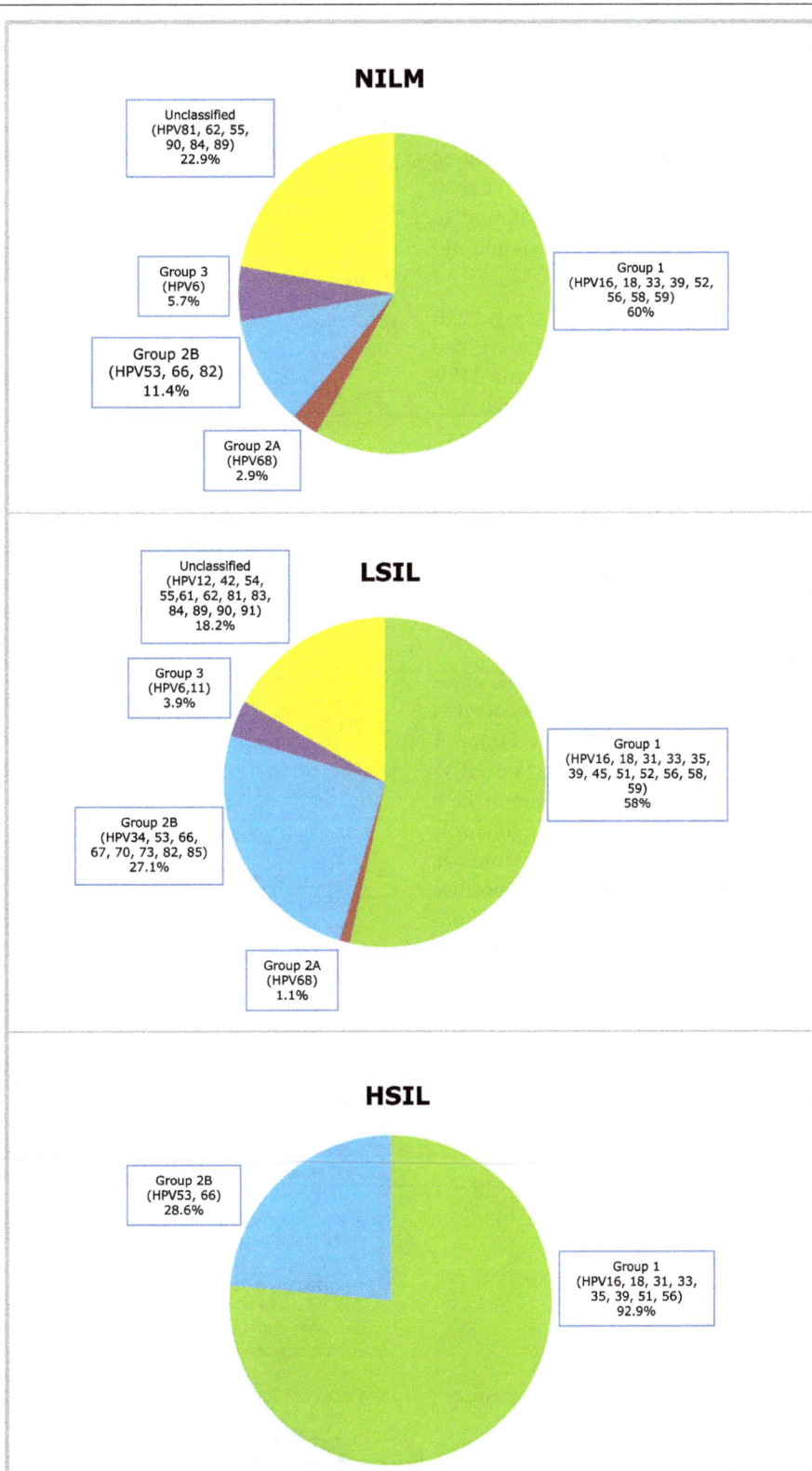

**Fig. 1** Distribution of Group 1, 2A, 2B, 3 and unclassified HPVs in NILM, low grade SIL (LSIL) and high grade SIL (HSIL). Representativeness of the genotypes contained in each Group is expressed as percentage of all HPV positive cases in each category

higher than in the Italian cervical cancer screening population. Moreover, the behavioral risk factors, such as the number of sexual partners and condom use, have not been considered, and the follow up of infected women has not been performed precluding the possibility to evaluate the persistence over the time of unclassified viruses. However, the use of broad spectrum consensus primers able to amplify all 62 mucosotropic HPV genotypes allowed to determine the global distribution of risk classified and unclassified HPVs in the study population.

The application of high-throughput sequencing technology and metagenomic analyses have recently enabled the discovery of many novel HPVs and that the HPV heterogeneity in healthy humans is very complex [37, 38]. It remains to be investigated whether the unclassified virus coinfections have a protecting role, by interfering with the activity of oncogenic viruses or by stimulating the immune cross-reaction, or have a synergistic effect with high risk HPVs facilitating cervical neoplasia development [38].

## Conclusions

Our results show that the majority of low and high grade SIL in women referred for colposcopy at gynecological outpatient clinic of our Center are caused by Group 1 HPVs. The relative high prevalence of unclassified HPVs in low grade SIL and NILM and their absence in high grade SIL suggests that these viruses have a marginal role in cervical neoplasia in the general population. However, the identification of unclassified HPVs in HIV positive women with high grade lesions observed in previous studies, suggests that uncommon and unclassified HPV genotypes need to be characterized in immune compromised patients to allow a correct clinical management.

## Abbreviations

HPV: Human papillomavirus; NILM: Negative for intraepithelial lesion or malignancy; PCR: Polymerase chain reaction; SIL: squamous intraepithelial lesion

## Acknowledgements
We are grateful to Immacolata Di Biase, Noemy Starita, Marianna Tortora for technical support.

## Funding
This project and the publication cost was supported by the research grant. Ricerca Corrente N. 2611892 from the Ministero della Salute.

## Authors' contributions
CA performed the experimental analysis and drafted the manuscript; GS and SG enrolled the patients and collected clinical samples; MPC, VS, SL and GB performed pathological evaluation; LB performed the statistical analysis; FMB obtained the grant and supervised the project; MLT designed the research project and wrote he manuscript. All authors reviewed the manuscript. All authors read and approved the final manuscript.

## Competing interests
The authors declare that they have no competing interests.

## Author details
[1]Molecular Biology and Viral Oncology Unit, Istituto Nazionale Tumori IRCCS "Fondazione G. Pascale", via M Semmola, 80131 Naples, Italy. [2]Gynecology Oncology Unit, Istituto Nazionale Tumori IRCCS "Fondazione G. Pascale", 80131 Naples, Italy. [3]Department of Pathology, Istituto Nazionale Tumori IRCCS "Fondazione G. Pascale", 80131 Naples, Italy.

## References
1.  Bravo IG, Felez-Sanchez M. Papillomaviruses: viral evolution, cancer and evolutionary medicine. Evol Med Public Health. 2015;2015:32–51.
2.  Bzhalava D, Guan P, Franceschi S, Dillner J, Clifford G. A systematic review of the prevalence of mucosal and cutaneous human papillomavirus types. Virology. 2013;445:224–31.
3.  Zur Hausen H, de Villiers EM. Reprint of: cancer "causation" by infections--individual contributions and synergistic networks. Semin Oncol. 2015;42:207–22.
4.  de Villiers EM, Fauquet C, Broker TR, Bernard HU, Zur Hausen H. Classification of papillomaviruses. Virology. 2004;324:17–27.
5.  Bernard HU, Burk RD, Chen Z, van DK, Zur Hausen H, de Villiers EM. Classification of papillomaviruses (PVs) based on 189 PV types and proposal of taxonomic amendments. Virology. 2010;401:70–9.
6.  Bzhalava D, Eklund C, Dillner J. International standardization and classification of human papillomavirus types. Virology. 2015;476:341–4.
7.  Guan P, Howell-Jones R, Li N, Bruni L, de Sanjosé S, Franceschi S, Clifford GM. Human papillomavirus types in 115,789 HPV-positive women: a meta-analysis from cervical infection to cancer. Int J Cancer. 2012;131:2349–59.
8.  Munoz N, Bosch FX, de Sanjose S, Herrero R, Castellsague X, Shah KV, Snijders PJ, Meijer CJ. Epidemiologic classification of human papillomavirus types associated with cervical cancer. N Engl J Med. 2003;348:518–27.
9.  IARC: IARC monographs on the evaluation of carcinogenic risks to humans. A Review of Human Carcinogens Part B: Biological Agents. Lyon, France; 2011.
10. Biological agents. Volume 100 B. A review of human carcinogens. IARC Monogr Eval Carcinog Risks Hum 2012, 100:1–441.
11. Schiffman M, Clifford G, Buonaguro FM. Classification of weakly carcinogenic human papillomavirus types: addressing the limits of epidemiology at the borderline. Infect Agent Cancer. 2009;4:8.
12. Mesplede T, Gagnon D, Bergeron-Labrecque F, Azar I, Senechal H, Coutlee F, Archambault J. p53 degradation activity, expression, and subcellular localization of E6 proteins from 29 human papillomavirus genotypes. J Virol. 2012;86:94–107.
13. Bruni L, Diaz M, Castellsague X, Ferrer E, Bosch FX, de Sanjosé S. Cervical human papillomavirus prevalence in 5 continents: Meta-analysis of 1 million women with normal cytological findings. J Infect Dis. 2010;
14. Baussano I, Franceschi S, Gillio-Tos A, Carozzi F, Confortini M, Dalla Palma P, De Lillo M, Del Mistro A, De Marco L, Naldoni C, Pierotti P, Schincaglia P, Segnan N, Zorzi M, Giorgi-Rossi P, Ronco G. Difference in overall and age-specific prevalence of high-risk human papillomavirus infection in Italy: evidence from NTCC trial. BMC Infect Dis. 2013;13:238.
15. Carozzi FM, Tornesello ML, Burroni E, Loquercio G, Carillo G, Angeloni C, Scalisi A, Macis R, Chini F, Buonaguro FM, Giorgi-Rossi P. Prevalence of human papillomavirus types in high-grade cervical intraepithelial neoplasia and Cancer in Italy. Cancer Epidemiol Biomark Prev. 2010;19:2389–400.
16. Tornesello ML, Duraturo ML, Botti G, Greggi S, Piccoli R, De Palo G, Montella M, Buonaguro L, Buonaguro FM. Prevalence of alpha-papillomavirus genotypes in cervical squamous intraepithelial lesions and invasive cervical carcinoma in the Italian population. J Med Virol. 2006;78:1663–72.
17. Giorgi Rossi P, Bisanzi S, Paganini I, Di Iasi A, Angeloni C, Scalisi A, Macis R, Pini MT, Chini F, Carozzi FM. Prevalence of HPV high and low risk types in

cervical samples from the Italian general population: a population based study. BMC Infect Dis. 2010;10:214.

18. Giorgi Rossi P, Sideri M, Carozzi FM, Vocaturo A, Buonaguro FM, Tornesello ML, Burroni E, Mariani L, Boveri S, Zaffina LM, Chini F. HPV type distribution in invasive cervical cancers in Italy: pooled analysis of three large studies. Infect Agent Cancer. 2012;7:26.

19. Galati L, Peronace C, Fiorillo MT, Masciari R, Giraldi C, Nistico S, Minchella P, Maiolo V, Barreca GS, Marascio N, Lamberti AG, Giancotti A, Lepore MG, Greco F, Mauro MV, Borelli A, Bocchiaro GL, Surace G, Liberto MC, Foca A. Six years genotype distribution of human papillomavirus in Calabria region, southern Italy: a retrospective study. Infect Agent Cancer. 2017;12:43.

20. Tornesello ML, Losito S, Benincasa G, Fulciniti F, Botti G, Greggi S, Buonaguro L, Buonaguro FM. Human papillomavirus (HPV) genotypes and HPV16 variants and risk of adenocarcinoma and squamous cell carcinoma of the cervix. Gynecol Oncol. 2011;121:32–42.

21. Del Prete R, Ronga L, Addati G, Magrone R, Di Carlo D, Miragliotta G. Prevalence, genotype distribution and temporal dynamics of human papillomavirus infection in a population in southern Italy. Infez Med. 2017; 25:247–57.

22. Tornesello ML, Cassese R, De Rosa N, Buonaguro L, Masucci A, Vallefuoco G, Palmieri S, Schiavone V, Piccoli R, Buonaguro FM. High prevalence of human papillomavirus infection in eastern European and west African women immigrants in South Italy. APMIS. 2011;119:701–9.

23. Resnick RM, Cornelissen MT, Wright DK, Eichinger GH, Fox HS, ter SJ, Manos MM. Detection and typing of human papillomavirus in archival cervical cancer specimens by DNA amplification with consensus primers. J Natl Cancer Inst. 1990;82:1477–84.

24. Soderlund-Strand A, Carlson J, Dillner J. Modified general primer PCR system for sensitive detection of multiple types of oncogenic human papillomavirus. J Clin Microbiol. 2009;47:541–6.

25. Tornesello ML, Loquercio G, Tagliamonte M, Rossano F, Buonaguro L, Buonaguro FM. Human papillomavirus infection in urine samples from male renal transplant patients. J Med Virol. 2010;82:1179–85.

26. Eklund C, Zhou T, Dillner J. Global proficiency study of human papillomavirus genotyping. J Clin Microbiol. 2010;48:4147–55.

27. de Roda Husman AM, Walboomers JM, Meijer CJ, Risse EK, Schipper ME, Helmerhorst TM, Bleker OP, Delius H, van den Brule AJ, Snijders PJ. Analysis of cytomorphologically abnormal cervical scrapes for the presence of 27 mucosotropic human papillomavirus genotypes, using polymerase chain reaction. Int J Cancer. 1994;56:802–6.

28. Giorgi Rossi P, Chini F, Bisanzi S, Burroni E, Carillo G, Lattanzi A, Angeloni C, Scalisi A, Macis R, Pini MT, Capparucci P, Guasticchi G, Carozzi FM, Prevalence Italian Working Group HPV. Distribution of high and low risk HPV types by cytological status: a population based study from Italy. Infect Agent Cancer. 2011;6:2.

29. Tornesello ML, Duraturo ML, Giorgi-Rossi P, Sansone M, Piccoli R, Buonaguro L, Buonaguro FM. Human papillomavirus (HPV) genotypes and HPV16 variants in human immunodeficiency virus-positive Italian women. J Gen Virol. 2008;89:1380–9.

30. Garbuglia AR, Piselli P, Lapa D, Sias C, Del Nonno F, Baiocchini A, Cimaglia C, Agresta A, Capobianchi MR. Frequency and multiplicity of human papillomavirus infection in HIV-1 positive women in Italy. J Clin Virol. 2012; 54:141–6.

31. Clifford GM, Goncalves MA, Franceschi S. Human papillomavirus types among women infected with HIV: a meta-analysis. AIDS. 2006;20:2337–44.

32. Clifford GM, Tully S, Franceschi S. Carcinogenicity of human papillomavirus (HPV) types in HIV-positive women: a Meta-analysis from HPV infection to cervical Cancer. Clin Infect Dis. 2017;64:1228–35.

33. Carrillo-García A, Ponce-de-León-Rosales S, Cantú-de-León D, Fragoso-Ontiveros V, Martínez-Ramírez I, Orozco-Colín A, Mohar A, Lizano M. Impact of human papillomavirus coinfections on the risk of high-grade squamous intraepithelial lesion and cervical cancer. Gynecol Oncol. 2014;134:534–9.

34. HPV vaccine works against nine viral types. Cancer Discov 2014, 4:OF2–8290.

35. de Sanjose S, Quint WG, Alemany L, Geraets DT, Klaustermeier JE, Lloveras B, Tous S, Felix A, Bravo LE, Shin HR, Vallejos CS, De Ruiz PA, Lima MA, Guimera N, Clavero O, Alejo M, Llombart-Bosch A, Cheng-Yang C, Tatti SA, Kasamatsu E, Iljazovic E, Odida M, Prado R, Seoud M, Grce M, Usubutun A, Jain A, Suarez GA, Lombardi LE, Banjo A, Menendez C, Domingo EJ, Velasco J, Nessa A, Chichareon SC, Qiao YL, Lerma E, Garland SM, Sasagawa T,

Ferrera A, Hammouda D, Mariani L, Pelayo A, Steiner I, Oliva E, Meijer CJ, Al-Jassar WF, Cruz E, Wright TC, Puras A, Llave CL, Tzardi M, Agorastos T, Garcia-Barriola V, Clavel C, Ordi J, Andujar M, Castellsague X, Sanchez GI, Nowakowski AM, Bornstein J, Munoz N, Bosch FX. Human papillomavirus genotype attribution in invasive cervical cancer: a retrospective cross-sectional worldwide study. Lancet Oncol. 2010;11:1048–56.

36. Li N, Franceschi S, Howell-Jones R, Snijders PJ, Clifford GM. Human papillomavirus type distribution in 30,848 invasive cervical cancers worldwide: variation by geographical region, histological type and year of publication. Int J Cancer. 2011;128:927–35.

37. Liu Z, Yang S, Wang Y, Shen Q, Yang Y, Deng X, Zhang W, Delwart E. Identification of a novel human papillomavirus by metagenomic analysis of vaginal swab samples from pregnant women. Virol J. 2016;13:122.

38. Ma Y, Madupu R, Karaoz U, Nossa CW, Yang L, Yooseph S, Yachimski PS, Brodie EL, Nelson KE, Pei Z. Human papillomavirus community in healthy persons, defined by metagenomics analysis of human microbiome project shotgun sequencing data sets. J Virol. 2014;88:4786–97.

# 24

# Immunogenicity of a Fap2 peptide mimotope of *Fusobacterium nucleatum* and its potential use in the diagnosis of colorectal cancer

Leonardo A. Guevarra Jr[1,2]*, Andrea Claudine F. Afable[1], Patricia Joyce O. Belza[1], Karen Joy S. Dy[1], Scott Justin Q. Lee[1], Teresa T. Sy-Ortin[3] and Pia Marie S. P. Albano[2,4]

## Abstract

**Background:** The role of *Fusobacterium nucleatum* Fap2 protein in the development of colorectal cancer has recently been explained. Fap2, when bound to the human inhibitory receptor, TIGIT, inhibits the cytotoxic activity of natural killer (NK) cells against cancer cells, thus, allowing proliferation of the latter eventually leading to tumor growth. The aim of the study was to identify the immunogenicity of a peptide mimotope of the Fap2 protein and to determine the reactivity of colorectal cancer patients' sera against the mimotope.

**Methods:** Immunogenic epitope of the Fap2 protein of *F. nucleatum* was selected using the B-cell epitope prediction of the Immune Epitope Database and Analysis Resource (IEDB). The immunogenicity of the synthetic peptide mimotope of the Fap2 protein was determined in animal models and reactivity of colorectal cancer patients' sera against the mimotope was done by indirect ELISA.

**Results:** Results show that the selected peptide mimotope, with sequence TELAYKHYFGT, of the outer membrane protein Fap2 of *F. nucleatum* is immunogenic. Increase in the absorbance readings of peptide-immunized rabbit sera was observed starting Week 1 which was sustained up to Week 10 in the indirect ELISA performed. Colorectal cancer cases ($n = 37$) were all reactive in an ELISA-based analysis using the mimotope as the capture antigen.

**Conclusions:** In this study, we identified an immunogenic epitope of the Fap2 protein of the *Fusobacterium nucleatum*. We demonstrated the reactivity of serum of histopathologically confirmed CRC patients in a peptide-capture indirect ELISA which may serve as proof of concept for the development of CRC diagnostics.

**Keywords:** Fap2 protein, *Fusobacterium nucleatum*, ELISA, Colorectal cancer, Immunodiagnostics

## Background

The composition of the gut microbiome has recently been implicated in the development of colorectal cancer (CRC) [1]. Dysbiosis, a condition characterized by a pathological imbalance in the microbial community, is shown to contribute in the growth and progression of colorectal tumors [2]. Several studies reported the high association of microorganisms belonging to the proteobacteria, such as *Pseudomonas*, *Helicobacter*, and *Acinetobacter*, with colon cancer [3]. The most current is that of *Fusobacterium nucleatum*, whose role in CRC progression has recently been described [4].

*F. nucleatum* is a non-spore forming, non-motile, gram-negative, spindle-shaped opportunistic anaerobic bacteria that can be found in the oral cavity and the gastrointestinal tract [5]. Its cell envelope is composed of outer and inner membranes flanking a periplasmic space and outer membrane proteins which comprise a third of its mass [6]. Originally identified as an oral commensal and a periodontal pathogen, *F. nucleatum* has recently been associated with several human illnesses

---

* Correspondence: laguevarra@ust.edu.ph
[1]Department of Biochemistry, Faculty of Pharmacy, University of Santo Tomas, Manila, Philippines
[2]Research Center for Natural and Applied Sciences, University of Santo Tomas, Manila, Philippines
Full list of author information is available at the end of the article

which include adverse pregnancy outcomes, cardiovascular disease, rheumatoid arthritis, respiratory tract infections, Lemierre's syndrome, Alzheimer's disease, and gastrointestinal disorders including CRC [7]. The association of *F. nucleatum* with CRC development is attributed to the ability of patients' infected cancer cells to inhibit the ability of the immune system to attack tumoral cells [7, 8].

Fap2 protein is a 390-kilodalton protein encoded by the *Fap2* gene of *F. nucleatum* [9]. It is an outer membrane protein composed of 3692 amino acid which is identified to induce apoptosis in human lymphocytes [9, 10]. Recently, Fap2 protein has been shown to be involved in the binding of *F. nucleatum* to cancer cells and to interact with the immunoglobulin and ITIM domain (TIGIT) receptor mainly expressed on NK, Treg, CD8+ and CD4+ T cells [11]. The binding of Fap2 to TIGIT was found to inhibit the activity of natural killer (NK) cells against the tumor cells, thus causing the growth and progression of CRC [12].

Given this role of the *F. nucleatum* Fap2 protein in CRC tumorigenesis and the lack of a reported Fap2 immunogenic epitope in the Immune Epitope Database (IEDB) Resource Analysis (www.iedb.org), this study, therefore, sought to search for an immunogenic epitope of the *F. nucleatum* Fap2 protein to test the immunogenicity of a peptide mimotope in vivo and to measure the reactivity of plasma samples from confirmed CRC patients and clinically healthy controls to the mimotope.

## Methods

### Immune epitope prediction and peptide mimotope synthesis

Prediction of the immune epitope of *Fusobacterium nucleatum* Fap2 protein was done in silico using the Immune Epitope Database (IEDB) Analysis Resource. The primary sequence of the Fap2 protein was taken from the National Center for Biotechnology Information (NCBI) Protein Database. The amino acid sequence of the epitope was selected using B-cell epitope prediction platform of the IEDB. Candidate immunogenic epitope was selected based on its antigenicity, surface accessibility, and hydrophilicity using Kolaskar & Tongaonkar Antigenicity Scale and Emini Surface Accessibility Scale. The predicted immunogenic mimotope was synthesized by Genscript (New York, USA).

### Immunization

Immunogen was prepared by conjugating the peptide mimotope to bovine serum albumin (BSA) following the methods of Coligan et al. [13]. Peptide conjugation in BSA (10:1) was done in the presence of glutaraldehyde in borate buffer (pH 10) [13]. The BSA-conjugated peptide solution was reconstituted with PBS to produce a 1 mg/mL stock solution, which was then dialyzed against 4 l of water for 24 h.

Immunogenicity of the peptides was tested in 10- to 12-week-old white male New Zealand rabbits. Animal care and immunization were done following the protocols described by Bio-Synthesis (http://www.biosyn.com/) and as approved by the Institutional Animal Care and Utilization Committee (IACUC) of the University of Santo Tomas, Philippines. Six rabbits were randomly assigned to negative control ($n = 2$) and experimental ($n = 4$) groups. Each rabbit from the experimental group was immunized with 1.0 mL solution containing 100 µg of peptide distributed to five subcutaneous sites and two intramuscular sites. The immunogen was prepared by reconstituting the previously prepared peptide-BSA stock solution with PBS emulsified with Complete Freund's Adjuvant (Sigma). Four booster doses of the same amount of peptide emulsified with Incomplete Freund's Adjuvant (Sigma) were given at two weeks interval. Rabbits in the negative controls were given the same treatment except that the solutions used in the immunization did not contain the peptide mimotope.

### Immunogenicity assay

Immunogenicity of the synthetic peptide mimotope of the Fap2 predicted epitope was analyzed by detecting presence of anti-peptide mimotope antibody in the sera of rabbits. Blood was collected through the marginal ear vein before immunization to serve as baseline, and after immunization at weekly intervals for 10 weeks for the immunogenicity assay. Serum was separated from the cells by centrifugation of the collected blood at 3400 × g. Collected serum was transferred to Eppendorf tubes and stored at – 20 °C until use.

Presence of anti-peptide mimotope antibody was detected by indirect ELISA. Wells were coated with 50 µL of coating buffer (0.05 M carbonate buffer, pH 9.6) containing 10 µg of peptides and blocked with 100 µL of blocking solution (2% gelatin in 0.01 M PBS containing 0.05% Tween 20). Fifty microliters of 1:100 diluted rabbit sera were then added to each well after washing with wash buffer (0.01 M PBS containing 0.05% Tween 20) and incubated for 1 h at 37 °C. The wells were washed again to remove the unbound rabbit antibodies. HRP-conjugated goat anti-rabbit antibody (Genscript, New York) was used to detect presence of anti-peptide mimotope rabbit antibody using TMB as substrate.

### Reactivity assay

Reactivity of sera collected from confirmed CRC cases ($n = 37$) and clinically healthy case-matched controls was also determined by indirect ELISA as previously mentioned. Patients' sera were also diluted 1:100 and the anti-peptide mimotope human antibody was detected using HRP-conjugated anti-human antibody (Koma Biotech, Seoul, Korea). Protocols on the use of left-over plasma samples were approved by the Ethics Review Board of the University of Santo Tomas Hospital.

## Statistical treatment and analysis

Comparison of the mean absorbance readings from the indirect ELISA of negative control and experimental groups from baseline up to 10 weeks after the initial immunization was done by multivariate analysis using IBM SPSS Statistics version 20. $P$-values less than 0.05 were considered statistically significant.

The ELISA cut-off values were computed based on the formula described by Frey et al. [14]. Values higher than the computed cut-off were assessed as reactive while those that were lower were evaluated as non-reactive.

## Results

In this study, selection of a candidate immune epitope was done using in silico analysis tools embedded in the Immune Epitope Database and Analysis Resource (IEDB). The sequence of the predicted immunogenic epitope was TELAYKHYFGT which is located at the 3596th to 3606th position of the Fap2 protein. Antigenicity and surface accessibility scores were 1.028 and 1.198, respectively, which were above the cut-off values 0.998 and 1.000, respectively. The synthetic peptide mimotope of the selected immunogenic epitope was also reported to be soluble in ultrapure water, 0.1 M PBS pH 7.1, and DMSO, at a gross peptide concentration of less than 15 mg/mL.

Immunogenicity of the synthetic peptide mimotope was evaluated by monitoring the weekly anti-peptide antibody titer in the animal models immunized with the peptide. Figure 1 presents the weekly mean absorbance readings of the negative control and peptide immunized groups.

The mean absorbance of the baseline blood samples of the peptide immunized and negative control groups were 0. 052 and 0.055, respectively. These readings were below the computed cut-off value of 0.072. An increase in the absorbance was observed in the peptide-immunized group but not in the negative control group starting a week after the

first immunization. A constant increase in anti-Fap2 titer was observed from Week 1 to Week 10 of immunization of the experimental rabbits. Independent $t$-test showed no significant difference in the absorbance readings of baseline blood samples collected from the normal control and peptide immunization group ($p$-value = 0.387). However, multivariate analysis revealed statistically significant increase in the absorbance readings starting Week 1 after immunization as compared to the negative control ($p$-values< 0.02).

After confirming the immunogenicity of the synthetic peptide, we tested for the reactivity of plasma samples from histologically confirmed colorectal cancer cases and their age- and sex- matched clinically healthy controls to the peptide by indirect ELISA. Figure 2 presents the $OD_{540}$ readings of CRC positive sera and their case-matched controls in contrast to the cut-off value of 0.05284.

All cases ($n$ = 37; 100%) showed reactivity to the Fap2 peptide mimotope. Twelve of the controls (32%) also tested positive for IgG against the peptide (Table 1). These results gave a sensitivity of 100% and a specificity of 68%. The positive predictive value and the negative predictive value are 76% and 100%, respectively.

## Discussion

In silico analysis tools provide a valuable platform in predicting and selecting candidate peptide sequences that can be used for immunodiagnostics and immunotherapeutics [15]. They have improved and greatly accelerated epitope design, which is a crucial step in vaccine as well as in diagnostic development [16]. When existing databases provide limited information on desired immunogenic epitopes, such as the case of the Fap2 protein of *F. nucleatum*, several immune epitope prediction tools, which are based on the physico-chemical properties of a portion of a polypeptide chain, can be used [17]. These physico-chemical properties include antigenicity,

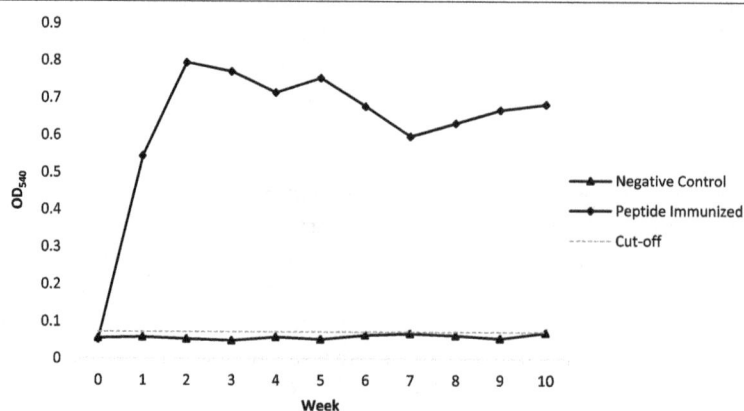

**Fig. 1** Immunogenicity of a Fap2 Peptide Mimotope. Indirect ELISA absorbance readings of peptide immunized group as compared to the negative control and computed cut-off value

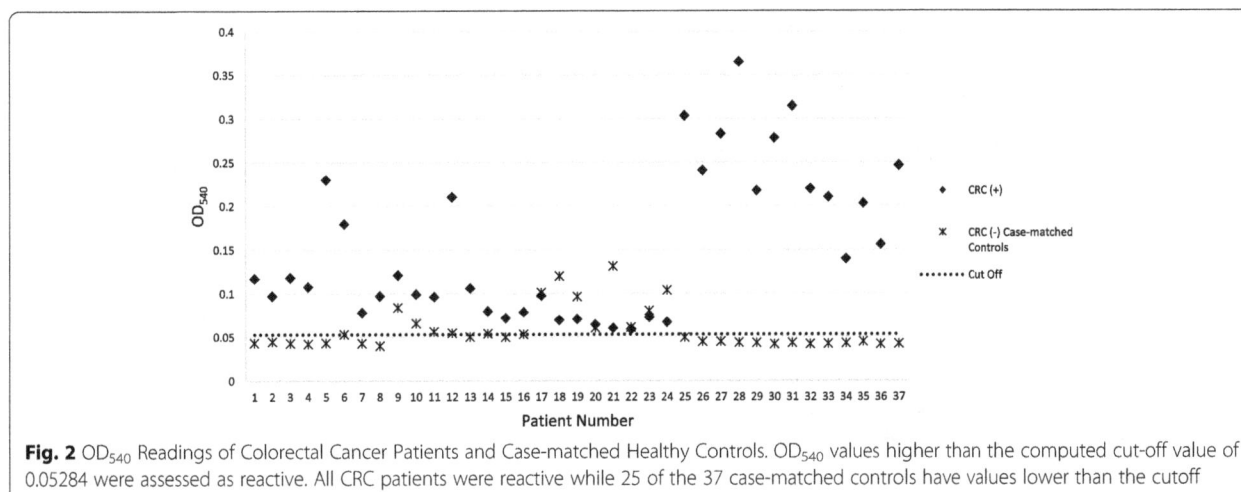

**Fig. 2** $OD_{540}$ Readings of Colorectal Cancer Patients and Case-matched Healthy Controls. $OD_{540}$ values higher than the computed cut-off value of 0.05284 were assessed as reactive. All CRC patients were reactive while 25 of the 37 case-matched controls have values lower than the cutoff

surface accessibility, and hydrophilicity based on the frequency of existing amino acids in the primary sequence of a target antigen [17–19].

In this study, we have shown in vivo the immunogenicity of the in silico-predicted immunogenic epitope of Fap2 antigen. The statistically significant increase in the absorbance readings in the ELISA of the mimotope-immunized rabbits, a pattern which was not observed in negative control group, is indicative of the production of an anti-peptide IgG.

Peptides have the ability to induce an immune response and prompt the cell to produce antibodies [20]. Synthetic peptides can excellently mimic proteins because they are exact copies of protein fragments which are responsible for the protein's activity [21]. Synthetic peptide immunogens can induce an immune response by mimicking the activity of the subunit of the whole protein antigen and be used as a promising tool in vaccine and immunodiagnostic tool development [22]. Because of the simplicity, ease of use, and target specificity of utilizing peptide mimotopes, this procedure is preferred over other existing methods [22, 23]. Although one major challenge in using peptides as immunogen is its weak immunogenic property, this can be solved by conjugating it with carrier proteins such as BSA and keyhole limpet hemocyanin [24].

Synthetic peptides mimicking immunogenic epitopes of protein antigens can initiate and activate the immune response by binding to either the Class I or Class II major histocompatibility complex (MHC) [25]. In 2005, Wang et al. demonstrated the ability of peptide mimotopes prepared from MHC Class I library of baculovirus to bind to T-cell and secret interleukin-2 [26]. In the same year, Gevorkian et al. were able to elicit polyclonal antibodies against a cell surface antigen of *Mycobacterium tuberculosis* in rabbits using a 15-mer chemically synthesized peptide [27]. Buchwald et al (2005), in their search for a potential vaccine against pneumococcus, observed that a 12-mer peptide elicited production of antibodies in mice models which were then seroprotected during the infection challenge [28]. The anti-tumor activity of peptide mimotopes through the production of anti-HBJ127, a tumor suppressing anti-CD98 heavy chain antibody, was observed by Saito et al. [29].

Synthetic peptides are also used in ELISA in the diagnosis of diseases [30]. Antibodies present in serum of immunized or previously infected individuals reacts to the peptides in immunoassays [31–33]. This was also observed in our experiments when we used the peptide as the capture antigen in the ELISA performed to detect presence of anti-peptide antibody in the sera of peptide-immunized rabbits as well as patients with colorectal carcinoma – a disease associated with the presence of harmful microbiota, such as *F. nucleatum*, in the gut.

The human gut is home to a complex system of microorganisms which play a vital role in the host's health homeostasis [2]. Recent studies suggest the role of the gut microbiota in the development in colorectal cancer due to their ability to interfere in the host's inflammatory and immunomodulatory activities, which subsequently favor carcinogenesis and tumorigenesis [33–36]. Among the recently studied and implicated in colorectal carcinoma

**Table 1** Seroreactivity to *Fusobacterium nucleatum* Fap2 Peptide Mimotope of Colorectal Cancer Cases and Clinically Healthy Controls

| Seroreactivity to Fap2 Peptide Mimotope | CRC Cases | | Healthy Controls | | Total | |
|---|---|---|---|---|---|---|
| | n | % | n | % | n | % |
| Reactive | 37 | 100% | 12 | 32 | 49 | 66% |
| Non-reactive | 0 | 0 | 25 | 68 | 25 | 34% |
| Total | 37 | 100% | 37 | 100% | 74 | 100% |

development is *F. nucleatum* [37, 38]. This bacterium has also been associated with chemoresistance of cancer cells during treatment [38]. Hence, there is the need to develop methods for their detection as well as determine the anti-*F. nucleatum* titer that is associated with CRC.

*F. nucleatum*'s outer membrane protein Fap2 is identified to adhere to host's cell surface and induce pro-inflammatory and pro-carcinogenic response [39]. Its association to the development of colorectal cancer and its role in immune evasion was first reported by Kaplan et al. [40] when they observed that *F. nucleatum* proteins induce lymphocyte apoptosis. This was further supported by Mima et al. [8] when they observed that the number of *F. nucleatum* cells in CRC cases was observed to be inversely associated with the density of CD3$^+$ T-cells. Recently, proposed roles and molecular mechanisms of *F. nucleatum* outer membrane proteins in immune evasion have been reported. The ability of *F. nucleatum* to bind colorectal adenocarcinoma cells was reported previously [41]. It was also observed that the binding of Fap2 to human inhibitory receptor TIGIT protects the cancer cells from the immunosurveillance activity of NK cells, which, in effect, would allow the cancer cells to grow and proliferate [11]. These studies serve as impetus in understanding the role and mechanism of Fap2 protein in the colorectal carcinogenesis.

The ability to identify the immunogenic epitopes of the Fap2 of *F. nucleatum* is relevant in developing immunodiagnostic and therapeutic methods for CRC. The immunogenicity of and the reactivity of the CRC patients' plasma samples to the peptide mimotope can serve as starting point in developing methods in the screening and detection CRC.

## Conclusions

We have identified an immunogenic epitope of the Fap2 protein of *F. nucleatum*. The peptide TELAYKHYFGT located at the 3596th to 3606th amino acid of the outer membrane protein Fap2 of the CRC-associated pathogen *F. nucleatum* proved to be immunogenic in animal models. Seroreactivity of CRC patients against the peptide mimotope in an indirect ELISA was also observed.

Identifying immunogenic epitopes of CRC-associated pathogens such as *F. nucleatum* may serve as impetus in the development of vaccine and immunodiagnostic tools against colorectal cancer. Future studies may use results from this study to pursue a pathogen-targeted control of cancer similar to the human papilloma virus (HPV) or as a biomarker for detection and determination of risks of cancer development similar to Eppstein Barr virus.

## Abbreviations

BSA: bovine serum albumin; CRC: Colorectal cancer; ELISA: Enzyme-linked immunosorbent assay; HRP: horseradish peroxidase; IACUC: Institutional Animal Care and Utilization Committee; IEDB: Immune epitope database; IgG: Immunoglobulin G; NCBI: National Center for Biotechnology Information; NK: Natural killer; PBS: phosphate buffered saline; TIGIT: T cell immunoglobulin and ITIM domain (TIGIT); TMB: 3,3',5,5'-Tetramethylbenzidine

## Acknowledgments

The authors would like to acknowledge the support of the Department of Biochemistry, Faculty of Pharmacy, University of Santo Tomas and the Research Center for Natural and Applied Sciences for allowing them to use their facilities.

## Funding

This research was done as an independent individual initiative of the authors. No funding was received from any research grant institution from the Philippines or abroad except for the in-house financial assistance provided by the Research Center for Natural and Applied Sciences (RCNAS) of the University of Santo Tomas to RCNAS-affiliated researchers.

## Authors' contributions

The following are the contributions of the individual authors: LAG. Corresponding author, primarily responsible for the preparation of the manuscript, design of the protocols used in the experiment and analysis of results. ACFA. Data collection and preliminary analysis of results. Primarily responsible in peptide selection. PJOB. Data collection and preliminary analysis of results, primarily responsible for animal care and utilization. Also involved in troubleshooting during optimization of ELISA protocols. KJSD. Data collection and preliminary analysis of results, primarily responsible in writing the preliminary manuscript. SJQL. Data collection and preliminary analysis of results, primarily responsible in performance of ELISA and troubleshooting during optimization.TTS. Data collection and review of the manuscript. PMSPA. PhD.Conceptualization, troubleshooting of the immuno-based assay, and internal review of the paper. All authors read and approved the final manuscript.

## Author's information

Mr. Leonardo A. Guevarra Jr., the principal investigator of this project and the corresponding author for this study, is a faculty member at the Department of Biochemistry, Faculty of Pharmacy and Research Faculty at the Research Center for Natural and Applied Sciences, University of Santo Tomas. He first got his interest in infectious disease, cancer, and diagnostics development when he was doing his research for the Master of Science in Biochemistry at the Department of Biochemistry and Molecular Biology, College of Medicine, University of the Philippines - Manila. His current organizational involvement includes the Philippine Society of Biochemistry and Molecular Biology (lifetime member), UK Biochemical Society, and the Japanese Peptide Society where he recently presented (poster presentation) the results in the paper being submitted for publication. Mr. Guevarra is establishing his research career in immune epitope prediction and its application in infectious disease and cancer diagnostics.

## Competing interests

The authors declare that they have no competing interests.

## Author details

[1]Department of Biochemistry, Faculty of Pharmacy, University of Santo Tomas, Manila, Philippines. [2]Research Center for Natural and Applied Sciences, University of Santo Tomas, Manila, Philippines. [3]Benavidez Cancer Institute, University of Santo Tomas Hospital, Manila, Philippines. [4]Department of Biological Sciences, College of Science, University of Santo Tomas, Manila, Philippines.

## References

1.  Lucas C, Barnich N, Nguyen HTT. Microbiota, inflammation and colorectal cancer. Int J Mol Sci. 2017;18(6). https://doi.org/10.3390/ijms18061310.
2.  Dulal SK, Keku TO. Gut microbiome and colorectal adenomas. Cancer J. 2015;20(3):225–31.
3.  Sanapareddy N, Legge RM, Jovov B, McCoy A, Burcal L, Araujo-Perez F, Keku TO. Increased rectal microbial richness is associated with the presence of colorectal adenomas in humans. ISME J. 2012;6(10):1858–68.
4.  Gholizadeh P, Eslami H, Kafil HS. Carcinogenesis mechanisms of *Fusobacterium nucleatum*. Biomed Pharmacother. 2017;89:918–25.
5.  Bakken V, Høgh BT, Jensen HB. Growth conditions and outer membrane proteins of *Fusobacterium nucleatum*. Scand J Dent Res. 1990;98:215–24.
6.  Bolstad AI, Jensen HB, Bakken V. Taxonomy, biology, and periodontal aspects of *Fusobacterium nucleatum*. Clin Microbiol Rev. 1996;9(1):55–71.
7.  Han YW. *Fusobacterium nucleatum*: a commensal-turned pathogen. Curr Opin Microbiol. 2015;23:141–7.
8.  Mima K, Sukawa Y, Nishihara R, Qian ZR, Yamauchi M, Inamura K, Ogino S. *Fusobacterium nucleatum* and T cells in colorectal carcinoma. JAMA Oncol. 2015;1(5):653.
9.  Coppenhagen-Glazer S, Sol A, Abed J, Naor R, Zhang X, Han YW, Bachrach G. Fap2 of fusobacterium nucleatum is a galactose-inhibitable adhesin involved in coaggregation, cell adhesion, and preterm birth. Infect Immun. 2015;83:1104–13. [PubMed: 25561710]
10. Nosho K, Sukawa Y, Adachi Y, Ito M, Mitsuhashi K, Kurihara H, et al. Association of *Fusobacterium nucleatum* with immunity and molecular alterations in colorectal cancer. World J Gastroenterol. 2016;22(2):557–66.
11. Kaplan CW, Ma X, Paranjpe A, Jewett A, Lux R, Kinder-Haake S, Shi W. *Fusobacterium nucleatum* outer membrane proteins Fap2 and RadD induce cell death in human lymphocytes. Infect Immun. 2010;78(11):4773–8.
12. Gur C, Ibrahim Y, Isaacson B, Yamin R, Abed J, Gamliel M, et al. Binding of the Fap2 protein of *Fusobacterium nucleatum* to human inhibitory receptor TIGIT protects tumors from immune cell attack. Immunity. 2015;42(2):344–55.
13. Coligan JE. Current Protocols in Immunology. New York: Wiley; 2001.
14. Frey A, Di Canzio J, Zurakowski D. A statistically defined endpoint titer determination method for immunoassays. J Immunol Methods. 1998;221(1–2):35–41.
15. Fleri W, Paul S, Dhanda SK, Mahajan S, Xu X, Peters B, Sette A. The immune epitope database and analysis resource in epitope discovery and synthetic vaccine design. Front Immunol. 2017;8(MAR):1–16. https://doi.org/10.3389/fimmu.2017.00278.
16. Flower DR. Designing immunogenic peptides. Nat Chem Biol. 2013;9(12):749–53.
17. Emini EA, Hughes JV, Perlow DS, Boger J. Induction of hepatitis a virus-neutralizing antibody by a virus-specific synthetic peptide. J Virol. 1985;55(3):836–9.
18. Kolaskar AS, Tongaonkar PC. A semi-empirical method for prediction of antigenic detetermininants on protein antigens. Febbs Lett. 1990;276(1,2):172–4.
19. Parker JMR, Guo D, Hodges RS. New hydrophilicity scale derived from high-performance liquid chromatography peptide retention data: correlation of predicted surface residues with antigenicity and X-ray-derived accessible sites. Biochemist. 1986;25(19):5425–32.
20. Wallach J. Peptide antigen: a practical approach. In: Wisdom GB, editor. Biochemistry and molecular biology education. Oxford: Oxford University Press; 1996. p. 244–52.
21. Groß A, Hashimoto C, Sticht H, Eichler J. Synthetic peptides as protein mimics. Front Bioeng Biotechnol. 2016;3:211. https://doi.org/10.3389/fbioe.2015.00211.
22. Meloen RH, Puyk WC, Meijer DJA, Lankhof H, Posthumus WPA, Antigenicity SWMM. Immunogenicity of synthetic peptides of foot and mouth disease. J Gen Virol. 1987;68:305–14.
23. Van Regenmortel MHV. Antigenicity and immunogenicity of synthetic peptides. Biologicals. 2001;29(3–4):209–13.
24. Azmi F, Fuaad AAHA, Skwarczynski M, Toth I. Recent progress in adjuvant discovery for peptide-based subunit vaccines. Hum Vaccin Immunother. 2014;10(3):778–96.
25. Blum J, Wearsch P, Cresswell P. Pathways of antigen processing. Annu Rev Immunol. 2013;31(1):443–73.
26. Wang Y, Rubtsov A, Heiser R, White J, et al. Using a baculovirus display library to identify MHC class I mimotopes. PNAS. 2005;102(7):2476–81.
27. Gevorkian G, Segura E, Acero G, Palma JP, et al. Peptide mimotopes of mycobacterium tuberculosis carbohydrate immunodeterminants. Biochem J. 2005;387(2):411–7.
28. Buchwald UK, Lees A, Steinitz M, Pirofski L. A peptide mimotope of type 8 pneumococcal capsular polysaccharide induces a protective immune response in mice. Infect Immun. 2005;73(1):325–33.
29. Saito M, Kondo M, Ohshima M, Deguchi K, et al. Identification of anti-CD98 antibody mimotopes for inducing antibodies with antitumor activity by mimotope immunization. Cancer Sci. 2014;105(4):396–401.
30. Ma F, Zhang L, Wang Y, Lu R, et al. Development of a peptide ELISA for the diagnosis of aleutian mink disease. PLoS ONE. 2016;11(11):e0165793. https://doi.org/10.1371/journal.pone.0165793.
31. Sharma A, Saha A, Bhattacharjee S, Majumdar S, Das Gupta SK. Specific and randomly derived immunoactive peptide mimotopes of mycobacterial antigens. Clin Vaccine Immunol. 2006;13(10):143–1154.
32. Chen J, Domingue JC, and Sears CL. Microbiota dysbiosis in select human cancers: evidence of association and causality. Semin Immunol. 2017; (July), 0–1. https://doi.org/10.1016/jsmim201708.001.
33. Kang M, Martin A. Microbiome and colorectal cancer: Unraveling host-microbiota interactions in colitis-associated colorectal cancer development. Semin Immunol. 2017;(February):0–1. https://doi.org/10.1016/jsmim201704.003.
34. Fardini Y, Wang X, Temoin S, Nithianantham S, Lee D, Shoham M, Han WY. *Fusobacterium nucleatum* adhesin FadA binds vascular- endothelial cadherin and alters endothelial integrity. Mol Microbiol. 2012;82(6):1468–80.
35. Van Raay T, Allen-Vercoe E. Microbial Interactions and Interventions in Colorectal Cancer. Microbiol Spect. 2017;5:3. https://doi.org/10.1128/microbiolspec.BAD-0004-2016. Review
36. Yoon H, Kim N, Park JH, Kim YS, Lee J, Kim HW, et al. Comparisons of gut microbiota among healthy control, patients with conventional adenoma, sessile serrated adenoma, and colorectal Cancer. J Cancer Prev. 2017;22(2):108–14.
37. Zeller G, Tap J, Voigt AY, Sunagawa S, Kultima JR, Costea PI, et al. Potential of fecal microbiota for early-stage detection of colorectal cancer. Mol Syst Biol. 2014;10(11):766.
38. Yu T, Guo F, Yu Y, Sun T, Ma D, Han J, et al. *Fusobacterium nucleatum* promotes chemoresistance to colorectal cancer by modulating autophagy. Cell. 2017;170(3):548–63.e16
39. Rubinstein MR, Wang X, Liu W, Hao Y, Cai G, Wan Y. *Fusobacterium nucleatum* promotes colorectal carcinogenesis by modulating E-cadgerin/β-catein signalling via its FadA adhesin. Cell Host Microbe. 2013;14(2):195–206.
40. Kaplan CW, Lux R, Huynh T, Jewett A, Shi W, Haake SK. *Fusobacterium nucleatum* apoptosis-inducing outer membrane protein. J Dent Res. 2005;84(8):700–4.
41. Abed J, Emgård JEM, Zamir G, Faroja M, Grenov A, Sol A, et al. Fap2 mediates *Fusobacterium nucleatum* colorectal adenocarcinoma enrichment by binding to tumor-expressed gal-GalNAc. Cell Host Microbe. 2017;20(2):215–25.

# Permissions

# List of Contributors

**Melissa A. Yow and Melissa C.Southey**
Genetic Epidemiology Laboratory, Department of Pathology, Faculty of Medicine, Dentistry and Health Sciences, University of Melbourne, VIC, Australia 3010

**Sepehr N. Tabrizi**
Department of Microbiology and Infectious Diseases, Royal Women's Hospital, Parkville, VIC, Australia 3052
Department of Obstetrics and Gynaecology, University of Melbourne, Parkville, VIC, Australia 3010
Murdoch Childrens Research Institute, Parkville, VIC, Australia 3052

**Graham G. Giles**
Cancer Epidemiology and Intelligence Division, Cancer Epidemiology Centre, Cancer Council Victoria, Level 2, 615 St Kilda Road, Melbourne, VIC, Australia 3004
Centre for Epidemiology and Biostatistics, Melbourne School of Population and Global Health, University of Melbourne, Level 3, 207 Bouverie Street, Carlton, VIC, Australia 3053

**Damien M. Bolton**
Department of Surgery, University of Melbourne, Austin Health, 145 Studley Road, Heidelberg, VIC, Australia 3084

**John Pedersen**
TissuPath, 92-96 Ricketts Road, Mount Waverley, VIC, Australia 3149

**Gianluca Severi**
Human Genetics Foundation (HuGeF), Via Nizza, 52-10126 Torino, Italy

**Australian Prostate Cancer Bio Resource**
Australian Prostate Cancer BioResource, the Prostate Cancer Research Program, Department of Anatomy and Developmental Biology, Monash University, Melbourne, VIC, Australia 3800

**Francesca Pezzuto, Luigi Buonaguro, Franco M. Buonaguro and Maria Lina Tornesello**
Molecular Biology and Viral Oncology Unit, Istituto Nazionale Tumori IRCCS "Fondazione G Pascale", 80131 Napoli, Italy

**Serena Delbue**
Department of Biomedical, Surgical and Dental Sciences, University of Milano, Via Pascal, 36-20133 Milan, Italy

**Pasquale Ferrante**
Department of Biomedical, Surgical and Dental Sciences, University of Milano, Via Pascal, 36-20133 Milan, Italy
Istituto Clinico Città Studi, Milan, Italy

**Manola Comar**
Department of Medical Sciences, University of Trieste, Trieste, Italy
Institute for Maternal and Child Health-IRCCS "Burlo Garofolo", 34137 Trieste, Italy

**Madina Shaimerdenova, Damel Mektepbayeva and Dana Akilbekova**
National Laboratory Astana, Nazarbayev University, Qabanbay Batyr Avenue 53, Astana 010000, Kazakhstan

**Orynbassar Karapina**
Nazarbayev University Research and Innovation System, Nazarbayev University, Astana, Kazakhstan

**Kenneth Alibek**
Locus Solutions LLC, Solon, OH, USA

**Edwin A. Afari**
Department of Epidemiology and Disease Control, School of Public Health, College of Health Sciences, University of Ghana, Accra, Ghana

**Adolf K. Awua**
Department of Epidemiology and Disease Control, School of Public Health, College of Health Sciences, University of Ghana, Accra, Ghana.
Cellular and Clinical Research Centre, Radiological and Medical Sciences Research Institute, GAEC, Accra, Ghana

**Richard M. K. Adanu**
Population, Family and Reproductive Health, School of Public Health, College of Health Sciences, University of Ghana, Accra, Ghana

**Edwin K. Wiredu**
Department of Pathology, School of Biomedical and Allied Health Science, College of Health Sciences, University of Ghana, Korle-Bu, Accra, Ghana

**Alberto Severini**
National Microbiology Laboratory, Public Health Agency of Canada, Winnipeg, MB, Canada
University of Manitoba, Winnipeg, MB, Canada

**Emilomo Ogbe**
International Centre for Reproductive health, Department of Obstetrics and Gynaecology, Ghent University, De Pintelaan 185 P3, 9000 Ghent, Belgium

**Hillary Mabeya**
International Centre for Reproductive health, Department of Obstetrics and Gynaecology, Ghent University, De Pintelaan 185 P3, 9000 Ghent, Belgium Moi University/Gynocare Fistula Centre, Eldoret, Kenya

**Davy van den Broeck**
International Centre for Reproductive health, Department of Obstetrics and Gynaecology, Ghent University, De Pintelaan 185 P3, 9000 Ghent, Belgium Faculty of Medicine and Health Sciences, Laboratory of Cell Biology and Histology, University of Antwerp, Antwerp, Belgium

**Sonia Menon**
International Centre for Reproductive health, Department of Obstetrics and Gynaecology, Ghent University, De Pintelaan 185 P3, 9000 Ghent, Belgium CDC Foundation Atlanta, Atlanta, USA

**Rodolfo Rossi**
AMBIOR (Applied Molecular Biology Research Group), Antwerpen, Belgium

**Sylwia Fołtyn, Anastazja Boguszewska and Małgorzata Polz-Dacewicz**
Department of Virology, Medical University of Lublin, Lublin, Poland

**Małgorzata Strycharz-Dudziak**
Chair and Department of Conservative Dentistry with Endodontics, Medical University of Lublin, Lublin, Poland

**Bartłomiej Drop**
Chair and Department of Public Health, Medical University of Lublin, Lublin, Poland

**Thar Htet San, Masayoshi Fujisawa, Teizo Yoshimura, Toshiaki Ohara, Xu Yang and Akihiro Matsukawa**
Department of Pathology and Experimental Medicine, Graduate School of Medicine, Dentistry and Pharmaceutical Sciences, Okayama University, 2-5-1 Shikata, Okayama 700-8558, Japan

**Soichiro Fushimi**
Department of Pathology and Experimental Medicine, Graduate School of Medicine, Dentistry and Pharmaceutical Sciences, Okayama University, 2-5-1 Shikata, Okayama 700-8558, Japan

Department of Pathology, Himeji Red Cross Hospital, Himeji, Japan

**Lamin Soe**
Department of Pathology, Myeik General Hospital, Myeik, Myanmar

**Ngu Wah Min**
Department of Pathology, Sakura Specialist Hospital, Yangon, Myanmar

**Ohnmar Kyaw**
Immunology Research Division, Department of Medical Research, Yangon, Myanmar

**Marco Cascella, Sabrina Bimonte and Arturo Cuomo**
Division of Anesthesia and Pain Medicine, Istituto Nazionale Tumori – IRCCS- "Fondazione G. Pascale", Via Mariano Semmola, 80131 Naples, Italy

**Maria Rosaria Muzio**
Division of Infantile Neuropsychiatry, UOMI - Maternal and Infant Health, ASL NA 3 SUD, Torre del Greco, Via Marconi, 80059 Naples, Italy

**Vincenzo Schiavone**
Division of Anesthesia and Intensive Care, Presidio Ospedaliero "Pineta Grande", Castel Voltuno, 81100 Caserta, Italy

**V. Vanderpuye**
National center for Radiotherapy and Nuclear Medicine, Korle-Bu Teaching Hospital, Accra, Ghana

**S. Grover**
Hospital of University of Pennsylvania, Department of Radiation Oncology, (Botswana-UPENN program), 3400 Civic Center Blvd., Philadelphia, PA 19104, USA

**N. Hammad**
Cancer Centre of Southeastern Ontario, Burr 2, Kingston General Hospital, 25 King Street W, Kingston, ON K7L 5P9, Canada

**Pooja Prabhakar**
University of Texas Southwestern Medical Center, Dallas, TX, USA

**H. Simonds**
Division of Radiation Oncology, Tygerberg Hospital/ University of Stellenbosch, Tygerberg, South Africa

**F. Olopade**
The University of Chicago, 5841 S Maryland Avenue, MC 2115, Chicago, IL 60637, USA

**D. C. Stefan**
Walter Sisulu University Nelson Mandela Dr, Nelson Mandela Drive, Mthatha 5100, Eastern Cape, South Africa

**Teiko Nartey, Stella Melana, James F. Holland and Beatriz G. T. Pogo**
Icahn School of Medicine at Mount Sinai, New York, NY, USA

**Chiara M. Mazzanti and Generoso Bevilacqua**
Department of Pathology, University of Pisa, Pisa, Italy.

**Wendy K. Glenn, Noel J. Whitaker and James S. Lawson**
School of Biotechnology and Biomolecular Sciences, University of New South Wales, Sydney, Australia

**Ming-Sian Wu, Fan-Chen Tseng, Yin-Chiu Lo, Yi-Ping Kuo, De-Jiun Tsai and Wan-Ting Tsai**
National Institute of Infectious Diseases and Vaccinology, National Health Research Institutes, 35 Keyan Road, Zhunan, Miaoli County 35053, Taiwan

**Guann-Yi Yu**
National Institute of Infectious Diseases and Vaccinology, National Health Research Institutes, 35 Keyan Road, Zhunan, Miaoli County 35053, Taiwan Center of Infectious Disease and Signaling Research, National Cheng-Kung University, Tainan 70101, Taiwan

**Chun-Hsiang Wang and Hsuan-Ju Yang**
Division of Gastroenterology, Tainan Municipal Hospital, Tainan 70173, Taiwan

**María Teresa Magaña-Torres, Luis Felipe Jave-Suárez and Adriana Aguilar-Lemarroy**
División de Inmunología, Centro de Investigación Biomédica de Occidente (CIBO), Instituto Mexicano del Seguro Social (IMSS), Guadalajara, Jalisco, Mexico

**Cristina Artaza-Irigaray and María Guadalupe Flores-Miramontes**
División de Inmunología, Centro de Investigación Biomédica de Occidente (CIBO), Instituto Mexicano del Seguro Social (IMSS), Guadalajara, Jalisco, Mexico Programa de Doctorado en Ciencias Biomédicas, Centro Universitario de Ciencias de la Salud (CUCS), Universidad de Guadalajara, Jalisco, Mexico

**Dominik Olszewski**
Institute of Pharmacy and Molecular Biotechnology, University of Heidelberg, Heidelberg, Germany

**María Guadalupe López-Cardona**
Unidad de Medicina Genómica y Genética, Hospital Regional Dr. Valentín Gómez Farías - ISSSTE, Guadalajara, Jalisco, Mexico

**Yelda Aurora Leal-Herrera**
Unidad de Investigación Médica Yucatán (UIMY)]-IMSS, Mérida, Yucatán, Mexico

**Patricia Piña-Sánchez**
Laboratorio de Oncología Molecular, Unidad de Investigación Médica en Enfermedades Oncológicas (UIMEO) -IMSS, Ciudad de Mexico, Mexico

**A. Nappi and M. Spatarella**
Pharmacy Unit, Hospital D. Cotugno – AORN Azienda dei Colli, Naples, Italy

**A. Perrella, P. Bellopede and C. Sbreglia**
VII Division Infectious Disease and Immunology, Hospital D. Cotugno –AORN Azienda dei Colli, Naples, Italy

**A. Lanza**
I Division Infectious Disease, Hospital D. Cotugno – AORN Azienda dei Colli, Naples, Italy

**A. Izzi**
Hepatology Unit, Hospital A. Cardarelli, Naples, Italy

**Xiu-Tao Fu, Ying-Hong Shi, Yuan-Fei Peng, Wei-Ren Liu, Guo-Ming Shi, Qiang Gao, Xiao-Ying Wang and Kang Song**
Liver Cancer Institute, Zhongshan Hospital, and Key Laboratory of Carcinogenesis and Cancer Invasion (Ministry of Education), Fudan University, Shanghai 200032, China

**Jian Zhou**
Liver Cancer Institute, Zhongshan Hospital, and Key Laboratory of Carcinogenesis and Cancer Invasion (Ministry of Education), Fudan University, Shanghai 200032, China Institute of Biomedical Sciences, Fudan University, Shanghai 200032, China

**Jia Fan**
Liver Cancer Institute, Zhongshan Hospital, and Key Laboratory of Carcinogenesis and Cancer Invasion (Ministry of Education), Fudan University, Shanghai 200032, China Institute of Biomedical Sciences, Fudan University, Shanghai 200032, China Department of Liver Surgery, Zhongshan Hospital, Fudan University, 1609 Xietu Road, Shanghai 200032, China

**Zhen-Bin Ding**
Liver Cancer Institute, Zhongshan Hospital, and Key Laboratory of Carcinogenesis and Cancer Invasion (Ministry of Education), Fudan University, Shanghai 200032, China
Department of Liver Surgery, Zhongshan Hospital, Fudan University, 1609 Xietu Road, Shanghai 200032, China

**Yang Shen**
Department of Hematology, Shanghai Institute of Hematology, Rui Jin Hospital Affiliated to Shanghai Jiao Tong University School of Medicine and Collaborative Innovation Center of Systems Biomedicine, Shanghai Jiao Tong University, Shanghai 200000, China

**Renfang Zhang, Li Liu, Yinzhong Shen, Wei Song, Tangkai Qi, Yang Tang, Zhenyan Wang, Liqian Guan and Hongzhou Lu**
Department of Infectious Diseases, Shanghai Public Health Clinical Center, Fudan University, Shanghai 201508, China

**Shingo Miyamoto, Koji Matsumoto, Akihiko Sekizawa and Mamiko Onuki**
Department of Obstetrics and Gynecology, Showa University School of Medicine, Tokyo, Japan

**Yuri Tenjimbayashi and Yusuke Hirose**
Department of Obstetrics and Gynecology, Showa University School of Medicine, Tokyo, Japan
Pathogen Genomics Center, National Institute of Infectious Diseases, 4-7-1 Gakuen, Musashi-murayama, Tokyo 208-0011, Japan

**Seiichiro Mori, Yoshiyuki Ishii, Takamasa Takeuchi and Iwao Kukimoto**
Pathogen Genomics Center, National Institute of Infectious Diseases, 4-7-1 Gakuen, Musashi-murayama, Tokyo 208-0011, Japan

**Nobutaka Tasaka and Toyomi Satoh**
Department of Obstetrics and Gynecology, Faculty of Medicine, University of Tsukuba, Tsukuba, Japan

**Tohru Morisada and Takashi Iwata**
Department of Obstetrics and Gynecology, Keio University School of Medicine, Tokyo, Japan

**Narongsak Rungsakulkij, Wikran Suragul, Somkit Mingphruedhi, Pongsatorn Tangtawee, Paramin Muangkaew and Suraida Aeesoa**
Department of Surgery, Faculty of Medicine, Ramathibodi Hospital, Mahidol University, 270 Praram VI Road, Ratchathewi, Bangkok 10400, Thailand

**Marco Cascella, Sabrina Bimonte, Domenico Caliendo and Arturo Cuomo**
Division of Anesthesia and Pain Medicine, Istituto Nazionale Tumori – IRCCS – "Fondazione G. Pascale", Via Mariano Semmola, 80131 Naples, Italy

**Antonio Barbieri, Vitale Del Vecchio and Claudio Arra**
S.S.D. Sperimentazione Animale, Istituto Nazionale Tumori - IRCCS - Fondazione "G. Pascale", Via Mariano Semmola, 80131 Naples, Italy

**Vincenzo Schiavone**
Division of Anesthesia and Intensive Care, Hospital "Pineta Grande", Castel Volturno, Caserta, Italy

**Roberta Fusco and Vincenza Granata**
Division of Radiology, "Istituto Nazionale Tumori - IRCCS - Fondazione G. Pascale", Via Mariano Semmola, 80131 Naples, Italy

**Jorge Levican, Mónica Acevedo, Oscar León and Aldo Gaggero**
Programa de Virología, Instituto de Ciencias Biomedicas, Facultad de Medicina, Universidad de Chile, Santiago, Chile

**Francisco Aguayo**
Departamento de Oncología Básico clínica, Facultad de Medicina, Universidad de Chile, Santiago, Chile
Advanced Center for Chronic Diseases (ACCDiS), Universidad de Chile, Santiago, Chile

**Mubarak M. Al-Mansour**
Princess Noorah Oncology Center, King Abdulaziz Medical City, Ministry of National Guard Health Affairs-Western Region (WR), Jeddah 21423, Kingdom of Saudi Arabia
College of Medicine (COM), King Saud Bin Abdulaziz University for Health Sciences (KSAU-HS), Jeddah, Saudi Arabia

**Saif A. Alghamdi, Musab A. Alsubaie, Abdullah A. Alesa and Muhammad A. Khan**
College of Medicine (COM), King Saud Bin Abdulaziz University for Health Sciences (KSAU-HS), Jeddah, Saudi Arabia

**Arnolfo Petruzziello, Samantha Marigliano, Giovanna Loquercio and Gerardo Botti**
Virology and Molecular Biology Unit, Department of Diagnostic Pathology, Istituto Nazionale Tumori, Fondazione "G. Pascale" IRCCS Italia, Via Mariano Semmola, 80131 Naples, Italy

**Nicola Coppola**
Section of Infectious Diseases, Department of Mental Health and Public Medicine, University of Naples "Luigi Vanvitelli", Naples, Italy

**Mauro Piccirillo, Maddalena Leongito and Francesco Izzo**
Hepatobiliar and Pancreatic Unit, Department of Surgical Oncology, Istituto Nazionale Tumori - Fondazione "G. Pascale", IRCCS Italia, Naples, Italy

**Rosa Azzaro**
Transfusion Service, Department of Hemathology, Istituto Nazionale Tumori - Fondazione "G. Pascale", IRCCS Italia, Naples, Italy

**Clorinda Annunziata, Luigi Buonaguro, Franco Maria Buonaguro and Maria Lina Tornesello**
Molecular Biology and Viral Oncology Unit, Istituto Nazionale Tumori IRCCS "Fondazione G. Pascale", via M Semmola, 80131 Naples, Italy

**Giovanni Stellato and Stefano Greggi**
Gynecology Oncology Unit, Istituto Nazionale Tumori IRCCS "Fondazione G. Pascale", 80131 Naples, Italy

**Veronica Sanna, Maria Pia Curcio, Simona Losito and Gerardo Botti**
Department of Pathology, Istituto Nazionale Tumori IRCCS "Fondazione G. Pascale", 80131 Naples, Italy

**Andrea Claudine F. Afable, Patricia Joyce O. Belza, Karen Joy S. Dy and Scott Justin Q. Lee**
Department of Biochemistry, Faculty of Pharmacy, University of Santo Tomas, Manila, Philippines

**Leonardo A. Guevarra Jr**
Department of Biochemistry, Faculty of Pharmacy, University of Santo Tomas, Manila, Philippines
Research Center for Natural and Applied Sciences, University of Santo Tomas, Manila, Philippines

**Pia Marie S. P. Albano**
Research Center for Natural and Applied Sciences, University of Santo Tomas, Manila, Philippines
Department of Biological Sciences, College of Science, University of Santo Tomas, Manila, Philippines

**Teresa T. Sy-Ortin**
Benavidez Cancer Institute, University of Santo Tomas Hospital, Manila, Philippines

# Index

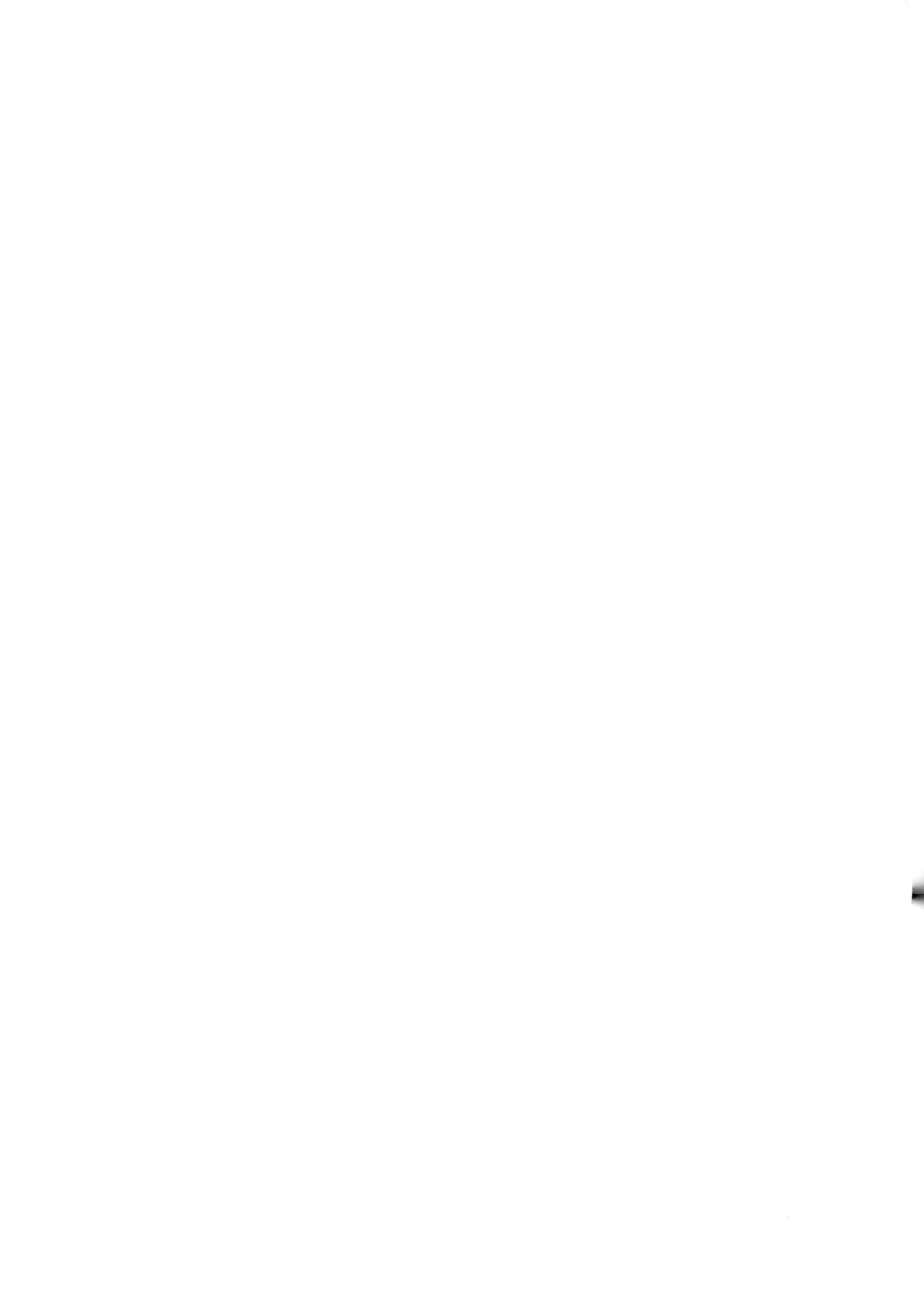